Medical Genetics

Medical Genetics

LYNN B. JORDE, PhD

Professor and Associate Chairman
Department of Human Genetics
University of Utah Health Sciences Center
Salt Lake City, Utah

JOHN C. CAREY, MD

Professor and Director, Division of Medical Genetics
Department of Pediatrics
University of Utah Health Sciences Center
Salt Lake City, Utah

MICHAEL J. BAMSHAD, MD

Assistant Professor
Department of Pediatrics
University of Utah Health Sciences Center
Salt Lake City, Utah

RAYMOND L. WHITE, PhD

Chairman, Department of Oncological Sciences
Executive Director, Huntsman Cancer Institute
University of Utah Health Sciences Center
Salt Lake City, Utah

SECOND EDITION

 Mosby

St. Louis Baltimore Boston Carlsbad Chicago Minneapolis New York Philadelphia Portland
London Milan Sydney Tokyo Toronto

Mosby

Dedicated to Publishing Excellence

A Times Mirror
Company

Publisher: Richard Furn
Editor: Beverly Copland
Senior Developmental Editor: Linda Caldwell
Project Manager: Patricia Tannian
Project Specialist: Ann E. Rogers
Book Design Manager: Gail Morey Hudson
Art Director: Pete Wilder
Illustration Manager: Danny Pyne
Cover Designer: Greg Wise
Manufacturing Manager: Dave Graybill
Product Manager: Julie Swanston

SECOND EDITION

Printed in the United States of America.
Composition, lithography, and color separation by Graphic World, Inc.
Printing/binding by Von Hoffmann Press, Inc.

Mosby, Inc.
11830 Westline Industrial Drive
St. Louis, Missouri 63146

Library of Congress Cataloging in Publication Data
Medical genetics / Lynn B. Jorde . . . [et al.]. — 2nd ed.
    p.   cm.
  Rev. ed. of: Medical genetics / Lynn B. Jorde, John C. Carey,
Raymond L. White. Rev. ed. 1997.
   Includes bibliographical references and index.
   ISBN 0-8151-4608-6
   1. Medical genetics   I. Jorde, Lynn B.
   [DNLM: 1. Hereditary Diseases—genetics. 2. Genetics, Medical.
QZ 50 M48848 1999]
RB155.J67 1999
616'.042—dc21
DNLM/DLC
for Library of Congress   98-7537
                                    CIP

98 99 00 01 02 / 9 8 7 6 5 4 3 2 1

To our families

Eileen and **Alton Jorde**
Leslie, Patrick, and **Andrew Carey**
Jerry and **Joanne Bamshad**
Joan, Juliette, and **Jeremy White**

Foreword

J.B.S. Haldane titled an anthology of some of his more dyspeptic writings, "Everything Has a History," and this is clearly applicable to the field of medical genetics. More than 200 years ago scientists such as Buffon, Lamarck, Goethe, and Kielmeyer reflected on how the developmental history of each organism related to the history of life on Earth. Based on these ideas, the discipline of biology was born in eighteenth-century Europe, enjoyed adolescence as morphology and comparative anatomy in the nineteenth century, and has reached adulthood in the twentieth century as the field of genetics. However, the late nineteenth century definition of genetics (heredity) as the science of variation (and its causes) is still valid. Thus, human genetics is the science of human variation, medical genetics the science of abnormal human variation, and clinical genetics that branch of medicine that cares for individuals and families with abnormal variation of structure and function.

In the late nineteenth and early twentieth century, the unity of morphology-based science was gradually replaced by a pluralistic view of biology that splintered the field into many different, and often rivalrous, disciplines. However, thanks to the application of novel molecular biological methods to the analysis of development and to the understanding of the materials of heredity (i.e., genes), the various branches of biology are being reunited. This new discipline, termed molecular morphology, may be defined as the study of the form, formation, transformation, and malformation of living organisms. Indeed, ignorant as they may be of the traditional methods of historiography, geneticists have developed their own brilliant and highly effective methods. Consequently, they have achieved a perspective remarkably longer and much better documented than that of historians. This nearly four-billion-year perspective unites living organisms into a single web of life related to each other in unbroken descent to a common ancestor. This makes the phylogenetic (i.e., the genetic relationships of different species to one another) and the ontogenetic perspectives of development (i.e., the genetic basis for the development of individual organ-

isms) not only complementary but inseparable. Thus, it is now possible to effectively explore a key question of biology of the nineteenth and twentieth centuries: what is the relationship between evolution and development?

In 1945 the University of Utah established the Laboratory for the Study of Hereditary and Metabolic Disorders (later called the Laboratory of Human Genetics). Here, an outstanding group of scientists performed pioneering studies on clefts of lips and palate, muscular dystrophy, albinism, deafness, hereditary polyposis of the colon (Gardner syndrome), and familial breast cancer. These predecessors would be enormously proud of their current peers at the University of Utah, whose successes have advanced knowledge in every aspect of the field of genetics.

In their attempts to synthesize the story of genetics and its applications to human variability, health and disease, development, and cancer, the authors of this text have succeeded admirably. In the second edition, the authors have extensively revised the previous twelve chapters by adding new research data and human applications. They have also added two new chapters that discuss the fundamental concepts and clinical applications of biochemical genetics and developmental genetics. Thus, this concise, well written and illustrated, carefully edited and indexed book is highly recommended to undergraduate students, new graduate students, medical students, genetic counseling students, nursing students, and students in the allied health sciences. Importantly, it is also a wonderful text for the practicing physician (primary care providers and specialists) who wants an authoritative introduction to the basis and principles of modern genetics as applied to human health and development. This text, by distinguished and internationally respected colleagues and friends who love to teach, is a joy to read in its expression of enthusiasm and of wonder, which Aristotle said was the beginning of all knowledge.

Einstein once said, "The most incomprehensible thing about the world is that it is comprehensible." When I began to work in the field of medical genetics, the gene was widely viewed as incomprehensible. Indeed, some scientists, such as Goldschmidt, cast doubt on the very existence of the gene, although the great American biologist E.B. Wilson had predicted its chemical nature more than 100 years previous. In this text, genes and their function in health and disease are made comprehensible in a manner that should have wide appeal to all.

John Opitz, MD
Salt Lake City, Utah

Preface

Medical genetics is a rapidly progressing field. No textbook can remain factually current for long, so we have attempted to emphasize the central principles of genetics and their clinical application. In particular, this textbook integrates recent developments in molecular genetics with clinical practice.

This new edition maintains the format and presentation that were well received in the first edition. Basic principles of molecular biology are introduced early in the book so that they can be discussed and applied in subsequent chapters. The chapters on autosomal and X-linked disorders include discussions of recent developments such as genomic imprinting, anticipation, and expanded trinucleotide repeats. The chapter on cytogenetics highlights recent molecular advances in this area. Gene mapping and cloning, a central focus of modern medical genetics, is treated at length. Chapters are included on the rapidly developing fields of immunogenetics and cancer genetics. Departing somewhat from tradition, this book gives special emphasis to the genetics of common adult diseases such as diabetes, cancer, and heart disease. Although such diseases are more refractory to genetic analysis than many of the pediatric diseases usually found in medical genetics textbooks, their impact on public health is enormous. Fortunately, they too are beginning to yield to newer methods of genetic analysis. The book concludes with chapters on genetic diagnosis (again emphasizing current molecular approaches) and clinical genetics and genetic counseling.

A new feature in this edition is the connection of content throughout the text with a Web site. To provide access to the continually changing information in medical genetics, we have developed an Internet Web page at the University of Utah School of Medicine (http://medgen.genetics.utah.edu). The Web page includes many additional patient photographs, other clinical images, hyperlinks to other relevant sites, recent research findings, and other up-to-the-minute changes in the field. The symbol **www** will be found throughout the text next to topics that are supplemented by information on the Web page.

Several pedagogical aids are incorporated in this book:
- Clinical Commentary boxes present detailed coverage of the most important genetic diseases and provide examples of modern clinical management.
- Mini-summaries highlighted in a second color are placed on nearly every page to help the reader understand and summarize important concepts.
- Study questions provided at the end of each chapter assist the reader in review and comprehension.
- A detailed glossary is included at the end of the book.
- Key terms are emphasized in boldface.
- Important references are listed at the end of each chapter.

Many major additions have been incorporated into this revision:
- A new chapter on the biochemical aspects of genetic disease (Chapter 7) provides expanded explanation of the concepts that underlie biochemical genetics.
- A new chapter on developmental genetics (Chapter 10) discusses the many recent advances in our understanding of gene regulation and their clinical consequences.
- Expanded content on gene cloning, gene therapy, and genetic diagnosis stresses some of the fastest growing clinical applications of genetics.
- Forty new clinical photographs have been added.
- Several "vignettes" from patients and families have been added to provide the patient's perspective on genetic disease.
- Additional study questions have been included in each chapter.
- An expanded comprehensive index includes all text citations of all diseases.

This textbook evolved from courses we teach for medical students, nursing students, and graduate and undergraduate students in human genetics. These students are the primary audience for this book, but it should also be useful for students in genetic counseling and biology and for house staff, physicians, and other health care professionals who wish to become more familiar with medical genetics.

ACKNOWLEDGMENTS

Many of our colleagues have generously donated their time and expertise in reading and commenting on portions of this book. We extend our sincere gratitude to Arthur Brothman, PhD; Peter Byers, MD; William Carroll, MD; Debbie Dubler, BS; Ruth Foltz, MS; Sandra Hasstedt, PhD; James Kushner, MD; Jean-Marc Lalouel, MD, DSc; Claire Leonard, MD; Mark Leppert, PhD; William McMahon, MD; James Metherall, PhD; Shige Sakonju, PhD; Carl Thummel, PhD; Thérèse Tuohy, PhD; Scott Watkins, BS; John Weis, PhD; H. Joseph Yost, PhD; Maxine J. Sutcliffe, PhD; Leslie R. Schover, PhD; and Craig Smith, medical student. In addition, a number of colleagues provided photographs; they are acknowledged individually in the figure captions. We wish to thank Peeches Cedarholm, RN, and Bridget Kramer, RN, for their help in obtaining and organizing the photographs. The karyotypes in Chapter 6 were provided by Arthur Brothman, PhD, and Bonnie Issa, BS. The illustrations were originally created by Carol Cassidy. Our editors at Mosby, Linda Caldwell and Beverly Copland, offered ample encouragement and understanding. Finally, we wish to acknowledge the thousands of students with whom we have interacted during the past two decades. Teaching involves communication in both directions, and we have undoubtedly learned as much from our students as they have learned from us.

Lynn B. Jorde
John C. Carey
Michael J. Bamshad
Raymond L. White

Contents

1
Background and History

Genetics is playing an increasingly important role in the practice of clinical medicine. Medical genetics, once largely confined to relatively rare diseases seen by only a few specialists, is now becoming a central component of our understanding of most major diseases. These include not only the pediatric diseases, but also common adult diseases such as heart disease, diabetes, many cancers, and many psychiatric disorders. Because all components of the human body are influenced by genes, genetic disease is relevant to all medical specialties. Today's health care practitioners must understand the science of medical genetics.

WHAT IS MEDICAL GENETICS?

Medical genetics involves any application of genetics to medical practice. It thus includes studies of the inheritance of diseases in families, the mapping of disease genes to specific locations on chromosomes, analyses of the molecular mechanisms through which genes cause disease, and the diagnosis and treatment of genetic disease. As a result of rapid progress in molecular genetics, gene therapy—the insertion of normal genes into patients in order to correct genetic diseases—has recently been initiated. Medical genetics also includes genetic counseling, which involves the communication of information regarding risks, prognoses, and treatment to patients and their families.

WHY IS A KNOWLEDGE OF MEDICAL GENETICS IMPORTANT FOR TODAY'S HEALTH CARE PRACTITIONER?

There are several answers to this question. Genetic diseases make up a large proportion of the total disease burden in both the pediatric and adult populations (Table 1-1). This proportion will continue to grow as

our understanding of the genetic basis of diseases grows. In addition, modern medicine is placing an increasing emphasis on the importance of prevention. Because genetics provides a basis for understanding the fundamental biological makeup of the organism, it naturally leads to a better understanding of the disease process. In many cases this knowledge can lead to the actual prevention of the disorder. It also leads to more effective disease treatment. Prevention and effective treatment are among the highest goals of medicine. In the chapters that follow, we shall see many examples of the ways in which genetics contributes to these goals. But first, we shall review the foundations upon which current practice is built.

A BRIEF HISTORY

The inheritance of physical traits has been a subject of curiosity and interest for thousands of years. The ancient Hebrews and Greeks, as well as later Medieval scholars, described many genetic phenomena and proposed theories to account for them. Many of these theories were incorrect. Gregor Mendel (Fig. 1-1), an Austrian monk who is usually considered to be the "father" of genetics, advanced the field significantly by performing a series of cleverly designed experiments on living organisms (garden peas). He then used this experimental information to formulate a series of fundamental principles of heredity.

Mendel published the results of his experiments in 1865 in a relatively obscure journal. It is one of the ironies of biological science that his discoveries, which still form the foundation of genetics, received virtually no recognition for 35 years. At about the same time, Charles Darwin formulated his theories of evolution, and his cousin, Francis Galton, performed an extensive series of family studies (concentrating especially on twins) in an effort to understand the influence of heredity on various

TABLE 1-1   A Partial List of Some Important Genetic Diseases

Disease	Approximate prevalence
Chromosome Abnormalities	
Down syndrome	1/700 to 1/1,000
Klinefelter syndrome	1/1,000 males
Trisomy 13	1/15,000 to 2/20,000
Trisomy 18	1/6,000
Turner syndrome	1/2,500 to 1/10,000 females
Single-Gene Disorders	
Adenomatous polyposis coli	1/6,000
Adult polycystic kidney disease	1/1,000
α-1-Antitrypsin deficiency	1/2,500 to 1/10,000 Caucasians
Cystic fibrosis	1/2,000 to 1/4,000 Caucasians
Duchenne muscular dystrophy	1/3,500 males
Familial hypercholesterolemia	1/500
Fragile X syndrome	1/1,500 males; 1/2,500 females
Hemochromatosis (hereditary; symptomatic)	1/5,000
Hemophilia A	1/10,000 males
Hereditary nonpolyposis colorectal cancer	Up to 1/200
Huntington disease	1/20,000 Caucasians
Marfan syndrome	1/10,000 to 1/20,000
Myotonic dystrophy	1/7,000 to 1/20,000 Caucasians
Neurofibromatosis type 1	1/3,000 to 1/5,000
Osteogenesis imperfecta	1/5,000 to 1/10,000
Phenylketonuria	1/10,000 to 1/15,000 Caucasians
Retinoblastoma	1/20,000
Sickle cell disease	1/400 to 1/600 African-Americans; up to 1/50 in central Africa
Tay-Sachs disease	1/3,000 Ashkenazi Jews
Thalassemia	1/50 to 1/100 (South Asian and circum-Mediterranean population)
Multifactorial Disorders	
Congenital malformations	
Cleft lip with/without cleft palate	1/500 to 1/1,000
Club foot (talipes equinovarus)	1/1,000
Congenital heart defects	1/200 to 1/500
Neural tube defects (spina bifida, anencephaly)	1/200 to 1/1,000
Pyloric stenosis	1/300
Adult diseases	
Alcoholism	1/10 to 1/20
Alzheimer disease	1/10 (Americans over age 65)
Bipolar affective disorder	1/100 to 1/200
Cancer (all types)	1/3
Diabetes (types I and II)	1/10
Heart disease/stroke	1/3 to 1/5
Schizophrenia	1/100
Mitochondrial diseases	
Kearns-Sayre disease	Rare
Leber hereditary optic neuropathy (LHON)	Rare
Mitochondrial encephalopathy, lactic acidosis, and strokelike episodes (MELAS)	Rare
Myoclonic epilepsy and ragged-red fiber disease (MERRF)	Rare

FIG. 1-1 Gregor Johann Mendel
(From Raven PH, Johnson GB [1992] Biology. Ed. 3. Mosby, St Louis. With permission of McGraw-Hill, NY.)

human traits. Neither scientist was aware of Mendel's work.

Genetics as we know it today is largely the result of research performed during the twentieth century. Mendel's principles were independently rediscovered in 1900 by three different scientists working in three different countries. This was also the year in which Landsteiner discovered the ABO blood group. In 1902, Archibald Garrod described alkaptonuria as the first "inborn error of metabolism." In 1909, Johannsen coined the term **gene** to denote the basic unit of heredity.

The next several decades were a period of considerable experimental and theoretical work. Several organisms, including *Drosophila* (fruit flies) and *Neurospora* (bread mold) served as useful experimental systems in which to study the actions and interactions of genes. For example, H.J. Muller demonstrated the genetic consequences of ionizing radiation in the fruit fly. During this period, much of the theoretical basis of population genetics was developed by three central figures: Ronald Fisher, J.B.S. Haldane, and Sewall Wright. In addition, the modes of inheritance of several important genetic diseases, including phenylketonuria, sickle cell disease, Huntington disease, and cystic fibrosis, were established. In 1944, Oswald Avery showed that genes are composed of **DNA (deoxyribonucleic acid).**

Probably the most significant achievement of the 1950s was the specification of the physical structure of DNA by James Watson and Francis Crick in 1953. Their seminal paper, which was only one page in length, formed the basis for what is now known as **molecular genetics** (the study of the structure and function of genes at the molecular level). Another significant accomplishment in this decade was the correct specification of the number of human chromosomes. Since the

early 1920s, it had been thought that humans had 48 chromosomes in each cell. Only in 1956 was the correct number, 46, finally determined. The ability to count and identify chromosomes led to a flurry of new findings in cytogenetics, including the discovery in 1959 that Down syndrome is caused by an extra copy of chromosome 21.

Technological developments since 1960 have brought about significant achievements at an ever-increasing rate. The most spectacular have occurred in the field of molecular genetics. During the past decade, nearly 6,000 genes have been mapped to specific chromosome locations. The Human Genome Project, a large collaborative venture begun in 1990, hopes to provide the complete human DNA sequence by the year 2005 (the term **genome** refers to all of the genes in an organism). Important developments in computer technology help to decipher the barrage of data being generated by this and related projects. In addition to mapping genes, molecular geneticists have pinpointed the molecular defects underlying a number of important genetic diseases. This research has contributed greatly to our understanding of the ways in which gene defects can cause diseases, opening the path to more effective treatment and potential cures. The next decade promises to be a time of great excitement and fulfillment.

TYPES OF GENETIC DISEASES

Each human is estimated to have approximately 50,000 to 100,000 different genes. Alterations in these genes, or in combinations of them, can produce genetic disorders. These disorders are classified into several major groups:

1. **Chromosome disorders**, in which entire chromosomes, or large segments of them, are missing, duplicated, or otherwise altered. These disorders include diseases such as Down syndrome and Turner syndrome.
2. Disorders in which single genes are altered (often termed "mendelian" conditions, or **single-gene disorders**). Well-known examples include cystic fibrosis, sickle cell disease, and hemophilia.
3. **Multifactorial disorders**, which are due to a combination of multiple genetic as well as environmental causes. Many birth defects, such as cleft lip and/or cleft palate, as well as many adult disorders, including heart disease and diabetes, belong in this category.
4. **Mitochondrial disorders**, a relatively small number of diseases caused by alterations in the small cytoplasmic mitochondrial chromosome.

Table 1-1 provides some examples of each of these types of diseases.

Of these major classes of diseases, the single-gene disorders have probably received the greatest amount of attention. These disorders are classified according to the way in which they are inherited in families (autosomal dominant, autosomal recessive, and X-linked). These modes of inheritance will be discussed extensively in Chapters 4 and 5. As Table 1-2 shows, the number of defined single-gene traits has grown considerably during recent years, with a total of more than 9,000 conditions presently defined. With continued advances, this number is certain to increase.

While some genetic disorders, particularly the single-gene conditions, are strongly determined by genes, many others are the result of multiple genetic and nongenetic factors. We can therefore think of genetic diseases as lying along a continuum (Fig. 1-2), with disorders such as cystic fibrosis and Duchenne muscular dystrophy situated at one end (strongly determined by genes), and conditions such as measles situated at the other (strongly determined by environment). Many of the most prevalent disorders, such as many birth defects and common diseases like diabetes, hypertension, heart disease, and cancer, lie somewhere in the middle of the continuum. These diseases are the products of varying degrees of both genetic and environmental influences.

THE CLINICAL IMPACT OF GENETIC DISEASE

Genetic diseases are sometimes perceived as being so rare that the average health care practitioner will seldom encounter them. This is far from the truth, which is becoming increasingly evident as our knowledge and technology progress. Less than a century ago, diseases of largely nongenetic causation (diseases caused by malnutrition, unsanitary conditions, and pathogens) accounted for the great majority of deaths in children. During the twentieth century, however, public health has vastly improved. As a result, genetic diseases have come to account for an ever-increasing proportion of pediatric deaths in developed countries. For example, the percentage of deaths due to genetic causes in various hospitals in the United Kingdom has increased from 16.5% in 1914 to 50% in 1976 (Table 1-3).

In addition to contributing to a large proportion of childhood deaths, genetic diseases also account for a large share of admissions into pediatric hospitals. For example, a survey of Seattle hospitals showed that 27% of all pediatric inpatients presented with a genetic disorder, and a survey of admissions into a major pediatric hospital in Mexico showed that 37.8% had a disease that was either genetic or "partly genetic."

Another way to assess the importance of genetic diseases is to ask, "What proportion of individuals in the population will be diagnosed with a genetic disorder?" This is not as simple a question as it may seem. A variety of factors can influence the answer. For example, some diseases are found more frequently in certain ethnic groups. Cystic fibrosis is especially common among Europeans, while sickle cell disease is especially common among Africans. Some diseases are more common in older individuals. Colon cancer, breast cancer, and Alzheimer disease, for instance, are each caused by dominant genes in a small proportion (5% to 10%) of cases

TABLE 1-2 **Number of Entries Representing Loci Identified Mainly by Mendelizing Phenotypes**

Mendelian Inheritance in Man edition	Autosomal dominant	Autosomal recessive	X-linked	Total	Grand total
1966 (ed 1)	269 (+568)*	237 (+294)	68 (+51)	574 (+913)	1487
1968 (ed 2)	344 (+449)	280 (+349)	68 (+55)	692 (+853)	1545
1971 (ed 3)	415 (+528)	365 (+418)	86 (+64)	866 (+1010)	1876
1975 (ed 4)	583 (+635)	466 (+481)	93 (+78)	1142 (+1194)	2336
1978 (ed 5)	736 (+753)	521 (+596)	107 (+98)	1364 (+1447)	2811
1983 (ed 6)	934 (+893)	588 (+710)	115 (+128)	1637 (+1731)	3368
1986 (ed 7)	1172 (+1029)	610 (+810)	124 (+162)	1906 (+2001)	3907
1988 (ed 8)	1442 (+1117)	626 (+851)	139 (+171)	2207 (+2139)	4346
1990 (ed 9)	1864 (+1183)	631 (+923)	161 (+175)	2656 (+2281)	4937
1992 (ed 10)	2470 (+1241)	647 (+984)	190 (+178)	3307 (+2403)	5710
1994 (ed 11)	4458	1730	412	6678[†]	6678
1996 (online edition)	7430[‡]		461	7975	7975
1998 (online edition)	8544[‡]		527	9158	9158

From McKusick VA (1994) Mendelian Inheritance in Man: Catalogs of Autosomal Dominant, Autosomal Recessive, and X-Linked Phenotypes. Ed. 11. Johns Hopkins University Press, Baltimore.
*Values in parentheses refer to loci not fully identified or validated. Increasingly loci identified by molecular and cellular genetic methods are included despite the lack of mendelian variation in the phenotype.
[†]The total for the 1994 edition includes 19 Y-linked loci and 59 mitochondrial loci not shown in the table.
[‡]This number includes both autosomal dominant and autosomal recessive traits, which are not separated in the online edition. The grand total for 1996 includes 24 Y-linked and 60 mitochondrial traits, and the grand total for 1998 includes 27 Y-linked and 60 mitochondrial traits.

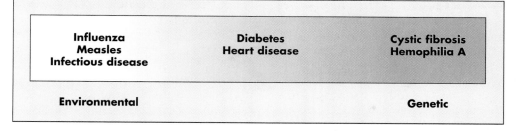

FIG. 1-2 Continuum of genetic diseases. Some diseases (e.g., cystic fibrosis) are strongly determined by genes, whereas others (e.g., infectious disease) are strongly determined by environment.

TABLE 1-3 Percentages of Childhood Deaths in United Kingdom Hospitals Attributable to Nongenetic (e.g., Infections) and Genetic Causes

Cause	London 1914	London 1954	Newcastle 1966	Edinburgh 1976
Nongenetic	83.5	62.5	58.0	50.0
Genetic				
Single gene	2.0	12.0	8.5	8.9
Chromosomal	—	—	2.5	2.9
Multifactorial	14.5	25.5	31.0	38.2

From Rimoin Dl, Connor JM, Pyeritz RE (1997) Emery and Rimoin's Principles and Practice of Medical Genetics. Churchill Livingstone, Edinburgh.

and are not usually seen until later in life. The prevalence estimates for these genetic diseases would be higher in a more aged population. Variations in diagnostic and recording practices can also cause prevalence estimates to vary. Accordingly, the prevalence figures shown in Table 1-4 are given as rather broad ranges. Keeping these sources of variation in mind, it is notable that 3% to 7% of the population will be diagnosed with a recognizable genetic disease. This tabulation does not include most cases of the more common adult diseases, such as heart disease, diabetes, and cancer. But it is known that these diseases also have genetic components. If we include these diseases in our assessment, the clinical impact of genetic disease is considerable indeed.

SUGGESTED READINGS

Baird PA, Anderson TW, Newcombe HB, Lowry RB (1988) Genetic disorders in children and young adults: a population study. Am. J. Hum. Genet. 42:677-693

Dunn LC (1965) A Short History of Genetics. McGraw-Hill, New York

McKusick VA (1993) Medical genetics: a 40-year perspective on the evolution of a medical specialty from a basic science. JAMA 270:2351-2356

McKusick VA (1994) Mendelian Inheritance in Man. Johns Hopkins University Press, Baltimore

McKusick VA (1997) History of medical genetics. In: Rimoin DL, Connor JM, Pyeritz RE (eds) Emery and Rimoin's Principles and Practice of Medical Genetics. Vol. 1. Churchill Livingstone, Edinburgh, pp 1-30

TABLE 1-4 Approximate Prevalence of Genetic Disease in the General Population

Type of genetic disease	Lifetime prevalence per 1,000
Autosomal Dominant	3 to 9.5
Autosomal Recessive	2 to 2.5
X-linked	0.5 to 2
Chromosome disorders*	6 to 9
Congenital malformation[†]	20 to 50
TOTAL	31.5 to 73

*The upper limit of this range is obtained when newer chromosome banding techniques (see Chapter 6) are used.
[†]"Congenital" means "present at birth." Most congenital malformations are thought to be multifactorial and thus likely have both genetic and environmental components.

Passarge E (1995) Color Atlas of Genetics. Georg Thieme Verlag, Stuttgart

Rimoin DL, Connor JM, Pyeritz RE (eds) (1997) Emery and Rimoin's Principles and Practice of Medical Genetics. Churchill Livingstone, Edinburgh

Scriver CR, Beaudet AL, Sly WS, Valle D (eds) (1995) The Metabolic Basis of Inherited Disease. McGraw-Hill, New York

Seashore MS, Wappner RS (1996) Genetics in Primary Care and Clinical Medicine. Appleton & Lange, Stamford, CT

Watson JD, Crick FHC (1953) Molecular structure of nucleic acids: a structure for deoxyribose nucleic acid. Nature 171:737

2

Basic Cell Biology: Structure and Function of Genes and Chromosomes

All genetic diseases involve defects at the level of the cell. For this reason, one must understand basic cell biology to understand genetic disease. Errors may occur in the replication of genetic material or in the translation of genes into proteins. These errors commonly produce single-gene disorders. In addition, errors occurring during cell division can lead to disorders involving entire chromosomes. To provide the basis for understanding these errors and their consequences, this chapter focuses on the processes through which genes are replicated and translated into proteins, as well as the process of cell division.

In the nineteenth century, microscopic studies of cells led scientists to suspect that the nucleus of the cell (Fig. 2-1) contained the important mechanisms of inheritance. They found that **chromatin**, the substance that gives the nucleus a granular appearance, is observable in the nuclei of nondividing cells. Just before a cell undergoes division, the chromatin condenses to form discrete, dark-staining bodies called **chromosomes** (from the Greek for "colored bodies"). With the rediscovery of Mendel's breeding experiments at the beginning of the twentieth century, it soon became apparent that chromosomes contained **genes**. Genes are transmitted from parent to offspring and are considered to be the basic unit of inheritance. It is through the transmission of genes that physical traits, such as eye color, are inherited in families. Diseases can also be transmitted through genetic inheritance.

Physically, genes are composed of **deoxyribonucleic acid (DNA).** DNA provides the genetic "blueprint" for all proteins in the body. Thus, genes ultimately influence all aspects of body structure and function. The human is estimated to have 50,000 to 100,000 **structural genes** (genes that code for proteins). An error (or **mutation**) in one of these genes

often leads to a recognizable genetic disease. To date, approximately 9,600 single-gene traits have been identified; most of these represent disease conditions (see Table 1-2 in Chapter 1).

▼ **Genes, the basic unit of inheritance, are contained in chromosomes and consist of DNA.** ▲

Each human **somatic cell** (cells other than the **gametes**, or sperm and egg cells) contains 23 pairs of different chromosomes, for a total of 46. One member of each pair is derived from the individual's father, while the other member is derived from the mother. One of the chromosome pairs consists of the **sex chromosomes**. In normal males, the sex chromosomes are a Y chromosome inherited from the father and an X chromosome inherited from the mother. Two X chromosomes are found in normal females, one inherited from each parent. The other 22 pairs of chromosomes are termed **autosomes**. The members of each pair of autosomes are said to be **homologs**, or **homologous**, because their DNA is very similar. The X and Y chromosomes are not homologs of one another.

Somatic cells, having two of each chromosome, are termed **diploid** cells. Human gametes have the **haploid** number of chromosomes, 23. The diploid number of chromosomes is maintained in successive generations of somatic cells by the process of **mitosis**, while the haploid number is obtained through a process known as **meiosis**. Both of these processes will be discussed in detail in the latter part of this chapter.

▼ **Somatic cells are diploid, having 23 pairs of chromosomes (22 pairs of autosomes and one pair of sex chromosomes). Gametes are haploid and have a total of 23 chromosomes.** ▲

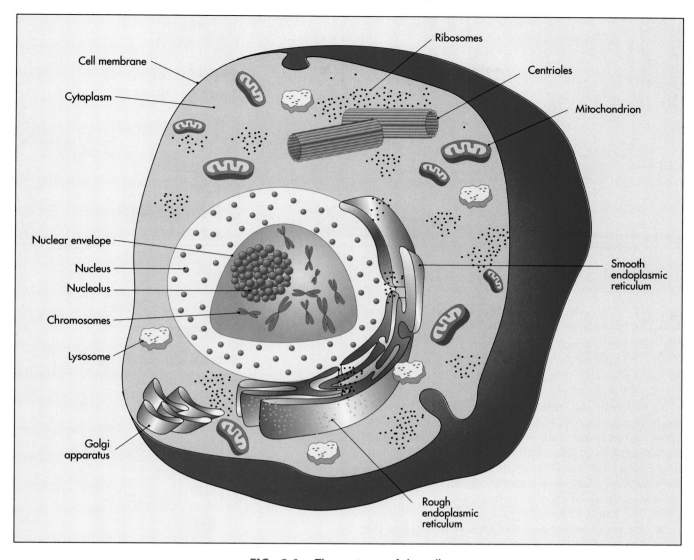

FIG. 2-1   The anatomy of the cell.

DNA, RNA, AND PROTEINS: HEREDITY AT THE MOLECULAR LEVEL

DNA

Composition and Structure of DNA

The DNA molecule has three basic components: the pentose sugar, deoxyribose; a phosphate group; and four types of nitrogenous **bases** (so named because they can combine with hydrogen ions in acidic solutions). Two of the bases, **cytosine and thymine**, are single carbon-nitrogen rings called **pyrimidines**. The other two bases, **adenine and guanine**, are double carbon-nitrogen rings called **purines** (Fig. 2-2). The four bases are commonly represented by their first letters: C, T, A, and G.

One of Watson and Crick's contributions was to demonstrate how these three components are physically assembled to form DNA. They proposed the now-famous **double helix** model, in which DNA can be envisioned as a twisted ladder with chemical bonds as its rungs (Fig. 2-3). The two sides of the ladder are composed of the sugar and phosphate components, held together by strong phosphodiester bonds. Projecting from each side of the ladder, at regular intervals, are the nitrogenous bases. The base projecting from one side is bound to the base projecting from the other by relatively weak hydrogen bonds. The paired nitrogenous bases therefore form the rungs of the ladder.

Fig. 2-3 illustrates the chemical bonds between bases and shows that the ends of the ladder terminate in either 3' or 5'. These labels are derived from the order in which the five carbon atoms composing deoxyribose are numbered. Each DNA subunit, consisting of one deoxyribose, one phosphate group, and one base, is called a **nucleotide**.

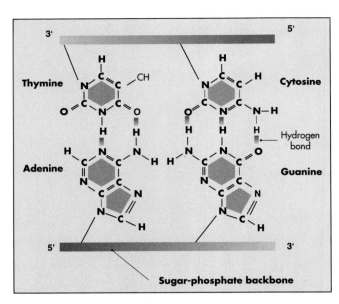

FIG. 2-2 Chemical structure of the four bases, showing hydrogen bonds between base pairs. Three hydrogen bonds are formed between cytosine-guanine pairs, and two bonds are formed between adenine-thymine pairs.

As we shall see, different sequences of nucleotide bases (e.g., ACCAAGTGC) specify different proteins. Specification of the body's many proteins must require a great deal of genetic information. Indeed, each haploid human cell contains approximately 3 billion nucleotide pairs, more than enough information to specify the composition of all of our proteins.

▼ **The most important constituent of DNA is the four nucleotide bases: adenine, thymine, cytosine, and guanine. DNA has a double helix structure.** ▲

DNA Coiling

Textbook illustrations usually depict DNA as a double-helix molecule that continues in a long, straight line. However, if the DNA in a cell were actually stretched out in this way, it would be about 2 meters in length. To package all of this DNA into a tiny cell nucleus, it is coiled at several levels. First, the DNA is wound around a **histone** protein core to form a **nucleosome** (Fig. 2-4). About 140 to 150 DNA bases are wound around each histone core, and then 20 to 60 bases form a "spacer" element before the next nucleosome complex. The nucleosomes in turn form a helical **solenoid**; each turn of the solenoid includes about six nucleosomes. The solenoids themselves are organized into **chromatin loops,** which are attached to a protein scaffold. Each of these loops contains approximately 100,000 base pairs (100 **kilobases,** or **kb**) of DNA. The end result of this coiling and looping is that the DNA, when at its maximum stage

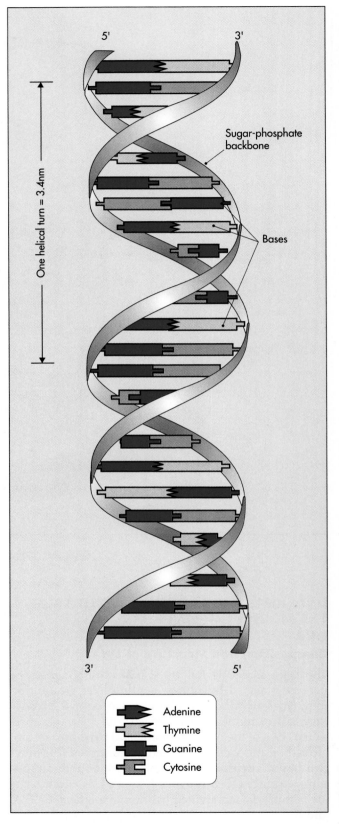

FIG. 2-3 The DNA double helix, with sugar-phosphate backbone and nitrogenous bases.

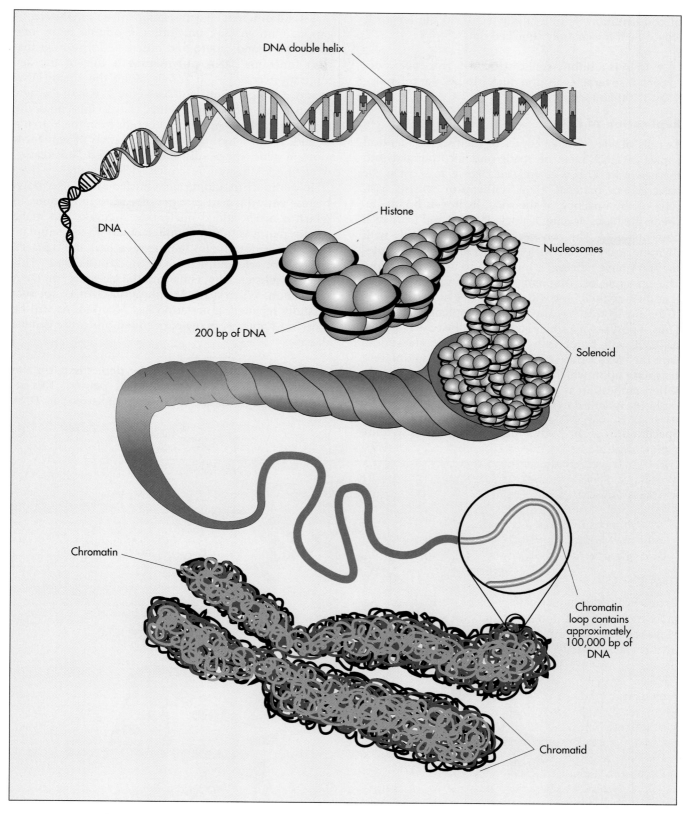

FIG. 2-4 Patterns of DNA coiling. DNA is wound around histones to form nucleosomes. These are organized into solenoids, which in turn compose chromatin loops.

of condensation, is only about 1/10,000 the length it would be if it were fully stretched out.

▼ DNA is a tightly coiled structure. This coiling occurs at several levels: the nucleosome, the solenoid, and 100-kb loops. ▲

Replication of DNA

As cells divide to make copies of themselves, identical copies of DNA must be made and incorporated into the new cells. This is essential if DNA is to serve as the basic genetic material. DNA **replication** consists basically of the breaking of the weak hydrogen bonds between the bases, leaving a single DNA strand with each base unpaired. The consistent pairing of adenine with thymine and guanine with cytosine, known as **complementary base pairing**, is the key to accurate replication. The principle of complementary base pairing dictates that the unpaired base will attract a free nucleotide only if the nucleotide has the proper complementary base. Thus, a portion of a single strand with the base sequence ATTGCT will bond with a series of free nucleotides with the bases TAACGA. The single strand is said to be a **template** upon which a complementary strand is built. When replication is complete, a new double-stranded molecule identical to the original is formed (Fig. 2-5).

Several different enzymes are involved in DNA replication. One enzyme unwinds the double helix, one holds the strands apart, and others perform other distinct functions. **DNA polymerase** is one of the key replication enzymes. It travels along the single DNA strand, adding free nucleotides to the 3′ end of the new strand. Nucleotides can be added only to this end of the strand, so replication always proceeds from the 5′ to the 3′ end. When referring to the orientation of sequences along a gene, the 5′ direction is termed "upstream," while the 3′ direction is termed "downstream."

In addition to adding new nucleotides, DNA polymerase performs part of a **proofreading** procedure, in which a newly added nucleotide is checked to make certain that it is in fact complementary to the template base. If it is not, the nucleotide is excised and replaced with a correct complementary nucleotide base. This process substantially enhances the accuracy of DNA replication. When a DNA replication error is not successfully repaired, a mutation has occurred. As will be seen in Chapter 3, many such mutations cause genetic diseases.

▼ DNA replication is critically dependent on the principle of complementary base pairing. This allows a single strand of the double-stranded DNA

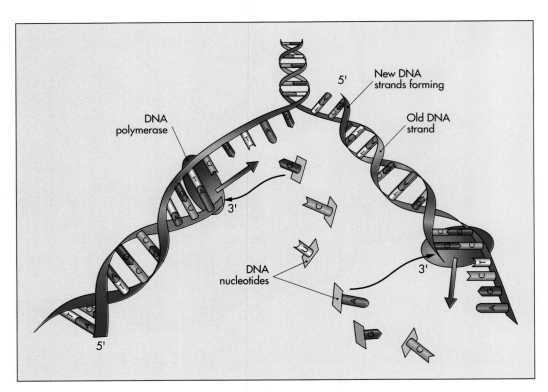

FIG. 2-5   DNA replication. The hydrogen bonds between the two original strands are broken, allowing the bases in each strand to undergo complementary base pairing with free bases. This process, which proceeds 5′ to 3′ on each strand, forms two new double strands of DNA.

molecule to form a template for the synthesis of a new, complementary strand. ▲

The rate of DNA replication in humans, about 40 to 50 nucleotides per second, is comparatively slow. In bacteria the rate is much higher, reaching 500 to 1,000 nucleotides per second. Given that some human chromosomes have as many as 250 million nucleotides, replication would be an extraordinarily time-consuming process if it proceeded linearly from one end of the chromosome to the other (for a chromosome of this size, a single round of replication would require nearly 2 months). Instead, replication begins at many different points along the chromosome, termed **replication origins**. The resulting multiple separations of the DNA strands are called **replication bubbles** (Fig. 2-6). By occurring simultaneously at many different sites along the chromosome, the replication process can proceed much more quickly.

▼ **Replication bubbles allow DNA replication to take place at multiple locations on the chromosome, greatly speeding the replication process.** ▲

From Genes to Proteins

While DNA is formed and replicated in the cell nucleus, protein synthesis takes place in the cytoplasm. The information contained in DNA must thus be transported to the cytoplasm and then used to dictate the composition of proteins. This involves two processes, **transcription** and **translation.** Briefly, the DNA code is **transcribed** into messenger RNA, which then leaves the nucleus to be **translated** into proteins. These

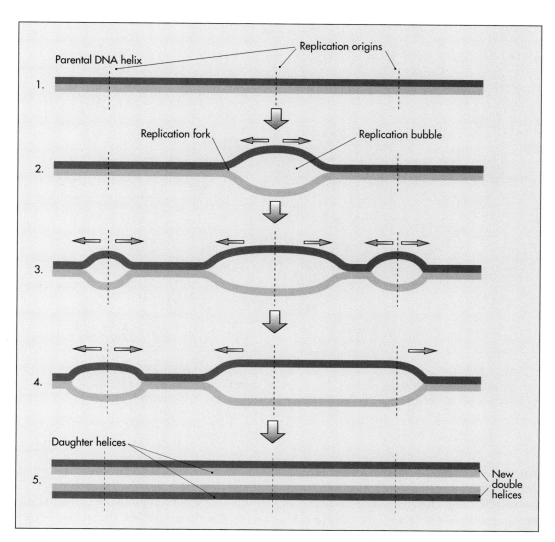

FIG. 2-6 Replication bubbles form at multiple points along the DNA strand, allowing replication to proceed more rapidly.

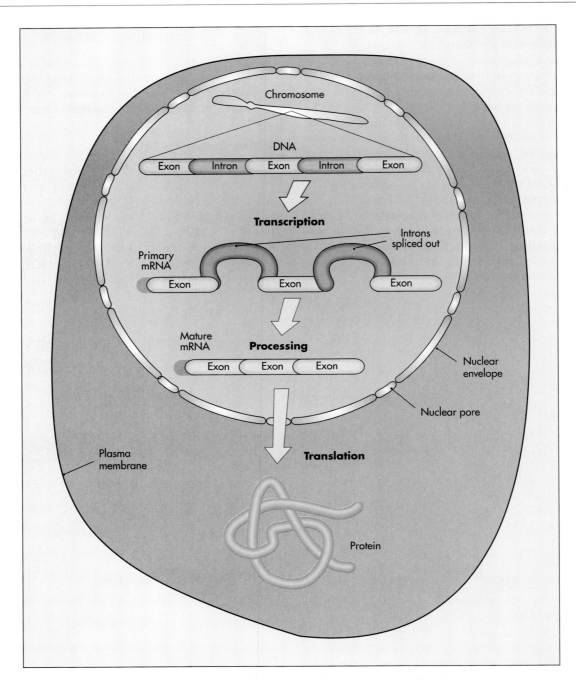

FIG. 2-7 A summary of the steps leading from DNA to proteins. Replication and transcription occur in the cell nucleus. The mRNA is then transported to the cytoplasm, where translation of the mRNA into amino acid sequences composing a protein occurs.

processes, summarized in Fig. 2-7, will be discussed at length later. Transcription and translation are both mediated by **ribonucleic acid (RNA),** a type of nucleic acid that is chemically similar to DNA. Like DNA, RNA is composed of sugars, phosphate groups, and nitrogenous bases. It differs from DNA in that the sugar is ribose instead of deoxyribose and in that uracil rather than thymine is one of the four bases. Uracil is structurally similar to thymine, so, like thymine, it can pair with adenine. Another difference between RNA and DNA is that whereas DNA usually occurs as a double strand, RNA usually occurs as a single strand.

▼ DNA sequences encode proteins through the processes of transcription and translation. These both involve ribonucleic acid, a single-stranded molecule similar to DNA except that it has a ribose sugar and a uracil base rather than thymine. ▲

Transcription

Transcription is the process by which an RNA sequence is formed from a DNA template (Fig. 2-8). The type of RNA produced by the transcription process is termed **messenger RNA** (**mRNA**). To initiate mRNA transcription, one of the **RNA polymerase** enzymes (RNA polymerase II) binds to a **promoter** site on the DNA (a promoter is a nucleotide sequence that lies just upstream of a gene). The RNA polymerase then pulls a portion of the DNA strands apart from one another, exposing unattached DNA bases. One of the two DNA strands provides the template for the sequence of mRNA nucleotides. Although either DNA strand could in principle serve as the template for mRNA synthesis, only one is chosen to do so in a given region of the chromosome. This choice is determined by the promoter sequence, which orients the RNA polymerase in a specific direction along the DNA sequence. Since mRNA can be synthesized only in the 5′ to 3′ direction, the promoter, by specifying directionality, determines which DNA strand serves as the template. RNA polymerase moves in the 3′ to 5′ direction along the DNA template strand, assembling the complementary mRNA strand from 5′ to 3′ (see Fig. 2-8). Because of complementary base pairing, the mRNA nucleotide sequence is identical to that of the DNA strand that does not serve as the template (except, of course, for the substitution of uracil for thymine).

Soon after RNA synthesis begins, the 5′ end of the growing RNA molecule is "capped" by the addition of a chemically modified guanine nucleotide. This **5′ cap** appears to help to prevent the RNA molecule from being degraded during synthesis, and later it helps to indicate the starting position for translation of the mRNA molecule into protein. Transcription continues until a group of bases called a **termination sequence** is reached. Near this point, a series of 100 to 200 adenine bases are added to the 3′ end of the RNA molecule. This structure, known as the poly-A tail, may be involved in stabilizing the mRNA molecule so that it is not degraded when it reaches the cytoplasm. RNA polymerase usually continues to transcribe DNA for several thousand additional bases, but the mRNA bases following the **poly-A tail** are eventually lost. Finally, the DNA strands and RNA polymerase separate from the RNA strand, leaving a transcribed single mRNA strand. This mRNA molecule is termed the **primary transcript.**

In some human genes, such as the one that can cause Duchenne muscular dystrophy, several different pro-

FIG. 2-8   Transcription of DNA to mRNA. RNA polymerase II proceeds along the DNA strand in the 3′ to 5′ direction, assembling a strand of mRNA nucleotides that is complementary to the DNA template strand.

moters exist and are located in different parts of the gene. Thus, transcription of the gene can start in different places, producing somewhat different proteins. This allows the same gene sequence to code for variations of a protein in different tissues (e.g., muscle tissue versus brain tissue).

▼ In the process of transcription, RNA polymerase II binds to a promoter site near the 5′ end of a gene on the non-template strand and, through complementary base pairing, helps to produce an mRNA strand from the template DNA strand. ▲

Transcription and the Regulation of Gene Expression

Some genes—a fairly small proportion—are transcribed in all cells of the body. These **housekeeping genes** encode products that are required for the cell's maintenance and metabolism. However, most genes are transcribed only in specific tissues at specific points in time. In most cells, then, only a small proportion of genes are actively transcribed. This specificity explains why there is a large variety of different cell types making different protein products, even though nearly all cells have exactly the same DNA sequence. For example, the globin genes are transcribed only in the progenitors of red blood cells (where they help to form hemoglobin), and the low-density lipoprotein (LDL) receptor genes are transcribed only in liver cells.

Many different proteins participate in the process of transcription. Some of these are required for the transcription of all structural genes and are termed **general transcription factors.** Others, labeled **specific transcription factors,** have more specialized roles, activating only certain genes at certain stages of development. A key transcriptional element is RNA polymerase II, which was described previously. Although this enzyme plays a vital role in initiating transcription by binding to the promoter region, it cannot locate the promoter region on its own. Furthermore, it is incapable of producing significant quantities of mRNA by itself. Effective transcription requires the interaction of a large complex of 50 or so different proteins. These include general transcription factors, which bind to RNA polymerase and to specific DNA sequences in the promoter region (sequences such as TATA and others needed for transcription initiation). The general transcription factors allow RNA polymerase to bind to the promoter region so that it can function effectively in transcription (Fig. 2-9).

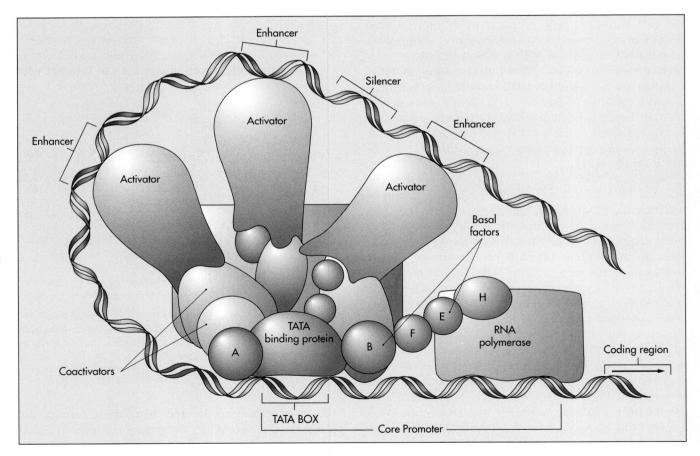

FIG. 2-9 Key elements of transcription control include general (basal) transcription factors and specific enhancers and silencers. The activity of enhancers is mediated by activators and co-activators, which are specific transcription factors.
(Adapted from Tjian R [1995] Molecular machines that control genes. Sci. Am. 272:54-61.)

The transcriptional activity of specific genes can be greatly increased by interaction with sequences called **enhancers,** which may be located thousands of bases upstream or downstream of the gene. Enhancers, however, do not interact directly with genes. Instead, they are bound by a class of specific transcription factors, termed **activators.** Activators bind to a second class of specific transcription factor, **co-activators**, which in turn bind to the general transcription factor complex described previously (see Fig. 2-9). This chain of interactions, from enhancer to activator to co-activator to the general transcription complex and finally to the gene itself, increases the transcription rate of specific genes at specific points in time. Whereas enhancers help to increase the transcriptional activity of genes, other DNA sequences, known as **silencers**, help to repress the transcription of genes through a similar series of interactions.

Mutations in enhancer, silencer, or promoter sequences, as well as mutations in the genes encoding transcription factors, can lead to faulty expression of vital genes and consequently to genetic disease. Many examples of such diseases are discussed in the following chapters.

▼ Transcription factors are required for the transcription of DNA to mRNA. These include general transcription factors that are utilized by all genes as well as specific transcription factors that help to initiate the transcription of genes in specific cell types at specific points in time. Transcription is also regulated by enhancer and silencer sequences that may be located thousands of bases away from the gene. ▲

The large number and complexity of transcription factors allows for fine-tuned regulation of gene expression. But how do the transcription factors locate specific DNA sequences? This is achieved by **DNA-binding motifs**: configurations in the protein that allow them to fit snugly and stably into a unique portion of the DNA double helix. Several examples of these binding motifs are listed in Table 2-1, and Fig. 2-10 illustrates the binding of one such motif to DNA. Each major motif contains many variations that allow specificity in DNA binding.

An intriguing type of DNA-binding motif is contained in the HMG (high-mobility group) class of proteins. These proteins are capable of bending DNA and thus may facilitate interactions between distantly located enhancers and the appropriate basal factors and promoters (see Fig. 2-9).

▼ Transcription factors contain DNA-binding motifs that allow them to interact with specific DNA sequences. In some cases, they can bend DNA so that distant enhancer sequences can interact with target genes. ▲

TABLE 2-1	The Major Classes of DNA-Binding Motifs Found in Transcription Factors	
Motif	**Description**	**Human disease examples**
Helix-turn-helix	Two α helices are connected by a short chain of amino acids, which constitute the "turn." The carboxyl-terminal helix is a recognition helix that binds to the DNA major groove.	Homeodomain proteins (HOX): mutations in human *HOXD13* and *HOXA13* cause synpolydactyly and hand-foot-genital syndrome, respectively.
Helix-loop-helix	Two α helices (one short and one long) are connected by a flexible loop. The loop allows the two helices to fold back and interact with one another. The helices can bind to DNA or to other helix-loop-helix structures.	Mutations in the *TWIST* gene cause Saethre-Chotzen syndrome (acrocephalosyndactyly type III)
Zinc finger	Zinc molecules are used to stabilize amino acid structures (e.g., α helices or β sheets), with binding of the α helix to the DNA major groove.	*BRCA1* (breast cancer gene); *WT1* (Wilms tumor gene); *GLI3* (Greig syndrome gene); vitamin D receptor gene (mutations cause rickets)
Leucine zipper	Two leucine-rich α helices are held together by amino acid side chains. The α helices form a Y-shaped structure whose side chains bind to the DNA major groove.	*RB1* (retinoblastoma gene); *JUN* and *FOS* oncogenes
β Sheets	Side chains extend from the 2-stranded β sheet to form contacts with the DNA helix.	TBX family of genes: *TBX5* (Holt-Oram syndrome); *TBX3* (ulnar-mammary syndrome)

FIG. 2-10 A helix-loop-helix motif binds tightly to a specific DNA sequence.

FIG. 2-11 Gene splicing. Introns are precisely removed from the primary mRNA transcript to produce a mature mRNA transcript. Consensus sequences mark the sites at which splicing occurs.

Gene activity can also be related to patterns of DNA coiling. For example, regions of DNA in which the chromatin is highly condensed are not easily accessible to transcription factors and are thus likely to be transcriptionally inactive.

Gene Splicing

The primary mRNA transcript is exactly complementary to the base sequence of the DNA template. In **eukaryotes,*** an important step takes place before this RNA transcript leaves the nucleus. Sections of the RNA are removed by nuclear enzymes, and the remaining sections are spliced together to form the functional mRNA that will migrate to the cytoplasm. The excised sequences are called **introns,** and the sequences that are left to code for proteins are called **exons** (Fig. 2-11). Only when gene splicing is completed does the **mature transcript** move out of the nucleus into the cytoplasm. Some genes contain **alternative splice sites,** which allow the same primary transcript to be spliced in different ways, ultimately producing different protein products from the same gene. Errors in gene splicing, like replication errors, are a form of mutation that can lead to genetic disease.

▼ Introns are spliced out of the primary mRNA transcript before the mature transcript leaves the nucleus. Exons contain the mRNA that specifies proteins. ▲

The Genetic Code

Proteins are composed of one or more **polypeptides**, which are in turn composed of sequences of **amino acids**. The body contains 20 different types of amino acids, and the amino acid sequences that make up

polypeptides must in some way be designated by the DNA after transcription into mRNA.

Because there are 20 different amino acids and only four different RNA bases, a single base could not specify each amino acid. Similarly, specific amino acids could not be defined by couplets of bases (e.g., adenine followed by guanine, or uracil followed by adenine) because only 16 (4 × 4) different couplets are possible. If triplet sets of bases are translated into amino acids, however, 64 (4 × 4 × 4) combinations can be achieved—more than enough to specify each amino acid. Conclusive proof that amino acids are specified by these triplets of bases, or **codons,** was obtained by manufacturing synthetic nucleotide sequences and allowing them to direct the formation of polypeptides in the laboratory. The correspondence between specific codons and amino acids, known as the **genetic code,** is shown in Table 2-2.

Of the 64 possible codons, 3 signal the end of a gene and are known as **stop codons**. These are UAA, UGA, and UAG. The remaining 61 all specify amino acids. This means that most amino acids can be specified by more than one codon, as Table 2-2 shows. The genetic code is thus said to be "degenerate." While a given

---

*Eukaryotes are organisms that have a defined cell nucleus, as opposed to **prokaryotes,** which lack a defined nucleus.

First Position (5' end) ↓	Second Position				Third Position (3' end) ↓
	U	**C**	**A**	**G**	
U	Phe	Ser	Tyr	Cys	U
U	Phe	Ser	Tyr	Cys	C
U	Leu	Ser	STOP	STOP	A
U	Leu	Ser	STOP	Trp	G
C	Leu	Pro	His	Arg	U
C	Leu	Pro	His	Arg	C
C	Leu	Pro	Gln	Arg	A
C	Leu	Pro	Gln	Arg	G
A	Ile	Thr	Asn	Ser	U
A	Ile	Thr	Asn	Ser	C
A	Ile	Thr	Lys	Arg	A
A	Met	Thr	Lys	Arg	G
G	Val	Ala	Asp	Gly	U
G	Val	Ala	Asp	Gly	C
G	Val	Ala	Glu	Gly	A
G	Val	Ala	Glu	Gly	G

TABLE 2-2   The Genetic Code*†

*Examples: UUG is translated into leucine; UAA is a stop codon; GGG is translated into glycine. Under some circumstances the UGA codon can specify an amino acid called *selenocysteine*. This is often termed the "21st" amino acid.

†*Ala*, Alanine; *Arg*, arginine; *Asn*, asparagine; *Asp*, aspartic acid; *Cys*, cysteine; *Gln*, glycine; *Glu*, glutamine; *Gly*, glutamic acid; *His*, histidine; *Ile*, isoleucine; *Leu*, leucine; *Lys*, lysine; *Met*, methionine; *Phe*, phenylalanine; *Pro*, proline; *Ser*, serine; *Thr*, threonine; *Trp*, tryptophan; *Tyr*, tyrosine; *Val*, valine.

FIG. 2-12 The structure of tRNA. In two dimensions, the tRNA has a cloverleaf shape. Note the 3' site of attachment for an amino acid. The anticodon pairs with a complementary mRNA codon.

amino acid may be specified by more than one codon, each codon can designate only one amino acid.

▼ Individual amino acids, which compose proteins, are encoded by units of three mRNA bases, termed "codons." There are 64 possible codons and only 20 amino acids, so the genetic code is degenerate. ▲

A significant feature of the genetic code is that it is universal: virtually all living organisms use the same DNA codes to specify amino acids. One known exception to this rule is in **mitochondria**, cytoplasmic organelles that are the sites of cellular respiration (see Fig. 2-1). The mitochondria have their own extranuclear DNA molecules. Several codons of mitochondrial DNA encode different amino acids than do the same nuclear DNA codons.

Translation

Translation is the process in which mRNA provides a template for the synthesis of a polypeptide. mRNA cannot, however, bind directly to amino acids. Instead, it interacts with **transfer RNA (tRNA)**, a cloverleaf-shaped RNA strand of about 80 nucleotides. As Fig. 2-12 illustrates, the tRNA molecule has a site at its 3' end for the attachment of an amino acid by a covalent bond. At the opposite end of the cloverleaf is a sequence of three nucleotides called the **anticodon**. This sequence undergoes complementary base pairing with an appropriate codon in the mRNA. mRNA thus specifies the sequence of amino acids by acting through tRNA.

The cytoplasmic site of protein synthesis is the **ribosome**, which consists of roughly equal parts of enzymatic proteins and **ribosomal RNA (rRNA)**. The function of rRNA is to help to bind mRNA and tRNA to the ribosome. During translation, depicted in Fig. 2-13, the ribosome first binds to an initiation site on the mRNA sequence. This site consists of a specific codon, AUG, which specifies the amino acid methionine (this amino acid is usually removed from the polypeptide before the completion of polypeptide synthesis). The ribosome then binds the tRNA to its surface so that base pairing can occur between tRNA and mRNA. The ribosome moves along the mRNA sequence, codon by codon, in

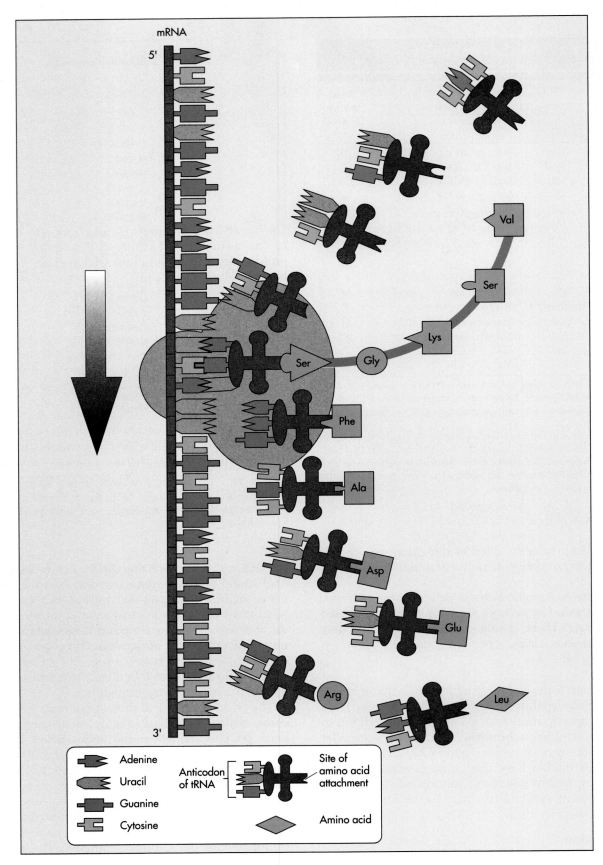

FIG. 2-13 Translation of mRNA to amino acids. The ribosome moves along the mRNA strand in the 5' to 3' direction, assembling a growing polypeptide chain. In this example the mRNA sequence GUG-AGC-AAG-GGU-UCA has assembled five amino acids, Val, Ser, Lys, Gly, and Ser, into a polypeptide.

the usual 5' to 3' direction. As each codon is processed, an amino acid is translated by the interaction of mRNA and tRNA.

In this process, the ribosome provides an enzyme that catalyzes the formation of covalent peptide bonds between the adjacent amino acids, resulting in a growing polypeptide. When the ribosome arrives at a stop codon on the mRNA sequence, translation and polypeptide formation cease. The amino (NH_2) terminus of the polypeptide corresponds to the 5' end of the mRNA strand, and the carboxyl (COOH) terminus corresponds to the 3' end. With synthesis completed, the mRNA, ribosome, and polypeptide separate from one another. The polypeptide is then released into the cytoplasm.

▼ **In the process of translation, the mRNA sequence serves as a template to specify sequences of amino acids. These sequences, which form polypeptides, are assembled by ribosomes. tRNA and rRNA interact with mRNA in the translation process.** ▲

Before a newly synthesized polypeptide can begin its existence as a functional protein, it often undergoes further processing, termed **posttranslational modification.** These modifications can take a variety of forms, including cleavage into smaller polypeptide units or combination with other polypeptides to form a larger protein. Other possible modifications include the addition of carbohydrate side chains to the polypeptide. These modifications are needed, for example, to produce proper folding of the mature protein or to stabilize its structure. An example of a clinically important protein that undergoes considerable posttranslational modification is given by type 1 collagen (Clinical Commentary 2-1).

▼ **Posttranslational modification consists of various chemical changes that occur in proteins shortly after they are translated.** ▲

THE STRUCTURE OF GENES AND THE GENOME

Some aspects of gene structure, such as the existence of introns and exons, have already been touched on. Alterations of different parts of genes can have quite distinct consequences in terms of genetic disease. It is therefore necessary to describe more fully the details of gene structure. A schematic diagram of gene structure is given in Fig. 2-14.

Introns and Exons

The intron-exon structure of genes, discovered in 1977, is one attribute that distinguishes eukaryotes from prokaryotes. Introns form the major portion of most eukaryotic genes. As noted previously, introns are spliced out of the mRNA before it leaves the nucleus. This splicing must be under very precise control, or there would be an intolerable amount of variation in the amino acid sequences produced from mRNA. Splicing is controlled by DNA sequences known as **consensus sequences** (so named because the sequences are common in all eukaryotic organisms) that are located adjacent to each exon.

Since most eukaryotic genes are composed primarily of introns, it is natural to ask whether introns might have some function. At present, this is largely material for speculation. One interesting hypothesis is that introns, by lengthening genes, encourage the shuffling of genes when homologous chromosomes exchange material during meiosis (see later discussion). It has also been suggested that introns have evolved to modify the amount of time required for DNA replication and transcription.

▼ **The intron-exon structure is a key feature of most eukaryotic genes. Presently, the function of introns, if any, is unknown.** ▲

Surprisingly, at least a few introns contain transcribed genes that are apparently unrelated to the gene in which

FIG. 2-14 Details of gene structure, showing promoter and upstream regulation (enhancer) sequences and a poly-A addition site.

CLINICAL COMMENTARY 2-1

OSTEOGENESIS IMPERFECTA, AN INHERITED COLLAGEN DISORDER

As its name implies, osteogenesis imperfecta is a disease caused by defects in the formation of bone. This disorder, sometimes known as "brittle bone disease," affects approximately 1/10,000 individuals in all ethnic groups. WWW

Nearly all cases of osteogenesis imperfecta are caused by defects in type I collagen, a major component of bone that provides much of its structural stability. The function of collagen in bone is analogous to that of the steel bars incorporated in reinforced concrete. This is perhaps an especially apt analogy because the tensile strength of collagen fibrils is roughly equivalent to that of steel wires.

When type I collagen is improperly formed, the bone loses much of its strength and thus fractures easily (Fig. 2-15). Patients with osteogenesis imperfecta may suffer hundreds of bone fractures, or they may suffer only a few. The disease is highly variable in its expression (reasons for this will be discussed in Chapter 4). In addition to bone fractures, patients may have short stature, hear-

ing loss, abnormal tooth development (dentinogenesis imperfecta), bluish sclerae, and various bone deformities. Osteogenesis imperfecta is commonly classified into four types, as shown in Table 2-3. There is currently no cure for this disease, and patient management consists largely of the repair of fractures and, in some cases, the use of external or internal bone support (e.g., surgically implanted rods). Physical rehabilitation also plays an important role in clinical management.

Type I collagen is a trimeric protein (having three subunits) with a triple helix structure (Fig. 2-16). It is formed from a precursor protein, type I procollagen. Two of the three subunits of type 1 procollagen (labeled proα1[I] chains) are encoded by a gene on chromosome 17 that is about 18,000 base pairs (18 kb) in length. The third subunit, the proα2(I) chain, is encoded by a gene on chromosome 7 that is 38 kb in size. Each of these genes contains more than 50 exons. After transcription and splicing, the mature mRNA formed from each gene is only 5 to 7 kb in length. The mature mRNAs proceed to the cytoplasm, where they are translated into polypeptide chains by the ribosomal machinery of the cell.

At this point, the polypeptide chains undergo a series of posttranslational modifications. Many of the proline

A

B

FIG. 2-15 **A,** A stillborn infant with type II osteogenesis imperfecta (the perinatal lethal form). The infant had a type I procollagen mutation and presents with short, slightly twisted limbs. **B,** Radiograph of the infant shown in part **A**. Note rib fractures and bowed, thickened femurs.

TABLE 2-3   Subtypes of Osteogenesis Imperfecta (OI)

OI type	Disease features
I	Mild bone fragility, blue sclerae, hearing loss in 50% of patients, normal stature, few bone deformities
II	Most severe form with extreme bone fragility, long bone deformities, compressed femurs; lethal in the perinatal period (most die of respiratory failure)
III	Severe bone fragility, very short stature, variably blue sclerae, progressive bone deformities, dentinogenesis imperfecta common
IV	Short stature, normal sclerae, mild to moderate bone deformity, hearing loss in some patients, dentinogenesis imperfecta common; bone fragility is variable

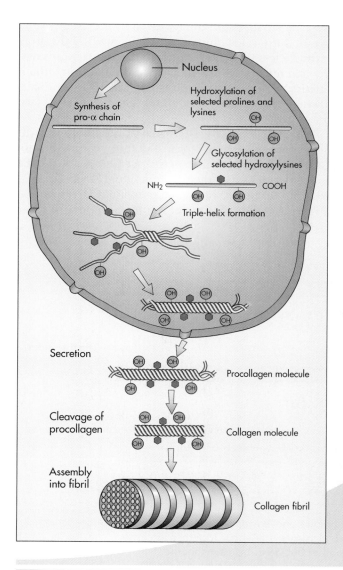

and lysine **residues*** are hydroxylated (i.e., hydroxyl groups are added) to form hydroxyproline and hydroxylysine, respectively. The three polypeptides, two proα1(I) chains and one proα2(I) chain, begin to associate with one another at their COOH termini. This association is stabilized by sulfide bonds that form between the chains near the COOH termini. The triple helix then forms, in zipper-like fashion, beginning at the COOH terminus and proceeding toward the NH$_2$ terminus. Some of the hydroxylysines are glycosylated: sugars are added, a modification that commonly occurs in the rough endoplasmic reticulum (see Fig. 2-1), where the chains reside for a time. The hydroxyl groups in the hydroxyprolines help to connect the three chains by forming hydrogen bonds, which then stabilize the triple helix. Critical to the proper folding of the helix is the presence of a glycine in every third position of each polypeptide. This is because every third residue must fit into the center of the helix, and only glycine is small enough to do so.

Once the protein has folded into a triple helix, it moves from the endoplasmic reticulum to the Golgi apparatus (see Fig. 2-1) and is secreted from the cell. Yet another modification then takes place: the procollagen is cleaved by proteases near both the NH$_2$ and COOH termini of the triple helix, removing some amino acids at each end. These amino acids performed essential functions earlier in the life of the protein (e.g., helping to form the triple helix structure, helping to thread the protein through the endoplasmic reticulum) but are no longer needed. This cleavage results in the mature protein, type I collagen. The collagen then assembles itself into fibrils, which react with adjacent molecules outside the cell, forming covalent cross-links that impart tensile strength to the fibrils.

The path from the DNA sequence to the mature collagen protein involves many steps. The complexity of this path provides many opportunities for mistakes (in replication, transcription, translation, or posttranslational modification) that can cause disease. One common mutation produces a replacement of glycine by another amino acid. Since only glycine is small enough to be accommodated in the center of the helix structure, substitution of a different amino acid will cause instability of the structure and thus poorly formed fibrils. This type of mutation is seen in most cases of type II osteogenesis imperfecta. Other mutations can cause excess posttranslational modification of the polypeptide chains, again producing abnormal fibrils. Other examples of disease-causing mutations are provided in the suggested readings at the end of this chapter.

---

*A residue is an amino acid that has been incorporated into a polypeptide chain.

FIG. 2-16   The process of collagen fibril formation. After the pro-α polypeptide chain is formed, a series of posttranslational modifications takes place, including hydroxylation and glycosylation. Three polypeptide chains assemble into a triple helix, which is secreted outside the cell. Portions of each end of the procollagen molecule are cleaved, resulting in the mature collagen molecule. These molecules then assemble into collagen fibrils.

the introns are contained. For example, introns of the human neurofibromatosis type 1 *(NF1)* gene contain three genes that are transcribed in the direction opposite that of the *NF1* gene itself. These genes appear to have no functional relationship to the *NF1* gene. Similar gene inserts have been found within the factor VIII gene on the human X chromosome.

Types of DNA

While most of the emphasis in genetics is given to DNA that encodes proteins, it is important to note that fewer than 10% of the three billion nucleotide pairs in the human genome actually perform this role. Most of our genetic material has no known function. To better understand the nature of all types of DNA, we will briefly review the several categories into which they are classified (Fig. 2-17).

The first, and most common, class of DNA is termed **single-copy DNA.** As the name implies, single-copy DNA sequences are seen only once (or possibly a few times) in the genome. Single-copy DNA composes about 75% of the genome and includes the protein-coding genes. However, protein-coding DNA represents only a small proportion of all single-copy DNA. Most of it is found in introns or in DNA sequences that lie between genes.

The remaining 25% of the genome consists of **repetitive DNA,** sequences that are repeated over and over again in the genome, often thousands of times. There are two major classes of repetitive DNA, **dispersed repetitive DNA** and **satellite DNA.** Satellite repeats are clustered together in certain chromosome locations, where they occur in tandem (i.e., the beginning of one

repeat occurs immediately adjacent to the end of another). Dispersed repeats, as the name implies, tend to be scattered singly throughout the genome (they do not occur in tandem).

The term "satellite" is derived from the fact that these sequences, because of their composition, can be easily separated by centrifugation in a cesium chloride density gradient. The DNA appears as a "satellite," separate from the other DNA in the gradient. This term is not to be confused with the "satellites" that can be observed microscopically on certain chromosomes (Chapter 6). Satellite DNA composes approximately 10% of the genome and can be further subdivided into several categories. **Alpha-satellite DNA** occurs as tandem repeats of a 171-bp (base pairs) sequence that can extend several million bp or more in length. This type of satellite DNA is found near the centromeres of chromosomes. **Minisatellites** are blocks of tandem repeats whose total length is much smaller. These repeats, which are 20 to 70 bp in length, usually have a total length of a few thousand base pairs or so. A final category, **microsatellites,** are smaller still: the repeat units are usually only 2, 3, or 4 bp in length, and the total length of the array is usually less than a few hundred base pairs. Minisatellites and microsatellites are of special interest in human genetics because they vary in length among individuals, making them highly useful for gene mapping (see Chapter 8).

Dispersed repetitive DNA makes up about 15% of the genome, and these repeats fall into two major categories, **SINEs** (short interspersed elements) and **LINEs** (long interspersed elements). Individual SINEs range in size from 90 to 500 bp, while individual LINEs can be as large as 7,000 kb. One of the most important types

Single-copy DNA (75%)

Dispersed repetitive DNA (15%)

Satellite DNA (10%)

FIG. 2-17 Single-copy DNA sequences are unique and are dispersed throughout the genome. Satellite DNA sequences are repetitive elements that occur together in clusters, whereas dispersed repeats are similar to one another but do not cluster together.

of SINEs is termed the "*Alu* repeats." The term "*Alu*" derives from the fact that these repeat units, which are about 300 bp in size, contain a DNA sequence that can be cut by the *Alu* restriction enzyme (see Chapter 3 for further discussion). The *Alu* repeats are a **family** of genes, meaning that all of them have highly similar DNA sequences. About 300,000 to 500,000 *Alu* repeats are scattered throughout the genome; these repeats thus constitute about 2% to 3% of all human DNA. A remarkable feature of *Alu* sequences is that they can generate copies of themselves, which can then insert into other parts of the genome. This insertion can sometimes interrupt a protein-coding gene, causing genetic disease (examples will be discussed in Chapter 4).

▼ There are several major types of DNA, including single-copy DNA, satellite DNA, and dispersed repetitive DNA. The latter two categories are both classes of repeated DNA sequences. Less than 10% of our DNA actually encodes proteins. ▲

THE CELL CYCLE

During the course of development, each human progresses from a single-cell **zygote** (an egg cell fertilized by a sperm cell) to a marvelously complex organism containing approximately 100 trillion (10^{14}) individual cells. Because few cells last for an individual's entire lifetime, new ones must be generated to replace those that die. Both of these processes, development and repair, require the manufacture of new cells. The cell division processes responsible for the creation of new diploid cells from existing ones are termed **mitosis** (nuclear division) and **cytokinesis** (cytoplasmic division). Before dividing, a cell must duplicate its contents, including its DNA; this occurs during **interphase.** The alternation of mitosis and interphase is referred to as the **cell cycle.**

As Fig. 2-18 shows, a typical cell spends most of its life in interphase. This portion of the cell cycle is divided into three phases, **G1, S,** and **G2.** During G1 ("gap 1," the interval between mitosis and the onset of DNA replication), synthesis of RNA and proteins takes place. DNA replication occurs during the S (synthesis) phase. During G2 (the interval between the S phase and the next mitosis), some DNA repair takes place, and the cell prepares for mitosis. By the time G2 has been reached, the cell contains 2 identical copies of each of the 46 chromosomes. These identical chromosomes are referred to as **sister chromatids.** Sister chromatids often exchange material during or after the S phase, a process known as **sister chromatid exchange.**

▼ The cell cycle consists of the alternation of cell division (mitosis and cytokinesis) and interphase. DNA replication and protein synthesis take place during interphase. ▲

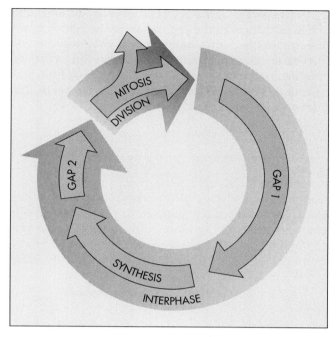

FIG. 2-18   Major phases of the mitotic cell cycle, showing the alternation of interphase and mitosis (division).

The length of the cell cycle varies considerably from one cell type to another. In rapidly dividing cells such as those of epithelial tissue (found in the lining of the intestines and lungs, for example), the cycle may be completed in fewer than 10 hours. Other cells, such as those of the liver, may divide only once each year or so. Some cell types, such as skeletal muscle cells and neurons, completely lose their ability to divide and replicate in adults. Although the lengths of all stages of the cell cycle vary somewhat, the great majority of this variation is due to differences in the length of the G1 phase. When cells stop dividing for a long period, they are often said to be in the G0 stage.

Cells divide in response to important internal and external cues. Before entering mitosis, for example, DNA replication has to be accurate and complete and the cell has to have achieved an appropriate size. The cell must respond to extracellular stimuli that require increased or decreased rates of division. Complex molecular interactions mediate this regulation. Among the most important of these molecules are **cyclin-dependent kinases** (CDKs), a family of kinases that phosphorylate other regulatory proteins at key stages of the cell cycle. In order to carry out this function, they must form complexes with various **cyclins**, proteins that are synthesized at specific cell-cycle stages and are then degraded when CDK action is no longer needed. The cyclins and CDKs, as well as the many proteins that interact with them, are the subjects of intense study because of their vital role in the cell cycle and because their malfunction can lead to cancer (Chapter 11).

▼ The length of the cell cycle varies in different cell types. Critical to the regulation of the cell cycle are cyclin-dependent kinases, which regulate the cell cycle by phosphorylating other proteins, and cyclins, which must form complexes with cyclin-dependent kinases. Faulty regulation of the cell cycle can lead to cancer. ▲

Mitosis

Although mitosis usually requires only 1 to 2 hours to complete, this portion of the cell cycle involves many critical and complex processes. Mitosis is divided into several phases (Fig. 2-19). During **prophase,** the first mitotic stage, the chromosomes become visible under a light microscope as they condense and coil (chromo-

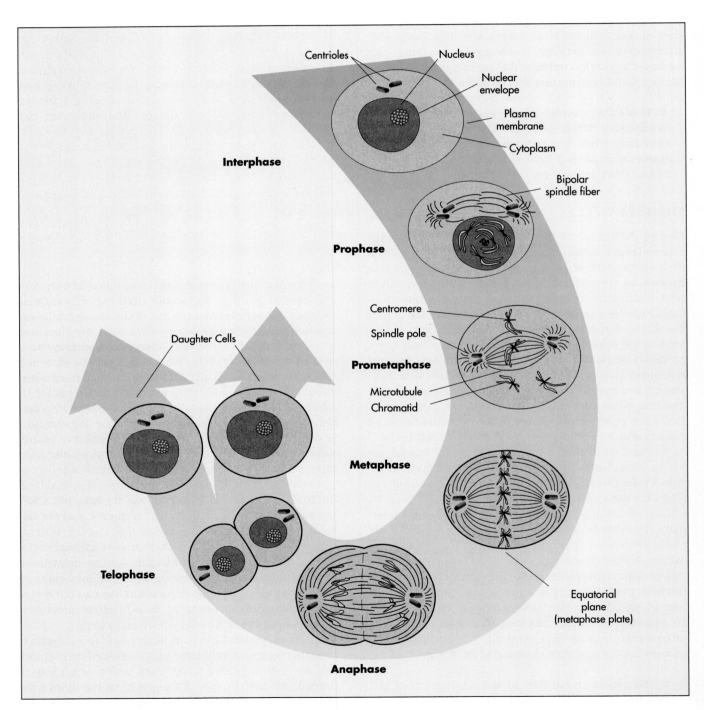

FIG. 2-19 The stages of mitosis, during which two identical diploid cells are formed from one original diploid cell.

somes are not clearly visible during interphase). The two sister chromatids of each chromosome lie together, attached at a point called the **centromere.** The nuclear membrane, which surrounds the nucleus, disappears during this stage. **Spindle fibers** begin to form. These radiate from two **centrioles** located on opposite sides of the cell. The spindle fibers become attached to the centromeres of each chromosome and eventually pull the two sister chromatids in opposite directions.

The chromosomes reach their most highly condensed state during **metaphase,** the next stage of mitosis. Because they are highly condensed, they are easiest to visualize microscopically during this phase. For this reason, clinical diagnosis of chromosome disorders is usually based on metaphase chromosomes. During metaphase the spindle fibers begin to contract and pull the centromeres of the chromosomes, which are now arranged along the middle of the spindle (the **equatorial plane** of the cell).

During **anaphase,** the next mitotic stage, the centromeres of each chromosome split, allowing the sister chromatids to separate. The chromatids are then pulled by the spindle fibers, centromere first, toward opposite sides of the cell. At the end of anaphase, the cell contains 92 separate chromosomes, half lying near one side of the cell and half lying near the other side. If all has proceeded correctly, the two sets of chromosomes are identical.

Telophase, the final stage of mitosis, is characterized by the formation of new nuclear membranes around each of the two sets of 46 chromosomes. Also, the spindle fibers disappear, and the chromosomes begin to decondense. Cytokinesis generally occurs after nuclear division and results in a roughly equal division of the cytoplasm into two parts. When telophase is completed, two diploid **daughter cells,** both identical to the original cell, have been formed.

▼ Mitosis is the process through which two identical diploid daughter cells are formed from a single diploid cell. ▲

Meiosis

When an egg cell and sperm cell unite to form a zygote, their chromosomes are combined into a single cell. Because humans are diploid organisms, there must be a mechanism to reduce the number of chromosomes in gametes to the haploid state. Otherwise the zygote would have 92, instead of the normal 46, chromosomes. The primary mechanism by which haploid gametes are formed from diploid precursor cells is termed **meiosis.**

Two cell divisions occur during meiosis. Each meiotic division has been divided into stages with the same names as those of mitosis, but the processes involved in some of the stages are quite different (Fig. 2-20). During meiosis I, often called the **reduction division stage,** two haploid cells are formed from a diploid cell. These diploid cells are the **oogonia** in females and the **spermatogonia** in males. Following meiosis I, a second meiosis, the **equational division,** takes place, and each haploid cell is replicated.

The first stage of meiosis is **interphase I.** During this phase, as in mitotic interphase, important processes such as replication of chromosomal DNA take place. The second phase of meiosis I, **prophase I,** is quite complex and includes many of the key events that distinguish meiosis from mitosis. Prophase I begins as the chromatin strands coil and condense, causing them to become visible as chromosomes. During a process called **synapsis,** the homologous chromosomes pair up, side by side, lying together in perfect alignment (in males, the X and Y chromosomes, being mostly nonhomologous, line up end to end). This pairing of homologous chromosomes is an important part of the cell cycle that does not occur in mitosis. As prophase I continues, the chromatids of the two chromosomes intertwine. Each pair of intertwined homologous chromosomes is called a **bivalent** (indicating two chromosomes in the unit) or **tetrad** (indicating four chromatids in the unit).

A second key feature of prophase I is the formation of **chiasmata** (plural of **chiasma**), cross-shaped structures that mark attachments between the homologous chromosomes (Fig. 2-21). Each chiasma indicates a point at which the homologous chromosomes exchange genetic material. This process, called **crossing over,** produces chromosomes consisting of combinations of parts of the original chromosomes. This chromosomal "shuffling" is important because it greatly increases the possible combinations of genes in each gamete and thereby increases the number of possible combinations of human traits. Also, as we shall see in Chapter 8, this phenomenon is critically important in assessing the order of genes along chromosomes. At the end of prophase I, the bivalents begin to move toward the equatorial plane, a spindle apparatus begins to form in the cytoplasm, and the nuclear membrane dissipates.

Metaphase I is the next phase. Like mitotic metaphase, this stage is characterized by the completion of spindle formation and the alignment of the bivalents, which are still attached at the chiasmata, in the equatorial plane. The two centromeres of each bivalent now lie on opposite sides of the equatorial plane.

During **anaphase I,** the next stage, the chiasmata disappear, and the homologous chromosomes are pulled by the spindle fibers toward opposite poles of the cell. The key feature of this phase is that, unlike the corresponding phase of mitosis, *the centromeres do not duplicate and divide,* so that only half of the original number of chromosomes migrate toward each pole. The

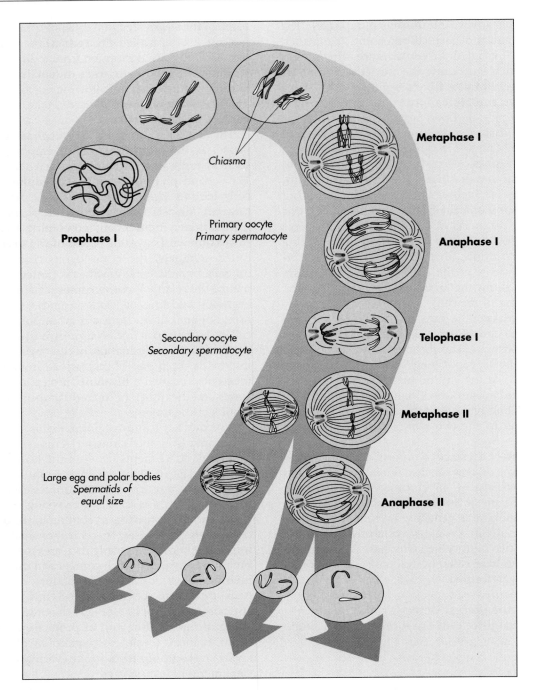

FIG. 2-20 The stages of meiosis, during which haploid gametes are formed from a diploid cell. For brevity, prophase II and telophase II are not shown. Note the relationship between meiosis and spermatogenesis and oogenesis.

chromosomes migrating toward each pole thereby consist of one member of each pair of autosomes and one of the sex chromosomes.

The next stage, **telophase I,** begins when the chromosomes reach opposite sides of the cell. The chromosomes uncoil slightly, and a new nuclear membrane begins to form. The two daughter cells each contain the haploid number of chromosomes, each having two sister chromatids. In humans, cytokinesis also occurs during this phase. The cytoplasm is divided approximately equally between the two daughter cells in the gametes formed in males. In those formed in females, nearly all of the cytoplasm goes into one daughter cell, which will later form the egg. The other daughter cell

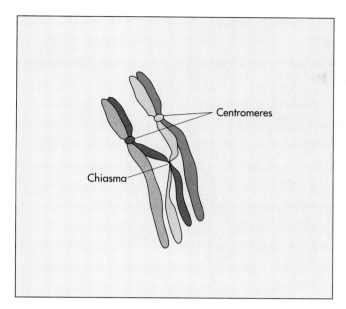

FIG. 2-21 The process of chiasma formation and crossing over results in the exchange of genetic material between homologous chromosomes.

becomes a **polar body,** a small nonfunctional cell that eventually degenerates.

▼ Meiosis I (reduction division) includes a prophase I stage in which homologous chromosomes line up and exchange material (crossing over). During anaphase I the centromeres do not duplicate and divide, so that only one member of each pair of chromosomes migrates to each daughter cell. ▲

The equational division, meiosis II, then begins with **interphase II**. This is a very brief phase. The important feature of interphase II is that, unlike interphase I and mitotic interphase, *no replication of DNA occurs.* **Prophase II**, the next stage, is quite similar to mitotic prophase, except that the cell nucleus contains only the haploid number of chromosomes. During prophase II the chromosomes thicken as they coil, the nuclear membrane disappears, and new spindle fibers are formed. Following this phase is **metaphase II**, during which the spindle fibers pull the chromosomes into alignment at the equatorial plane.

Anaphase II then follows. This stage resembles mitotic anaphase in that the centromeres split, each carrying a single chromatid toward a pole of the cell. The chromatids have now separated, but as Fig. 2-20 shows, chiasma formation and crossing over produce newly separated sister chromatids that may not be identical.

Telophase II, like telophase I, begins when the chromosomes reach opposite poles of the cell. There they begin to uncoil. New nuclear membranes are formed around each group of chromosomes, and cytokinesis

occurs. In gametes formed in males, the cytoplasm is again divided equally between the two daughter cells. The end result of male meiosis is thus four functional daughter cells, each of which has an equal amount of cytoplasm. In female gametes, unequal division of the cytoplasm again occurs, forming the egg cell and another polar body. The polar body formed during meiosis I sometimes undergoes a second division, so three polar bodies may be present when the second stage of meiosis is completed.

▼ Meiosis is a specialized cell division process in which a diploid cell gives rise to haploid gametes. This is accomplished by combining two rounds of division with only one round of DNA replication. ▲

Most chromosome disorders are caused by errors that occur in meiosis. Gametes can be created that contain missing or additional chromosomes or chromosomes with altered structures. In addition, mitotic errors that occur early in the life of the embryo can affect enough of the body's cells to produce clinically significant disease. Mitotic errors occurring at any point in one's lifetime can, under some circumstances, cause cancer. Cancer genetics will be discussed in Chapter 11, and chromosome disorders will be the subject of Chapter 6.

The Relationship Between Meiosis and Gametogenesis

The stages of meiosis can be related directly to stages in **gametogenesis,** the formation of gametes (see Fig. 2-20). In mature males, the seminiferous tubules of the testes are populated by spermatogonia, which are diploid cells. After going through several mitotic divisions, the spermatogonia produce **primary spermatocytes.** Each primary spermatocyte, which is also diploid, undergoes meiosis I to produce a pair of **secondary spermatocytes,** each of which contains 23 double-stranded chromosomes. These undergo meiosis II, and each produces a pair of **spermatids** that contain 23 single-stranded chromosomes. The spermatids then lose most of their cytoplasm and develop tails for swimming as they become mature **sperm** cells. This process, known as **spermatogenesis,** continues throughout the life of the mature male.

▼ In spermatogenesis, each diploid spermatogonium produces four haploid sperm cells. ▲

Oogenesis, the process in which female gametes are formed, differs in several important ways from spermatogenesis. Whereas the cycle of spermatogenesis is constantly recurring in males, much of female oogenesis is completed before birth. Diploid oogonia divide mitotically to produce **primary oocytes** by the third month of fetal development. More than 2 million primary oocytes are formed during gestation, and these are suspended in prophase I by the time the female is born. Meiosis continues only when a mature primary oocyte is ovulated. In meiosis I, the primary oocyte produces one **secondary oocyte** (containing the cytoplasm) and one polar body. The secondary oocyte then emerges from the follicle and proceeds down the fallopian tube, with the polar body attached to it. Meiosis II begins only if the secondary oocyte is fertilized by a sperm cell. If this occurs, one haploid **mature ovum**, containing the cytoplasm, and another haploid polar body are produced. The polar bodies eventually disintegrate. About an hour after fertilization, the nuclei of the sperm cell and ovum fuse, forming a diploid zygote. The zygote then begins its development into an embryo through a series of mitotic divisions.

▼ In oogenesis, one haploid ovum and three haploid polar bodies are produced meiotically from a diploid oogonium. Unlike spermatogenesis, which continues throughout the mature male's life, the first phase of oogenesis is completed before the female is born; oogenesis is then halted until ovulation occurs. ▲

SUGGESTED READINGS

Alberts B, Bray D, Lewis J, Raff M, Roberts K, Watson JD (1994) Molecular Biology of the Cell. Garland Publishing, New York

Byers PH (1995) Disorders of collagen biosynthesis and structure. In: Scriver CR, Beaudet AL, Sly WS, Valle D (eds) The Metabolic and Molecular Bases of Inherited Disease. Vol. 3. McGraw-Hill, New York, pp 4029-4077

Dynlacht BD (1997) Regulation of transcription by proteins that control the cell cycle. Nature 389:149-152

Engelkamp D, van Heyningen V (1996) Transcription factors in disease. Curr. Opin. Genet. Dev. 6:334-342

Gao CY, Zelenka PS (1997) Cyclins, cyclin-dependent kinases and differentiation. BioEssays 19:307-315

Gardiner K (1996) Base composition and gene distribution: critical patterns in mammalian genome organization. Trends Genet. 12:519-524

Lewin B (1997) Genes VI. Oxford University Press, Oxford

Murray A, Hunt T (1994) The Cell Cycle: An Introduction. Oxford University Press, Oxford

Papavassiliou AG (1995) Transcription factors. N. Eng. J. Med. 332:45-47

Sauer F, Tjian R (1997) Mechanisms of transcriptional activation: differences and similarities between yeast, *Drosophila*, and man. Curr. Opin. Genet. Dev. 7:176-181

Tjian R (1995) Molecular machines that control genes. Sci. Am. 272:54-61

STUDY QUESTIONS

1. Consider the following double-stranded DNA sequence:
   5'-CAG AAG AAA ATT AAC ATG TAA-3'
   3'-GTC TTC TTT TAA TTG TAC ATT-5'
   What is the mRNA sequence produced by transcription of this DNA sequence? What is the amino acid sequence produced by translation of the mRNA sequence?

2. Arrange the following terms according to their hierarchical relationship to one another: genes, chromosomes, exons, codons, nucleotides, genome.

3. Less than 10% of our DNA encodes proteins. Furthermore, in a given cell type only 10% of the coding DNA actively encodes proteins. Explain these statements.

4. What are the major differences between mitosis and meiosis?

5. The human body contains approximately 10^{14} cells. Starting with a single-cell zygote, how many mitotic cell divisions, on average, would be required to produce this number of cells?

6. How many mature sperm cells will be produced by 100 primary spermatocytes? How many mature egg cells will be produced by 100 primary oocytes?

3
Genetic Variation: Its Origin and Detection

Humans display a remarkable degree of genetic variation. This is seen in traits such as height, blood pressure, and skin color. Included in the spectrum of genetic variation are disease states, such as cystic fibrosis or type 1 neurofibromatosis (see Chapter 4). This aspect of genetic variation is the focus of medical genetics.

All genetic variation originates from the process known as **mutation**, which is defined as a change in DNA sequence. Mutations can affect either somatic or **germline** cells (cells that produce gametes). Mutations in **somatic** cells (all cells other than germline cells) can lead to cancer and are thus of significant concern. However, our attention in this chapter will be directed primarily to germline mutations because these can be transmitted from one generation to the next.

As a result of mutations, a gene may differ among individuals in terms of its DNA sequence. The differing sequences are referred to as **alleles**. A gene's location on a chromosome is termed a **locus** (from the Latin for "place"). Thus, we might say that an individual has a certain allele at the β-globin locus on chromosome 11. If an individual has the same allele on both members of a chromosome pair, he or she is said to be a **homozygote**. If the alleles differ in DNA sequence, the individual is a **heterozygote**. The alleles that are present at a given locus are referred to as the individual's **genotype**. Some **loci** (plural of locus) vary considerably among individuals. If a locus has two or more alleles whose frequencies each exceed 1% in a population, the locus is said to be **polymorphic** ("many forms"). The polymorphic locus is often termed a **polymorphism**.

In this chapter, we will examine mutation as the source of genetic variation. We will discuss the different types of mutations, as well as the causes and consequences of mutation. In addition, we will discuss biochemical and molecular techniques that are now used to detect genetic variation in human populations.

MUTATION—THE SOURCE OF GENETIC VARIATION
Types of Mutation

Some mutations consist of an alteration of the number or structure of chromosomes in a cell. These major chromosome abnormalities can be observed microscopically and will be the subject of Chapter 6. Here, we will focus on mutations that affect only single genes and are not microscopically observable. Most of our discussion will center on mutations that take place in coding DNA or in regulatory sequences, since mutations occurring in other parts of the genome usually have no clinical consequences.

One important type of **single-gene mutation** is the **base pair substitution**, in which one base pair is replaced by another.* This can result in a change in amino acid sequence; however, because of the redundancy of the genetic code, many of these mutations do not change the amino acid sequence and thus have no consequence. These mutations are called **silent substitutions**. Nonsilent base pair substitutions consist of two basic types: **missense** mutations produce a change in a single amino acid, while **nonsense** mutations produce one of the three stop codons in the mRNA (UAA, UAG, or UGA) (Fig. 3-1). These codons terminate translation of the mRNA and thus result in a premature termination of the polypeptide chain. Conversely, when a stop codon is altered so that it encodes an amino acid, an abnormally elongated polypeptide is produced. Alterations of amino acid sequences can have profound consequences, and many of the serious genetic diseases to be discussed later are the result of such alterations.

---

*In molecular genetics, base pair substitutions are also termed **point mutations**. The latter term, however, was used in classical genetics to denote any mutation small enough to be unobservable under a microscope.

FIG. 3-1 Missense mutations **(A)** produce a single amino acid change, whereas nonsense mutations **(B)** produce a stop codon in the mRNA. Stop codons terminate translation of the polypeptide.

A second major type of mutation consists of **deletions** or **insertions** of one or more base pairs. These mutations, which can produce extra or missing amino acids in a protein, are often detrimental. An example of such a mutation is a three-base-pair deletion that causes most cases of cystic fibrosis seen in Europeans (see Chapter 4). Deletions and insertions tend to be especially harmful when the number of missing or extra base pairs is not a multiple of three. Since codons consist of groups of three base pairs, such insertions or deletions can alter all of the downstream codons. This is termed a **frameshift mutation** (Fig. 3-2). For example, a single-base insertion (an A in the second codon) could convert a sequence read as 5'-ACT GAT TGC GTT-3' to 5'-ACT GA<u>A</u> TTG CGT-3'. This would convert an amino acid sequence from Thr-Asp-Cys-Val to Thr-Glu-Leu-Arg. Frequently, a frameshift mutation produces a stop codon downstream of the insertion or deletion, resulting in a truncated polypeptide.

On a larger scale, **duplications** of whole genes can also lead to genetic disease. The best current example is given by Charcot-Marie-Tooth disease. This disorder, named after the three physicians who described it a century ago, is a peripheral nervous system disease that leads to progressive atrophy of the distal limb muscles.

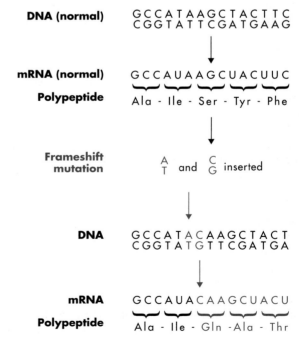

FIG. 3-2 Frameshift mutations result from the addition or deletion of a number of bases that is not a multiple of three. This alters all of the codons downstream from the site of insertion or deletion.

It affects approximately one in 2,500 individuals and exists in several different forms. About 70% of patients who have the most common form (type 1) display a 1.5 million bp duplication on one copy of chromosome 17. As a result, they have three, rather than two, copies of the genes in this region. One of these genes, *PMP22*, encodes a peripheral myelin protein. The increased dosage of the gene product contributes in some way to the demyelination that is characteristic of this form of the disorder. Interestingly, a deletion of this same region produces a distinct disease, hereditary neuropathy with liability to pressure palsies (paralysis). Because a reduction (to 50%) or an increase (to 150%) of the gene product produces disease, this gene is said to display **dosage sensitivity.** Point mutations in *PMP22* itself can produce yet another disease, Dejerine-Sottas syndrome (distal muscle weakness, sensory alterations, muscular atrophy, enlarged spinal nerve roots). **www**

Other types of mutations can alter the regulation of transcription or translation. A **promoter mutation** can decrease the affinity of RNA polymerase for a promoter site, often resulting in reduced production of mRNA. The final result is decreased production of a protein. Mutations of transcription factor genes or enhancer sequences can have similar effects.

Mutations may also interfere with the splicing of introns as mature mRNA is formed from the primary mRNA transcript. **Splice site mutations,** occurring at intron-exon boundaries, alter the splicing signal necessary for proper excision of an intron. These may occur at the GT sequence that always defines the 5′ **donor site** or at the AG sequence that defines the 3′ **acceptor site.** They may also take place in the sequences that lie near the donor and acceptor sites (i.e., the consensus sequences defined in Chapter 2). When such mutations occur, the excision will often be made within the next exon, at a splice site located in the exon. These splice sites, whose DNA sequences differ slightly from those of normal splice sites, are ordinarily unused and "hidden" within the exon. They are thus termed **cryptic splice sites.** The use of a cryptic site for splicing results in partial deletion of the exon. In other cases, an entire exon can be deleted. As Fig. 3-3 shows, splice site mutations can also result in the abnormal inclusion of part or all of an intron in the mature mRNA. Finally, a mutation may occur at a cryptic splice site, causing it to appear as a normal splice site, thus competing with the normal splice site.

Several types of DNA sequences are capable of propagating copies of themselves; these copies are then inserted in other locations on chromosomes. The insertion of these **transposons** (or **mobile elements**) can cause frameshift mutations. Until recently, it was not clear whether this phenomenon, which has been well documented in experimental animals such as fruit flies, occurred in humans. The insertion of mobile elements has now been shown to cause isolated cases of type 1

neurofibromatosis, familial breast cancer, familial polyposis (colon cancer), and hemophilia A and B (clotting disorders) in humans.

The final type of mutation to be considered here has been discovered quite recently and affects tandem repeated DNA sequences (see Chapter 2) that occur within or near certain disease genes. The repeat units are three bases long, so a typical example would be CAGCAGCAG. A normal individual will have a relatively small number of these tandem repeats (e.g., 20 to 30) at a specific chromosome location. For reasons that are not yet understood, the number of repeats can increase dramatically during meiosis or possibly during early fetal development, so that a newborn may have hundreds or even thousands of repeats. When this occurs in certain regions of the genome, it causes genetic disease. Like other mutations, these **expanded repeats** can be transmitted to the patient's offspring. More than a dozen genetic diseases are now known to be caused by expanded repeats. These will be discussed further in Chapter 4.

▼ Mutations are the ultimate source of genetic variation. Some mutations result in genetic disease, whereas others have no physical effects. The principal types of mutations include missense, nonsense, frameshift, deletion, duplication, promoter, and splice site mutations. There is also evidence for mutations caused by the random insertion of mobile elements, and some genetic diseases are known to be caused by expanded repeats. ▲

Molecular Consequences of Mutation

It is useful to think of mutations in terms of their effects on the protein product. Broadly speaking, mutations can result in either a **gain of function** or a **loss of function** of the protein product. Gain-of-function mutations occasionally result in a completely novel protein product. More commonly, they result in over-expression of the product or inappropriate expression (i.e., in the wrong tissue or in the wrong stage of development). Gain-of-function mutations produce a **dominant** disorder.* Charcot-Marie-Tooth disease, mentioned previously, results from overexpression of the protein product and is considered a gain-of-function mutation. Huntington disease, to be discussed in Chapter 4, is thought to be another example.

Loss-of-function mutations are often seen in **recessive** diseases. Here, a mutation results in the loss of 50% of the protein product (e.g., a metabolic enzyme), but the 50% that remains is sufficient for normal

---

*The terms "dominant" and "recessive" are discussed fully in Chapter 4. Briefly, a dominant disease is caused by a single copy of a mutation (i.e., heterozygotes are affected), while a recessive disease requires that both copies of the allele are mutated (only homozygotes are affected).

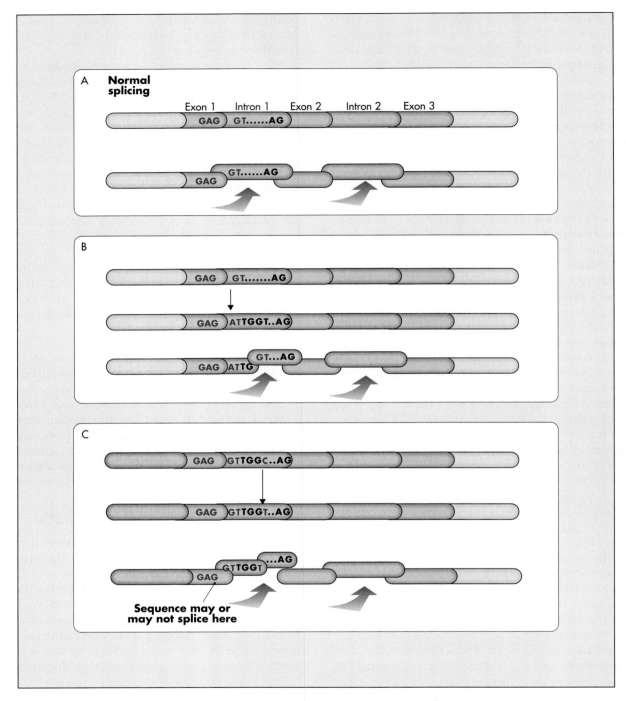

FIG. 3-3   In the first splice site mutation shown here **(B),** the donor sequence, GT, is replaced with AT. This results in an incorrect splice that leaves part of the intron in the mature mRNA transcript. In the second mutation **(C),** a second GT donor site is created in the first intron, resulting in a combination of abnormally and normally spliced mRNA products.

function. The heterozygote is thus unaffected. In some cases, however, 50% of the protein product is not sufficient for normal function **(haploinsufficiency),** and a dominant disorder can result. Haploinsufficiency is seen, for example, in the autosomal dominant disorder familial hypercholesterolemia (see Chapter 12). A single copy of the mutation (heterozygosity) reduces the number of low-density lipoprotein (LDL) receptors by 50%. Cholesterol levels in heterozygotes are approximately double those of normal homozygotes, producing a substantial increase in the risk of heart disease. As with most disorders involving haploinsufficiency, affected homozygotes, having few, if any, functional LDL receptors, suffer more serious disease than do heterozygotes. Both haploinsufficiency and gain-of-function mutations are examples of dosage sensitivity, mentioned previously.

Another type of loss of function is seen in the **dominant negative** mutation. This type of mutation results in a protein product that is not only nonfunctional but also inhibits the function of the protein produced by the normal allele in the heterozygote. Typically, dominant negative mutations are seen in genes that encode multimeric proteins (i.e., proteins composed of two or more subunits). Type 1 collagen (see Chapter 2), which is composed of three helical subunits, is an example of such a protein. An abnormal helix, created by a single mutation, may combine with the other helices, distorting them and producing a seriously compromised triple helix protein.

▼ Mutations can result in either a gain of function or a loss of function of the protein product. Gain-of-function mutations are sometimes seen in dominant diseases. Loss of function is seen in (1) recessive diseases; (2) diseases involving haploinsufficiency, in which 50% of the gene product is insufficient for normal function; and (3) dominant negative mutations, in which the abnormal protein product interferes with the normal protein product. ▲

Clinical Consequences of Mutation: The Hemoglobin Disorders

Genetic disorders of human hemoglobin are the most common group of single-gene disorders: an estimated 5% of the world's population carries one or more mutations of the genes involved in hemoglobin synthesis. Because nearly all of the types of mutation described in this chapter have been observed in the hemoglobin disorders, these disorders serve as an important illustration of the clinical consequences of mutation.

The hemoglobin molecule is a tetramer composed of four polypeptide chains, two of which are labeled α and two of which are labeled β. The β chains are encoded by a gene on chromosome 11, and the α chains are encoded by two genes on chromosome 16 that are very similar to one another. A normal individual would thus have two normal β genes and four normal α genes (Fig. 3-4). Ordinarily, tight regulation of these genes ensures that roughly equal numbers of α and β chains are produced. Each of these **globin** chains is associated with a **heme** group, which contains an iron atom and binds with oxygen. This property allows hemoglobin to perform the vital function of transporting oxygen in erythrocytes (red blood cells).

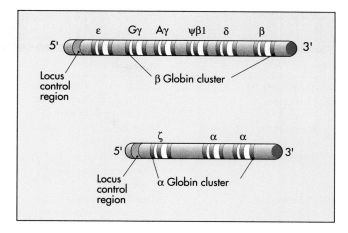

FIG. 3-4   The α-globin gene cluster on chromosome 16 and the β-globin gene cluster on chromosome 11. The β-globin cluster includes the ε-globin gene that encodes embryonic globin and the γ-globin genes that encode fetal globin. The ψβ1 and δ genes are not expressed. The α-globin cluster includes the ζ-globin gene, which encodes embryonic α-globin.

The hemoglobin disorders can be classified into two broad categories: *structural abnormalities*, in which the hemoglobin molecule is altered, and *thalassemias*, a group of conditions in which the hemoglobin is structurally normal but reduced in quantity. Another condition, hereditary persistence of fetal hemoglobin (HPFH), occurs when fetal hemoglobin, encoded by the α-globin genes and by two β-globin-like genes called ^Aγ and ^Gγ (see Fig. 3-4), continues to be produced after birth (normally, γ-chain production ceases and β-chain production begins at the time of birth). HPFH does not cause disease but instead can compensate for a lack of normal adult hemoglobin.

A large array of different hemoglobin disorders have been identified. The discussion that follows is a greatly simplified presentation of the major forms of these disorders. The hemoglobin disorders, the mutations that cause them, and their major features are summarized in Table 3-1.

Sickle Cell Disease

The most important of the structural hemoglobin abnormalities is sickle cell disease, a disorder that affects approximately 1/400 to 1/600 African-American births. It is even more common in parts of Africa, where it can affect up to one in 50 births, and it is also seen occasionally in Mediterranean and Mideastern populations. Sickle cell disease is caused by a single missense mutation that effects a substitution of valine for glutamic acid at position six of the β-globin polypeptide chain. In homozygous form, this amino acid substitution alters the characteristics of

TABLE 3-1   Summary of the Major Hemoglobin Disorders

Disease	Mutation type	Major disease features
Sickle cell disease	β-globin missense mutation	Anemia, tissue infarctions, infections
Hb H disease	Deletion or abnormality of three of the four α-globin genes	Moderately severe anemia, splenomegaly
Hydrops fetalis (Hb Barts)	Deletion or abnormality of all four α-globin genes	Severe anemia or hypoxemia, congestive heart failure; stillbirth or neonatal death
$β^0$-Thalassemia	Usually nonsense, frameshift, or splice site donor or acceptor mutations; no β-globin produced	Severe anemia, splenomegaly, skeletal abnormalities, infections; often fatal during first decade if untreated
$β^+$-Thalassemia	Usually missense, regulatory, or splice site consensus sequence or cryptic splice site mutations; small amount of β-globin produced	Features similar to those of $β^0$-thalassemia but often somewhat milder

A   B

FIG. 3-5 Erythrocytes from sickle cell patients assume a characteristic shape under conditions of low oxygen tension **(A).** Compare with normal erythrocytes **(B).**

the hemoglobin molecule such that the erythrocytes assume a characteristic "sickle" shape under conditions of low oxygen tension (Fig. 3-5, *A*). These conditions are experienced in capillaries, the tiny vessels whose diameter is smaller than that of the erythrocyte.

Normal erythrocytes (Fig. 3-5, *B*) can squeeze through capillaries, but sickled erythrocytes are less flexible and are unable to do so. The resultant vascular obstruction produces localized hypoxemia (lack of oxygen), painful sickling "crises," and infarctions of various tissues, including bone, spleen, kidneys, and lungs (an infarction is tissue death due to hypoxemia). Premature destruction of the sickled erythrocytes decreases the number of circulating erythrocytes and the hemoglobin level, producing **anemia**. The spleen becomes enlarged (splenomegaly), but infarctions eventually destroy this organ, producing some loss of immune function. This contributes to the recurrent bacterial infections (especially pneumonia) that are commonly seen in individuals with sickle cell disease and that frequently cause death. In North America, it is estimated that about 15% of children with sickle cell disease die before the age of 5 years. **WWW**

▼ Sickle cell disease, which causes anemia, tissue infarctions, and multiple infections, is the result of a single missense mutation that produces an amino acid substitution in the β-globin chain. ▲

Thalassemia

The term "thalassemia" is derived from the Greek word for "sea," *thalassa*. This refers to the fact that thalassemia was first described in populations living near the Mediterranean Sea, although it is also common in portions of Africa, the Mideast, India, and Southeast Asia. Thalassemia can be divided into two major groups, α-*thalassemia* and β-*thalassemia*, depending on the globin chain that is reduced in quantity. When one type of chain is decreased in number, the other chain type, unable to participate in normal tetramer formation, tends to form molecules consisting of four chains of the excess type only (these are termed **homotetramers,** in contrast to the **heterotetramers** normally formed by α and β chains). In α-thalassemia, the α-globin chains are deficient, so the β chains (or γ chains in the fetus) are found in excess. They form homotetramers that have a greatly reduced oxygen-binding capacity, producing hypoxemia. In β-thalassemia, the excess α-chains form homotetramers that precipitate and damage the cell membranes of red cell precursors (i.e., the cells that form circulating erythrocytes). This leads to premature erythrocyte destruction and anemia. **WWW**

Most cases of α-thalassemia are caused by deletions of the α-globin genes. A loss of one or two of these genes has no clinical effect. The loss or abnormality of three of the α genes produces moderately severe anemia and splenomegaly (Hb H disease). Loss of all four α genes, a condition seen primarily among Southeast Asians, produces hypoxemia in the fetus and *hydrops fetalis* (a condition in which there is a massive buildup of fluid). Severe hypoxemia invariably causes stillbirth or neonatal death.

▼ The α-thalassemia conditions are usually caused by deletions of α-globin genes. The loss of three of these genes leads to moderately severe anemia, and the loss of all four is fatal. ▲

Individuals with a β-globin mutation in one copy of chromosome 11 (heterozygotes) are said to have β-thalassemia minor, a condition that involves little or no anemia and does not ordinarily require clinical management. Those in whom both copies of the chromosome carry a β-globin mutation develop β-thalassemia major (also called Cooley's anemia) or the less serious condition, β-thalassemia intermedia. β-globin may be completely absent (β^0-thalassemia) or reduced to about 10% to 30% of the normal amount (β^+-thalassemia).

Because β-globin is not produced until after birth, the effects of β-thalassemia major are not seen clinically until the age of 2 to 6 months. These patients develop severe anemia. If the condition is left untreated, substantial growth retardation can occur. The anemia causes bone marrow expansion, which in turn produces skeletal changes, including a protuberant upper jaw and cheekbones and thinning of the long bones (making them susceptible to fracture). Splenomegaly (Fig. 3-6) and infections are common, and untreated β-thalassemia major patients often die during the first decade of life. β-thalassemia can vary considerably in severity, depending on the precise nature of the responsible mutation.

In contrast to α-thalassemia, gene deletions are relatively rare in β-thalassemia. Instead, most cases are

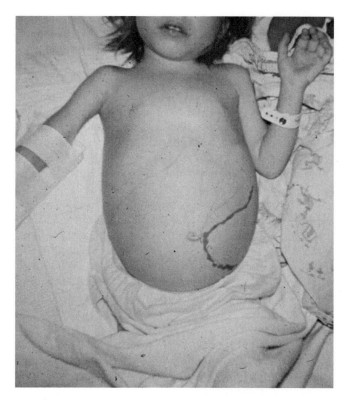

FIG. 3-6 A child with β-thalassemia major who has severe splenomegaly.

caused by single-base mutations. Nonsense mutations, which result in premature termination of translation of the β-globin chain, usually produce β⁰-thalassemia. Frameshift mutations also typically produce the β⁰ form. In addition to mutations in the β-globin gene itself, alterations in regulatory sequences are often seen. β-globin transcription is regulated by a promoter, two enhancers, and an upstream region known as the **locus control region** (LCR) (see Fig. 3-4). Mutations in these regulatory regions usually result in reduced synthesis of mRNA and a reduction, but not complete absence, of β-globin (β⁺-thalassemia). Several types of splice site mutations have also been observed. When a point mutation occurs at the donor or acceptor sites, normal splicing is destroyed completely, producing β⁰-thalassemia. Mutations in the surrounding consensus sequences usually produce β⁺-thalassemia. Mutations also occur in the cryptic splice sites found in introns or exons of the β-globin gene, causing these sites to be available to the splicing mechanism. These additional splice sites then compete with the normal splice sites, producing some normal and some abnormal β-globin chains. The result is usually β⁺-thalassemia.

▼ **Many different types of mutations can produce β-thalassemia conditions. Nonsense, frameshift, and splice site donor and acceptor mutations tend to produce more severe disease. Regulatory mutations and those involving splice site consensus sequences and cryptic splice sites tend to produce less severe disease.** ▲

More than 300 different β-globin mutations have been reported. Consequently, most β-thalassemia patients are not "homozygotes" in the strict sense: they usually have a *different* β-globin mutation on each copy of chromosome 11 and are termed **compound heterozygotes.** Even though the mutations differ, each of the two β-globin genes is altered, producing a disease state. It is quite common to apply the term "homozygote" loosely to compound heterozygotes.

Sickle cell and β-thalassemia major patients are sometimes treated with blood transfusions and with chelating agents that remove excess iron introduced by the transfusions. Prophylactic administration of antibiotics and antipneumococcal vaccination are used to diminish bacterial infections in sickle cell disease patients, and analgesics are administered for pain relief during sickling crises. Bone marrow transplants, which provide donor stem cells that produce genetically normal erythrocytes, have been performed on patients with severe β-thalassemia and sickle cell disease. However, it is often impossible to find a suitably matched donor, and the mortality rate from these transplants is still fairly high (approximately 5% to 30%, depending

on the severity of disease and the age of the patient). A lack of normal adult β-globin can be compensated by re-activating the genes that encode fetal β-globin (the γ-globin genes discussed previously). Agents such as hydroxyurea and butyrate can re-activate these genes and are being investigated. Also, the hemoglobin disorders are a possible candidate for gene therapy (see Chapter 13).

Causes of Mutation

A large number of agents are known to cause **induced mutations.** These mutations, which can be attributed to a known environmental cause, can be contrasted with **spontaneous mutations,** which arise naturally during the process of DNA replication. Agents that cause induced mutations are known collectively as **mutagens.** Animal studies have shown that **radiation** is an important class of mutagen (Clinical Commentary 3-1). **Ionizing radiation,** such as that produced by x-rays and nuclear fallout, can eject electrons from atoms, forming electrically charged ions. When these ions are situated within or near the DNA molecule, they can promote chemical reactions that change DNA bases. Ionizing radiation can also break double-stranded DNA. This form of radiation can reach all cells of the body, including the germ line.

Nonionizing radiation does not form charged ions but can move electrons from inner to outer orbits in the atom. The atom becomes chemically unstable. Ultraviolet (UV) radiation, which occurs naturally in sunlight, is an example of nonionizing radiation. UV radiation causes the formation of covalent bonds between adjacent pyrimidine bases (i.e., cytosine or thymine). These **pyrimidine dimers** (a dimer is a molecule having two subunits) are unable to pair properly with purines during DNA replication; this results in a base pair substitution (Fig. 3-7). Because UV radiation is absorbed by the epidermis, it does not reach the germ line but can cause skin cancer (see Clinical Commentary 3-2).

A variety of chemicals can also induce mutations, sometimes because of their chemical similarity to DNA bases. Because of this similarity, these **base analogs**, such as 5-bromouracil, can be substituted for a true DNA base during replication. The analog is not exactly the same as the base it replaces, so it can cause pairing errors during subsequent replications. Other chemical mutagens, such as acridine dyes, can physically insert themselves between existing bases, distorting the DNA helix and causing frameshift mutations. Still other mutagens can directly alter DNA bases, causing replication errors. An example of the latter is nitrous acid, which removes an amino group from cytosine, converting it to uracil. Although uracil is normally found in RNA, it mimics the pairing action of thymine in DNA. Thus,

CLINICAL COMMENTARY 3-1
THE EFFECTS OF RADIATION ON MUTATION RATES

Because mutation is a rare event, occurring less than once per 10,000 genes per generation, it is difficult to measure directly in humans. The relationship between radiation exposure and mutation is similarly difficult to assess. For a person living in a developed country, a typical lifetime exposure to ionizing radiation is about 6 to 7 rem.* About one third of this amount is thought to originate from medical and dental x-rays.

Certain unfortunate situations have arisen in which specific human populations have received much larger radiation doses. The most thoroughly studied such population consists of the survivors of the atomic bomb blasts that occurred in Hiroshima and Nagasaki, Japan, at the close of World War II. Many of those who were exposed to high doses of radiation died of radiation sickness. Others, however, survived, and many produced offspring.

To study the effects of radiation exposure in this population, a large team of Japanese and American scientists conducted medical and genetic investigations of many of the survivors. A significant number of those exposed developed cancers and chromosome abnormalities in their somatic cells, probably as a consequence of radiation exposure. To assess the effects of radiation exposure on the subjects' germ lines, the scientists compared the offspring of those who suffered substantial radiation exposures with the offspring of those who did not. While it is difficult to establish radiation doses with precision, there is no doubt that, in general, those who were situated closer to the blasts suffered much greater exposure levels. It is estimated that the exposed group received roughly 30 to 60 rem of radiation, many times the average lifetime radiation exposure.

In a series of more than 76,000 offspring of these individuals, a large number of factors was assessed. These included stillbirths, chromosome abnormalities, birth defects, cancer before age 20, death before age 26, and various measures of growth and development, including intelligence quotient (IQ). There were no statistically significant differences between the offspring of individuals who were exposed to radiation and those who were not. In addition, direct genetic studies of mutations have been carried out using minisatellite polymorphisms and protein electrophoresis, a technique that detects mutations that lead to amino acid changes (see following discussion). Parents and offspring were compared to determine whether germline mutations had occurred in these loci. The numbers of mutations detected in the exposed and unexposed groups were statistically equivalent.

More recently, a study of those who were exposed to radiation from the Chernobyl nuclear power plant accident indicated a two-fold increase in germline mutation rates. It is difficult to compare this result with the Japanese studies, because the types of radiation are quite different, the Chernobyl sample size was much smaller (79 families), and the unexposed control group for the Chernobyl study was sampled from a British population. Additional studies of the Chernobyl population will be necessary to determine conclusively whether these individuals have suffered radiation-induced germline mutations.

A number of other studies of the effects of radiation on humans have been reported, including investigations of those who live near nuclear power plants. The radiation doses received by these individuals are substantially smaller than those discussed earlier, and the results of these studies are equivocal.

It is remarkable that, even though there was substantial evidence for radiation effects on somatic cells in the Hiroshima-Nagasaki studies, no detectable effect could be seen for germ cells. What could account for this? It is likely that DNA repair is at least in part responsible. Also, we must recognize that, even with a large sample of individuals who received relatively high doses of radiation, increased mutation levels are difficult to detect.

These results argue that radiation danger should not be taken lightly. Above-ground nuclear testing in the American Southwest has produced increased rates of leukemia and thyroid cancer in a segment of the population. Radon, a radioactive gas that is produced by the decay of naturally occurring uranium, can be found at dangerously high levels in some homes and poses a risk for lung cancer. Any unnecessary exposure to radiation, particularly to the gonads or to developing fetuses, should be avoided if at all possible.

---

*A rem is a standard unit for measuring radiation exposure. It is roughly equal to 0.01 joule of absorbed energy per kilogram of tissue.

---

it pairs with adenine, instead of pairing with guanine, as the original cytosine would have done. The end result is a base pair substitution.

Hundreds of chemicals are now known to be mutagenic in laboratory animals. Among these are nitrogen mustard, vinyl chloride, alkylating agents, formaldehyde, sodium nitrite, and saccharin. It should be emphasized that some of these chemicals are much more potent mutagens than others. Nitrogen mustard, for example, is a powerful mutagen, whereas saccharin is a relatively weak one. Although some mutagenic chemicals are produced by humans, many occur naturally in the environment (e.g., aflatoxin B1, a common contaminant of foods).

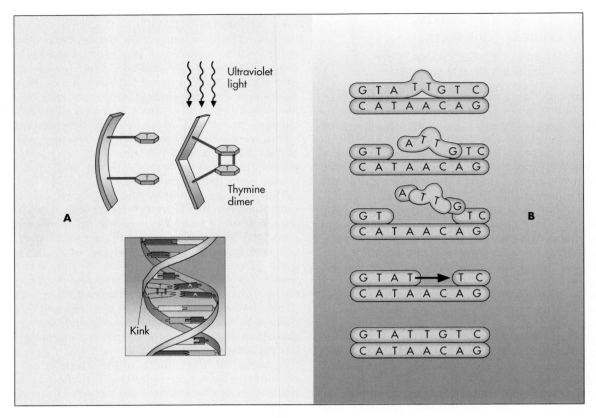

FIG. 3-7 Pyrimidine dimers originate when covalent bonds form between adjacent pyrimidine (cytosine or thymine) bases. This deforms the DNA, interfering with normal base pairing **(A).** The dimer and bases on either side of it are removed and replaced, using the complementary DNA strand as a template **(B).**

▼ Many substances in our environment are known to be mutagenic. These include ionizing and nonionizing radiation, as well as hundreds of different chemicals. These mutagens are capable of causing base substitutions, deletions, and frameshifts. Ionizing radiation can induce double-stranded DNA breaks. Some mutagens occur naturally, while others are generated by humans. ▲

DNA Repair

Considering that 3 billion DNA base pairs must be replicated in each cell division, and considering the large number of mutagens to which we are exposed, DNA replication is surprisingly accurate. A primary reason for this accuracy is the process of **DNA repair**, which takes place in all normal cells of higher organisms. Several dozen different enzymes are involved in repairing damaged DNA. They collectively recognize an altered base, excise it by cutting the DNA strand, replace it with the correct base (determined from the complementary strand), and reseal the DNA. It is estimated that these repair mechanisms correct 99.9% of initial errors.

Because DNA repair is essential for the accurate replication of DNA, defects in DNA repair systems can lead to many types of disease. For example, inherited mutations in genes responsible for **DNA mismatch repair** result in the persistence of cells with replication errors (i.e., mismatches) and can lead to some types of cancers (see Chapter 11). A compromised ability to repair **double-stranded DNA breaks** can lead to ovarian and breast cancer. **Nucleotide excision repair** is necessary for the removal of larger changes in the DNA helix (e.g., pyrimidine dimers). Defects in excision repair lead to a number of diseases, of which xeroderma pigmentosum is an important example (Clinical Commentary 3-2).

▼ DNA repair helps to ensure the accuracy of the DNA sequence by correcting replication errors (mismatches), repairing double-stranded DNA breaks, and excising damaged nucleotides. ▲

Mutation Rates

How often do spontaneous mutations occur? At the nucleotide level, the mutation rate is usually estimated

XERODERMA PIGMENTOSUM, A DISEASE OF FAULTY DNA REPAIR

An inevitable consequence of exposure to ultraviolet radiation is the formation of potentially dangerous pyrimidine dimers in the DNA of skin cells. Fortunately, a highly efficient system of enzymes usually repairs these dimers in normal individuals. Among those affected with the rare disease xeroderma pigmentosum (XP), this system does not work properly, and the resulting replication errors lead to base pair substitutions in skin cells. Varying substantially in severity, XP usually begins within the first 10 years of life. The skin is dry and scaly (xeroderma), and extensive freckling and abnormal skin pigmentation (pigmentosum) are followed by numerous skin tumors (Fig. 3-8). Neurological abnormalities are seen in some cases. It is estimated that the risk of skin tumors in individuals with XP is elevated approximately 1000-fold. These cancers are concentrated primarily in sun-exposed parts of the body. Patients are advised to avoid ultraviolet light sources (such as sunlight), and cancerous growths are removed surgically. XP patients can develop severe malignancies, sometimes causing death before age 20.

Several different repair enzymes are involved in correcting pyrimidine dimers. They include helicases that unwind the double-stranded DNA helix, an endonuclease that cuts the DNA at the site of the dimer, an exonuclease that removes the dimer and nearby nucleotides, a polymerase that fills the gap with DNA bases (using the complementary DNA strand as a template), and a ligase that rejoins the corrected portion of DNA to the original strand. An inherited mutation in any of seven repair enzyme genes can produce xeroderma pigmentosum.

FIG. 3-8   A child with xeroderma pigmentosum, showing the multiple skin tumors characteristic of this disease. (From Raven PH, Johnson GB [1992] Biology. Ed 3. Mosby, St Louis. With permission of McGraw-Hill, NY.)

It must be emphasized that our discussion involves two distinct classes of mutations. The repair-enzyme mutations occur in the germ line and thus can be transmitted from one generation to the next. Because they result in deficient DNA repair, they in turn permit skin cell mutations to persist, resulting in tumors. The skin cell mutations themselves cannot, of course, be inherited.

Although XP is probably the best-known disease that results from deficient DNA repair, it is not the only one. Other examples are given in Table 3-2.

TABLE 3-2   Examples of Diseases That Are Caused by a Defect in DNA Repair

Disease	Features	Type of repair defect
Xeroderma pigmentosum	Skin tumors, photosensitivity, cataracts, neurological abnormalities	Nucleotide excision repair defects, including mutations in helicase and endonuclease genes
Cockayne syndrome	Reduced stature, skeletal abnormalities, optic atrophy, deafness, photosensitivity, mental retardation	Defective repair of UV-induced damage in transcriptionally active DNA; considerable etiological and symptomatic overlap with xeroderma pigmentosum and trichothiodystrophy
Fanconi anemia	Anemia; leukemia susceptibility; limb, kidney, and heart malformations; chromosome instability	As many as eight different genes may be involved, but their exact role in DNA repair is not yet known
Bloom syndrome	Growth deficiency, immunodeficiency, chromosome instability, increased cancer incidence	Mutations in the reqQ helicase family
Werner syndrome	Cataracts, osteoporosis, atherosclerosis, loss of skin elasticity, short stature, diabetes, increased cancer incidence; sometimes described as "premature aging"	Mutations in the reqQ helicase family
Ataxia telangiectasia	Cerebellar ataxia, telangiectases,* immune deficiency, increased cancer incidence, chromosome instability	Normal gene product is likely to be involved in halting the cell cycle after DNA damage occurs
Hereditary nonpolyposis colorectal cancer	Proximal bowel tumors, increased susceptibility to several other types of cancers	Mutations in any of four DNA mismatch repair genes

*Telangiectases are vascular lesions caused by the dilatation of small blood vessels. This typically produces discoloration of the skin.

to be about 10^{-9} per base pair per cell division (these represent mutations that have escaped the process of DNA repair). At the level of the gene, the mutation rate is quite variable, ranging from 10^{-4} to 10^{-7} per locus per cell division. There are at least two reasons for this large range of variation.

1. Genes vary tremendously in size. The somatostatin gene, for example, is quite small, containing 1,480 bp. In contrast, the gene responsible for Duchenne muscular dystrophy (DMD) spans more than 2 million bp. As might be expected, larger genes present larger "targets" for mutation and usually experience mutation more frequently than do smaller genes. The DMD gene, as well as the genes for hemophilia A and type 1 neurofibromatosis, are all very large and have high mutation rates.

2. It is well established that certain nucleotide sequences are especially susceptible to mutation. These are termed **mutation hot spots**. The best-known example is the two-base (dinucleotide) sequence CG. In mammals, about 80% of CG dinucleotides are **methylated**: a methyl group is attached to the cytosine base. The methylated cytosine, 5-methylcytosine, easily loses an amino group, converting it to thymine. The end result is a mutation from cytosine to thymine (Fig. 3-9). Surveys of mutations in human genetic diseases have shown that the mutation rate at CG dinucleotides is about 12 times higher than at other dinucleotide sequences. Mutation hot spots, in the form of CG dinucleotides, have been identified in a number of important human disease genes, including the procollagen genes responsible for osteogenesis imperfecta (see Chapter 2). Other disease examples are discussed in Chapters 4 and 5.

Mutation rates also vary considerably with the age of the parent. Some chromosome abnormalities increase dramatically with elevated maternal age (see Chapter 6). In addition, single-gene mutations can increase with elevated paternal age. This increase is seen in several single-gene disorders, including Marfan syndrome and achondroplasia. As Fig. 3-10 shows, the risk of producing a child with Marfan syndrome is approximately five times higher for a male over age 40 than for a male in his 20s. This paternal age effect is usually attributed to the fact that the stem cells giving rise to sperm cells continue to divide throughout the life of males, allowing a progressive buildup of DNA replication errors.

▼ Mutation rates vary substantially in different parts of the genome. Large genes, because of their size, are generally more likely to experience mutations than are small genes. Mutation hot spots, particularly in the form of CG dinucleotides, are also known to occur. For some single-gene disorders, there is a substantial increase in mutation risk with advanced paternal age. ▲

DETECTION AND MEASUREMENT OF GENETIC VARIATION

For centuries, humans have been intrigued by the differences that can be seen among individuals. Attention was long focused on observable differences, such as skin coloration and body shape and size. Only in the twentieth century did it become possible to examine variation in genes, the consequence of mutations accumulated through time. The evaluation and measurement of this variation in populations and families are important in mapping genes to specific locations on

FIG. 3-9 Cytosine methylation. The addition of a methyl group (CH_3) to a cytosine base forms 5-methylcytosine. The subsequent loss of an amino group (deamination) forms thymine, thus resulting in a cytosine→thymine substitution.

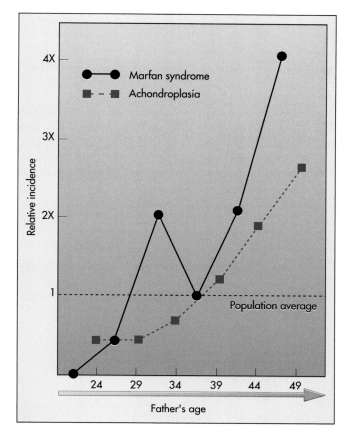

FIG. 3-10 The risk of producing a child with the single-gene diseases achondroplasia and Marfan syndrome (Y axis) increases with the father's age (X axis).
(Data from Vogel F, Rathenberg R [1975] Adv. Hum. Genet. 5:223-318.)

TABLE 3-3 The Relationship Between ABO Genotype and Blood Type

Genotype	Blood type	Antibodies present
$I^A I^A$	A	Anti-B
$I^A I^O$	A	Anti-B
$I^B I^B$	B	Anti-A
$I^B I^O$	B	Anti-A
$I^A I^B$	AB	None
$I^O I^O$	O	Anti-A and anti-B

chromosomes, a key step in determining gene function (see Chapter 8). The evaluation of genetic variation also provides the basis for much of genetic diagnosis, and it is highly useful in medical forensics. In this section, we will discuss several key approaches to detecting genetic variation in humans.

Blood Groups

Several dozen **blood group** systems have been defined on the basis of antigens located on the surfaces of erythrocytes. Some are involved in determining whether a given individual can receive a blood transfusion from a given donor. Because individuals differ extensively in terms of blood groups, these systems provided an important early means of assessing genetic variation.

Each of the blood group systems is determined by a different gene or set of genes. The various antigens that can be expressed within a system are the result of different DNA sequences in these genes. Two blood group systems that have special medical significance, the ABO and Rh systems, will be discussed here.

The ABO System

Human blood transfusions were carried out as early as 1818, but they were often unsuccessful. After transfusions, some recipients would suffer a massive, sometimes fatal, hemolytic reaction. In 1900 Karl Landsteiner discovered that this reaction was due to the ABO antigens located on erythrocyte surfaces. The ABO system consists of two major antigens, labeled A and B. Individuals can have one of four blood types: blood type A individuals carry the A antigen on their erythrocytes, type B individuals carry the B antigen, type AB individuals carry both A and B, and type O individuals carry neither antigen. Each individual will have antibodies that react against any antigens that are not found on their own red blood cell surfaces. Thus, a person with type A blood has anti-B antibodies, and transfusing type B blood into this individual would provoke a severe antibody reaction. It is straightforward to determine ABO blood type in the laboratory by mixing a small sample of a person's blood with solutions containing different antibodies and then observing which combinations cause the clumping characteristic of an antibody-antigen interaction.

The ABO system, which is encoded by a single gene on chromosome 9, consists of three primary alleles, labeled I^A, I^B, and I^O. In addition, there are subtypes of both the I^A and I^B alleles, but they will not be addressed here. Individuals who have the I^A allele have the A antigen on their erythrocyte surfaces (blood type A), while those with I^B have the B antigen on their cell surfaces (blood type B). Those with both alleles express both antigens (blood type AB), and those having only two copies of the I^O allele have neither antigen (type O blood). Because the I^O allele produces no antigen, those who are $I^A I^O$ or $I^B I^O$ heterozygotes have blood types A and B, respectively (Table 3-3).

Since populations vary substantially in terms of the frequency with which the ABO alleles occur, the ABO locus was the first blood group system used extensively in studies of genetic variation among individuals. For example, early studies showed that the A antigen is relatively common in western European populations, while the B antigen is especially common among Asians. Neither antigen is common among Native South American populations, the great majority of whom have blood type O.

The Rh System

Like the ABO system, the Rh system is defined on the basis of antigens that are present on erythrocyte surfaces. This system is named after the Rhesus monkey, the experimental animal in which it was first isolated by Landsteiner in the late 1930s. It is typed in the laboratory using a procedure similar to the one described for the ABO system. The Rh system varies considerably among individuals and populations and thus has been another highly useful tool for assessing genetic variation. Recently, the molecular basis of variation in both the ABO and the Rh systems has been elucidated (for further details, see the suggested readings at the end of this chapter).

The ABO and Rh systems are both of key importance in determining the compatibility of blood transfusions and tissue grafts. Some combinations of these systems can produce maternal-fetal incompatibility, sometimes with serious results for the fetus. These issues are discussed in detail in Chapter 9.

▼ **The blood groups, of which the ABO and Rh systems are examples, have provided an important means of studying human genetic variation. Blood group variation is the result of antigens that occur on the surfaces of erythrocytes.** ▲

Protein Electrophoresis

Although the blood group systems have been a useful means of measuring genetic variation, their number is quite limited. **Protein electrophoresis**, developed first in the 1930s and applied widely to humans in the 1950s and 1960s, increased the number of detectable polymorphic systems considerably. This technique makes use of the fact that a single amino acid difference in a protein (the result of a mutation in the corresponding DNA sequence) can cause a slight difference in the electrical charge of the protein. An example is the common sickle cell disease mutation discussed earlier. The replacement of glutamic acid with valine in the β-globin chain produces a difference in electrical charge because glutamic acid has two carboxyl groups, whereas valine has only one carboxyl group.

Electrophoresis can be used to determine whether an individual has normal hemoglobin (HbA) or the mutation that causes sickle cell disease (HbS). The hemoglobin is placed in an electrically charged gel composed of starch, agarose, or polyacrylamide (Fig. 3-11, A). The

FIG. 3-11 The process of protein electrophoresis. A tissue sample is loaded in the slot at the top of the gel, and an electrical current is run though the gel **(A)**. After staining, distinct bands, representing molecules with different electrical charges and thus different amino acid sequences, are visible. HbA homozygotes show a single band closer to the negative pole, while HbS homozygotes show a single band closer to the positive pole **(B)**. Heterozygotes, having both alleles, show two bands.

slight difference in charge resulting from the amino acid difference will cause the HbA and HbS forms to migrate at different rates through the gel. After allowing the protein molecules to migrate through the gel for several hours, they can be stained with chemical solutions so that their positions can be seen (Fig. 3-11, *B*). It can then be determined whether an individual is an HbA homozygote, HbS homozygote, or a heterozygote having HbA on one chromosome and HbS on the other.

Protein electrophoresis has been used to detect amino acid variation in hundreds of human proteins. However, silent substitutions, which do not alter amino acids, cannot be detected using this approach. In addition, some amino acid substitutions do not alter the electrical charge of the protein molecule. Thus, it is estimated that protein electrophoresis detects only about one third of mutations occurring in coding DNA. Single-base substitutions in noncoding DNA are not usually detected by protein electrophoresis.

▼ Protein electrophoresis detects variation in genes that encode certain serum proteins. This variation is observable because proteins with slight variations in their amino acid sequence will migrate at different rates through electrically charged gels. ▲

Detection of Variation at the DNA Level

It is estimated that humans vary at approximately 1/300 to 1/500 bp. Thus, approximately 10 million polymorphisms may exist among the 3 billion base pairs that compose the human genome. Since there are only 100 or so blood group and protein electrophoretic polymorphisms, these approaches have detected only a tiny proportion of our DNA variation. Yet the assessment of this variation is critical to gene mapping and genetic diagnosis, as is shown in Chapters 8 and 13. Fortunately, new molecular techniques have evolved during the past 20 years to enable the detection of thousands of new polymorphisms at the DNA level. These techniques, which have revolutionized both the practice and the potential of medical genetics, are discussed next.

Restriction Fragment Length Polymorphisms (RFLPs)

The earliest major approach to detecting genetic variation at the DNA level took advantage of the existence of bacterial enzymes known as **restriction endonucleases**, or **restriction enzymes**. These enzymes are produced by various bacteria species to "restrict" the entry of foreign DNA into the bacterium by cutting, or cleaving, the DNA at specifically recognized sequences. These sequences are referred to as **restriction sites**, or **recognition sites**. For example, the intestinal bacterium *Escherichia coli* produces a restriction enzyme, *Eco*RI, which recognizes the DNA sequence GAATTC. Each time this sequence is encountered, the enzyme cleaves the sequence between the G and the A. This produces DNA **restriction fragments**.

Now imagine a region of DNA that is several thousand bases in length and includes three recognition sites for *Eco*RI. Suppose that a polymorphism exists within the middle restriction site (e.g., some individuals might have the sequence GAATT instead of the GAATTC sequence recognized by *Eco*RI). The enzyme will not cleave the GAATTT sequence, although it will cleave the normal restriction sites that are located on either side of the polymorphic sequence. This specific DNA fragment will be longer in the individual who lacks the restriction site than in the individual who has it (Fig. 3-12). If these differing lengths could be visualized directly, it would be possible to observe DNA sequence differences among individuals (i.e., DNA polymorphism).

A series of steps has been devised that permits this visualization (Fig. 3-13). First, DNA is extracted from a tissue sample, usually blood. Then the DNA is exposed to a restriction enzyme such as *Eco*RI. This process is termed a **restriction digest**. The digest produces more than 1 million DNA fragments. To assess length variation, these fragments are subjected to gel

FIG. 3-12   Cleavage of DNA by the *Eco*RI restriction enzyme. The enzyme cleaves the three GAATTC recognition sequences in **B,** producing two smaller fragments. In **A,** the middle sequence is GAATTT instead of GAATTC, so it cannot be cleaved by the enzyme. The result is a single, longer fragment.

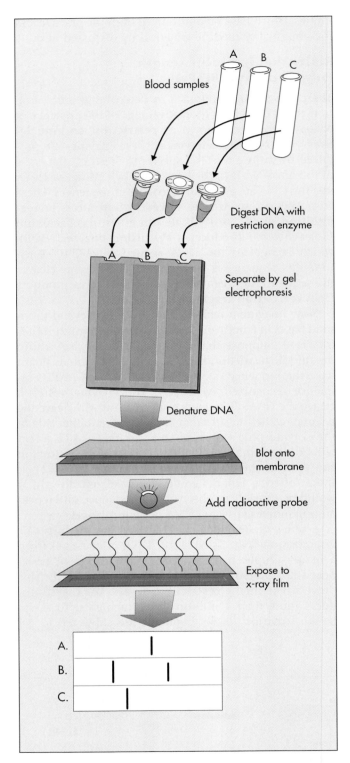

Blood samples

Digest DNA with restriction enzyme

Separate by gel electrophoresis

Denature DNA

Blot onto membrane

Add radioactive probe

Expose to x-ray film

A.

B.

C.

FIG. 3-13 The RFLP process. DNA is extracted from blood samples from subjects A, B, and C; digested by a restriction enzyme; and loaded on a gel. Electrophoresis separates the DNA fragments according to their size. The DNA is denatured and transferred to a solid membrane, where it is hybridized with a radioactive probe. Exposure to x-ray film (autoradiography) reveals specific DNA fragments (bands) of different sizes in individuals A, B, and C.

electrophoresis. This procedure is similar to the protein electrophoresis described previously, except that the DNA fragments migrate down the gel according to size rather than electrical charge. The smaller fragments migrate more quickly than the larger ones. The DNA is denatured (i.e., converted from double-stranded to single-stranded form) by exposing it to alkaline chemical solutions. In order to fix the positions of the DNA fragments permanently, they are transferred from the gel to a solid membrane, such as nitrocellulose (this is termed a **Southern transfer**, after the man who invented the process in the mid-1970s). At this point, the solid membrane, often called a "Southern blot," contains many thousands of fragments arrayed according to their size. If one looked at all of these fragments at once, it would be impossible to distinguish one from another because of their large number. How do we pick out specific DNA fragments?

Here, it is possible to exploit the principle of complementary DNA base pairing. A **probe** is constructed using recombinant DNA techniques (Box 3-1). This probe consists of a small piece of single-stranded human DNA (a few kilobases in length) that has been inserted into a vector such as a phage, plasmid, or cosmid. The probe is labeled, often with a radioactive isotope. The blot is exposed to thousands of copies of the labeled probe, which under proper conditions will then undergo complementary base pairing only with the appropriate single-stranded DNA fragments on the blot (a large number of probe copies is required so that a strong signal can be visualized). Because it is only a few kilobases in size, the probe identifies a specific portion of the DNA, usually just one or two fragments. To visualize the position of the hybridized probe, the blot is exposed to x-ray film, which darkens at the probe's position due to the emission of radioactive particles from the labeled probe. These darkened positions are usually referred to as "bands," and the film is termed an **autoradiogram** (Fig. 3-15).

Having thought through this sequence of steps, the term "restriction fragment length polymorphism" (usually abbreviated RFLP) should now be self-explanatory. These are *polymorphisms* revealed by variation in the *lengths* of *restriction fragments*.

▼ RFLPs result from variations in DNA sequence at specific restriction sites. These produce variations in DNA fragment lengths, which are sorted by electrophoresis and visualized through the use of labeled probes. ▲

The process can be illustrated using the example of sickle cell disease. As discussed previously, normal individuals have glutamic acid at position six of the β-globin polypeptide. Glutamic acid is encoded by the DNA sequence GAG. If the DNA sequence is instead GTG, valine is substituted for glutamic acid. The restriction enzyme *Mst*II recognizes the DNA sequence CCTNAGG (the N signifies that the enzyme will recognize any DNA base in this position). Thus, it cleaves the DNA sequence of the "normal" chromosome at this site, as well as at the restriction sites on either side of it (Fig. 3-16). This produces two fragments of DNA, one that is 1100 bp long and another that is only 200 bp long. In chromosomes with the valine substitution, *Mst*II can no longer recognize this particular site, so this DNA is not cleaved. The result is a longer DNA fragment, now 1300 bp in size instead of 1100. (The restriction sites flanking the site of interest do not vary, so they are always cut by the enzyme.) The shorter fragment will migrate further on a gel, so the two different sizes can easily be distinguished after hybridizing the blot with a probe containing DNA from the β-globin gene. In this case, the RFLP approach

permits direct detection of the mutation causing the disease. In current practice, more efficient methods are now used to test for sickle-cell mutations (see Chapter 13). However, the approach outlined here remains useful in detecting many polymorphisms and disease-causing mutations.

There are several thousand known restriction enzymes, most of which recognize a distinct DNA sequence. In addition, thousands of different probes have been created, each representing a different small piece of the human DNA sequence. By combining these various probes and enzymes, thousands of polymorphic sites were detected in the human genome. These polymorphisms were instrumental in localizing many important disease genes, including those for cystic fibrosis, Huntington disease, and type 1 neurofibromatosis (see Chapter 8).

BOX 3-1
GENETIC ENGINEERING, RECOMBINANT DNA, AND CLONING

In the last two decades, most of the lay public has acquired at least a passing familiarity with the terms "recombinant DNA," "cloning," and "genetic engineering." Indeed, these techniques lie at the heart of what is often called the "new genetics."

Genetic engineering refers to the laboratory alteration of genes. A number of various alterations can be made. Here, we discuss one that is of special importance in medical genetics, the manufacturing of **clones**. Briefly, a clone is an identical copy of a DNA sequence. We will outline one approach to the artificial cloning of human genes.

Our goal is to insert human DNA into a rapidly reproducing organism so that copies (clones) of the DNA can be made quickly. One system commonly used for this purpose is the **plasmid**, which is a small, circular, self-replicating piece of DNA that resides in many bacteria. Plasmids can be removed from bacteria or inserted into them without seriously disrupting bacterial growth or reproduction.

To insert human DNA into the plasmid, we need a way to cut DNA into pieces so that it can be manipulated. Restriction enzymes, discussed earlier in the text, perform this function efficiently. The DNA sequence recognized by the restriction enzyme *Eco*RI, GAATTC, has the convenient property that its complementary sequence, CTTAAG, is the same sequence, except backwards. Such sequences are called **palindromes**. When plasmid or human DNA is cleaved with *Eco*RI, the DNA fragments have "sticky ends," as shown in Fig. 3-14. This means that if we cut both human and plasmid DNA with this enzyme, both DNA fragments will have exposed ends that can undergo complementary base pairing with one another. Then, when the human and plasmid DNA are mixed together, they *recombine* (hence the term **recombinant DNA**). The plas-

mids now contain human DNA **inserts**. They are then inserted back into bacteria, where they can reproduce rapidly through natural cell division. The human DNA sequence, which is reproduced along with the other plasmid DNA, is thus cloned.

The plasmid is referred to as a **vector.** Several other types of vectors may also be used as cloning vehicles. These include **bacteriophages** (viruses that infect bacteria), **cosmids** (a phage-plasmid hybrid that is capable of carrying relatively large DNA inserts), **yeast artificial chromosomes** (YACs, vectors that are inserted into yeast cells and that behave much like ordinary yeast chromosomes), **bacterial artificial chromosomes** (BACs), and, most recently, **human artificial chromosomes** (see Chapters 8 and 13). While plasmids and bacteriophages can accommodate only relatively small inserts (about 10 and 20 kb, respectively), cosmids can carry inserts of approximately 50 kb, and YACs can carry inserts up to 1,000 kb in length.

Cloning is typically used to create the thousands of copies of human DNA needed for Southern blotting and other experimental applications. In addition, this approach is now being used to produce genetically engineered therapeutic products, such as insulin, interferon, human growth hormone, clotting factor VIII (used in the treatment of hemophilia A, a coagulation disorder), and tissue plasminogen activator (a blood clot–dissolving protein that helps to prevent heart attacks and strokes). When these genes are cloned into bacteria or other organisms, the organism produces the human gene product along with its own gene products. In the past, these products were obtained from donor blood or from other animals. Obtaining and purifying them was slow and costly. Genetically engineered gene products are rapidly becoming a cheaper and more efficient alternative.

Continued

BOX 3-1—cont'd

GENETIC ENGINEERING, RECOMBINANT DNA, AND CLONING—cont'd

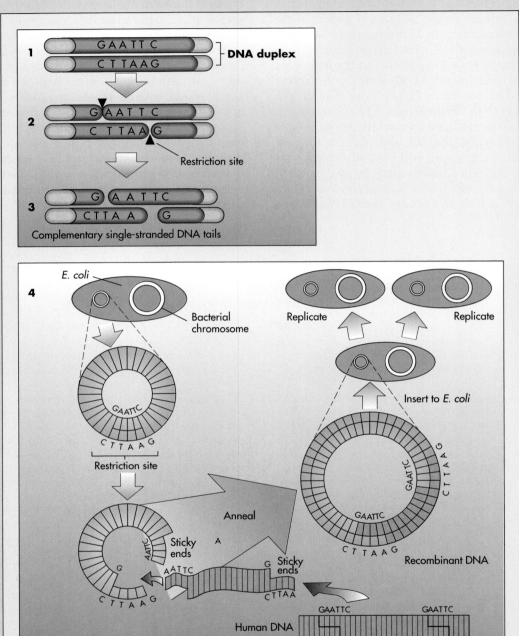

FIG. 3-14 Recombinant DNA technology. Human and circular plasmid DNA are both cleaved by a restriction enzyme, producing sticky ends (1-3). This allows the human DNA to anneal and recombine with the plasmid DNA. Inserted into the plasmid DNA, the human DNA is now replicated when the plasmid is inserted into a bacterium, such as *E. coli* (4).

FIG. 3-15 An autoradiogram, showing the positions of a 4.1-kb band and a 3.3-kb band. Each lane represents DNA from a subject in the family shown above the autoradiogram.

Variable Number of Tandem Repeat Polymorphisms

The approach just described usually detects the *presence* or *absence* of a restriction site; these polymorphisms are often termed **restriction site polymorphisms** (RSPs). In this case, a polymorphism has only two possible alleles, placing a limit on the amount of genetic diversity that can be seen. More diversity could be observed if a polymorphic system had many alleles, rather than just two. A variation on the RFLP approach has provided just such a system. This particular variation exploits the minisatellites that exist throughout the genome. Recall from Chapter 2 that minisatellites are regions in which the same DNA sequence is repeated over and over again, in tandem. The genetic variation measured here is in the *number* of repeats in a given region, which varies substantially from individual to individual (hence the term "**variable number of tandem repeats**," or **VNTRs**).

VNTRs are detected using an approach similar to that used for conventional RFLPs. DNA is digested with a restriction enzyme, and the fragments are electrophoresed, denatured, and transferred to a solid medium. The principal difference is that special probes are used that hybridize only to a given minisatellite region.

FIG. 3-16 Cleavage of β-globin DNA by the *Mst*II restriction enzyme. The sickle cell mutation removes an *Mst*II recognition site, producing a longer 1.3-kb fragment. The normal DNA sequence includes the restriction site (i.e., CCTGAG becomes CCTGTG), so a shorter 1.1-kb fragment is produced. Sickle cell homozygotes thus have a single 1.3-kb band, whereas normal homozygotes have a single 1.1-kb band. Heterozygotes have both the 1.1-kb and 1.3-kb bands. Note that the banding pattern here, based on DNA sequence differences, resembles the banding pattern shown in Fig. 3-11, which is based on amino acid sequence detected by protein electrophoresis.

FIG. 3-17   VNTR polymorphisms. Bands of differing lengths, A and B, are created by different numbers of tandem repeats in the DNA on two different chromosomes. Restriction sites are found on either side of the repeat region, and a radioactively labeled probe hybridizes to the DNA, allowing the different fragment lengths to be visualized on an autoradiogram.

While RSPs reveal polymorphisms because of the presence or absence of a restriction site, VNTRs reveal polymorphisms because of different numbers of repeats located between two restriction sites (Fig. 3-17). The number of these repeats can vary considerably in populations: a minisatellite region could have as few as two or three repeats or as many as 20 or more. These polymorphisms can therefore reveal a high degree of genetic variation. This is especially useful for mapping genes using the process of linkage analysis, to be discussed in Chapter 8.

> ▼ **VNTRs are a form of RFLP that arise from variation in the numbers of tandem repeats in a DNA region. Because VNTR loci can have many different alleles, they are especially useful in medical genetic and other applications.** ▲

Just as minisatellite regions can vary in length, microsatellites can also vary in length as a result of differing numbers of repeats (see Chapter 2). Each microsatellite repeat is substantially smaller than a minisatellite repeat (2, 3, or 4 bp in length). These are referred to as **dinucleotide**, **trinucleotide**, and **tetranucleotide repeats**, respectively. A microsatellite repeat may occur in tandem as many as several hundred times, and this number varies considerably among individuals (and usually between the two homologous chromosomes of an individual). These **microsatellite repeat polymorphisms** differ from the VNTRs just discussed in terms of their size and also in that they are not defined by restriction sites that flank the repeat region. Instead, the polymerase chain reaction technique, discussed next, is used to isolate them. Like VNTRs, microsatellite repeat polymorphisms are highly useful for gene mapping. They are more abundant than VNTRs, more evenly distributed in the genome, and easier to assay in the laboratory. Thus, they have become the

polymorphism of choice in most gene mapping studies. Both types of polymorphisms are useful in forensic applications, such as paternity testing and the identification of criminal suspects (Box 3-2).

DNA Amplification Using the Polymerase Chain Reaction (PCR)

The RFLP and VNTR approaches, which have been useful in many applications, originally depended on Southern blotting and cloning procedures. These techniques suffer from certain limitations. Cloning is time consuming, often requiring a week or more of laboratory time. In addition, the standard Southern blotting approach requires relatively large amounts of purified DNA, usually several micrograms (up to 1 ml of fresh blood would be needed to produce this much DNA). A newer approach to making copies of DNA, the **polymerase chain reaction** (**PCR**), has made the detection of genetic variation at the DNA level much more efficient. Essentially, PCR is an artificial means of replicating a short specific DNA sequence (several kb or less) very quickly, so that millions of copies of the sequence are made.

The PCR process, summarized in Fig. 3-19, requires four components:

1. Two **primers**, consisting of 15 to 20 bases of DNA each. These small DNA sequences are termed **oligonucleotides**, *oligo* meaning "a few." The primers correspond to the DNA sequences immediately adjacent to the sequence of interest (e.g., this sequence may contain a mutation that causes disease or it could contain a microsatellite repeat polymorphism). These oligonucleotide primers are synthesized using a laboratory instrument.

2. DNA polymerase. A thermally stable form of this enzyme, initially derived from the bacterium *Thermus aquaticus*, performs the vital process of DNA replication (here termed **primer extension**).

BOX 3-2

DNA PROFILES IN THE FORENSIC SETTING

Because of the large number of polymorphisms observed in the human, it is virtually certain that each of us is genetically unique (with the exception of identical twins). It follows that genetic variation could be used to identify individuals, much as a conventional fingerprint does. Since DNA can be found in any tissue sample, including blood, semen, and even hair, genetic variation could have substantial potential in forensic applications (criminal cases, paternity suits, identification of accident victims, and so forth).* VNTR and microsatellite repeat polymorphisms, with their many alleles, are very useful in establishing a highly specific **DNA profile**.

The principle underlying a DNA profile is quite simple. If we examine enough polymorphisms in a given individual, the probability that any other individual in the population would have the same alleles at each locus becomes extremely small. DNA left at the scene of a crime in the form of blood or semen, for example, can be typed for a series of VNTRs and/or microsatellite polymorphisms. Because of the extreme sensitivity of the PCR approach, even a tiny, several-year-old sample can yield enough DNA for laboratory analysis (but extreme care must be taken to avoid contamination when using PCR with such samples). These alleles are then compared with the alleles of a suspect (Fig. 3-18). If the alleles in the two samples match, then the suspect is implicated.

A key question is whether another person in the general population might have the same alleles as the suspect. Could the DNA profile then falsely implicate the wrong person? In criminal cases, the probability of obtaining an allele match with a random member of the population is calculated. Because of the high degree of allelic variation in VNTRs and microsatellite polymorphisms, these probabilities are usually very small. A set of just four VNTR loci will typically provide random match probabilities in the neighborhood of one in one million. The use of additional loci will make this probability smaller. Provided that a large enough number of loci are used under well-controlled laboratory conditions, and provided that the data are collected

A   B   C

FIG. 3-18 DNA profiles. The autoradiogram shows that the band pattern of suspect A's DNA does not match the DNA taken from the crime scene (C), whereas the band pattern of suspect B's DNA does match. In practice, several such VNTR or microsatellite systems are assayed to reduce the possibility of a false match.

(Courtesy Jay Henry, Criminalistics Laboratory, Department of Public Safety, State of Utah.)

and evaluated carefully, these DNA profiles can furnish highly useful forensic evidence.

While we tend to think of such evidence in terms of identifying the guilty party, it should be kept in mind that when a match is not obtained, a suspect may be exonerated. It has been reported that, among approximately one third of the rape cases in which DNA profiles were used, the suspect was freed because his DNA did not match that of the evidentiary sample. Thus, DNA profiles can also benefit those who are falsely accused.

---

*It was recently reported that fingerprints left at a crime scene often contain enough DNA for PCR amplification and DNA profiling.

3. A large number of free DNA nucleotides.
4. Genomic DNA from an individual. Because of the extreme sensitivity of PCR, the quantity of this DNA can be very small.

The genomic DNA is first heated to a relatively high temperature (95° C or so) so that it denatures and becomes single-stranded. This DNA is then exposed to large quantities of primers, which hybridize, or anneal,

to the appropriate complementary bases in the genomic DNA as it is cooled to an annealing temperature of approximately 35° to 65° C. The DNA is then heated to an intermediate temperature (70° to 75° C). In the presence of a large number of free DNA bases, a new DNA strand is synthesized by the DNA polymerase at this temperature, extending from the primer sequence. The newly synthesized DNA consists of a double strand

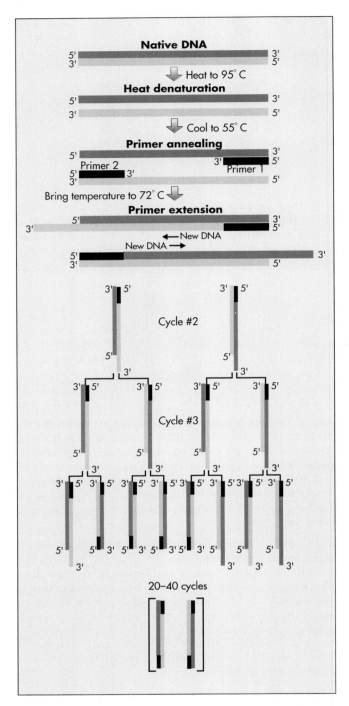

FIG. 3-19 The PCR process. Genomic DNA is first heated and denatured to form single strands. In the annealing phase, the DNA is cooled, allowing hybridization with primer sequences that flank the region of interest. Then the reaction is heated to an intermediate primer extension temperature, in which DNA polymerase adds free bases in the 3' direction along each single strand, starting at the primer. Blunt-ended DNA fragments are formed, and these provide a template for the next cycle of heating and cooling. Repeated cycling produces a large number of DNA fragments bounded on each end by the primer sequence.

that has the 5' end of the primer at one end, followed by the bases added through primer extension by DNA polymerase. The double-stranded DNA is then heated to a high temperature again, causing it to denature. The heating-cooling cycle is then repeated. Now, the newly synthesized DNA serves as the template for further synthesis. As the cooling-heating cycles are repeated, the primer-bounded DNA products are amplified geometrically: the number of copies doubles in each cycle (i.e., 2, 4, 8, 16, and so on). This is why the process is termed a "chain reaction." Typically, the cycles are repeated 20 to 30 times, producing millions of copies of the original DNA. In summary, the PCR process consists of three basic steps: DNA denaturing at high temperature, primer hybridization at a low temperature, and primer extension at an intermediate temperature. The result is a product that consists almost entirely of a defined DNA sequence.

Since each heating-cooling cycle requires only a few minutes or less, a single molecule of DNA can be amplified to make millions of copies in only a few hours. Because the procedure is simple and entirely self-contained, inexpensive machines have been developed to automate it completely. Once the DNA is amplified, it can be analyzed in a variety of ways.

PCR has several advantages over older techniques. First, it can be used with extremely small quantities of DNA (nanogram or even picogram amounts, as opposed to the micrograms required for cloning). The amount of DNA in a several-year-old blood stain, a single hair, or even the back of a licked postage stamp, is often sufficient for analysis. Second, because it does not require gene cloning, the procedure is much faster than older techniques. The genetic diagnosis of sickle cell disease, which required a week or more using older techniques, can be done in a single day with PCR. Finally, because PCR can make large quantities of very pure DNA, it is less often necessary to use radioactive probes to detect specific DNA sequences or mutations. Instead, safer nonradioactive labeling substances, such as biotin, can be used.

PCR does have some disadvantages. First, primer synthesis obviously requires knowledge of the DNA sequence flanking the DNA of interest. When no sequence information is available, other techniques must be used. Second, the extreme sensitivity of PCR makes it susceptible to contamination in the laboratory. A number of precautions are commonly taken in order to guard against contamination. Finally, it is difficult to apply PCR to sequences longer than one or a few kb. Thus, it cannot be used to detect deletions larger than this (i.e., it is difficult or impossible to amplify the longer, normal sequence). Southern blotting techniques are typically used instead.

Because PCR is such a powerful and versatile technique, it is now used extensively in genetic disease diagnosis, forensic medicine, and evolutionary genetics. It has supplanted the Southern blotting technique in many applications and is now often used to assay RFLPs and VNTRs. PCR is so sensitive that it has been used to analyze DNA from ancient mummies and even from a 30,000-year-old Neandertal specimen. Analysis of this specimen showed that modern humans are genetically quite distinct from Neandertals and are thus unlikely to have descended directly from them.

▼ PCR provides a convenient and efficient means of making millions of copies of a short DNA sequence. Heating-cooling cycles are used to denature DNA and then build new copies of a specific, primer-bounded sequence. Because of its speed and ease of use, this technique is now widely used for assessing genetic variation, diagnosing genetic diseases, and for forensic purposes. ▲

DNA Sequencing

In many genetic studies, a primary goal is to determine the actual array of DNA base pairs that composes a gene or part of a gene. This **DNA sequence** can indicate a great deal about the nature of a specific mutation, the function of a gene, and the gene's degree of similarity to other known genes. We will discuss one technique that is widely used to determine DNA sequences.

The **dideoxy method** of DNA sequencing, invented by Frederick Sanger, makes use of chain-terminating dideoxynucleotides. These are chemically quite similar to ordinary deoxynucleotides, except that they are missing one hydroxyl group. This prevents the subsequent formation of phosphodiester bonds with free DNA bases. Thus, although dideoxynucleotides can be incorporated into a growing DNA helix, no additional nucleotides can be added once they are included. Four different dideoxynucleotides are used, each one corresponding to one of the four nucleotides (A, C, G, and T). The single-stranded DNA whose sequence we wish to determine is mixed with radioactively labeled primers, DNA polymerase, ordinary nucleotides, and one type of dideoxynucleotide (Fig. 3-20). The primer hybridizes to the appropriate complementary position in the single-stranded DNA, and DNA polymerase adds free bases to the growing DNA molecule, as in the PCR process. The dideoxynucleotides are incorporated into the chain just as a corresponding nucleotide is. However, once the dideoxynucleotide is incorporated, the chain is terminated. At any given position, either an ordinary nucleotide or the corresponding dideoxynucleotide may be added; this is a random process. The procedure thus yields DNA fragments of varying lengths, each ending with the same dideoxynucleotide. The DNA fragments can be separated according to length by electrophoresis, as discussed previ-

ously. Four different sequencing reactions are run, one for each base. The fragments obtained from each reaction are electrophoresed side by side on the same gel, so that the position of each fragment can be compared. Since each band corresponds to a DNA chain terminating with a unique base, the DNA sequence can be read by observing the order of the bands on the gel after autoradiography (the radioactive primer indicates the position of the fragment on the film). Several hundred base pairs can usually be sequenced in one reaction series.

▼ DNA sequencing can be accomplished using the dideoxy method. This method depends on the fact that dideoxynucleotides behave in a fashion similar to ordinary deoxynucleotides, except that, once incorporated into the DNA chain, they terminate it. They thus mark the positions of specific bases. ▲

It should be apparent that sequencing DNA in this way is a relatively slow, laborious, and error-prone process. More recently, strategies for **automated DNA sequencing** using fluorescent, chemiluminescent, or colorimetric detection systems have been developed. The use of fluorochrome-labeled primers or dideoxynucleotides has become the most popular of these methods, partly because it can easily be adapted for rapid automation.

Typically, a DNA template is sequenced using a method similar to the primer extension step in PCR. Each of the four different nucleotides can be labeled with a fluorochrome that emits a distinct spectrum of light. The fluorochrome-labeled reaction products are electrophoresed through a very thin polyacrylamide gel, and as they migrate past a window, they are excited by a beam of light from a laser. The emitted light is captured by a digital camera for translation into an electronic signal, and a composite gel image is generated. This gel image is analyzed to produce a graph in which each of the four different nucleotides is depicted by a different-colored peak (see Color Plate 1 following p. 116). Up to 500 bp of DNA from 64 individuals can be analyzed on a single gel in 2 to 4 hours. Automated sequencers can also be adapted to assay microsatellite polymorphisms, *Alu* elements, and single nucleotide polymorphisms (see Chapter 8).

By using computers and advanced automated technology, approaches such as this have greatly increased the potential speed of DNA sequencing. Eventually, these techniques will permit the sequencing of the entire three-billion-base human genome.

▼ Automated DNA sequencing, using fluorescent labels and laser detection, greatly increases the speed and efficiency of the sequencing process. ▲

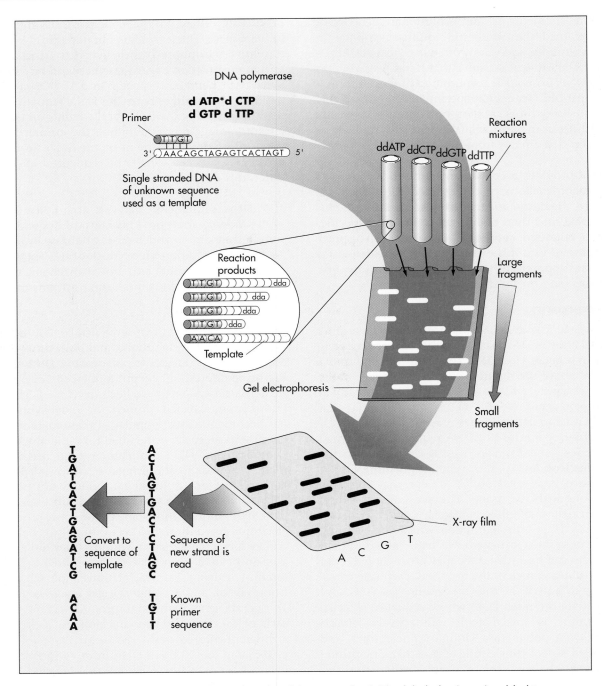

FIG. 3-20 DNA sequencing using the dideoxy method. The labeled primer is added to the single-stranded DNA whose sequence is unknown. DNA polymerase adds free bases to the single strand, using complementary base pairing. Four different reactions are carried out, corresponding to the four different dideoxynucleotides (ddATP, ddCTP, ddGTP, and ddTTP). These terminate the DNA sequence whenever they are incorporated instead of the normal deoxynucleotide (dATP, dCTP, dGTP, and dTTP, corresponding to the bases A, C, G, and T, respectively). This produces fragments of varying length, which can be separated by electrophoresis. The position of each fragment is indicated by the emission of radioactive particles from the label. This then allows the DNA sequence to be read directly.

Detection of Mutations at the DNA Level

The detection of mutations in DNA sequences is often a critical step in understanding how a gene causes a specific disease. The molecular methods developed during the past decade have spawned a number of new techniques for detecting mutation at the DNA level. The Southern blotting approach permits the detection of relatively large deletions. Those smaller than 50 bp cannot be seen on Southern blots because of the limited resolution of this technique. Mutations that alter a restriction site can also be recognized using the Southern blotting approach, but most mutations do not occur at known restriction sites. After using PCR to amplify a specific region of DNA, it can be sequenced directly using the technique described previously. Mutations are then detected by comparing the DNA sequence of a patient with that of an unaffected individual.

Although direct sequencing is a useful and accurate means of detecting mutations, it can be very time consuming. Other techniques provide a more rapid approach to surveying large numbers of patients for mutations. These techniques can indirectly indicate the existence and location of a mutation, after which the DNA in the indicated region can be sequenced to identify the specific mutation (Table 3-4).

Two approaches to be mentioned here make use of the fact that, under certain conditions, mutations alter the mobility of DNA fragments in gel electrophoresis. **Denaturing gradient gel electrophoresis (DGGE)** employs a gel in which there is an increasing gradient of a denaturing factor, such as temperature. **Single-strand**

TABLE 3-4   Methods of Mutation Detection

Technique	Brief description	Application
Southern blotting	Digestion of test DNA with restriction enzyme; resolution of fragments with agarose gel electrophoresis; transfer of DNA to nylon membrane and hybridization of labeled probe to DNA fragments	Detection of insertions, deletions, and rearrangements; ordering of DNA fragments into physical map
Direct DNA sequencing	Determination of linear order of nucleotides of test DNA; specific nucleotide detected by chemical cleavage, dideoxy-chain termination, or fluorochrome dye	Detection of insertions, deletions, point mutations, rearrangements
Single-strand conformational polymorphism (SSCP) analysis	Differential electrophoretic mobility of single-stranded test DNA with different secondary structures (conformations) through a non-denaturing gel	Detection of small insertions or deletions, and point mutations
Denaturing gradient gel electrophoresis (DGGE) analysis	Migration of DNA duplexes through an electrophoretic gel with increasing amounts of a denaturant (e.g., chemical, temperature) until DNA strands separate; resolution of alleles by PAGE	Detection of small insertions or deletions, and point mutations
DNA mismatch cleavage	Hybridization of a labeled probe to test DNA; cleavage of DNA at site of base-pairing mismatch	Detection of small insertions or deletions, and point mutations
Allele-specific oligonucleotide (ASO) hybridization	Preferential hybridization of labeled probe to test DNA with uniquely complementary base composition	Detection of alleles of known composition
Mass spectrometry	Detection of physical mass of sense and anti-sense strands of test DNA	Detection of small insertions or deletions, and point mutations
DNA chip hybridization	Hybridization of test DNA to arrays of oligonucleotides ordered on silicone chip	Detection of test DNA of known composition
Protein truncation	Test RNA used to make cDNA by RT-PCR with 5' primer containing T7 promoter; cDNA translated and product resolved by SDS-PAGE	Detection of frameshift, splice site, or nonsense mutations that truncate the protein product

PAGE, Polyacrylamide gel electrophoresis; *RT-PCR*, reverse transcriptase-PCR; *SDS*, sodium dodecyl sulfate.

BOX 3-3
THE CAUSES OF GENETIC VARIATION

While mutation is the ultimate source of genetic variation, it cannot alone account for the substantial differences in the incidence of many genetic diseases among different ethnic groups. Why, for example, is sickle cell disease seen in approximately 1/600 African-Americans, but almost never in northern Europeans? Why is cystic fibrosis 40 times more common in Europeans than in Asians? Although mutation is the process that introduces diseases into populations, several evolutionary factors determine how common the disease genes become in a population. These include natural selection, genetic drift, and gene flow. These forces change **gene frequencies** in populations (a gene frequency is defined as the proportion of a population's chromosomes having a specific allele, a concept discussed further in Chapter 4).

Natural selection is often described as the "editor" of genetic variation. It increases the population frequency of favorable mutations (i.e., those who carry the mutation will produce more surviving offspring), and it decreases the frequency of genes that are unfavorable in a given environment (gene carriers produce fewer surviving offspring). Typically, disease mutations are continually introduced into a population through the error processes described earlier, while natural selection removes the mutations. Certain environments, however, may result in a selective advantage for a disease mutation. We can turn again to sickle cell disease for an example. As discussed previously, those who are homozygotes for the sickle cell mutation are much more likely to die early. Heterozygotes ordinarily have no particular advantage or disadvantage. However, it has been shown that sickle cell heterozygotes have a distinct survival advantage in environments in which *Plasmodium falciparum* malaria is common (as in west-central Africa) (Fig. 3-21). This is because the malaria parasite does not survive well in the erythrocytes of sickle cell heterozygotes. Thus, heterozygotes are less likely to succumb to malaria than are the normal homozygotes, conferring a selective advantage on the sickle-cell gene in this environment. While there is selection *against* the gene in sickle-cell homozygotes, there is selection *for* the gene in heterozygotes. The result is that the disease gene persists at a relatively high frequency in African populations. In non-malarial environments (such as northern Europe), the gene has no advantage, so natural selection acts strongly against it by eliminating homozygotes. This example illustrates the concept that variation in genetic disease incidence among populations can be caused by natural selection operating differentially in different environments.

Genetic drift is another force that can cause disease genes to vary in frequency among populations. To understand the process of genetic drift, consider a coin-tossing exercise in which 10 coins are tossed. Since heads and tails are equally likely, the expected number of heads and tails in this exercise would be 5 each. However, it is intuitively clear that, by chance, we could observe a substantial departure from this expectation. We would not be surprised to see seven heads and three tails, for example. If, however, we toss 1,000 coins, the degree of departure from the expected proportion of 50% heads and 50% tails is much smaller. A reasonable outcome might be 470 heads and 530 tails, but it would be quite unlikely to obtain 700 heads and 300 tails. Thus, we see less random fluctuation in larger samples.

Frequency of sickle cell gene

- 10%–20%
- 5%–10%
- 1%–5%

Distribution of *falciparum* malaria

FIG. 3-21 Correspondence between frequency of the sickle cell allele and the distribution of *Plasmodium falciparum* malaria.

Continued

The same principle applies to gene frequencies in populations. In a very small population, a gene frequency can deviate substantially from one generation to the next, but this is unlikely in a large population. Thus, genetic drift is greater in smaller populations. This means that genetic diseases that are otherwise uncommon may be seen fairly frequently in a small population. For example, Ellis–van Creveld syndrome, a rare disorder that involves reduced stature, polydactyly (extra digits), and congenital heart disease, is seen with greatly elevated frequency among the Old Order Amish population of Pennsylvania. The Amish population was founded in the United States by about 50 couples. There was thus great potential for genetic drift, resulting in the elevation of certain disease gene frequencies.

It is common to observe the effect of genetic drift in small, isolated populations throughout the world. Even relatively large populations may have experienced drift effects in the recent past if they underwent severe population bottlenecks or were established by a small number of founders (**founder effect**). For example, more than 30 otherwise rare genetic diseases are found with elevated frequency in Finland's population, which is thought to have been founded primarily by a small number of individuals some 100 generations ago. Phenylketonuria and cystic fibrosis, which are common in other Caucasian populations, are relatively rare in Finland, illustrating the fact that genetic drift can both increase and decrease the frequency of disease genes. Several genetic diseases (e.g., torsion dystonia, Tay-Sachs disease, Gaucher disease; see Chapter 7) occur with increased frequency in the Ashkenazi Jewish population; this may be due to population bottlenecks that have occurred in the history of this population.

Gene flow occurs when populations exchange migrants who mate with one another. Through time, gene flow between populations tends to make them genetically more similar to one another. One reason why sickle-cell disease is less common among African-Americans than among many African populations is because of gene flow with Caucasians in North America (this same process is likely to have increased the frequency of cystic fibrosis in the African-American population). In addition, because *Plasmodium falciparum* malaria is not found in North America, the African-American population does not experience selection in favor of the sickle-cell mutation.

The forces of mutation, natural selection, genetic drift, and gene flow interact in complex and sometimes unexpected ways to influence the distribution and prevalence of genetic diseases in populations. The study of the ways in which these processes influence genetic evolution is referred to as **population genetics**.

---

conformation polymorphism (SSCP) analysis makes use of the fact that the secondary structure of a DNA segment can be altered by a mutation in DNA sequence. This will change the rate of migration of a single-stranded DNA segment in a non-denaturing gel. Using either of these two techniques, sequence differences between a patient's DNA and that of a normal control can be identified (Fig. 3-22). Once a difference is detected, the patient's DNA can be sequenced in order to determine the precise nature of the mutation.

Another mutation-detection approach employs chemicals or enzymes that cleave DNA when there is a mismatch between two otherwise complementary hybridized DNA sequences (i.e., one strand contains the normal sequence, while the other strand contains an altered base). This **mismatch cleavage** will produce fragments of differing lengths that can then be detected on a gel. The mismatch cleavage method has been adapted for use with automated sequencers, greatly increasing the efficiency and speed of this method.

A great deal of progress is now being made in fabricating **DNA chips** and using them for mutation detection. As the name implies, these are computer chips that contain arrays of thousands of different oligonucleotides. These oligonucleotides consist of normal DNA sequences as well as DNA sequences that con-

FIG. 3-22 Single-stranded conformational polymorphism (SSCP) analysis is a method used to rapidly screen a region of DNA for differences between individuals. Depending on its nucleotide sequence, the conformation of each DNA strand varies in a non-denaturing gel, altering its mobility through the gel. This permits the differentiation between a normal allele (*small arrow*) and a mutant allele (*large arrow*) in this family with an autosomal dominant disorder.

tain known disease-causing mutations. Fluorescently labeled DNA from a subject is hybridized with the oligonucleotides on the chip to determine whether the DNA hybridizes with the normal or mutation-containing oligonucleotides. This approach offers the extraordinary speed, miniaturization, and accuracy of computer-based mutation analysis. Tests for specific mutations, an important aspect of genetic diagnosis, will be discussed further in Chapter 13.

▼ Many techniques can be used to detect mutations at the DNA sequence level. These include Southern blotting, direct DNA sequencing, and electrophoretic techniques such as denaturing gradient gel electrophoresis, single-strand conformation polymorphism analysis, and mismatch cleavage analysis. In addition, DNA chips are beginning to be used in mutation detection. ▲

STUDY QUESTIONS

1. In the following amino acid sequences, the normal sequence is given first, followed by sequences that are produced by different types of mutations. Identify the type of mutation most likely to cause each altered amino acid sequence.

Normal:	Phe-Asn-Pro-Thr-Arg
Mutation 1:	Phe-Asn-Pro
Mutation 2:	Phe-Asn-Ala-His-Thr
Mutation 3:	Phe-His-Pro-Thr-Arg

2. Missense and transcription (promoter, enhancer, transcription factor) mutations often produce milder disease conditions than do frameshift, donor/acceptor site, and nonsense mutations. Using the globin genes as examples, explain why this is so.

3. Individuals who have mutations that lower their production of both α-globin and β-globin often present with milder disease symptoms than do those who have mutations lowering the production of only one type of chain. Why?

4. Outline the major differences between restriction site polymorphisms, VNTRs, and microsatellite repeat polymorphisms. Which of these three types of polymorphisms is represented in the autoradiogram in Fig. 3-23?

5. α-1-antitrypsin deficiency is a disease that arises when both copies of the α-1-antitrypsin gene are altered by mutations. Liver disease, chronic emphysema, and pulmonary failure can result. One of the mutations that causes α-1-antitrypsin deficiency occurs in exon 3 of the gene and destroys a recognition site for the restriction enzyme *Bst*EII. RFLP analysis was performed on three members of a family, producing the autoradiogram in Fig. 3-24. Determine the disease status of each individual.

FIG. 3-23 Autoradiogram for study question 4.

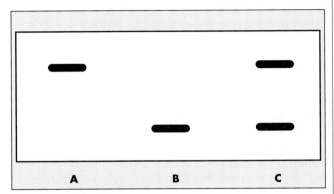

FIG. 3-24 Autoradiogram for study question 5.

SUGGESTED READINGS

Antonarakis SE (1997) Mutations in human diseases: nature and consequences. In: Rimoin DL, Connor JM, Pyeritz RE (eds) Emery and Rimoin's Principles and Practice of Medical Genetics. Vol. 1. Churchill Livingstone, New York, pp 53-66

Arnheim N, Shibata D (1997) DNA mismatch repair in mammals: role in disease and meiosis. Curr. Opin. Genet. Dev. 7:364-370

Bunn HF (1997) Pathogenesis and treatment of sickle cell disease. N. Eng. J. Med. 337:762-769

Clark SJ, Harrison J, Frommer M (1995) CpNpG methylation in mammalian cells. Nature Genet. 10:20-27

Cooper DN, Krawczak M (1993) Human Gene Mutation. Bios Scientific, Oxford

Cooper DN, Krawczak M, Antonarakis SE (1995) The nature and mechanisms of human mutation. In: Scriver CR, Beaudet AL, Sly WS, Valle D (eds) The Metabolic and Molecular Basis of Inherited Disease. Vol. 1. McGraw-Hill, New York, pp 259-292

Copeland NE, Hanke CW, Michalak JA (1997) The molecular basis of xeroderma pigmentosum. Dermatol. Surg. 23:447-455

Cotton RGH (1997) Slowly but surely towards better scanning for mutations. Trends Genet. 13:43-46

Dubrova YE, Nesterov VN, Krouchinsky NG, Ostapenko VA, Neumann R, Neil DL, Jeffreys AJ (1996) Human minisatellite mutation rate after the Chernobyl accident. Nature 380: 683-686

Ginot F (1997) Oligonucleotide micro-arrays for identification of unknown mutations: how far from reality? Hum. Mutation 10:1-10

Housman D (1995) Human DNA polymorphism. N. Eng. J. Med. 332:318-320

Jorde LB (1996) Population-specific genetic markers and disease. In: Meyers RA (ed) Encyclopedia of Molecular Biology and Molecular Medicine. Vol. 5. VCH Publishers, New York, pp 44-49

Krontiris TG (1995) Minisatellites and human disease. Science 269:1682-1683

Lupski JR (1997) Charcot-Marie-Tooth disease: a gene-dosage effect. Hosp. Practice 32:83-122

Martin DIK, Fiering S, Groudine M (1996) Regulation of β-globin gene expression: straightening out the locus. Curr. Opin. Genet. Dev. 6:488-495

Mashal RD, Sklar J (1996) Practical methods of mutation detection. Curr. Opin. Genet. Dev. 6:275-280

Mouro I, Colin Y, Cherif-Zahar B, Cartron J, Le Van Kim C (1993) Molecular genetic basis of the human Rhesus blood group system. Nature Genet. 5:62-65

Mullis KB, Ferre F, Gibbs RA (1994) PCR—the Polymerase Chain Reaction. Birkhauser Verlag AG

Neel JV (1991) Update on the genetic effects of ionizing radiation. JAMA 266:698-701

Neel JV (1995) New approaches to evaluating the genetic effects of the atomic bombs. Am. J. Hum. Genet. 57:1263-1266

Risch N, Reich EW, Wishnick MM, McCarthy JG (1987) Spontaneous mutation and parental age in humans. Am. J. Hum. Genet. 41:218-248

Rosenthal N (1994) Tools of the trade—recombinant DNA. N. Eng. J. Med. 331:315-317

Rosenthal N (1995) Fine structure of a gene—DNA sequencing. N. Eng. J. Med. 332:589-591

Sankaranarayanan K (1993) Ionizing radiation, genetic risk estimation and molecular biology: impact and inferences. Trends Genet. 9:79-84

Schwartz RS (1995) Jumping genes. N. Eng. J. Med. 332:941-944

Weatherall DJ (1997) The thalassaemias. Brit. Med. J. 314:1675-1678

Weatherall DJ, Clegg JB, Higgs DR, Wood WG (1995) The hemoglobinopathies. In: Scriver CR, Beaudet AL, Sly WS, Valle D (eds) The Metabolic and Molecular Basis of Inherited Disease. Vol. 3. McGraw-Hill, New York, pp 3417-3484

Weiss KM (1993) Genetic Variation and Human Disease: Principles and Evolutionary Approaches. Cambridge University Press, Cambridge

Yamamoto F, Clausen H, White T, Marken J, Hakomori S (1990) Molecular genetic basis of the histo-blood group ABO system. Nature 345:229-233

4

Autosomal Dominant and Recessive Inheritance

Many important and well-understood genetic diseases are the result of a mutation at a single gene. The 1998 on-line edition of McKusick's *Mendelian Inheritance in Man* lists 8,855 known **single-gene, or monogenic,** traits defined thus far in the human. Of these, 8,249 are located on autosomes, and 519 are located on the X chromosome. Single-gene traits are the focus of much of the rapid progress now being made in medical genetics. In many cases these genes have been mapped to specific chromosome locations, cloned, and sequenced. This leads to new and exciting insights not only in genetics but also in the basic pathophysiology of disease.

In this chapter we focus on single-gene disorders caused by mutations on the autosomes. Single-gene disorders caused by mutations on the sex chromosomes are the subject of Chapter 5. We discuss the patterns of inheritance of these diseases in families, as well as factors that complicate these patterns. When appropriate, the molecular basis for genetic disease processes will be addressed. We also discuss the risks of transmitting single-gene diseases to one's offspring, since this is usually an important concern for at-risk couples.

BASIC CONCEPTS OF FORMAL GENETICS
Gregor Mendel's Contributions

Monogenic traits are also known as **mendelian** traits, after Gregor Mendel, a nineteenth-century Austrian monk who deduced several important genetic principles from his well-designed experiments with garden peas. Mendel studied seven traits in the pea, each of which is determined by a single gene. These traits included attributes such as height (tall plants vs. short plants) and seed shape (rounded vs. wrinkled). The variation in each of these traits is caused by different alleles at individual loci.

Two central principles emerged from Mendel's work. The first is the **principle of segregation**, which states that sexually reproducing organisms possess genes that occur in pairs and that only one member of this pair is transmitted to the offspring (i.e., it segregates). The prevalent thinking during Mendel's time was that hereditary factors from the two parents are "blended" in the offspring. In contrast, the principle of segregation states that genes remain intact and distinct. An allele for "rounded" seed shape can be transmitted to an offspring who can, in turn, transmit the same allele to its own offspring. If, instead of remaining distinct, genes were somehow blended in offspring, it would be impossible to trace genetic inheritance from one generation to the next. Thus, the principle of segregation was a key development in modern genetics.

Mendel's **principle of independent assortment** is his second great contribution to genetics. This principle states that genes at different loci are transmitted independently. Consider the two loci mentioned previously. One locus can have either the "rounded" or "wrinkled" allele, and the other can have either the "tall" or the "short" allele. In a reproductive event, a parent will transmit one allele from each locus to its offspring. The principle of independent assortment dictates that the allele transmitted at one locus ("rounded" or "wrinkled") has no effect on which allele is transmitted at the other locus ("tall" or "short").

Mendel's experiments also showed that the effects of one allele may mask those of another. He performed **crosses** (matings) between pea plants homozygous for the "tall" gene (i.e., they had two identical copies of an allele we will label H) and plants homozygous for the "short" gene (having two copies of an allele labeled h). This cross, which can produce only heterozygous (Hh) offspring, is illustrated in the **Punnett square** shown in Fig. 4-1. Mendel found that the offspring

FIG. 4-1   Punnett square illustrating a cross between HH and hh homozygote parents.

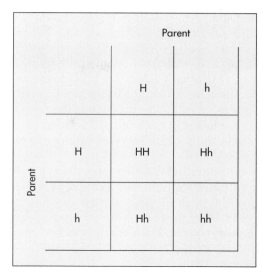

FIG. 4-2   Punnett square illustrating a cross between two Hh heterozygotes.

of these crosses, even though they were heterozygotes, were all tall. This reflects the fact that the *H* allele is **dominant**, while the *h* allele is **recessive** (it is conventional to label the dominant allele in upper case and the recessive allele in lower case). The term "recessive" comes from a Latin root meaning "to hide." This describes the behavior of recessive alleles well: in heterozygotes, the consequences of a recessive allele are hidden. Whereas a dominant allele exerts its effect both in the homozygote (*HH*) and heterozygote (*Hh*), the presence of the recessive allele is detected only when it occurs in homozygous form (*hh*). Thus, short pea plants could be created only by crossing parent plants that each carry at least one *h* allele. An example would be a heterozygote × heterozygote cross, shown in Fig. 4-2.

The principle of segregation describes the behavior of chromosomes in meiosis. The genes on chromosomes segregate during meiosis, and they are transmitted as distinct entities from one generation to the next. When Mendel performed his critical experiments, he had no direct knowledge of chromosomes, meiosis, or genes (indeed, the latter term was not coined until 1909, long after Mendel's death). Although his work was published in 1865 and cited occasionally, its fundamental significance was unrecognized for several decades. Yet Mendel's research, which was eventually replicated by other researchers at the turn of the twentieth century, forms the foundation of much of modern genetics.

▼ Mendel's key contributions were the principles of segregation and independent assortment, and his definition of dominance and recessiveness. ▲

Basic Concepts of Probability

Risk assessment is an important part of medical genetics. For example, the physician or genetic counselor commonly informs couples of their risk of producing a child with a genetic disorder. In order to understand how such risks are estimated, some basic concepts of probability must be presented. A **probability** is defined as the proportion of times that a specific outcome occurs in a series of events. Thus, we may speak of the probability of obtaining a 4 when a die is tossed, or the probability that a couple will produce a son versus a daughter. Since probabilities are proportions, they lie between 0 and 1, inclusive.

During meiosis, one member of a chromosome pair is transmitted to a given sperm or egg cell. The probability that one member of the pair is transmitted is $\frac{1}{2}$, and the probability that the other member of the pair is transmitted is also $\frac{1}{2}$ (note that the probabilities of all possible events must add to 1 for any given experiment). Since this is directly analogous to coin tossing, in which the probabilities of obtaining heads or tails are each $\frac{1}{2}$, we will use coin tossing as our illustrative example.

When a coin is tossed repeatedly, the outcome of each toss has no effect on subsequent outcomes. The events are thus said to be **independent**. Even if we have obtained ten heads in a row, the probability of obtaining heads or tails on the next toss remains $\frac{1}{2}$. Similarly, the probability that a parent will transmit one of the two alleles at a locus is independent from one reproductive event to the next.

The independence principle allows us to deduce two fundamental concepts of probability, the **multiplication rule** and the **addition rule**. The multiplication rule states that if two trials are independent, then the probability of obtaining a given outcome in both trials is the product of the probabilities of each outcome. For example, we may wish to know the probability that an individual will obtain heads on both tosses of a fair coin. Because the tosses are independent events, this probability is given by the product of the probabilities of obtaining heads in each individual toss: $1/2 \times 1/2 = 1/4$. Similarly, the probability of obtaining two tails in a row is $1/2 \times 1/2 = 1/4$.

The multiplication rule can be extended for any number of trials. Suppose that a couple wants to know the probability that all three of their planned children will be girls. Since the probability of producing a girl is approximately $1/2$, and since reproductive events are independent of one another, the probability of producing three girls is $1/2 \times 1/2 \times 1/2 = 1/8$. However, if the couple has already produced two girls and *then* wants to know the probability of producing a third girl, it is simply $1/2$. This is because the previous two events are no longer probabilities; they have actually occurred. Because of independence, these events have no effect on the outcome of the third event.

The addition rule states that if we want to know the probability of either one outcome *or* another, we can simply add the respective probabilities together. For example, the probability of getting two heads in a row ($1/2 \times 1/2$, or $1/4$) *or* the probability of getting two tails in a row ($1/4$) is given by adding the two probabilities together: $1/4 + 1/4 = 1/2$. As another example, imagine that a couple plans to have three children, and they have a strong aversion to having three children all of the same sex. They can be reassured somewhat by knowing that the probability of producing three girls ($1/8$) or three boys ($1/8$) is only $1/4$ ($1/8 + 1/8$). The probability that they will have some combination of boys and girls is thus $3/4$, since the sum of the probabilities of all possible outcomes must add to 1.

▼ **Basic probability enables us to understand and estimate genetic risks. The multiplication rule is used to estimate the probability that two events will occur together. The addition rule is used to estimate the probability that one event *or* another will occur.** ▲

Gene and Genotype Frequencies

The prevalence of many genetic diseases can vary considerably from one population to another. For example, cystic fibrosis, a severe respiratory disorder (Clinical Commentary 4-1), is quite common among Caucasians, affecting approximately 1/2,500 births. It is rare in Asian populations, affecting only 1/90,000 births. As discussed in Chapter 3, sickle cell disease is common among African-Americans, affecting approximately 1/600 births. Yet it is almost never seen among individuals of

northern European descent. The concepts of **genotype frequency** and **gene frequency** help us to measure and understand population variation in disease genes.

Imagine that we have typed 200 individuals in a population for the MN blood group. This blood group, which is encoded by a locus on chromosome two, has two major alleles, labeled *M* and *N*. In the MN system the effects of both alleles can be observed in the heterozygote. *M* and *N* are thus said to be **codominant**; the heterozygote can be distinguished from both homozygotes. Any individual in the population can have one of three possible genotypes (recall from Chapter 3 that the genotype is one's genetic makeup at a locus): he or she could be homozygous for *M* (genotype *MM*), heterozygous (*MN*), or homozygous for *N* (*NN*). After typing each person in our sample, we find the following distribution of genotypes: *MM*, 64; *MN*, 120; *NN*, 16. The genotype frequency is obtained simply by dividing each genotype count by the total number of subjects. The frequency of *MM* is 64/200 ($= 0.32$), the frequency of *MN* is 120/200 ($= 0.60$), and the frequency of *NN* is 16/200 ($= 0.08$). The sum of these frequencies must, of course, equal 1.

The gene frequency for each allele, *M* and *N*, can be obtained here by the process of **gene counting**. Each *MM* homozygote has two *M* alleles, while each heterozygote has one *M* allele. Similarly, *NN* homozygotes have two *N* alleles, and heterozygotes have one *N* allele. In the sample measured here, there are:

$$(64 \times 2) + 120 = 248 \text{ } M \text{ genes}$$
$$(16 \times 2) + 120 = 152 \text{ } N \text{ genes}$$

In total, there are 400 genes at the *MN* locus (i.e., twice the number of subjects, since each has two alleles). To obtain the frequency of *M*, we then calculate $248/400 = 0.62$. The frequency of *N*, 152/400, is 0.38. The sum of the two frequencies must equal 1.

▼ **Gene and genotype frequencies specify the proportions of each allele and each genotype, respectively, in a population. Under simple conditions these frequencies can be estimated by direct counting.** ▲

The Hardy-Weinberg Principle

The example given for the MN locus presents an ideal situation for gene frequency estimation, since, because of codominance, the three genotypes can easily be distinguished and counted. What happens when one of the homozygotes is indistinguishable from the heterozygote (i.e., when there is dominance)? Here the basic concepts of probability can be used to specify a predictable relationship between gene frequencies and genotype frequencies.

Imagine a locus having two alleles, labeled *A* and *a*. Suppose that, in a population, we know the frequency

CLINICAL COMMENTARY 4-1
CYSTIC FIBROSIS

Cystic fibrosis (CF) is one of the most common single-gene disorders in North America, affecting approximately 1/2,000 to 1/4,000 Caucasian newborns. It is less common in other ethnic groups. The prevalence among African-Americans is about 1/17,000, and it is very rare among Asians (one study of Pacific Islanders yielded a prevalence of 1/90,000 births). Approximately 30,000 Americans suffer from this disease. **WWW**

CF was first identified as a distinct disease entity in 1938, and its earlier name was "cystic fibrosis of the pancreas." This refers to the fibrotic lesions that develop in the pancreas, one of the principal organs affected by this disorder (Fig. 4-3, *A* and *B*). Approximately 85% of CF patients have pancreatic insufficiency (i.e., the pancreas is unable to secrete digestive enzymes, resulting in chronic malnutrition). The intestinal tract is also affected, and approximately 10% to 20% of newborns with CF have meconium ileus (a thick plug that blocks the colon). The sweat glands of CF patients are abnormal, resulting in high levels of chloride in the sweat. This is the basis for the sweat chloride test, commonly used in the diagnosis of this disease. More than 95% of males with CF are sterile due to absence or obstruction of the vas deferens. The most serious problem facing CF patients is obstruction of the lungs by heavy, thick mucus. Because this mucus cannot be cleared effectively, the lungs are highly susceptible to infection by bacteria such as *Staphylococcus aureus* and *Pseudomonas aeruginosa*. Chronic obstruction and infection lead to destruction of the lung tissue, resulting eventually in death from pulmonary disease in more than 90% of CF patients (Fig. 4-3, *C* and *D*).

As a result of improved antibiotics, aggressive chest physical therapy, and pancreatic enzyme replacement therapy, the survival rates of CF patients have improved substantially during the past three decades. Median survival is now about 30 years of age. This disease has highly variable expression, with some patients experiencing relatively little respiratory difficulty and nearly normal survival. Others may have much more severe respiratory problems and survive for only a few years.

The CF gene was mapped to chromosome 7q in 1985 by investigators in London, Toronto, and Salt Lake City, and it was cloned 4 years later by investigators in Michigan and Toronto. It is a large gene, spanning 250 kb and including 27 exons. The CF gene encodes a protein product, labeled the "cystic fibrosis transmembrane regulator" (CFTR). CFTR forms cyclic-AMP regulated chloride ion channels that span the membranes of specialized epithelial cells, such as those that line the bowel and lung. In addition, CFTR is involved in regulating the transport of sodium ions across epithelial cell membranes.

The fact that CFTR is involved in sodium and chloride transport helps us to understand the multiple effects of mutations at the CF locus. Defective ion transport results in salt imbalances, depleting the airway of water and producing the thick, obstructive secretions seen in the lungs. The pancreas is also obstructed by thick secretions, leading to fibrosis and pancreatic insufficiency. The chloride ion transport defect explains the abnormally high concentrations of chloride in the sweat secretions of CF patients: chloride is secreted instead of being reabsorbed by the sweat gland.

DNA sequence analysis has revealed more than 700 different mutations at the CF locus. The most common of these is a three-base deletion resulting in a loss of a phenylalanine at position 508 of the CFTR protein. This mutation is labeled "ΔF508" (i.e., deletion of phenylalanine at position 508). ΔF508 accounts for nearly 70% of all CF mutations. This mutation, along with several other relatively common ones, is assayed in the genetic diagnosis of CF (see Chapter 13).

Identification of the specific mutation(s) responsible for CF in a patient can be useful in predicting the course

FIG. 4-3 **A,** Normal pancreas. **B,** Pancreas from a cystic fibrosis patient, showing infiltration of fat and fibrotic lesions.
Continued

CLINICAL COMMENTARY 4-1
CYSTIC FIBROSIS—cont'd

of the disease. For example, the most severe classes of mutations (of which ΔF508 is an example) result in a complete lack of chloride ion channel production or in channels that cannot migrate to the cell membrane. Patients homozygous for these mutations nearly always have pancreatic insufficiency. In contrast, other mutations (e.g., R117H) result in ion channels that do proceed to the cell membrane but respond poorly to cyclic AMP and consequently do not remain open as long as they should. The phenotype is thus milder: patients who have this mutation are less likely to have pancreatic insufficiency. Patients with other "mild" CFTR mutations tend to have less severe pulmonary disease. The correlation between genotype and phenotype is far from perfect, however, indicating that additional factors (possibly other loci and environmental factors) must influence the expression of the disease.

In general, there is a reasonably good correlation between genotype and pancreatic function and a more variable relationship between genotype and pulmonary function.

In addition to enhancing our understanding of the pathophysiology of CF, cloning the CF gene has opened the possibility of gene therapy (see Chapter 13). Research in experimental systems has shown that insertion of normal CF genes into cells with defective chloride ion transport can correct the defect. This and other research have led to the initiation of clinical trials in which normal CF genes are inserted into adenoviruses or similar vectors, which then may be introduced into the lungs of CF patients. It is hoped that the adenoviruses will insert the normal gene into airway epithelial cells, inducing normal chloride channel function in these cells. Although many difficulties present themselves (e.g., the adenoviruses themselves lead to lung disease), gene therapy could eventually lead to a cure for this usually fatal disease.

FIG. 4-3, cont'd   C, Normal lung tissue. **D,** Lung tissue from a cystic fibrosis patient, showing extensive destruction as a result of obstruction and infection.
(Courtesy Dr. Edward Klatt, University of Utah Health Sciences Center.)

of allele *A*, which we will call *p*, and the frequency of allele *a*, which we will call *q*. From this we wish to determine the expected population frequencies of each genotype, *AA*, *Aa*, and *aa*. We will assume that individuals in the population mate at random with regard to their genotype at this locus (**random mating** is also referred to as **panmixia**). Thus, the genotype has no effect on mate selection. If men and women mate at random, then the assumption of independence is fulfilled. This allows us to apply the addition and multiplication rules to estimate genotype frequencies.

Suppose that the frequency, *p*, of allele *A* in our population is 0.7. Then 70% of the sperm cells in the population must have allele *A*, and 70% of the egg cells must have allele *A*. Since *p* and *q* must sum to 1, 30% of the egg and sperm cells must carry allele *a* (i.e., $q = 0.30$). Under panmixia, the probability that a sperm cell carrying *A* unites with an egg cell carrying *A* is given by the product of the gene frequencies: $p \times p = p^2 = 0.49$ (multiplication rule). This is the probability of producing an offspring with the *AA* genotype. Using the same reasoning, the probability of producing an offspring with the *aa* genotype is given by $q \times q = q^2 = 0.09$.

What about the frequency of heterozygotes in the population? There are two ways a heterozygote can be formed. Either a sperm cell carrying *A* can unite with an egg carrying *a*, or a sperm cell carrying *a* can unite with an egg carrying *A*. The probability of each of these two outcomes is given by the product of the gene frequencies, *pq*. Since we want to know the overall probability of obtaining a heterozygote (i.e., the first event *or* the second), we can apply the addition rule, adding the probabilities to obtain a heterozygote frequency of *2pq*. These operations are summarized in Fig. 4-4. The relationship between gene frequencies and genotype frequencies was established independently by two men, Godfrey Hardy and Wilhelm Weinberg and is termed the **Hardy-Weinberg principle**.

As already mentioned, we can use this principle to estimate gene and genotype frequencies when dominant homozygotes and heterozygotes are indistinguishable. This is often the case for recessive diseases such as cystic fibrosis. Only the affected homozygotes, with genotype *aa*, are distinguishable. The Hardy-Weinberg principle tells us that the frequency of *aa* should be q^2. For cystic fibrosis in the Caucasian population, $q^2 = 1/2,500$ (i.e., the prevalence of the disease among newborns). To estimate *q*, we take the square root of both sides of this equation: $q = \sqrt{1/2,500} = 1/50 = 0.02$. Since $p + q = 1$, $p = 0.98$. We can then estimate the genotype frequencies of *AA* and *Aa*. The latter genotype, which represents heterozygous **carriers** of the disease allele, is of particular interest. We find that $2pq = 1/25$ (note that, since *p* is nearly 1.0, we can simplify this

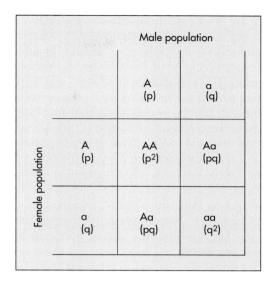

FIG. 4-4   The Hardy-Weinberg principle. The population frequencies of genotypes *AA*, *Aa*, and *aa* are predicted on the basis of gene frequencies (*p* and *q*). It is assumed that the gene frequencies are the same in males and females.

calculation by rounding *p* up to 1.0; then, without a significant loss of accuracy, $2q = 2/50 = 1/25$). This tells us something rather remarkable about cystic fibrosis and about recessive diseases in general. While the incidence of affected homozygotes is only 1/2,500, heterozygous carriers of the disease gene are much more common (1 in 25 individuals). The vast majority of recessive disease alleles, then, are effectively "hidden" in the genomes of heterozygotes.

▼ **Under panmixia, the Hardy-Weinberg principle specifies the relationship between gene frequencies and genotype frequencies. It is useful in estimating gene frequencies from disease prevalence data and in estimating the incidence of heterozygous carriers of recessive disease genes.** ▲

The Concept of Phenotype

The term "genotype" has been defined as an individual's genetic constitution at a locus. The **phenotype** is what we actually observe physically or clinically. Genotypes do not uniquely correspond to phenotypes. Two different genotypes, a dominant homozygote and a heterozygote, may have the same phenotype. An example would be cystic fibrosis. Conversely, the same genotype may produce different phenotypes in different environments. An example of this is the recessive disease phenylketonuria (commonly abbreviated as PKU), seen in approximately 1/10,000 Caucasian births. Mutations at the locus encoding the metabolic enzyme phenylalanine hydroxylase render the homozygote unable to metabolize the amino acid phenylalanine. While babies with PKU are normal at birth, their metabolic deficiency produces a buildup of phenylalanine and various toxic metabolites. This is highly destructive to the central nervous system, and it eventually produces severe mental retardation. It has been estimated that untreated PKU babies lose, on average, one to two IQ points per week during the first year of life. Thus, the PKU genotype can produce a severe disease phenotype. However, it is easy to screen for PKU at birth (see Chapter 13), and the disease can be avoided by initiating a low-phenylalanine diet within 1 month after birth. The individual still has the PKU genotype, but the phenotype of mental retardation has been profoundly altered by environmental modification. WWW

This example shows that the phenotype is the result of the *interaction* of genotype and environmental factors. It should be emphasized that "environment" can include the genetic environment (i.e., genes at other loci whose products may interact with a specific gene or its product).

▼ The phenotype, which is physically observable, results from the interaction of genotype and environment. ▲

Basic Pedigree Structure

The **pedigree** is one of the most commonly used tools in medical genetics. It illustrates the relationships among family members, and it shows which family members are affected or unaffected by a genetic disease. Typically, an arrow denotes the **proband**, the first individual diagnosed in the pedigree. The proband is sometimes also referred to as the **index case** or **propositus** (**proposita** for females). Fig. 4-5 describes the features of pedigree notation.

When discussing relatives in families, one often refers to degrees of relationship. First-degree relatives are those who are related at the parent-offspring or sibling (brother and sister) level. Second-degree relatives are those who are removed by one additional generational "step" (e.g., grandparents and grandchildren, uncles/aunts and nieces/nephews). Continuing this logic, third-degree relatives would include, for example, first cousins, great-grandchildren, and so on.

AUTOSOMAL DOMINANT INHERITANCE
Characteristics of Autosomal Dominant Inheritance

Currently, there are more than 4,400 known autosomal dominant traits, most of which are diseases. Individually, each autosomal dominant disease is rather rare in populations, with the most common ones having gene

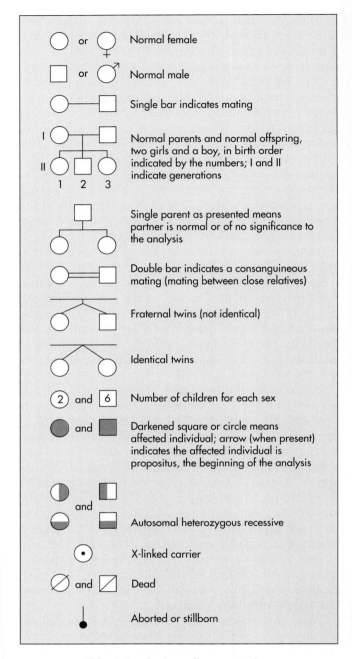

FIG. 4-5 Basic pedigree notation.

frequencies of about 0.001. Matings between two individuals both affected by the same autosomal dominant disease are thus uncommon. Most often, affected offspring are produced by the union of a normal parent with an affected heterozygote. The Punnett square in Fig. 4-6 illustrates this mating. The affected parent can pass either a disease gene or a normal gene to his or her children. Each event has a probability of 0.5. Thus, on the average, half of the children will be heterozygotes and will express the disease, while half will be normal homozygotes.

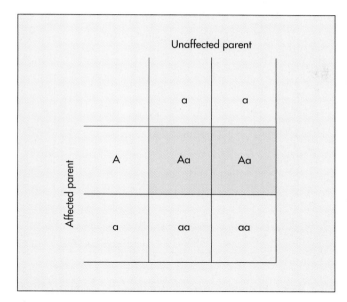

FIG. 4-6 Punnett square illustrating the mating of an unaffected individual (*aa*) with an individual who is heterozygous for an autosomal dominant disease gene (*Aa*). The genotypes of affected offspring are shaded.

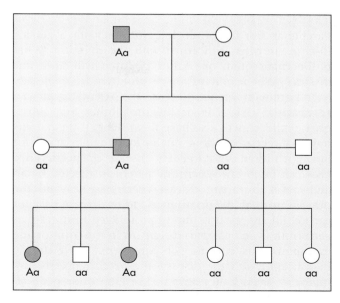

FIG. 4-8 A pedigree illustrating the inheritance pattern of postaxial polydactyly, an autosomal dominant disorder. Affected individuals are represented by shading.

FIG. 4-7 Postaxial polydactyly. An extra digit is located next to the fifth digit.

Postaxial polydactyly, the presence of an extra digit next to the fifth digit (Fig. 4-7), can be inherited as an autosomal dominant trait. Let *A* symbolize the gene for polydactyly, and let *a* symbolize the normal allele. An idealized pedigree for this disease is shown in Fig. 4-8. This pedigree illustrates several important characteristics of autosomal dominant inheritance. First, the two

sexes exhibit the trait in approximately equal proportions, and males and females are equally likely to transmit the trait to their offspring. This reflects the fact that this is an *autosomal* disease (as opposed to a disease caused by an X chromosome mutation, in which these proportions typically differ). Second, there is no skipping of generations: if an individual has polydactyly, one parent must also have it. This leads to a vertical transmission pattern, in which the disease phenotype is usually seen in one generation after another. Also, if neither parent has the trait, none of the children have it. Third, father-son transmission of the disease gene is observed. Although father-son transmission is not *required* to establish autosomal dominant inheritance, its presence in a pedigree excludes certain other modes of inheritance (particularly X-linked inheritance; see Chapter 5). Finally, as we have already seen, an affected heterozygote transmits the trait to approximately half of his or her children. However, since gamete transmission, like coin tossing, is subject to chance fluctuations, it is possible that all or none of the children of an affected parent will have the trait. When large numbers of matings of this type are studied, the proportion of affected children will closely approach one half. **WWW**

▼ Autosomal dominant inheritance is characterized by vertical transmission of the disease phenotype, a lack of skipped generations, and roughly equal numbers of affected males and females. Father-son transmission may be observed. ▲

Recurrence Risks

Parents at risk for producing children with a genetic disease are often concerned with the question: What is the chance that our future children will have this disease? When one or more children have already been born with a genetic disease, the parents are given a **recurrence risk**. This is the probability that subsequent children will also have the disease. If the parents have not yet had children, but are known to be at risk for having children with a genetic disease, an **occurrence risk** can be given. When one parent is affected by an autosomal dominant disease (heterozygote) and the other is normal, the occurrence and recurrence risks for each child are $1/2$. It is important to keep in mind that each birth is an *independent event*, as in the coin-tossing examples. Thus, even though parents may have already had a child with the disease, their recurrence risk remains $1/2$. Even if they have had several children, all affected (or all unaffected) with the disease, the law of independence dictates that the probability that their next child will have the disease is still $1/2$. While this concept may seem intuitively obvious, it is frequently misunderstood by the lay population. Further aspects of communicating risks to families will be discussed in Chapter 14.

▼ The recurrence risk for autosomal dominant disorders is 50%. Because of independence, this risk remains constant no matter how many affected or unaffected children are born. ▲

AUTOSOMAL RECESSIVE INHERITANCE

Like autosomal dominant diseases, autosomal recessive diseases are fairly rare in populations. As shown previously, heterozygous carriers for recessive disease genes are much more common than affected homozygotes. Consequently, the parents of individuals affected with autosomal recessive diseases are usually both heterozygous carriers. As the Punnett square in Fig. 4-9 demonstrates, one fourth of their offspring will be normal homozygotes, half will be phenotypically normal heterozygous carriers, and one fourth will be homozygotes affected with the disease (on average).

Characteristics of Autosomal Recessive Inheritance

Fig. 4-10 is a pedigree showing the inheritance of an autosomal recessive form of albinism that results from mutations in the gene that encodes tyrosinase, a tyrosine-metabolizing enzyme.* The resulting tyrosinase defi-

*This form of albinism, termed "tyrosinase-negative albinism," is distinguished from a second, milder form termed "tyrosinase-positive albinism." The latter form is typically caused by mutations in a gene on chromosome 15 that appears to affect tyrosine transport.

FIG. 4-9 Punnett square illustrating the mating of two heterozygous carriers of an autosomal recessive gene. The genotype of the affected offspring is shaded.

ciency creates a block in the metabolic pathway that normally leads to the synthesis of melanin pigment. Consequently, the affected individual has very little pigment in the skin, hair, and eyes (see Color Plate 2 following p. 116). Because melanin is also required for the normal development of the optic fibers, albinos may also display nystagmus (rapid uncontrolled eye movement), strabismus (deviation of the eye from its normal axis), and reduced visual acuity. The pedigree demonstrates most of the important criteria for distinguishing autosomal recessive inheritance (these criteria, along with those of autosomal dominant inheritance, are summarized in Table 4-1). First, unlike autosomal dominant diseases, in which the disease phenotype is seen in one generation after another, autosomal recessive diseases are usually seen in one or more siblings but not in earlier generations. Second, as in autosomal dominant inheritance, males and females are affected in equal proportions. Third, on average, one fourth of the offspring of two heterozygous carriers will be affected with the disorder. Finally, **consanguinity** is present more often in pedigrees involving autosomal recessive diseases than in those involving other types of inheritance (see Fig. 4-10). The term "consanguinity" (Latin, "with blood") refers to the mating of related individuals. It is often a factor in recessive disease because related individuals are more likely to share the same disease genes. Consanguinity will be discussed in greater detail later. www

▼ Autosomal recessive inheritance is characterized by clustering of the disease phenotype among siblings, but the disease is not usually seen among par-

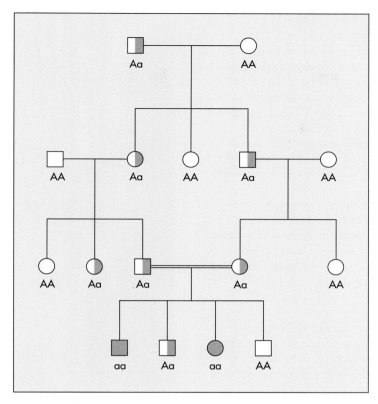

FIG. 4-10   Pedigree showing the inheritance pattern of tyrosinase-negative albinism, an autosomal recessive disease. Consanguinity in this pedigree is denoted by a double bar connecting the parents of the affected individuals.

TABLE 4-1   A Comparison of the Major Attributes of Autosomal Dominant and Autosomal Recessive Inheritance Patterns

Attribute	Autosomal Dominant	Autosomal Recessive
Usual recurrence risk	50%	25%
Transmission pattern	Vertical; disease phenotype seen in generation after generation	Horizontal; disease phenotype seen in multiple siblings, but usually no earlier generations affected
Sex ratio	Equal number of affected males and females (usually)	Equal number of affected males and females (usually)
Other	Father-son transmission of disease gene is possible	Consanguinity is sometimes seen, especially for rare recessive diseases

ents or other ancestors. Equal numbers of affected males and females are usually seen, and consanguinity may be present. ▲

Recurrence Risks

As already discussed, the most common mating type seen in recessive disease involves two heterozygous carrier parents. This reflects the relative commonness of heterozygous carriers and the fact that many autosomal recessive diseases are severe enough that affected individuals are less likely to become parents.

The Punnett square in Fig. 4-9 demonstrates that one fourth of the offspring from this mating will be homozygous for the disease gene and therefore affected. The recurrence risk for the offspring of carrier parents is then 25%. As before, these are *average* figures. In any given family there will likely be chance fluctuations, but a study of a large number of families would yield a figure quite close to this proportion.

Occasionally, a carrier of a recessive disease gene mates with an individual homozygous for the disease gene. In this case, roughly half of their children will be affected, while half will be heterozygous carriers. The recurrence risk is 50%. Because this pattern of inheritance mimics that of an autosomal dominant trait, it is sometimes referred to as **quasi-dominant** inheritance. With extended studies of pedigrees, in which carrier matings are observed, it can be distinguished from true dominant inheritance.

When two individuals affected by a recessive disease mate, all of their children must also be affected. This observation helps to distinguish recessive from dominant inheritance, since two parents both affected by a dominant disease will nearly always both be heterozygotes and thus one fourth of their children will be unaffected.

▼ The recurrence risk for autosomal recessive diseases is usually 25%. Quasi-dominant inheritance, with a recurrence risk of 50%, is seen when an affected homozygote mates with a heterozygote. ▲

"Dominant" Versus "Recessive": Some Cautions

The preceding discussion has treated dominant and recessive disorders as though they belong in rigid categories. However, these distinctions are becoming less strict as our understanding of these diseases increases. Many (probably most) "dominant" diseases are actually more severe in affected homozygotes than in heterozygotes. An example is achondroplasia, an autosomal dominant disorder in which heterozygotes have reduced stature (Fig. 4-11). Heterozygotes enjoy a nearly normal life span, estimated to be only about 10 years less than average. Affected homozygotes are much more severely affected and usually die in infancy of respiratory failure. **WWW**

Although heterozygous carriers of recessive disease genes are clinically normal, the effects of recessive genes can often be detected in heterozygotes because they result in reduced levels of enzyme activity. This is usually the basis for biochemical carrier detection tests (see Chapter 13). A useful and valid way to distinguish dominant and recessive disorders is that heterozygotes are clinically affected in most cases of dominant disorders, whereas they are nearly always clinically normal in recessive disorders.

▼ While the distinction between dominant and recessive diseases is not rigid, a dominant disease allele will produce disease in a heterozygote, whereas a recessive disease allele will not. ▲

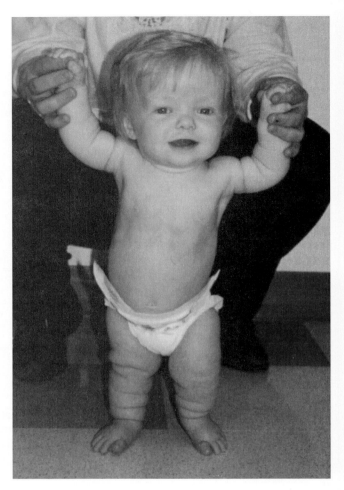

FIG. 4-11 Achondroplasia. This girl has short limbs relative to trunk length. She also has a prominent forehead, low nasal root, and redundant skin folds in the arms and legs.

Another caution is that a disease may be inherited in autosomal dominant fashion in some cases and autosomal recessive fashion in others. Familial isolated growth hormone deficiency (IGHD), another reduced stature disorder, is an example of one such disease. DNA sequencing of a pituitary growth hormone gene on chromosome 17 *(GH1)* has revealed a number of different mutations that can produce IGHD. *Recessive* IGHD can be caused by nonsense and splice site mutations that apparently alter the protein product (pituitary growth hormone) such that it cannot proceed to the secretory granules of the cell (cytoplasmic structures that secrete growth hormone and other products from the cell). Because they have one normal chromosome, heterozygotes still produce half of the normal amount of growth hormone. This is sufficient for normal stature. Homozygotes for these mutations produce no GH1 product and have reduced stature.

How, then, can a mutation at this locus produce *dominant* inheritance? In one form of dominantly inherited IGHD, a splice site mutation deletes the third exon of the *GH1* gene, producing a protein product that does proceed to the secretory granules. Here, the abnormal *GH1* product encoded by the mutated chromosome forms disulfide bonds with the normal product encoded by the normal chromosome. Acting as a dominant negative (see Chapter 3), the abnormal molecules disable the normal growth hormone molecules, resulting in greatly reduced production of GH1 product and thus reduced stature. This example illustrates some of the difficulties in applying the terms "dominant" and "recessive," and it also shows how molecular analysis of a gene can help to explain important disease features.

▼ In some cases, a disease may be inherited in either autosomal dominant or autosomal recessive fashion, depending on the nature of the mutation that alters the gene product. ▲

A final caution is that the terms "dominant" and "recessive," strictly speaking, apply to traits, not genes. To see why, consider the sickle cell mutation, discussed in Chapter 3. Homozygotes for this mutation develop sickle cell disease. Heterozygotes, said to have sickle cell *trait*, are usually clinically normal. However, a heterozygote has an increased risk for splenic infarctions at very high altitude. Is the mutant gene then dominant or recessive? Clearly, it makes more sense to refer to sickle cell *disease* as recessive and sickle cell *trait* as dominant. Nonetheless, it is common (and often convenient) to apply the terms "dominant" and "recessive" to genes.

FACTORS THAT MAY COMPLICATE INHERITANCE PATTERNS

The inheritance patterns described previously for postaxial polydactyly and albinism are quite straightforward. However, many autosomal diseases display more complex patterns. Some of these complexities are described next.

New Mutation

If a child has been born with a genetic disease and there is no history of the disease in the family, it is possible that the child is the product of a **new mutation** (this is especially likely if the disease in question is autosomal dominant). That is, the gene transmitted by one of the parents underwent a change in DNA resulting in a mutation from a normal to a disease-causing allele. The genes at this locus in the parent's other germ cells would still be normal. In this case the recurrence risk for the parents' subsequent offspring is not elevated above that of the general population. However, the offspring of the affected child may have a substantially elevated occurrence risk (e.g., it would be 50% for an autosomal dom-

inant disease). A large proportion of the observed cases of many autosomal dominant diseases are the result of new mutations. For example, it is estimated that $7/8$ of all cases of achondroplasia are due to new mutations, while only $1/8$ are transmitted by achondroplastic parents. This is primarily because the disease tends to limit the potential for reproduction. In order to provide accurate risk estimates, it is essential to know whether an observed case is due to an inherited disease gene or a new mutation. This can be done only if an adequate family history has been taken.

▼ New mutations are a frequent cause of the appearance of a genetic disease in an individual with no previous family history of the disorder. The recurrence risk for the individual's siblings is very low, but it may be substantially elevated for the individual's offspring. ▲

Germline Mosaicism

Occasionally, two or more offspring will present with an autosomal dominant disease when there is no family history of the disease. Since mutation is a rare event, it is unlikely that this would be due to multiple mutations in the same family. The mechanism most likely to be responsible is termed **germline mosaicism** (mosaicism describes the presence of more than one genetically distinct cell line in the body). During the embryonic development of one of the parents, a mutation occurred that affected all or part of the germline but few or none of the somatic cells of the embryo. Thus, the parent carries the mutation in his or her germline but does not actually express the disease. As a result, he or she can transmit the mutation to multiple offspring. This phenomenon, while relatively rare, can have significant effects on recurrence risks when it occurs.

Germline mosaicism has been studied extensively in the lethal perinatal form of osteogenesis imperfecta (OI type II, see Chapter 2), which is caused by mutations in the type 1 procollagen genes. The fact that unaffected parents sometimes produced multiple offspring affected with this disease led to the conclusion that type II OI was an autosomal recessive trait. This has been disputed by recent studies in which the PCR technique was used to amplify DNA from the sperm of a father of two type II OI cases. This DNA was compared with DNA extracted from his somatic cells (skin fibroblasts). Although procollagen mutations were not detected in the fibroblast DNA, they were found in approximately one in eight sperm cells. This is a direct demonstration of germline mosaicism in this individual. Although germline mosaicism has thus been demonstrated for type II OI, most cases are thought to be caused by isolated new mutations, and a few cases of true autosomal recessive inheritance have also been documented.

Other diseases in which germline mosaicism has been observed include achondroplasia, neurofibromatosis type 1, Duchenne muscular dystrophy, and hemophilia A (see Chapter 5 for further discussion of the latter two diseases).

▼ Germline mosaicism occurs when all or part of a parent's germ line is affected by a disease mutation but the somatic cells are not. It elevates the recurrence risk for future offspring of the mosaic parent. ▲

Delayed Age of Onset

While some genetic diseases are expressed at birth or shortly afterward, many others do not become apparent until well into adulthood. This is known as **delayed age of onset**. One of the best-known examples is Huntington disease, a neurological disorder whose main features are progressive dementia and increasingly uncontrollable movements of the limbs (see Clinical Commentary 4-2). The latter feature is known as chorea (from the Greek word for dance, *khoreia*), and the disease is sometimes called Huntington's chorea. This autosomal dominant disorder is named after Dr. George Huntington, who first described the disease in 1872. Symptoms are not usually seen until age 30 or later (Fig. 4-12). Thus, those who develop the disease have often had children before they are aware that they carry the gene. If the disease were present at birth, nearly all affected persons would die before reaching reproductive age, and the frequency of the gene in the population would be much lower. Delaying the age of onset thus reduces natural selection against a disease

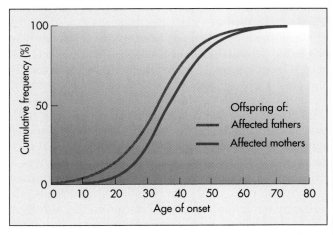

FIG. 4-12 Distribution of the age of onset for Huntington disease. The age of onset tends to be somewhat earlier when the affected parent is male.
(Based on data from Conneally PM [1984] Am. J. Hum. Genet. 36:520.)

gene, increasing its frequency in a population. Delayed age of onset can cause difficulties in deducing the mode of inheritance of a disease because it is not possible to determine until later in life whether an individual carries the disease gene. **WWW**

A person whose parent has Huntington disease has a 50% chance of inheriting the disease gene. Until fairly recently, this individual would be confronted with a torturous question: should I have children, knowing that there is a 50% chance that I might have this disease gene and then pass it to half of my children? With the identification of the mutation responsible for Huntington disease, it is now possible for at-risk individuals to know with a high degree of certainty whether or not they carry a disease-causing allele.

As mentioned previously, a number of important genetic diseases have a delayed age of onset. These include hemochromatosis, a potentially fatal recessive disorder of iron storage (see Chapter 7); familial Alzheimer disease (see Chapter 12); and many inherited cancers, including autosomal dominant breast cancer.*

▼ Delayed age of onset is observed in many genetic diseases. It complicates the interpretation of inheritance patterns in families. ▲

Reduced Penetrance

Another important characteristic of many genetic diseases is reduced **penetrance**: an individual who has the genotype for a disease may not exhibit the disease phenotype at all, even though he or she can transmit the disease gene to the next generation. Retinoblastoma, a malignant eye tumor (Clinical Commentary 4-3), is a good example of an autosomal dominant disorder in which reduced penetrance is seen. The transmission pattern of this disorder is illustrated in Fig. 4-15. Family studies have shown that about 10% of the **obligate carriers** of the retinoblastoma susceptibility gene (i.e., those who have an affected parent and affected children and therefore must themselves carry the gene) do not have the disease. The penetrance of the gene is then said to be 90%. Penetrance rates are usually estimated by examining a large number of families and determining what proportion of the obligate carriers or obligate homozygotes (in the case of recessive disorders) develop the disease phenotype. **WWW**

▼ Diseases genes in which an individual may have the disease genotype without expressing the disease phenotype are said to have reduced penetrance. ▲

---

*Epidemiological studies indicate that about 5% of breast cancer cases in the United States are caused by genes inherited in autosomal dominant fashion. See Chapters 11 and 12 for further discussion.

CLINICAL COMMENTARY 4-2
HUNTINGTON DISEASE

Huntington disease affects approximately one in 20,000 persons of European descent. It is substantially less common among Japanese and Africans. The disorder usually presents between ages 30 and 50, although it has been observed as early as 2 years of age and as late as 80 years of age.

Huntington disease is characterized by a progressive loss of motor control ("chorea") and by psychiatric problems, including dementia and affective disorder. There is a substantial loss of neurons in the brain, detectable by imaging techniques such as magnetic resonance imaging. Decreased glucose uptake in the brain, an early sign of the disorder, can be demonstrated by positron-emission tomography (PET). While many parts of the brain are affected, the area most noticeably damaged is the corpus striatum. In some patients the disease leads to a loss of 25% or more of total brain weight (Fig. 4-13).

The clinical course of Huntington disease is protracted. Typically, the interval from initial diagnosis to death is approximately 15 years. As in many neurological disorders, patients with Huntington disease experience difficulties in swallowing; aspiration pneumonia is the most common cause of death. Cardiorespiratory failure and subdural hematoma (due to head trauma) are other frequent causes of death. The suicide rate among Huntington disease patients is several times higher than that in the general population. Treatment includes the use of drugs such as benzodiazepines to help control the choreic movements. Affective disturbances are sometimes controlled with antipsychotic drugs and tricyclic antidepressants. Although these drugs help to control some of the symptoms of Huntington disease, there is currently no way to alter the outcome of the disease.

Huntington disease has one of the lowest known mutation rates of all human disease genes, estimated at approximately one per million (per locus per generation). There are currently only a few well-documented examples of individuals in whom the disease arose as a new mutation. This disorder is also notable in that affected homozygotes appear to display exactly the same clinical course as heterozygotes (in contrast to most dominant disorders, in which homozygotes are more severely affected). This attribute, and the fact that mouse models in which one copy of the gene is inactivated are perfectly normal, support the hypothesis that the mutation causes a gain of function (see Chapter 3). The Huntington disease has the distinction of being the first genetic disease mapped to a specific chromosome using an RFLP marker. James Gusella and colleagues mapped the disease gene to a region on the distal short arm of chromosome 4 in 1983.

After 10 years of work by a large number of investigators, the disease gene was cloned. DNA sequence analysis shows that the mutation is a CAG expanded repeat (see Chapter 3) located within the coding portion of the gene. Unaffected individuals typically have 11 to 35 copies of this repeat; those with Huntington disease may have from 36 to more than 100 copies of the repeat. Incomplete penetrance of the disease phenotype is seen in those who have 36 to 38 repeats. As in many disorders caused by trinucleotide repeat expansion, a larger number of repeats is correlated with earlier age of onset of the disorder. Also, there is a tendency for greater repeat expansion when the parent transmitting the disease gene is a male. This helps to explain the difference in ages of onset for maternally and paternally transmitted disease seen in Fig. 4-12. In particular, 80% of cases with onset before 20 years (termed "juvenile Huntington disease") are paternally transmitted, and these cases are accompanied by especially large repeat expansions. It remains to be seen why the degree of repeat instability in the Huntington gene is greater in paternal transmission than in maternal transmission.

Cloning the Huntington disease gene led quickly to the identification of the gene product, huntingtin. The CAG repeat expansion produces a lengthened series of glutamine residues near huntingtin's amino terminal. Although the role of the expanded glutamine tract in disease causation is unknown, recent studies show that it leads to a buildup of toxic protein aggregates within and near neuronal nuclei, causing early neuronal death. In addition, normal huntingtin interacts with several other proteins, including GAPDH (glyceraldehyde-3-phosphate dehydrogenase), an enzyme required for neuronal glycolysis. The expanded glutamine series may impede these interactions. Further study of huntingtin will increase our understanding of Huntington disease and may ultimately lead to more effective treatment.

FIG. 4-13 Cross section of a brain of an adult with Huntington disease, illustrating marked striatal atrophy. (Courtesy Dr. Jeanette Townsend, University of Utah Health Sciences Center.)

CLINICAL COMMENTARY 4-3
RETINOBLASTOMA

Retinoblastoma (Fig. 4-14) is the most common childhood eye tumor, affecting approximately 1 in 20,000 children. The tumor begins during embryonic development, when retinal cells are actively dividing and proliferating. It nearly always presents clinically by age 5.

Approximately 40% of retinoblastoma cases are familial (the remainder are **sporadic** and are not transmitted from one generation to the next). Before this gene was mapped to chromosome 13 and subjected to molecular analyses in the early 1980s, the cause of reduced penetrance in familial retinoblastoma was the subject of much speculation. The ability to examine changes in DNA near the disease gene finally explained the mechanism responsible for reduced penetrance. Briefly, an affected individual will transmit the disease gene to half of his or her children, on average. Thus, the offspring has inherited a mutation on one member of the chromosome 13 pair in every cell of his or her body. However, this is not sufficient to cause tumor formation (if it were, every cell in the body would give rise to a tumor). A *second* event must occur in the same region of the normal, homologous chromosome 13 in a fetus's developing retinal cell to initiate a tumor (this "two-hit" process is discussed further in Chapter 11). The second event, which can be considered a somatic mutation, has a relatively low probability of occurring. However, there are at least one million retinal cells in the developing fetus, each representing a potential "target" for the event. Usually, a fetus who has inherited a copy of the retinoblastoma disease gene will experience a second "hit" in several different retinal cells, giving rise to several tumors. Familial retinoblastoma is thus usually multifocal (consisting of several tumor foci) and bilateral (affecting both eyes). Since the second hits are random events, a small proportion of individuals who inherit the disease allele never experience a second hit in any retinal cell. They do not develop a retinoblastoma. The requirement for a second hit thus explains the reduced penetrance seen in this disorder.

The retinoblastoma gene has been cloned and sequenced, and the function of its gene product, pRb, has been studied closely. A major function of pRb, when hypophosphorylated, is to bind and inactivate E2F, a nuclear transcription factor. The cell requires active E2F to proceed from the G1 to the S phase of mitosis. By inactivating E2F, pRb applies a "brake" to the cell cycle. When cell division is required, pRb is phosphorylated by cyclin-dependent kinases (see Chapter 2). Consequently, E2F is released by pRb and thus activated. A mutation in pRb can cause a permanent loss of E2F-binding capacity, and the cell, having lost its brake, will undergo uncontrolled proliferation leading to a tumor. Because of its controlling effect on the cell cycle, the Rb gene belongs to a class of genes known as **tumor suppressors** (see Chapter 11).

If untreated, retinoblastomas can grow to considerable size. Reports from the nineteenth century described tumors achieving the size of "two fists." Fortunately, these tumors are now usually detected and treated before they become large. If found early enough through ophthalmological examination, the tumor may be treated successfully with radiation or cryotherapy (freezing). In more advanced cases enucleation (removal) of the eye is necessary. Because individuals with familial retinoblastoma have inherited a chromosome 13 mutation in all cells of their body, they are also susceptible to other types of cancers later in life. In particular, about 15% of those who inherit the mutation later develop osteosarcomas (malignant bone tumors). Careful monitoring for subsequent tumors, and avoidance of agents that could produce a second hit, such as radiation, are thus important aspects of managing the retinoblastoma patient.

FIG. 4-14   Bilateral retinoblastoma, showing presence of neoplastic tissue.
(From Rosai J [1996] Ackerman's Surgical Pathology. Ed 8. Mosby, St Louis.)

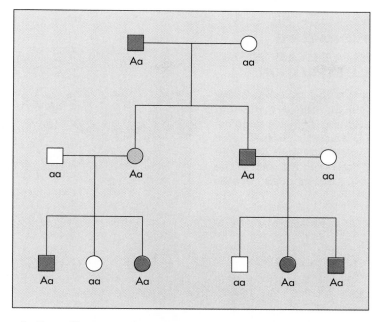

FIG. 4-15   Pedigree illustrating the inheritance pattern of retinoblastoma, a disorder with reduced penetrance. The unaffected obligate carrier is lightly shaded, and affected individuals are heavily shaded.

Variable Expression

A similar complication is **variable expression**. Here, the penetrance may be complete, but the severity of the disease can vary greatly. A well-studied example of variable expression in an autosomal dominant disease is neurofibromatosis type 1, or von Recklinghausen disease (after the German physician who described the disorder in 1882). Clinical Commentary 4-4 provides further discussion of this disorder. A parent with mild expression of the disease—so mild that he or she is not aware of it—can transmit the gene to a child who may have severe expression. As with delayed age of onset and reduced penetrance, variable expression provides a mechanism for disease genes to survive at higher frequencies in populations. **www**

It should be emphasized that penetrance and expression are distinct entities. Penetrance is an all-or-none phenomenon: one either has the disease phenotype or does not. Variable expression refers to the *extent* of expression of the disease phenotype.

The causes of variable expression are usually not known. Environmental effects can sometimes be responsible: in the absence of a certain environmental factor, the gene is expressed with diminished severity or not at all. Another possible cause is the interaction of other genes, called **modifier genes,** with the disease gene. Finally, as the molecular basis of mutation becomes better understood, it is clear that some cases of variable

expression are due to different types of mutations (i.e., different alleles) at the same disease locus. This is termed **allelic heterogeneity.** In some cases, clinically distinct diseases may be the result of allelic heterogeneity (e.g., as in the β-globin mutations that can cause sickle cell disease or various β-thalassemias).

Osteogenesis imperfecta is one disease in which genetic studies have helped to explain variable expression. Mutations that affect amino acids near the carboxyl terminal of the procollagen molecule generally cause more severe consequences than do mutations affecting the molecule near its amino terminal. It is also well documented that affected members of the same family, having the same mutation, can manifest large differences in disease severity. This may be due to different genetic "backgrounds" (i.e., modifier genes) in related individuals. And nongenetic events, such as an accidental bone fracture, can influence the severity of the disorder. Once a fracture occurs, casting and immobilization leads to a loss of bone mass, which further predisposes the patient to future fractures. Thus, a chance environmental event (such as trauma leading to a fracture in a baby during delivery) can cause a significant increase in severity of expression. Osteogenesis imperfecta thus provides examples of each factor thought to influence variable expression: environmental events, modifier genes, and allelic heterogeneity.

CLINICAL COMMENTARY 4-4

NEUROFIBROMATOSIS, A DISEASE WITH HIGHLY VARIABLE EXPRESSION

Neurofibromatosis type 1 (NF1) (Fig. 4-16) is one of the most common autosomal dominant disorders, affecting approximately 1 in 3,000 individuals. It offers a good example of variable expression in a genetic disease. Some patients will have only a few *café-au-lait* spots (from the French for "coffee with milk," describing the color of the hyperpigmented skin patches), Lisch nodules (benign

FIG. 4-16 Neurofibromatosis type 1. **A,** A young adult with multiple dermal neurofibromas of the trunk. A *café-au-lait* spot can be seen in the right upper abdomen. **B,** In a second patient with NF1, a large plexiform neurofibroma hangs from the lower right back, causing considerable inconvenience and discomfort. This was substantially improved by surgical removal of the tumor.

(*B,* Courtesy Dr. David Viskochil, University of Utah Health Sciences Center.)

▼ Variable expression of a genetic disease may be caused by environmental effects, modifier genes, or allelic heterogeneity. ▲

Pleiotropy and Heterogeneity

Genes having more than one discernible effect on the body are said to be **pleiotropic**. A good example of a gene with pleiotropic effects is given by Marfan syndrome. First described in 1896 by Antoine Marfan, a French pediatrician, this autosomal dominant disorder affects the eye, the skeleton, and the cardiovascular system (Clinical Commentary 4-5). All of the observed features of Marfan syndrome are due to unusually stretchable connective tissue. The gene for Marfan syndrome has been mapped to chromosome 15q, and it has been

demonstrated that mutations in the gene encoding fibrillin, a component of connective tissue, are responsible for the multiple defects seen in this disorder. We have discussed several other single-gene diseases in which pleiotropy is seen (e.g., cystic fibrosis, in which sweat glands, lungs, and pancreas can be affected; osteogenesis imperfecta, in which bones, teeth, and sclerae can be affected; and albinism, in which pigmentation and optic fiber development are affected). **WWW**

▼ Genes that exert effects on multiple aspects of physiology or anatomy are pleiotropic. Pleiotropy is a common feature of human genes. ▲

Just as a single gene may have multiple effects, a single disease phenotype may be caused by mutations at difgrowths on the iris), and perhaps a few neurofibromas (nonmalignant peripheral nerve tumors). These individuals are often unaware that they have the condition. Other patients may have a much more severe expression of the disorder, including hundreds to thousands of neurofibromas, optic gliomas (benign tumors of the optic nerve), learning disabilities, hypertension, scoliosis (lateral curvature of the spine), and malignancies (e.g., neurofibrosarcomas). Fortunately, about two thirds of patients have only a mild cutaneous involvement. Fewer than 10% develop malignancies as a result of the disorder. Expression can vary significantly within the same family: a mildly affected parent can produce severely affected offspring.

A standard set of diagnostic criteria for neurofibromatosis type 1 has been developed. The criteria are that two or more of the following must be present:

1. Six or more café-au-lait spots greater than 5 mm in diameter in prepubertal subjects and greater than 15 mm in postpubertal subjects
2. Freckling in the armpits or groin area
3. Two or more neurofibromas of any type or one plexiform neurofibroma (i.e., an extensive growth that occurs along a large nerve sheath)
4. Two or more Lisch nodules
5. Optic glioma
6. Distinctive bone lesions, particularly an abnormally formed sphenoid bone or tibial pseudarthrosis*
7. A first-degree relative diagnosed with neurofibromatosis using the previous six criteria

Although NF1 has highly variable expression, the

*Pseudarthrosis may occur when a long bone, such as the tibia, undergoes a loss of bone cortex, leading to weakening and fracture. Abnormal callus formation causes a "false joint" in the bone, leading to the term ("arthron" = joint).

penetrance of this gene is virtually 100%. It has one of the highest known mutation rates, about 1 in 10,000 per generation. Approximately 50% of NF1 cases are the result of new mutations. In 1987 the gene was mapped to chromosome 17q by researchers in Salt Lake City, and it was isolated and cloned 3 years later. It is a large gene, spanning approximately 350 kb of DNA. Its large size, which presents a sizable "target" for mutation, may help to account for the high mutation rate. The gene encodes a 13-kb mRNA transcript, and the gene product, termed neurofibromin, acts as a tumor suppressor (see Chapter 11).

A mutation in the NF1 gene occurring during embryonic development will affect only some cells of the individual, resulting in somatic mosaicism. In this case, disease features may be confined to only one part of the body (segmental neurofibromatosis). Neurofibromatosis type 2 (NF2) is much rarer than NF1 and involves café-au-lait spots and bilateral acoustic neuromas (tumors affecting the eighth cranial nerve). It does not, however, involve true neurofibromas. The term "neurofibromatosis type 2" is thus a misnomer. The NF2 gene has been mapped to chromosome 22 and subsequently cloned.

Mild cases of neurofibromatosis may involve very little clinical management. However, surgery may be required if malignancies develop or if benign tumors interfere with normal function. Scoliosis, tibial pseudarthrosis, and/or tibial bowing, seen in fewer than 5% of cases, may require orthopedic management. Hypertension may develop and is often secondary to a pheochromocytoma or a stenosis (narrowing) of the renal artery. The most common clinical problems in children are learning disabilities, short stature, and optic gliomas (which can lead to visual loss). Close follow-up can help to detect these problems and minimize their effects.

ferent loci in different families. The causation of the same disease phenotype by mutations at distinct loci is termed **locus heterogeneity** (compare with allelic heterogeneity, discussed previously). A good example is adult polycystic kidney disease (APKD), an autosomal dominant disorder in which a progressive accumulation of renal cysts is seen. Patients may also develop liver cysts, hypertension, cerebral aneurysms, and cardiac valvular defects. Occurring in about 1/1,000 Caucasians, this disorder is responsible for 8% to 10% of end-stage renal disease in North America. APKD can be caused by mutations in genes on either chromosome 16 (PKD1) or chromosome 4 (PKD2).* Both of these genes encode membrane-

*There is also evidence for a third, as yet unidentified, gene for APKD.

spanning glycoproteins that interact with one another and may be involved in cellular signaling (when this signaling goes awry, it is thought that cellular growth regulation is compromised, resulting in cyst formation). In one family, the disease may be caused by a PKD1 mutation, whereas in another family it may be caused by a PKD2 mutation. The disease states produced by mutations in these two genes may be clinically indistinguishable.

Osteogenesis imperfecta provides a second example of locus heterogeneity. Recall from Chapter 2 that the subunits of the procollagen triple helix are encoded by two genes, one on chromosome 17 and the other on chromosome 7 (Fig. 4-18). A mutation occurring in either of these genes can alter the normal structure of the triple helix, resulting ultimately in osteogenesis

CLINICAL COMMENTARY 4-5
MARFAN SYNDROME, AN EXAMPLE OF PLEIOTROPY

Marfan syndrome (Fig. 4-17) is an autosomal dominant condition seen in approximately 1/10,000 North Americans. It is characterized by defects in three major systems: the ocular, skeletal, and cardiovascular. The ocular defects include myopia, present in most Marfan patients, and detached lens (ectopia lentis), observed in about half of Marfan patients. The skeletal defects include dolichostenomelia (unusually long and slender limbs), pectus excavatum ("hollow chest"), pectus carinatum ("pigeon chest"), scoliosis, and arachnodactyly (literally "spider fingers," denoting the characteristically long, slender fingers). Marfan patients also typically exhibit joint hypermobility. The most life-threatening defects are those of the cardiovascular system. Most Marfan patients develop a prolapse of the mitral valve, a condition in which the cusps of the mitral valve protrude upward into the left atrium during systole. This can result in mitral regurgitation (leakage of blood

FIG. 4-17 **A**, A young man with Marfan syndrome, showing characteristically long limbs and narrow face. **B**, Arachnodactyly in an 8-year-old girl with Marfan syndrome.

back into the left atrium from the left ventricle). Mitral valve prolapse, however, is seen in 2% to 5% of the general population and is often of little consequence. Much more serious is dilatation (widening) of the ascending aorta, which is seen in 90% of Marfan patients. As dilatation increases, the aorta becomes susceptible to dissection or rupture, particularly when cardiac output is high (as in heavy exercise or pregnancy). As the aorta widens, the left ventricle enlarges, and cardiomyopathy (damage to the heart muscle) ensues. The end result is congestive heart failure, a frequent cause of death among Marfan patients.

All of these defects involve excessively "stretchy" connective tissue. The role of connective tissue is apparent for defects such as aortic dilatation and detached lens. Its role in skeletal defects is mediated by the periosteum, the connective tissue that covers bone and provides an oppositional force in normal bone growth. When the periosteum is more elastic than it should be, overgrowth of bone occurs, resulting in skeletal defects.

What is the basis of the connective tissue disorder? Answers are being provided by the discovery that Marfan patients have mutations of the chromosome 15 gene encoding fibrillin, a connective tissue protein. Fibrillin, a major component of microfibrils, is found in the aorta, the suspensory ligament of the lens, and the periosteum. The location of the gene product and its role as a component of connective tissue nicely explain the pleiotropic effects causing disturbances in the eye, the skeleton, and the cardiovascular system.

More than 100 different fibrillin mutations have been identified in Marfan syndrome patients. Most of these are missense mutations, but frameshifts and nonsense mutations producing a truncated fibrillin protein are also seen. In many cases, the missense mutations produce a more severe disease phenotype because of a dominant negative effect (i.e., the abnormal fibrillin proteins bind to and disable many of the normal fibrillin proteins produced by the normal allele in a heterozygote). A severe neonatal form of the disease is produced by mutations in exons 24 to 32. At least one Marfan syndrome compound heterozygote has been reported. This infant, who inherited a disease-causing allele from each of its affected heterozygous parents, had severe congestive heart failure and died of cardiac arrest at the age of 4 months.

Mutations in a second fibrillin gene, located on chromosome 5, cause a disease called "congenital contractural arachnodactyly." This condition shares many of the skeletal features of Marfan syndrome but does not involve cardiac or ocular defects.

Treatment for Marfan syndrome includes regular ophthalmological examinations and, for individuals with aortic dilatation, the avoidance of heavy exercise and contact sports. In addition, β-adrenergic blockers, such as propranolol, can be administered to decrease the strength and abruptness of heart contractions. This reduces stress on the aorta. In some cases, the aorta and aortic valve are surgically replaced with a synthetic tube and artificial valve.

A number of historical figures are thought to have possibly had Marfan syndrome, including Niccolo Paganini, the violinist, and Sergei Rachmaninoff, the composer and pianist. Most controversial is the proposal that Abraham Lincoln may have had Marfan syndrome. He had skeletal features consistent with the disorder, and examination of his medical records has shown that he may well have had aortic dilatation. Some have suggested that he was in congestive heart failure at the time of his death and that, had he not been assassinated, he still would not have survived his second term of office. Lincoln has no living descendants that could be evaluated for Marfan syndrome. However, samples of his blood, bone, and hair have been preserved. Once the specific mutations for Marfan syndrome are better characterized, it may be possible, using PCR, to amplify DNA from these specimens. DNA sequencing could then be used to determine whether indeed Lincoln had Marfan syndrome.

While this may seem like a silly exercise to some, it should be pointed out that genetic diseases such as Marfan syndrome are frequently viewed as serious impediments to success. To find that one of the greatest Presidents in United States history had this disorder would be an eloquent reply.

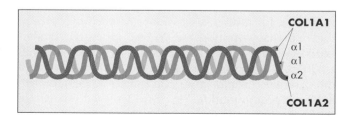

FIG. 4-18 Structure of the triple helix type 1 collagen protein. The two α1 chains are encoded by a gene on chromosome 17, and the α2 chain is encoded by a gene on chromosome 7.

imperfecta. Table 4-2 lists some additional examples of diseases in which there is locus heterogeneity.

▼ A disease that can be caused by mutations at different loci in different families is said to exhibit locus heterogeneity. ▲

Genomic Imprinting

Mendel's experimental work with garden peas established that the phenotype is the same whether a given

TABLE 4-2   Some Examples of Diseases in Which There Is Locus Heterogeneity

Disease	Description	Chromosomes on which known loci are located
Retinitis pigmentosa	Progressive retinopathy and loss of vision (see Chapter 8)	More than 20 chromosome regions identified
Osteogenesis imperfecta	Brittle bone disease	7, 17
Charcot-Marie-Tooth disease	Peripheral neuropathy	1, 5, 8, 11, 17, X
Familial Alzheimer disease	Progressive dementia	1, 14, 19, 21
Familial melanoma	Autosomal dominant melanoma (skin cancer)	1, 9
Hereditary nonpolyposis colorectal cancer	Autosomal dominant colorectal cancer	2p, 2q, 3, 7
Autosomal dominant breast cancer	Predisposition to early-onset breast and ovarian cancer (chromosome 17 form)	13, 17
Tuberous sclerosis	Seizures, facial angiofibromas, hypopigmented macules, mental retardation	9, 16
Adult polycystic kidney disease	Accumulation of renal cysts leading to kidney failure	4, 16

allele is inherited from the mother or the father. Indeed, this principle has been part of the central dogma of genetics. Recently, however, it has become increasingly apparent that this principle does not always hold. A striking example is provided by a deletion of 3 to 4 Mb on the long arm of chromosome 15. When this deletion is inherited from the father, the offspring manifest a disease known as Prader-Willi syndrome. The disease phenotype includes short stature, hypotonia (poor muscle tone), small hands and feet, obesity, mild to moderate mental retardation, and hypogonadism (Fig. 4-19, *A*). When the deletion is inherited from the mother, the offspring develop Angelman syndrome, which is characterized by severe mental retardation, seizures, and an ataxic gait (Fig. 4-19, *B*). Both diseases are seen in about 1/15,000 individuals, and in both about 70% of cases are caused by chromosome deletions. In most cases, the deletions that cause Prader-Willi and Angelman syndromes are microscopically indistinguishable. **www**

What could cause these differences? The 3 to 4 Mb portion of chromosome 15 that is deleted in both syndromes is known as the "critical region." Within this region several genes are transcriptionally active only on the chromosome inherited from the father, and they are inactive on the chromosome inherited from the mother. Similarly, other genes are transcriptionally active only on the chromosome inherited from the mother and inactive on the chromosome inherited from the father. Thus, there are several genes in the critical region that are active on only one chromosome (Fig. 4-19, *C*). If the single active copy of one of these genes is lost through a chromosome deletion, then no gene product is produced at all, and disease results. The differential activa-

tion of genes, depending on the parent from which they are inherited, is known as **genomic imprinting**.

Molecular analysis using many of the tools and techniques outlined in Chapter 3 (RFLPs, microsatellite polymorphisms, cloning, and DNA sequencing) has identified several specific genes in the critical region of chromosome 15. The gene that causes Angelman syndrome encodes a protein involved in ubiquitin-mediated protein degradation during brain development (consistent with the mental retardation and ataxia observed in this disorder). This gene is active only on the chromosome inherited from the mother; thus, a maternally inherited deletion removes the single active copy of this gene. Several genes appear to be involved in Prader-Willi syndrome, and they are active only on the chromosome inherited from the father. One of these genes, *SNRPN*, encodes a small nuclear riboprotein that is expressed in the brain.

Several mechanisms in addition to chromosome deletions can cause Prader-Willi and Angelman syndrome. One of these is uniparental disomy, a condition in which the individual inherits two copies of a chromosome from one parent and none from the other (see Chapter 6 for further discussion). When two copies of the maternal chromosome 15 are inherited, Prader-Willi syndrome results because no active paternal genes are present in the critical region. Conversely, disomy of the paternal chromosome 15 produces Angelman syndrome. Point mutations in the identified Angelman syndrome gene can also produce disease. Finally, about 1% of Prader-Willi syndrome cases result from a small deletion of the region that contains an **imprinting center** on chromosome 15. This is the DNA sequence

FIG. 4-19   Illustration of the effect of imprinting on chromosome 15 deletions. **A,** Inheritance of the deletion from the father produces Prader-Willi syndrome (note the inverted V-shaped upper lip, small hands, and truncal obesity). **B,** Inheritance of the deletion from the mother produces Angelman syndrome (note the characteristic posture).   *Continued.*

that apparently helps to set and reset the imprint itself. Box 4-1 presents clinical issues of Prader-Willi syndrome from the perspective of a patient's family.

A second example of imprinting in the human is given by Beckwith-Wiedemann syndrome, a disorder that involves large size for gestational age, large tongue, omphalocele (an abdominal wall defect), and a predisposition to Wilms tumor, a kidney cancer (see Chapter 14). Like Angelman syndrome, a minority of Beckwith-Wiedemann syndrome cases are caused by the inheri-

tance of two copies of a chromosome from the father and no copy of the chromosome from the mother (uniparental disomy, in this case affecting chromosome 11). Some genes on chromosome 11 are imprinted, including insulin-like growth factor 2 *(IGF2)*. This gene is imprinted on the maternally derived chromosome and active only on the paternal chromosome. When two copies of the paternal chromosome are inherited, the active *IGF2* gene is present in double dose. Two active copies can also result from a loss of the maternal imprint,

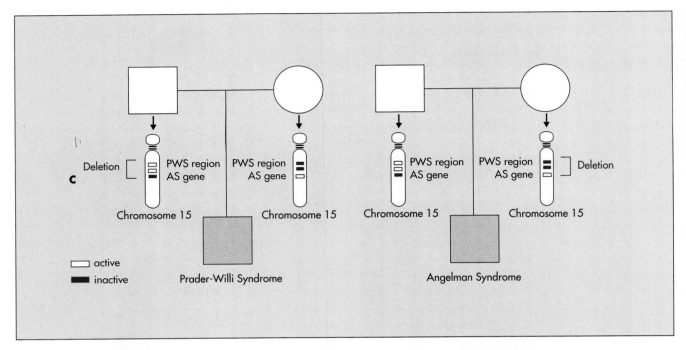

FIG. 4-19, cont'd   C, Pedigrees illustrate the inheritance pattern of this deletion and the activation status of genes in the critical region.

activating the maternally inherited gene. It is thought that increased levels of the growth factor gene lead to the overgrowth features of Beckwith-Wiedemann syndrome and to Wilms tumor. In contrast to Prader-Willi and Angelman syndromes, which are produced by a *missing* gene product, Beckwith-Wiedemann syndrome is caused, at least in part, by *over-expression* of a gene product. **www**

The molecular basis of imprinting remains unclear. In the 16 genes now known to be imprinted in mice or humans, there is a consistent association between methylation and transcriptional inactivation. The attachment of methyl groups to DNA may inhibit the binding of proteins that promote transcription. It is not yet known, however, whether methylation is the primary imprinting signal or whether it serves merely to maintain the imprinting signal once it is established by other mechanisms (e.g., alteration in chromatin structure).

▼ **Some disease genes may be expressed differently when inherited from one sex versus the other. This is genomic imprinting. It is associated with, and possibly caused by, methylation of DNA.** ▲

Anticipation and Repeat Expansion

Since the early part of the twentieth century, it has been observed that some genetic diseases seem to display an earlier age of onset and/or more severe expression in the more recent generations of a pedigree. This pattern was termed **anticipation**, and it has been the subject of considerable controversy and speculation. Many researchers believed that it was an artifact of better observation and clinical diagnosis in more recent times: a disorder that previously may have been undiagnosed until age 60 might now be diagnosed at age 40 simply because of better diagnostic tools. Others, however, believed that anticipation could be a real biological phenomenon, although evidence for the actual mechanism remained elusive.

Recently, molecular genetics has provided good evidence that anticipation does in fact have a biological basis. This has come in part from studies of myotonic dystrophy, an autosomal dominant disease that involves progressive muscle deterioration (Fig. 4-20). Seen in approximately one in 8,000 individuals, myotonic dystrophy is the most common muscular dystrophy that affects adults. In addition to affecting skeletal muscles, this disorder produces cardiac arrhythmias (abnormal heart rhythms), testicular atrophy, and cataracts. The disease-causing gene, which has been mapped to chromosome 19 and subsequently cloned, encodes a protein kinase. **www**

Analysis of the gene has produced some interesting results. The disease mutation is an expanded CTG trinucleotide repeat (see Chapter 3) that lies in the 3′ untrans-

BOX 4-1

A MOTHER'S PERSPECTIVE OF PRADER-WILLI SYNDROME

We have a 3½-year-old son, John, who has Prader-Willi syndrome. Months before John was born, we were concerned about his well-being because he wasn't as active in utero compared to his older siblings. At the first sight of John, the doctors suspected that things "weren't quite right." John opened his eyes but made no other movements. He couldn't adequately suck, required supplemental oxygen, and he was "puffy." He remained hospitalized for nearly 3 weeks. The following 3 years were filled with visits to occupational therapists, physical therapists, home health care aids, early childhood service providers, and speech therapists.

From the day John was born, we searched diligently for a diagnosis. His father insisted that we need only love and help him. However, I wanted specifics on how to help him and knowledge from other parents who might have traveled a similar path. After extensive testing and three "chromosome checks," John was diagnosed with Prader-Willi syndrome. We were glad to be provided with some direction and decided we would deal with further challenges as they came upon us. We used what we learned about PWS to get started helping John reach his potential. We were not going to worry about all the potential problems John could have because of his PWS.

John attends a special education preschool at the local elementary school 4 days a week. The bus ride takes about 5 minutes, but is long enough for John to very much anticipate it each day. If he is ill, we have to tell him that the bus is broken. He attends a Sunday school class with children of a similar age. He misbehaves by saying "hi" and "bye" very loudly to each participant. He receives speech therapy once a week, and I spend at least 30 minutes each day with John, practicing speech, cognitive, and play skills. John has not yet experienced the feeding difficulties commonly observed in children with PWS. However, excessive eating and weight gain are more common in older children with PWS.

Compared with other 3-year-old children, John struggles with speech and motor developmental milestones. Yet, he loves to play with his siblings and their friends and to look at books. In fact, we struggle to keep people from doing too many things for John because they might prevent him from attaining the same goal independently. We feel very privileged to have him in our family.

Our expectations for John are that he achieves everything that is possible for him plus a little bit more. Indeed, some of his care providers are already impressed with his capabilities. I hope that his success is partly because of the care and support that we have given to him. Moreover, I hope that John continues to overcome the daily challenges that face him.

FIG. 4-20 A three-generation family affected with myotonic dystrophy. The degree of severity increases in each generation. The grandmother (right) is only slightly affected, but the mother (left) has a characteristic narrow face and somewhat limited facial expression. The baby is more severely affected and has the facial features of children with neonatal-onset myotonic dystrophy, including an open, triangle-shaped mouth. The infant has more than 1000 copies of the trinucleotide repeat, whereas the mother and grandmother each have approximately 100 repeats.

lated portion of the gene (i.e., a region transcribed into mRNA but not translated into protein). The *number* of these repeats is strongly correlated with severity of the disease. Unaffected individuals typically have 5 to 30 copies of the repeat. Those with 50 to 100 copies of the repeat may be mildly affected or have no symptoms. Those with full-blown myotonic dystrophy may have anywhere from 100 to several thousand copies of the repeat sequence. The number of repeats often increases with succeeding generations: a mildly affected parent with 80 repeats may produce a severely affected offspring with more than 1,000 repeats (Fig. 4-21). Many families have now been documented in which the number of

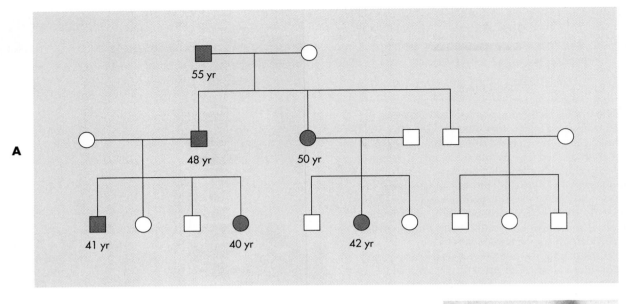

FIG. 4-21 **A,** Myotonic dystrophy pedigree illustrating anticipation. In this case, the age of onset for family members affected with an autosomal dominant disease is lower in more recent generations. **B,** An autoradiogram from a Southern blot analysis of the myotonic dystrophy gene in three individuals. Individual A is homozygous for a four- to five-repeat allele and is normal. Individual B has one normal allele and one disease allele of 175 repeats; this individual has myotonic dystrophy. Individual C is also affected with myotonic dystrophy and has one normal allele and a disease-causing allele of approximately 900 repeats.

(*B,* Courtesy Dr. Kenneth Ward and Dr. Elaine Lyon, University of Utah Health Sciences Center.)

repeats increases through successive generations, accompanied by increasing severity of the disorder. There is thus strong evidence that expansion of this trinucleotide repeat is the cause of anticipation in myotonic dystrophy.

Much remains to be discovered about this phenomenon. How does repeat expansion occur? How does it affect the gene product? Why does the severe congenital form of myotonic dystrophy arise only when the disease gene is inherited from the mother? It is especially mystifying that the repeated sequence lies *outside* of the translated portion of the gene. It is possible that mRNA stability is affected by the 3' mutation. There is also

TABLE 4-3   Diseases Associated With Trinucleotide Repeat Expansions

Disease	Description	Repeat sequence	Normal and abnormal range	Parent in which expansion usually occurs	Location of expansion
Category 1					
Huntington disease	Loss of motor control, dementia, affective disorder	CAG	6 to 34; 36 to 100 or more	More often through father	Exon
Spinal and bulbar muscular atrophy	Adult-onset motor-neuron disease associated with androgen insensitivity	CAG	11 to 34; 40 to 62	More often through father	Exon
Spinocerebellar ataxia type 1	Progressive ataxia, dysarthria, dysmetria	CAG	6 to 39; 41 to 81	More often through father	Exon
Spinocerebellar ataxia type 2	Progressive ataxia, dysarthria	CAG	15 to 29; 35 to 59		Exon
Spinocerebellar ataxia type 3 (Machado-Joseph disease)	Dystonia, distal muscular atrophy, ataxia, external ophthalmoplegia	CAG	13 to 36; 68 to 79	More often through father	Exon
Spinocerebellar ataxia type 6	Progressive ataxia, dysarthria, nystagmus	CAG	4 to 16; 21 to 27		Exon
Dentatorubral-pallidoluysian atrophy/Haw River syndrome	Cerebellar atrophy, ataxia, myoclonic epilepsy, choreoathetosis, dementia	CAG	7 to 25; 49 to 88	More often through father	Exon
Category 2					
Myotonic dystrophy	Muscle loss, cardiac arrhythmia, cataracts, frontal balding	CTG	5 to 37; 100 to several thousand	Either parent, but expansion to congenital form through mother	3' Untranslated region
Friedreich's ataxia	Progressive limb ataxia, dysarthria, hypertrophic cardiomyopathy, pyramidal weakness in legs	GAA	7 to 22; 200 to 900 or more	Disorder is autosomal recessive, so disease alleles are inherited from both parents	Intron
Fragile X syndrome (FRAXA)	Mental retardation, large ears and jaws, macro-orchidism in males	CGG	6 to 52; 200 to 2,000 or more	Exclusively through mother	5' Untranslated region
Fragile site FRAXE	Mild mental retardation	GCC	6 to 35; 200 or more	More often through mother	Unknown

increasing evidence that other genes located just 3' of the myotonic dystrophy gene are affected by the trinucleotide expansion, and this may account for some of the variability in phenotypic expression of the disease.

As discussed in Clinical Commentary 4-2, trinucleotide repeat expansion is also associated with anticipation in Huntington disease. It has also been observed in the fragile X syndrome, a leading genetic cause of men-tal retardation to be discussed in Chapter 5. Trinucleotide repeat expansions have now been identified as the cause of more than a dozen genetic diseases (Table 4-3), and anticipation is observed in most of these diseases.

As more repeat expansion diseases have been identified, some general patterns have begun to emerge. These diseases can be grouped into two categories, as indicated in Table 4-3. The first category consists of neurological diseases, such as Huntington disease and the spinocerebellar ataxias, that are caused by a CAG repeat expansion in a protein-coding portion of the gene. The repeats generally expand in number from a normal range of 10 to 35 to a disease-causing range of approximately 50 to 100. Expansions tend to be larger when transmitted through the father than through the mother, and the mutations have a gain-of-function effect. The second group consists of phenotypically more diverse diseases and includes fragile X syndrome, myotonic dystrophy, and Friedreich ataxia (the latter is the only recessive disease known to be caused by trinucleotide expansions). The repeat expansions are much larger than in the first category: the normal range is generally 5 to 50 trinucleotides, but the disease-causing range varies from 200 to several thousand trinucleotides. The repeats are located outside the protein-coding regions of the gene in all three of these disorders, and the mutations have a loss-of-function effect in each disease. Repeat expansions are larger when they are transmitted through the mother. Anticipation is seen in nearly all of the diseases in both categories.

Recently a new type of expansion has been seen in which a 12-base repeat expands in size from two to three repeats to approximately 60 repeats to cause myoclonus epilepsy, an autosomal recessive disorder. The repeat unit is located in the 5' untranslated portion of the gene, and the expansion has a loss-of-function effect. Repeat expansion diseases are now the focus of intense investigation, and they promise to reveal further insights into the molecular basis of genetic disease.

> ▼ Anticipation refers to progressively earlier or more severe expression of a disease in more recent times. Expansion of DNA repeats has been shown to cause anticipation in some genetic diseases. These diseases can be divided into two major categories, depending on the size of the expansion, the location of the repeat, the phenotypic consequences of the expansion, the effect of the mutation, and the parent in which large expansions typically occur. ▲

CONSANGUINITY IN HUMAN POPULATIONS

While relatively rare in Western populations, consanguinity is common in many populations of the world. For example, first-cousin unions are seen in 20% to 50% of marriages in many countries of the Mideast, and uncle-niece and first-cousin marriages are common in some parts of India. Because relatives more often share disease genes inherited from a common ancestor, consanguineous unions are more likely to produce offspring affected by autosomal recessive disorders. It is possible to quantify the proportion of genes shared by a pair of relatives by estimating the **coefficient of relationship** (Box 4-2). Estimation of this quantity shows, for example, that siblings share $1/2$ of their genes on average, first cousins share $1/8$, first cousins once removed share $1/16$, second cousins share $1/32$, and so on.*

Consanguinity and the Frequency of Recessive Diseases

Recall that about 1 in 25 Caucasians is a heterozygous carrier of the cystic fibrosis gene. A man who carries this gene thus has a 1 in 25 chance of meeting another carrier if he mates with somebody in the general population. He only triples his chance of meeting another carrier when he mates with a first cousin, who has a $1/8$ chance of carrying the same gene. In contrast, a carrier of a relatively rare recessive disease, such as classical galactosemia (a metabolic disorder discussed in Chapter 7), has only a 1/170 chance of meeting another carrier in the general population. Because he shares $1/8$ of his genes with his first cousin, the chance that his first cousin also has the galactosemia gene is still $1/8$. With this rarer disease, a carrier is 21 times more likely to mate with another carrier in a first-cousin marriage than in a marriage with an unrelated individual. This illustrates an important principle: the rarer the recessive disease, the more likely that the parents of the case are consanguineous.

This principle has been substantiated empirically. It has been estimated that only about 5% of cases of PKU, in which the carrier frequency is about 1/50 in Caucasians, are due to consanguineous matings. However, Wilson disease (see Chapter 7) is much rarer, with an estimated carrier frequency between 1/110 and 1/160. Here, approximately 50% of cases are the result of consanguineous matings.

> ▼ Consanguinity increases the chance that a mating couple will both carry the same disease gene. It is seen more frequently in pedigrees involving rare recessive diseases than in those involving common recessive diseases. ▲

Health Consequences of Consanguinity

It has been estimated that each person carries the equivalent of one to five recessive genes that would be lethal to offspring if matched with another copy of the gene (i.e., homozygosity). It would therefore be expected that matings between relatives would more often produce offspring with genetic diseases. In fact, most empirical

---

*First cousins are the offspring of two siblings and thus share a set of grandparents. A first cousin once removed is the offspring of one's first cousin. Second cousins are the offspring of two different first cousins and thus share a set of great-grandparents.

BOX 4-2
MEASUREMENT OF CONSANGUINITY: THE COEFFICIENT OF RELATIONSHIP

To determine the possible consequences of a consanguineous mating, it is useful to know what proportion of genes are shared by two related individuals. The **coefficient of relationship** is a measure of this proportion. Clearly, individuals who are more closely related must share a greater proportion of their genes. To begin with a simple example, an individual receives half of his or her genes from each parent. Thus, the coefficient of relationship between a parent and offspring is $1/2$. This also means that the *probability* that the parent and offspring share a given gene (for example, a disease allele) is $1/2$.

To continue with a more complex example, suppose that a man is known to be a heterozygous carrier for galactosemia, a relatively rare autosomal recessive metabolic disorder. If he mates with his first cousin, what is the probability that she also carries this disease gene? We know that this probability must be higher than that of the general population, because first cousins share one set of grandparents. There is thus a possibility that the grandparent who transmitted the galactosemia gene to the known carrier also transmitted it to the carrier's cousin. The coefficient of relationship specifies this probability. A pedigree for a first-cousin mating is shown in Fig. 4-22, A. The carrier is labeled A, and his cousin is labeled E. Since we are interested only in the family members who are related to both the man and his cousin, the pedigree is condensed in Fig. 4-22, B, to include only the individuals who form a "path" between the man and his cousin.

To estimate the coefficient of relationship, we begin with the carrier and ascend the pedigree. We know that there is

a probability of $1/2$ that the known carrier inherited the gene from the parent in the path, labeled B. There is also a probability of $1/2$ that he inherited the gene from his other parent, who is not related to his cousin and is thus not included in the diagram. By similar reasoning, the probability that individual B inherited the disease gene from his parent, individual C, is also $1/2$. The probability that individual C in turn passed on the disease gene to his offspring, D, is $1/2$, and the probability that D passed the disease gene to E is also $1/2$. Thus, for E to share a disease gene with A, each of these four events must have taken place. The multiplication rule dictates that, to find the probability that all four events have taken place, we take the product of all four probabilities. Since each of these probabilities is $1/2$, this gives $(1/2)^4 = 1/16$.

If individuals A and E shared only one grandparent, the coefficient of relationship would be $1/16$. But, as with most first cousins, they share a common grandfather *and* grandmother. Thus, there are two paths through which the disease gene could have passed. To obtain the probability that the gene passed through the second path, we use the same procedure as in the previous paragraph and obtain a probability of $1/16$. Now we need to estimate the probability that the gene went through either the first path *or* the second (i.e., through one grandparent or the other). The addition rule states that we can add these two probabilities together to get the overall probability that A and E share a disease gene: $1/16 + 1/16 = 1/8$. The probability that the carrier's cousin shares his disease allele, as a result of their descent from a common set of grandparents, is

FIG. 4-22   A, Pedigree for a first-cousin mating. **B,** This pedigree is condensed to show only those individuals in the pedigree who are related to both of the first cousins.

Continued

BOX 4-2—cont'd

MEASUREMENT OF CONSANGUINITY: THE COEFFICIENT OF RELATIONSHIP

thus $1/8$. This is the coefficient of relationship for first cousins.*

It should be recognized that individual E could also inherit a disease allele from an ancestor not included in either of these paths. However, for disease alleles, which are

---

*A related quantity, frequently used in population genetics, is the **inbreeding coefficient.** This coefficient is the probability that an individual is homozygous at a locus as a result of consanguinity in his or her parents. For a given type of mating, the inbreeding coefficient of an individual always equals the parents' coefficient of relationship multiplied by one half (e.g., the inbreeding coefficient for the offspring of a first-cousin mating is $1/16$).

relatively rare in populations, this probability is small and can usually be disregarded.

The rules for calculating the coefficient of relationship can be summarized as follows:

1. Each individual can appear in a route only once.
2. Always begin with one individual, proceed *up* the pedigree to the common ancestor, then *down* the pedigree to the other individual.
3. The coefficient of relationship for one route is given by $(1/2)^{n-1}$, where n is the number of individuals in the route.
4. If there are multiple routes (i.e., multiple common ancestors), the probabilities estimated for each route are added together.

TABLE 4-4 Mortality Levels Among Cousin and Unrelated Control Marriages in Selected Human Populations

Population	Mortality type	1.0 Cousin %	1.0 Cousin N	1.5 Cousin* %	1.5 Cousin* N	2.0 Cousin %	2.0 Cousin N	Unrelated %	Unrelated N
Amish (Old Order)	Prereproductive	14.4	1,218†	—	—	13.3	6,064	8.2	17,200
Bombay, India	Perinatal	4.8	3,309	2.8	176	0	30	2.8	35,620
France (Loir-et-Cher)	Prereproductive	17.7	282	6.7	105	11.7	240	8.6	1,117
Fukuoka, Japan	0 to 6 years	10.0	3,442	8.3	1,048	9.2	1,066	6.4	5,224
Hirado, Japan	Prereproductive	18.9	2,301	15.3	764	14.7	1,209	14.3	28,569
Kerala, India	Prereproductive	18.6	391	—	—	11.8	34	8.7	770
Punjab, Pakistan	Prereproductive	22.1	3,532	22.9	1,114	20.1	57	16.4	4,731
Sweden	Prereproductive	14.1	185	13.7	227	11.4	79	8.6	625
Utah Mormons	Prereproductive	22.4	1,048	15.3	517	12.2	1,129	13.2	302,454

Modified from Jorde LB (1991) In Delbecco R (ed.) Encyclopedia of Human Biology. Vol 4. Academic Press, San Diego.
*First cousins once removed.
†Includes 1.5 cousins.

studies show that mortality rates among the offspring of first-cousin marriages are substantially greater than those of the general population (Table 4-4). Similarly, the prevalence of genetic disease is roughly twice as high among the offspring of first-cousin marriages as among the offspring of unrelated individuals. First-cousin marriages are illegal in most states of the United States. Marriages between closer relatives (except double first cousins, who share both sets of grandparents) are prohibited throughout the United States.

Very few data exist for matings beween first-degree relatives (defined as **incest**). The limited data indicate that the proportion of abnormal offspring produced by

incestuous matings is very high: between $1/4$ and $1/2$. Mental retardation is particularly common among these offspring. Because of small sample sizes in these studies, it is difficult to separate the effects of genetics and substandard environment. It is likely that the problems experienced by the offspring of incestuous matings are due to both genetic and environmental influences.

▼ At the population level, consanguinity increases the frequency of genetic disease and mortality. The closer the degree of consanguinity, the greater the increase. ▲

STUDY QUESTIONS

1. Using protein electrophoresis, 100 members of a population have been studied to determine whether they carry genes for normal hemoglobin *(HbA)* or sickle hemoglobin *(HbS)*. The following genotypes were observed:
   HbA/HbA   88
   HbA/HbS   10
   Hbs/Hbs   2
   What are the gene frequencies of *HbA* and *HbS*? What are the observed genotype frequencies? Assuming Hardy-Weinberg proportions, what are the *expected* genotype frequencies?

2. Approximately 1/10,000 Caucasians is born with PKU. What is the frequency of the disease gene? What is the frequency of heterozygous carriers in the population?

3. A man who has achondroplasia marries a phenotypically normal woman. If they have four children, what is the probability that *none* of them will be affected with this disorder? What is the probability that *all* of them will be affected?

4. The estimated penetrance for familial retinoblastoma is approximately 90%. If a man has had familial retinoblastoma and mates with a woman who does not have a retinoblastoma mutation, what is the risk that their offspring will develop retinoblastoma?

5. A 30-year-old woman had a sister who died from infantile Tay-Sachs disease, an autosomal recessive disorder that is fatal by age 6. What is the probability that this woman is a heterozygous carrier of the Tay-Sachs gene?

6. Consider a woman who is a known heterozygous carrier of a mutation that causes PKU (autosomal recessive). What is the probability that her two grandchildren, who are first cousins, are *both* heterozygous carriers of this PKU-causing allele?

7. It is possible to create a zygote from two copies of the maternal genome alone. In amphibians, the zygote will then develop and mature into an adult without fertilization by a sperm cell (this process is known as parthenogenesis). The same experiment has been attempted in mice, but it always results in early prenatal death. Explain this.

8. Two mating individuals, labeled A and B in Fig. 4-23, share a single great-grandparent. What is their coefficient of relationship? Suppose that one member of this couple is a heterozygous carrier for PKU. What is the probability that this couple will produce a child affected with PKU?

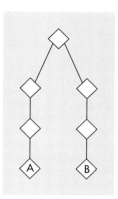

FIG. 4-23   Diagram for study question 8.

9. A suspect in a rape case has been typed for three VNTR systems. His alleles match those of the evidentiary sample (semen taken from the rape victim) for each system. He is a heterozygote for the first two systems, and a homozygote for the third. The allele frequencies for system one in the general population are 0.05 and 0.10. For system two, they are 0.07 and 0.02. For system three, the allele frequency in the general population is 0.08. What is the *probability* that a random individual in the general population would match the evidentiary sample?

10. A man implicated in a paternity suit has had his DNA tested to establish whether or not he is the father of a baby. Four microsatellite polymorphisms were tested for him, the mother, and the baby in question. The baby's alleles and his match for all four loci. The frequencies of these alleles in the general population are 0.05, 0.01, 0.01, and 0.02. What is the *probability* that someone else in the general population could be the father of the baby?

SUGGESTED READINGS

Barsh GS (1996) The genetics of pigmentation: from fancy genes to complex traits. Trends Genet. 12:299-305

Bates GP, Mangiarini L, Mahal A, Davies SW (1997) Transgenic models of Huntington's disease. Hum. Molec. Genet. 6:1633-1637

Bernards A, Gusella JF (1994) The importance of genetic mosaicism in human disease. N. Eng. J. Med. 331:1447-1449

Cassidy SB (1997) Prader-Willi syndrome. J. Med. Genet. 34:917-923

Francomano CA (1995) The genetic basis of dwarfism. N. Eng. J. Med. 332:58-59

Germino GG (1997) Autosomal dominant polycystic kidney disease: a two-hit model. Hosp. Practice 32:81-102

Hall JG (1997) Genomic imprinting: nature and clinical relevance. Ann. Rev. Med. 48:35-44

Hamshere MG, Brook JD (1996) Myotonic dystrophy, knockouts, warts and all. Trends Genet. 12:332-334

Harper PS, Harley HG, Reardon W, Shaw DJ (1992) Anticipation in myotonic dystrophy: new light on an old problem. Am. J. Hum. Genet. 51:10-16

Huson SM (1994) Neurofibromatosis 1: a clinical and genetic overview. In: Huson SM, Hughes RAC (eds) The Neurofibromatoses: a Pathogenetic and Clinical Overview. Chapman & Hall Medical, London, pp 160-203

Jorde LB (1997) Inbreeding in human populations. In: Dulbecco R (ed) Encyclopedia of Human Biology. Vol. 5. Academic Press, New York, pp 1-13

Kelsey G, Reik W (1997) Imprint switch mechanism indicated by mutations in Prader-Willi and Angelman syndromes. BioEssays 19:361-365

Phillips JA, Cogan JD (1994) Genetic basis of endocrine disease 6. Molecular basis of familial human growth hormone deficiency. J. Clin. Endocrinol. Metab. 78:11-16

Reddy PS, Housman DE (1997) The complex pathology of trinucleotide repeats. Curr. Opin. Genet. Dev. 9:364-372

Shen MH, Harper PS, Upadhyaya M (1996) Molecular genetics of neurofibromatosis type 1 (NF1). J. Med. Genet. 33:2-17

Spritz RA, Hearing VJ (1994) Genetic disorders of pigmentation. Adv. Hum. Genet. 22:1-45

Tsui L-C, Durie P (1997) Genotype and phenotype in cystic fibrosis. Hosp. Practice 32:115-140

Warren ST (1996) The expanding world of trinucleotide repeats. Science 271:1374-1375

Weinberg RA (1995) The retinoblastoma protein and cell cycle control. Cell 81:323-330

Welsh MJ, Smith AE (1995) Cystic fibrosis. Sci. Amer. 273:52-59

Wilkie AOM (1994) The molecular basis of dominance. J. Med. Genet. 31:89-98

5

Sex-Linked and Mitochondrial Inheritance

The previous chapter dealt with disease genes located on the 22 autosomes. In this chapter we discuss disease genes located in the sex chromosomes and in the mitochondria. The human X chromosome is a large chromosome, containing about 5% of the nuclear genome's DNA (approximately 160 million base pairs, or 160 Mb). More than 500 coding genes have been localized to the X chromosome. Diseases caused by genes on this chromosome are said to be **X-linked**. The great majority of known X-linked diseases are recessive, although there are also a few X-linked dominant diseases. In contrast to the X chromosome, the Y chromosome is quite small (70 Mb) and contains very few known genes. More than a dozen diseases are now known to be caused by mutations in mitochondrial DNA; these are discussed at the end of this chapter.

X INACTIVATION

It has long been known that human females have two X chromosomes while males have only one. It has also been known for most of the twentieth century that the X chromosome contains many important protein-coding genes. Thus, females have two copies of each X-linked gene, while males have only one copy. Yet males and females do not differ in terms of the products (such as enzyme levels) encoded by most of these genes. What could account for this?

In the early 1960s Mary Lyon hypothesized that one X chromosome in each somatic cell of the female is inactivated. This would result in **dosage compensation**, an equalization of X-linked gene products in males and females. The **Lyon hypothesis** stated that X inactivation occurs early in female embryonic development and that the X chromosome contributed by the father is inactivated in some cells, whereas in other cells the X chromosome contributed by the mother is inactivated.

This inactivation process is *random*, so the maternally and paternally derived X chromosomes will each be inactivated in about half of the embryo's cells. Thus, inactivation, like gamete transmission, is analogous to a coin-tossing experiment. Once an X chromosome is inactivated in a cell, it will remain inactive in all descendants of the cell. X inactivation is therefore said to be randomly determined, but *fixed*. As a result of X inactivation, all normal females have two distinct populations of cells: one population has an active paternally derived X chromosome, and the other has an active maternally derived X chromosome (Fig. 5-1 provides a summary of this process). With two populations of cells, females are mosaics (see Chapter 4) for the X chromosome. Males, having only one copy of the X chromosome, are not mosaics but are **hemizygous** for the X chromosome (hemi = "half").

▼ The Lyon hypothesis states that one X chromosome in each cell is randomly inactivated early in the embryonic development of females. This ensures that females, who have two copies of the X chromosome, will produce X-linked gene products in quantities roughly similar to those in males (dosage compensation). ▲

The Lyon hypothesis relied on several pieces of evidence, most of which were derived from animal studies. First, it was known that females are typically mosaics for some X-linked traits while males are not. For example, female mice heterozygous for certain X-linked coat-color genes exhibit a dappled coloring of their fur, whereas male mice do not. A similar example is given by the "calico cat." These female cats have alternating black and orange patches of fur that correspond to two populations of cells: one that contains X chromosomes in which the "orange" allele is active and one containing X chromosomes in which the "black" allele is active.

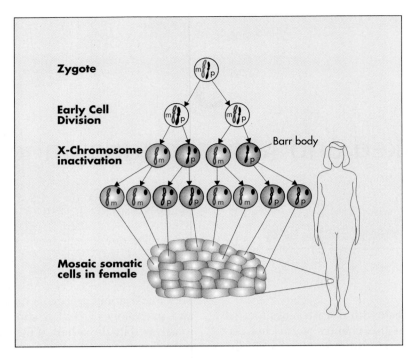

FIG. 5-1   The X inactivation process. The maternal (m) and paternal (p) X chromosomes are both active in the zygote and in early embryonic cells. X inactivation then takes place, resulting in cells having *either* an active paternal X or an active maternal X. Females are thus X chromosome mosaics, as shown in the tissue sample at the bottom of the figure.

Male cats of this breed do not exhibit alternating colors. A final example, seen in humans, is X-linked ocular albinism. This is an X-linked recessive condition characterized by a lack of melanin production in the retina and ocular problems such as nystagmus (rapid involuntary eye movements) and decreased visual acuity. Males who inherit the mutation show a uniform lack of melanin in their retinas, while female heterozygotes exhibit alternating patches of pigmented and nonpigmented tissue (Color Plate 3 following p. 116).

The Lyon hypothesis was also supported by biochemical evidence. The enzyme glucose-6-phosphate dehydrogenase (G6PD) is encoded by a gene on the X chromosome and is present in equal quantities in males and females (dosage compensation). In females heterozygous for two common G6PD alleles (labeled A and B), some skin cells produced only the A variant of the enzyme and others produced only the B variant. This is further proof of X chromosome mosaicism in females.

Finally, cytogenetic studies in the 1940s had shown that interphase cells of female cats often contained a densely staining chromatin mass in their nuclei (Fig. 5-2). These masses were never seen in males. They were termed **Barr bodies**, after Murray Barr, one of the scientists who described them. Barr and his colleague, Ewart Bertram, hypothesized that the Barr body, also

termed **sex chromatin**, represented a highly condensed X chromosome. It is now known that Barr and Bertram were correct, and that the inactive X chromosome is observable as a Barr body in the somatic cells of normal females. Its condensed state reflects the fact that its DNA is replicated later in the S phase than that of other chromosomes.

▼ The Lyon hypothesis is supported by cytogenetic evidence: Barr bodies, which are inactive X chromosomes, are seen only in cells with two or more X chromosomes. It is also supported by biochemical and animal studies that revealed mosaicism of X-linked traits in female heterozygotes. ▲

Further study has largely verified the Lyon hypothesis. mRNA is transcribed from only one X chromosome in each somatic cell of a normal female. The inactivation process takes place within approximately 2 weeks after fertilization, when the embryo consists of approximately several hundred cells. Inactivation is initiated at a single location on the X chromosome long arm (the **X inactivation center**) and then spreads along the chromosome. Although inactivation is random among cells that make up the embryo itself, only the paternally derived X chromosome is inactivated in cells that will become extraembryonic tissue (e.g., the placenta).

FIG. 5-2 A Barr body, which is the inactive X chromosome, is visible as a densely staining chromatin mass in the interphase nucleus of a normal female's somatic cell. DNA-based tools have now supplanted Barr body assays as a means of sex determination.

X inactivation is permanent for all somatic cells in the female, but the inactive X chromosome must become *reactivated* in the female's germ line so that each egg cell will receive one active copy of the chromosome.

An important implication of the Lyon hypothesis is that the number of Barr bodies in somatic cells is always one less than the number of X chromosomes. Normal females have one Barr body in each somatic cell, while normal males have none. Females with Turner syndrome (see Chapter 6), having only one X chromosome, have no Barr bodies. Males with Klinefelter syndrome (two X chromosomes and a Y chromosome) have one Barr body in their somatic cells, and females who have three X chromosomes per cell have two Barr bodies in each somatic cell. This pattern leads to another question: if the extra X chromosomes are inactivated, why aren't people with extra (or missing) X chromosomes phenotypically normal?

The answer to this question is that X inactivation is *incomplete*. Several regions of the X chromosome remain active in all copies. In particular, the tips of the short and long arms of the X chromosome do not undergo inactivation. The tip of the short arm of the X chromosome is highly homologous to the distal short arm of the Y chromosome (see Chapter 6). Other regions that escape inactivation include those that contain the genes for steroid sulfatase, the Xg blood group, and Kallman syndrome (a disorder that causes hypogonadism and an inability to perceive odor). Many of the X-linked genes

that escape inactivation have homologs on the Y chromosome, preserving equal gene dosage in males and females. Having extra (or missing) copies of active portions of the X chromosome must contribute to phenotypic abnormality.

▼ **X inactivation is random, fixed, and incomplete. The latter fact helps to explain why, in spite of X inactivation, most individuals with abnormal numbers of sex chromosomes are not phenotypically normal.** ▲

The X inactivation center contains at least one gene required for inactivation, *XIST*. As expected, *XIST* is transcribed only on the inactive X chromosome, and its 15 to 17 kb mRNA transcripts are detected in normal females but not in normal males. The RNA transcript, however, is not translated into a protein. Instead, it remains in the nucleus and coats the inactive X chromosome. This coating process may act as a signal that leads to other aspects of inactivation, including late replication and condensation of the inactive X chromosome.

Methylation is another feature of the inactive X chromosome. Many CG dinucleotides in the 5′ regions of genes on the inactive X are heavily methylated, and administration of demethylating agents, such as 5-azacytidine, can partially reactivate an inactive X chromosome in vitro. However, methylation does not appear to be involved in spreading the inactivation signal from the inactivation center to the remainder of the X chromosome. It is more likely to be responsible for maintaining the inactivation of a specific X chromosome in a cell and all of its descendants.

▼ **The *XIST* gene is located in the X inactivation center and is required for X inactivation. It encodes an RNA product that coats the inactive X chromosome. X inactivation is also associated with methylation of the inactive X chromosome, a process that may help to ensure the long-term stability of inactivation.** ▲

SEX-LINKED INHERITANCE

Sex-linked genes are those that are located on either the X or the Y chromosomes. Because few genes are known to be located on the human Y chromosome, our attention will be focused on X-linked diseases.

X-Linked Recessive Inheritance

A number of well-known diseases and traits are caused by X-linked recessive genes. These include hemophilia A (Clinical Commentary 5-1), Duchenne muscular dystrophy (see Clinical Commentary 5-2), and red-green color blindness (see Box 5-1). The inheritance patterns and recurrence risks for X-linked recessive diseases differ

CLINICAL COMMENTARY 5-1
HEMOPHILIA A

Hemophilia A, or "classical" hemophilia, affects approximately 1/5 to 1/10,000 males worldwide. It is the most common of the severe bleeding disorders and has been recognized as a familial disorder for centuries. The Talmud states that boys whose brothers or cousins bled to death during circumcision are exempt from the procedure (this may well be the first recorded example of genetic counseling). Queen Victoria carried the gene for hemophilia A, transmitting it to one son and two carrier daughters. They in turn transmitted the gene to many members of the royal families of Germany, Spain, and Russia (Fig. 5-3). One of the males affected by the disease was the Tsarevitch Alexis of Russia, the son of Tsar Nicholas II and Alexandra. Grigori Rasputin, the so-called "mad monk," had an unusual ability to calm the Tsarevitch during bleeding episodes, probably through hypnosis. As a result, he came to have considerable influence in the royal court, and some historians feel that his destabilizing effect helped to bring about the 1917 Bolshevik revolution. (Recently, the Russian royal family was again touched by genetics. Using PCR, autosomal DNA microsatellites and mitochondrial DNA sequences were assayed in the remains of several bodies exhumed near Yekaterinberg, the reputed murder site of the royal family. Analysis of this genetic variation, and comparison with living maternal relatives, showed that the bodies were indeed those of the Russian royal family.)

Hemophilia A is caused by deficient or defective factor VIII, a key component of the clotting cascade. Fibrin formation is affected, resulting in prolonged and often severe bleeding from wounds and hemorrhages in the joints and muscles. Bruising is frequently seen. Hemarthroses (bleeding into the joints) are common in joints such as the ankles, knees, hips, and elbows (Fig. 5-4). They are often painful, and repeated episodes can lead to destruction of the synovium and diminished joint function. Intracranial bleeding is also quite common, and, before the advent of effective treatment for bleeding episodes, it was the leading cause of death among hemophiliacs. It should be emphasized that platelet activity is normal in hemophiliacs, so minor lacerations and abrasions do not usually lead to excessive bleeding. WWW

Hemophilia A varies considerably in its severity, and this variation is correlated directly with factor VIII level. About half of hemophilia A patients fall into the "severe" category, with factor VIII levels that are less than 1% of normal. These individuals experience relatively frequent bleeding episodes, often several per month. Moderate hemophiliacs (1% to 5% of normal factor VIII) generally have bleeding episodes only after mild trauma and typically experience one to several episodes per year. Mild hemophiliacs have 5% to 25% of the normal factor VIII level and usually experience bleeding episodes only after surgery or relatively severe trauma.

Until about 35 years ago, hemophilia A was often fatal by about age 20. Then it became possible to purify factor

FIG. 5-3 A pedigree showing the inheritance of hemophilia A in the European royal families. The first known carrier in the family was Queen Victoria. Note that all of the affected individuals are male.

(Modified from Raven PH, Johnson GB [1992] Biology. Ed 3. Mosby, St. Louis. With permission of McGraw-Hill, NY.)

VIII from donor plasma. Factor VIII is usually administered at the first sign of a bleeding episode and is a highly effective treatment. Prophylactic factor VIII administration in severe hemophiliacs is effective in avoiding loss of joint function. By the 1970s the median age of death of hemophiliacs had increased to 68 years. The major drawback of donor-derived factor VIII was the fact that, because a typical infusion contained plasma products from hundreds or thousands of different donors, it was frequently contaminated by viruses. Consequently, hemophiliacs often suffered from hepatitis B and C. More seriously, human immunodeficiency virus (HIV) can be transmitted in this manner, and it is estimated that half of American hemophiliacs treated with donor-derived factor VIII between 1978 and 1985 became infected with HIV. Acquired immune deficiency syndrome (AIDS) is now the most common cause of death among hemophiliacs, and this disease produced a decrease in the median age of death to 49 years in the 1980s. Donor blood has been screened for HIV since 1985, and heat treatment of donor-derived factor VIII kills HIV and hepatitis B virus, nearly eliminating the threat of infection. Approximately 10% to 15% of hemophiliacs develop "inhibitor" antibodies to factor VIII itself, which further complicates treatment.

The factor VIII gene has been mapped to the distal long arm of the X chromosome and cloned. It contains 186 kb of DNA and 26 exons. The 9-kb mRNA transcript encodes a mature protein consisting of 2,332 amino acids. Cloning and sequencing the gene has led to a number of insights. Patients with nonsense mutations

FIG. 5-4   Hemophilia A. **A,** The enlarged right knee joint of a patient with hemophilia A, demonstrating the effects of hemarthrosis. **B,** Extensive bruising of the left forearm and hand.

(Courtesy Dr. Richard O'Brien, Primary Children's Medical Center, Salt Lake City, Utah.)

Continued

HEMOPHILIA A

usually develop severe hemophilia, while those with missense mutations usually have relatively mild disease. This is expected because nonsense mutations produce a truncated protein, while missense mutations produce a single amino acid substitution without a dominant negative effect. Many of the point mutations take place at CG sequences, which are hot spots for mutation (see Chapter 3). About 45% of severe cases of hemophilia A are caused by a chromosome inversion (see Chapter 6) that disrupts the factor VIII gene. An additional 5% of patients have deletions, which usually lead to relatively severe disease.

Cloning of the factor VIII gene has enabled the production of human factor VIII using recombinant DNA techniques. Extensive clinical testing showed that recombinant factor VIII works as effectively as the donor-derived form, and it was approved for commercial use in 1994. Recombinant factor VIII has, of course, the advantage that there is no possibility of viral contami-

nation. However, as with other forms of factor VIII, recombinant factor VIII does generate inhibitor antibody production in a minority of patients.

There are two other major bleeding disorders, hemophilia B and von Willebrand disease. Hemophilia B, sometimes called "Christmas disease,"* is also an X-linked recessive disorder and is caused by a deficiency of clotting factor IX. It is less severe than hemophilia A, and it is only about one fifth as common. The factor IX gene has also been cloned, and it consists of 34 kb of DNA and eight exons. The disorder can be treated with donor-derived factor IX. von Willebrand disease is an autosomal dominant disorder that is highly variable in expression. While it may affect as many as 1% of Caucasians, it reaches severe expression in fewer than 1/10,000. The von Willebrand factor, which is encoded by a gene on chromosome 12, acts as a carrier protein for factor VIII. In addition, it binds to platelets and damaged blood vessel endothelium, thus promoting the adhesion of platelets to damaged vessel walls.

*"Christmas" was the name of the first reported patient.

---

substantially from those of diseases caused by autosomal genes.

Because females inherit two copies of the X chromosome, they can be homozygous for a disease allele at a given locus, heterozygous, or homozygous for the normal allele at the locus. In females, an X-linked recessive trait behaves much like an autosomal recessive trait. However, only one X chromosome is active in an individual somatic cell. This means that about half of the cells in a heterozygous female will express a disease allele and half of the cells will express the normal allele. Thus, as with autosomal recessive traits, the heterozygote will produce about 50% of the normal level of gene product. Ordinarily this is sufficient for a normal phenotype. The situation is different for males, who are hemizygous for the X chromosome. If a male inherits a recessive disease gene on the X chromosome, he will be affected by the disease because the Y chromosome does not carry a normal allele to compensate for the effects of the disease gene. Hence, in X-linked inheritance, the terms "dominant" and "recessive" really apply only to females.

An X-linked recessive disease with gene frequency q will be seen in a proportion q of males. This is because of the fact that all males having the mutation will manifest the disease. Females, needing two copies of the mutant allele to express the disease, will have a disease frequency of only q^2, as in autosomal recessive diseases. For example, hemophilia A ("classical" hemophilia; see Clinical Commentary 5-1) is seen in about 1/10,000 males ($q = 0.0001$). Affected female homozy-

gotes are almost never seen, since $q^2 = 0.00000001$, or 1/100,000,000. This example shows that, in general, males are more frequently affected with X-linked recessive diseases than females, with this difference becoming more pronounced as the disease becomes rarer.

▼ Because females have two copies of the X chromosome and males have only one (hemizygosity), X-linked recessive diseases are much more common among males than females. ▲

Pedigrees for X-linked recessive diseases display several characteristics that distinguish them from pedigrees for autosomal dominant and recessive diseases (Fig. 5-5). As just mentioned, the trait is seen much more frequently in males than in females. Since a father can transmit only a Y chromosome to his son, X-linked genes are not passed from father to son. In contrast, father-son transmission *can* be observed for autosomal disease genes. An X-linked disease allele can be transmitted through a series of phenotypically normal heterozygous females, causing the appearance of "skipped" generations. The gene is passed from an affected father to all of his daughters, who, as carriers, transmit it to approximately half of their sons, who are affected.

▼ X-linked recessive inheritance is characterized by an absence of father-son transmission, "skipped" generations when genes are passed through female carriers, and a preponderance of affected males. ▲

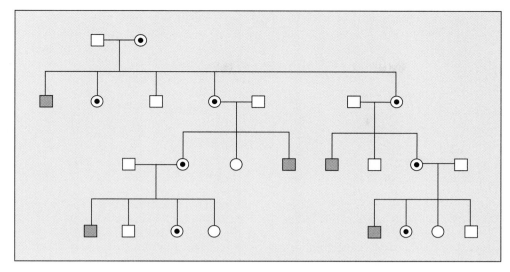

FIG. 5-5 A pedigree showing the inheritance of an X-linked recessive trait. Solid symbols represent affected individuals, and dotted symbols represent heterozygous carriers.

The most common mating type involving X-linked recessive genes is the combination of a carrier female and a normal male. The carrier mother will transmit the disease gene to half of her sons and half of her daughters. As Fig. 5-6 shows, half of the daughters in such a mating will be carriers, while half will be normal (on the average). Half of the sons will be normal, while half, on average, will have the disease.

The other common mating type is an affected father and a normal mother (Fig. 5-7). Here, all of the sons must be normal, since the father can transmit only his Y chromosome to them. Because all of the daughters must receive the father's X chromosome, they will all be heterozygous carriers. None of the children will manifest the disease, however. Since the father *must* transmit his X chromosome to his daughters and cannot transmit it to his sons, these risks, unlike those in the previous paragraph, are exact figures rather than probability estimates.

A much less common mating type is that of an affected father and a carrier mother (Fig. 5-8). Half of the daughters will be heterozygous carriers, while half, on average, will be homozygous for the disease gene and thus affected. Half of the sons will be normal, and half will be affected. Note that it may appear that father-son transmission of the disease has occurred, but the affected son has actually received the disease allele from his mother.

▼ **Recurrence risks for X-linked recessive disorders are more complex than for autosomal disorders. The risks depend on the genotype of each parent and the sex of the offspring.** ▲

Occasionally, females who inherit only a single copy of an X-linked recessive disease gene can be affected with the disease. Imagine a female embryo that has received

FIG. 5-6 Punnett square representation of the mating of a heterozygous female who carries an X-linked recessive disease gene with a normal male. In this and the following two figures, X_1 is the chromosome with the normal allele, and X_2 is the chromosome with the disease allele.

a normal factor VIII gene from one parent and a mutated factor VIII gene from the other. Ordinarily, X inactivation will result in approximately equal numbers of cells having active paternal and maternal X chromosomes. In this case the female carrier would produce about 50% of the normal level of factor VIII and would be phenotypically normal. However, because X inactivation is a random process, it will occasionally result in a heterozygous female in whom nearly all of the active X chromosomes happen to be the ones carrying the disease mutation. These females exhibit the disorder

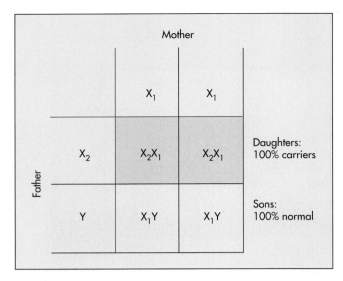

FIG. 5-7 Punnett square representation of the mating of a normal female with a male who is affected by an X-linked recessive disease.

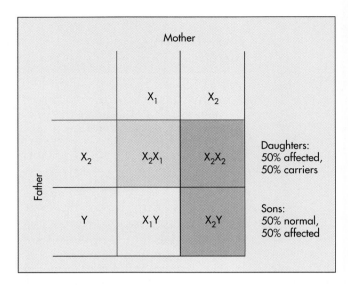

FIG. 5-8 Punnett square representation of the mating of a carrier female with a male affected with an X-linked recessive disease.

and are termed **manifesting heterozygotes**. Because such females usually maintain at least a small proportion of active normal X chromosomes, they tend to be relatively mildly affected. For example, approximately 5% of females who are heterozygous for hemophilia A have factor VIII levels low enough to be classified as mild hemophiliacs.

▼ Because X inactivation is a random process, some female heterozygotes may experience inactivation of most of the normal X chromosomes in their cells. These manifesting heterozygotes are usually mildly affected. ▲

Less commonly, females having only a single X chromosome (Turner syndrome) have been seen with X-linked recessive diseases such as hemophilia A. Females can also be affected with X-linked recessive diseases as a result of translocations or deletions of X chromosome material (see Chapter 6). These events are rare.

X-Linked Dominant Inheritance

With the important exception of fragile X syndrome (discussed later), X-linked dominant diseases are fewer in number and less clinically significant than are X-linked recessive diseases. An example of an X-linked dominant disease is hypophosphatemic rickets, a disease in which the kidneys are impaired in their ability to reabsorb phosphate. This results in abnormal ossification, with bending and distortion of the bones. Another example is incontinentia pigmenti type 1, a disorder characterized by abnormal skin pigmentation, conical or missing teeth, and ocular and neurological

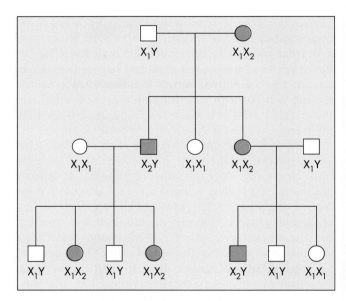

FIG. 5-9 Pedigree demonstrating the inheritance of an X-linked dominant trait. X_1 is the normal allele; X_2 is the disease allele.

abnormalities. This disorder is seen only in females. It is thought that hemizygous males are so severely affected that they do not survive to term. Heterozygous females, having one normal X chromosome, tend generally to have milder expression of X-linked dominant traits (just as heterozygotes for most autosomal dominant disease genes are less severely affected than are homozygotes). WWW

Fig. 5-9 illustrates a pedigree for X-linked dominant inheritance. As with autosomal dominant diseases, an individual need inherit only a single copy of

CLINICAL COMMENTARY 5-2
DUCHENNE MUSCULAR DYSTROPHY

Muscular dystrophy, defined as a progressive weakness and loss of muscle, exists in at least a dozen different forms. Of these, Duchenne muscular dystrophy (DMD), named after the French neurologist who first described the disease in 1868, is the most severe and the most common. It affects approximately 1/3,500 males; this prevalence figure is similar among all ethnic groups studied thus far.

The symptoms of *DMD* are usually seen before the age of 5 years, with parents often noticing clumsiness and muscle weakness. Pseudohypertrophy of the calves, the result of infiltration of muscle by fat and connective tissue, is often seen early in the course of the disease. All skeletal muscle degenerates eventually (Fig. 5-10), and most DMD patients are confined to wheelchairs by age 11. The heart and respiratory musculature become impaired, and death usually results from respiratory or cardiac failure. Survival beyond age 25 is uncommon. Despite much effort, there is no effective treatment for this disease. www

As muscle cells die, the enzyme creatine kinase (CK) leaks into the bloodstream. Serum CK assays show that in DMD patients it is elevated at least 20 times above the upper limit of the normal range. This elevation can be observed presymptomatically (i.e., before clinical symptoms such as muscle wasting are seen). Other diagnostic tools include electromyography, which reveals reduced action potentials, and muscle biopsy (Fig. 5-11).

Female heterozygous carriers of the *DMD* gene are usually free of disease, although 8% to 10% have some degree of muscle weakness. In addition, serum CK exceeds the 95th percentile in approximately two thirds of heterozygotes.

Until the *DMD* gene was isolated and cloned in 1986, little was known about the mechanism responsible for muscle deterioration. Cloning of the gene and identification of its protein product have advanced our knowledge tremendously. The *DMD* gene covers approximately 2.3 million base pairs of DNA, making it by far the largest gene known in the human. It contains at least 79 exons that produce a 14-kb mRNA transcript

FIG. 5-10 A patient with late-stage Duchenne muscular dystrophy, showing severe muscle loss.

FIG. 5-11 Transverse section of gastrocnemius muscle from (A) a normal boy and (B) a boy with Duchenne muscular dystrophy. Normal muscle fiber is replaced with fat and connective tissue.

Continued

CLINICAL COMMENTARY 5-2—cont'd
DUCHENNE MUSCULAR DYSTROPHY

(because of this gene's huge size, transcription of an mRNA molecule may take as long as 24 hours). The mRNA is translated into a mature protein of 3,685 amino acids. The protein product, named **dystrophin,** was unknown before the cloning of the *DMD* gene. Dystrophin accounts for only about 0.002% of a striated muscle cell's protein mass and is localized on the cytoplasmic side of the cell membrane. While its function is still being explored, it is likely to be involved in maintaining the structural integrity of the cell's cytoskeleton. The amino terminal of the protein binds F-actin, a key cytoskeletal protein. The carboxyl terminal of dystrophin binds a complex of glycoproteins, known as the dystroglycan-sarcoglycan complex, that spans the cell membrane and binds to extracellular proteins (Fig. 5-12). Dystrophin thus links these two cellular components and plays a key role in maintaining the structural integrity of the muscle cell. Lacking dystrophin, the muscle cells of the DMD patient gradually die as they are stressed by muscle contractions.

The large size of the *DMD* gene helps to explain its high mutation rate, about 10^{-4}. As with neurofibromatosis type 1, the *DMD* gene presents a large target for mutation. A slightly altered form of the *DMD* gene product is normally found in brain cells. Its absence in DMD patients helps to explain why approximately 25% have an intelligence quotient (IQ) below 75. In brain cells the transcription initiation site is further downstream in the gene, and a different promoter is used. Thus, the mRNA transcript, and the resulting gene product, differ from the gene product found in muscle cells. A third promoter has been identified for DMD transcripts expressed in cerebellar Purkinje cells. This is an intriguing example of a single gene that can produce different gene products as a result of modified transcription.

Becker muscular dystrophy (BMD), another X-linked recessive dystrophic condition, is less severe than the Duchenne form. The progression is also much slower, with onset at 11 years of age, on average. One study showed that while 95% of DMD cases are confined to wheelchairs before 11 years of age, 95% of BMD cases become wheelchair bound after 11 years of age. Some never lose their ability to walk. BMD is considerably less common than DMD, affecting only about 1/18,000 male births.

For some time, it was known that the BMD gene was located close to DMD on the X chromosome. It was unclear, however, whether the two diseases were caused by distinct loci or by different mutations at the same locus. Cloning the gene has shown that the two diseases are in fact caused by different mutations at the same locus and thus represent another example of allelic heterogeneity. Both diseases usually result from deletions (65% of DMD cases and 85% of BMD cases) or duplications (6% to 7% of DMD and BMD cases). But, whereas the great majority of DMD deletions and duplications

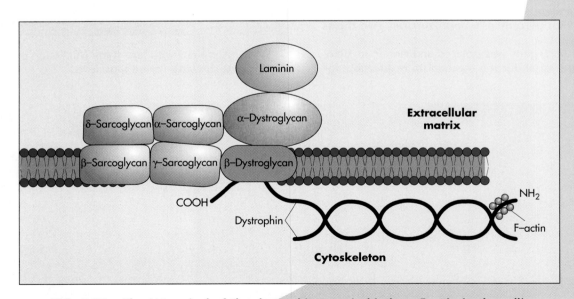

FIG. 5-12 The N-terminal of the dystrophin protein binds to F-actin in the cell's cytoskeleton, and dystrophin's C-terminal binds to elements of the dystroglycan-sarcoglycan complex. The latter complex of glycoproteins spans the cell membrane and binds to proteins in the extracellular matrix, such as laminin.

produce frameshifts, the majority of BMD mutations are in-frame alterations (i.e., a multiple of three bases is deleted or duplicated). One would expect that a frameshift, which is likely to alter the protein substantially (see Chapter 3), would produce a more severe disease than would an in-frame alteration.

The consequences of these different mutations can be observed in the gene product. While dystrophin is absent in nearly all DMD patients, it is usually present in reduced quantity (or as a shortened form of the protein) in BMD patients. Thus, a dystrophin assay can help to distinguish between the two diseases. It also helps to distinguish both diseases from other forms of muscular dystrophy, since several of these forms (e.g., various limb-girdle muscular dystrophies) result from mutations in genes encoding proteins of the dystroglycan-sarcoglycan complex, whereas dystrophin appears to be affected only in BMD and DMD.

Precise identification of the DMD gene has led to animal models for the disease (a mouse model and a dog model). Animal research is contributing considerably to our understanding of the human form of the disease. In addition, work is progressing on gene therapy for DMD (see Chapter 13). However, because all muscles of the body, including the heart, are affected, this type of therapy faces formidable challenges.

TABLE 5-1 A Comparison of the Major Attributes of X-Linked Dominant and X-Linked Recessive Inheritance Patterns*

Attribute	X-linked dominant	X-linked recessive
Recurrence risk for heterozygous female × normal male mating	50% Sons affected; 50% daughters affected	50% Sons affected; 50% daughters heterozygous carriers
Recurrence risk for affected male × normal female mating	0% Sons affected; 100% daughters affected	0% Sons affected; 100% daughters heterozygous carriers
Transmission pattern	Vertical; disease phenotype seen in generation after generation	Skipped generations may be seen, representing transmission through carrier females
Sex ratio	Twice as many affected females as affected males (unless disease is lethal in males)	Much greater prevalence of affected males; affected homozygous females are rare
Other	Male-male transmission not seen; expression less severe in female heterozygotes than in affected males	Male-male transmission not seen; manifesting heterozygotes may be seen in females

*Compare with the inheritance patterns for autosomal diseases shown in Table 4-1.

an X-linked dominant disease gene to manifest the disorder. Because females have two X chromosomes, either of which can potentially carry the disease gene, they are about twice as commonly affected as males (unless the disorder is lethal in males, as in incontinentia pigmenti). Affected fathers cannot transmit the trait to their sons. All of their daughters must inherit the disease gene, so all are affected. Affected females are usually heterozygotes and thus have a 50% chance of passing the disease allele to their daughters and sons. The characteristics of X-linked dominant and X-linked recessive inheritance are summarized in Table 5-1.

▼ X-linked dominant diseases display characteristic patterns of inheritance. They are about twice as common in females as males, skipped generations are uncommon, and father-son transmission is not seen. ▲

The Fragile X Story: Molecular Genetics Explains a Puzzling Pattern of Inheritance

Since the nineteenth century, it has been observed that there is an approximate 25% excess of males among the institutionalized mentally retarded. This excess is partly explained by several X-linked conditions causing mental retardation. The fragile X syndrome is the most common of these, accounting for approximately 40% of all X-linked mental retardation. Seen in approximately 1/1250 males and 1/2500 females, the fragile X syndrome is the single most common inherited cause of mental retardation. In addition to mental retardation, fragile X syndrome is characterized by a distinctive facial appearance, with large ears and long face (Fig. 5-13), hypermobile joints, and macroorchidism (increased testicular volume) in postpubertal males. The degree of mental retardation tends to be milder and more

FIG. 5-13 Boys with fragile X syndrome. Note the long faces, prominent jaws, and large ears and the similar characteristics of children from different ethnic groups. **A,** Caucasian. **B,** Asian. **C,** Hispanic.

variable in females than in males. The term "fragile X" is derived from the fact that the X chromosomes of affected individuals, when cultured in a medium that is deficient in folic acid, sometimes exhibit breaks and gaps near the tip of the long arm (Fig. 5-14). **www**

Fragile X syndrome is an X-linked dominant condition with 80% penetrance in males and only 30% pen-

etrance in females. The lower degree of penetrance in females, as well as variability in expression, is thought to be related to X-inactivation. Males who carry the gene but do not express the disease are termed "normal transmitting males." In the mid-1980s, studies of fragile X pedigrees revealed a perplexing pattern: whereas only about 9% of the brothers of transmitting males have the

FIG. 5-14   An X chromosome from a male with fragile X syndrome, showing an elongated, condensed region near the tip of the long arm.

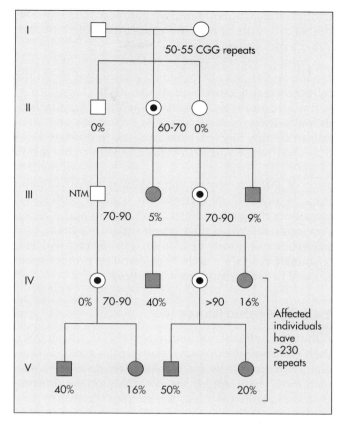

FIG. 5-15   A pedigree showing the inheritance of the fragile X syndrome. Females who carry a premutation (50 to 230 CGG repeats) are dotted. Affected individuals are represented by solid symbols. A normal transmitting male, who carries a premutation of 70 to 90 repeat units, is designated NTM. Note that the number of repeats increases each time the mutation is passed through another female. Also, only 5% of the NTM's sisters are affected, and only 9% of his brothers are affected, while 40% of his grandsons and 16% of his granddaughters are affected. This is the Sherman paradox.

fragile X syndrome, 40% of their grandsons and 50% of their great-grandsons have the syndrome (Fig. 5-15). Daughters of transmitting males are never affected with the disorder, but *their* sons can be affected. This pattern, dubbed the "Sherman paradox," is inconsistent with the rules of X-linked inheritance, which dictate equal penetrance in males who inherit the disease gene.

Many mechanisms were proposed to explain this pattern, including autosomal and mitochondrial modifier loci. Resolution of the Sherman paradox came only with the cloning of the disease gene, labeled *FMR1*. This gene is 38 kb in length, contains 17 exons, and produces a 4.8 kb mRNA transcript. The gene product, FMRP, binds to RNA and is capable of shuttling back and forth between the nucleus and cytoplasm. DNA sequence analysis showed that the 5' untranslated region of the gene contains a CGG repeat unit that is present in 6 to 50 copies in normal individuals. Those with fragile X syndrome have 230 to 1,000 or more CGG repeats (a "full mutation"). An intermediate number of repeats, ranging approximately from 50 to 230, is seen in normal transmitting males and their female offspring. When these female offspring transmit the gene to their offspring, there is often an expansion from this "premutation" of 50 to 230 repeats to the full mutation of more than 230 repeats. These expansions do not occur in male transmission. Furthermore, premutations tend to become larger in successive generations, and larger premutations are more likely to expand to a full mutation. These findings explain the Sherman paradox. They show why males with the premutation cannot transmit the disease to their daughters, and they explain why grandsons and great-grandsons of transmitting males are more likely to be affected with the disorder.

Measurement of mRNA transcribed from *FMR1* has shown that the highest mRNA expression levels are in the brain, as would be expected. Individuals with normal and premutation *FMR1* genes have equal levels of

mRNA expression. However, those with full mutations have no *FMR1* mRNA in their cells, indicating that transcription of the gene has been eliminated. The CGG repeat is heavily methylated among those with the full mutation, as is a series of CG sequences 5' of the gene. In addition, the degree of methylation is correlated with severity of expression of the disorder. These correlations indicate that methylation may influence the transcription rate of *FMR1*.

Further study of this region has revealed the presence of another fragile site distal to the fragile X site. This fragile site, termed *FRAXE*, is also associated with mental retardation and, like fragile X syndrome, is caused by the expansion of a CGG trinucleotide repeat. Repeat expansion at this locus is also associated with increased methylation. Unlike fragile X syndrome, the CGG repeat at this locus can expand when transmitted through either males or females.

Cloning the *FMR1* gene and identification of a repeat expansion has already explained a great deal about the inheritance and expression of the fragile X syndrome. It has also improved diagnostic accuracy for the condition, since cytogenetic analysis of chromosomes often fails to identify fragile X heterozygotes. In contrast, DNA diagnosis, which consists of measurement of the length of the CGG repeat sequence and the degree of methylation of *FMR1*, is very accurate. Many questions remain: What is the role of methylation in gene expression? How does the gene product affect mental and physical development? When does repeat expansion occur, during meiosis or during early mitosis in the embryo? Further analysis of the fragile X gene and its protein product will help to answer these questions.

Y-Linked Inheritance

Although it consists of approximately 70 Mb of DNA, the Y chromosome contains relatively few genes. To date, about two dozen Y-linked, or **holandric**, genes have been identified. These include the gene that initiates differentiation of the embryo into a male (see Chapter 6), several genes encoding testis-specific spermatogenesis factors, and a minor histocompatibility antigen, termed *HY*. Several housekeeping genes are located on the Y chromosome, and these all have inactivation-escaping ho-

mologs on the X chromosome. Transmission of Y-linked traits is strictly father-son (Fig. 5-16).

SEX-LIMITED AND SEX-INFLUENCED TRAITS

Confusion sometimes exists regarding traits that are *sex-linked* and those that are **sex-limited** or **sex-influenced**. A sex-limited trait occurs in only one of the sexes, due, for instance, to anatomical differences. Inherited uterine or testicular defects would be examples. A good example of a sex-influenced trait is male-pattern baldness, which occurs in both males and females, but much more commonly in males. Contrary to oft-stated belief, male-pattern baldness is not X-linked. It is thought to be inherited as an autosomal dominant trait in males, whereas in females it is inherited as an autosomal recessive trait. Female heterozygotes can transmit the trait to their offspring but do not manifest it. Females display the trait only when they inherit two copies of the gene. Even then, they are more likely to display marked thinning of the hair, rather than complete baldness.

MITOCHONDRIAL INHERITANCE

The great majority of genetic diseases are caused by defects in the nuclear genome. However, a small but significant number of diseases are the result of mitochondrial mutations. Because of the unique properties of the mitochondria, these diseases display characteristic modes of inheritance and a large degree of phenotypic variability.

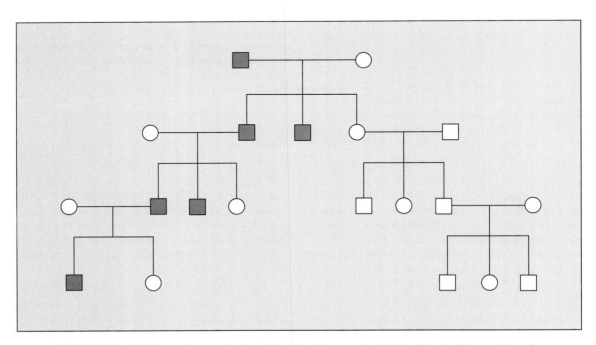

FIG. 5-16 Pedigree demonstrating the inheritance of a Y-linked trait. Transmission is exclusively male-male.

BOX 5-1
COLOR VISION: MOLECULAR BIOLOGY AND EVOLUTION

Human vision depends on a system of photoreceptors located in the retina. About 95% of these photoreceptor cells are termed **rod cells**, which contain the light-absorbing protein **rhodopsin** and allow us to see in conditions of dim light. In addition, the retina contains three classes of **cone cells**, which contain light-absorbing proteins (opsins) that react to the three primary colors, red, green, and blue. Color vision depends on the presence of all four of these cell types. Since three major colors are involved, normal color vision is said to be **trichromatic**.

There are many recognized defects of human color vision. The most common of these involve red and green color perception and have been known since 1911 to be inherited in X-linked recessive fashion. Thus, they are much more common in males than in females. Various forms of "red-green colorblindness" are seen in about 8% of Caucasian males, 4% to 5% of Asian males, and 1% to 4% of African and Native American males. Among Caucasian males, 2% are **dichromatic**: they are unable to perceive one of the primary colors, usually red or green. The inability to perceive green is termed **deuteranopia**, while the inability to perceive red is termed **protanopia**. About 6% of Caucasian males can detect green and red, but with altered perception of the relative shades of these colors. These are respectively termed **deuteranomalous** and **protanomalous** conditions.

It should be apparent that dichromats are not really color *blind*, since they can still perceive a fairly large array of different colors. True colorblindness (**monochromacy**, the ability to perceive only one color) is much less common, affecting approximately 1/100,000 individuals. There are two major forms of monochromatic vision. **Rod monochromacy** is an autosomal recessive condition in which all visual function is carried out by rod cells. **Blue cone monochromacy** is an X-linked recessive condition in which both the red and green cone cells are absent.

Cloning of the genes responsible for color perception has revealed a number of interesting facts about both the biology and evolution of color vision in humans. About 15 years ago, Jeremy Nathans and colleagues reasoned that the opsins in all four types of photoreceptor cells might have similar amino acid sequences because they carry out similar functions. Thus, the DNA sequences of the genes encoding these proteins should also be similar. But none of these genes had been located, and the precise nature of the protein products was unknown. How could they locate these genes? Fortunately, the gene encoding rhodopsin in cattle had been cloned. Even though humans and cattle are separated by millions of years of evolution, their rhodopsin proteins still share about 40% of the same amino acid sequence. Thus, the cattle (bovine) rhodopsin gene could be used as a probe to search for a homolog in the human genome. A portion of the bovine rhodopsin gene was converted to single-strand form, radioactively labeled, and

hybridized with human DNA (much in the same way that a probe is used in Southern blotting [see Chapter 3]). Low-stringency hybridization conditions were used: temperature and other conditions were manipulated so that complementary base pairing would occur despite some sequence differences between the two species. In this way, the human rhodopsin gene was identified and mapped to chromosome 3.

The next step was to use the human rhodopsin gene as a probe to identify the cone cell opsin genes. Each of the cone cell opsin amino acid sequences shares 40% to 45% similarity with the human rhodopsin amino acid sequence. By probing with the rhodopsin gene, the gene for blue-sensitive opsin was identified and mapped to chromosome 7. This gene was expected to map to an autosome because variants in blue sensitivity are inherited as an autosomal recessive trait. The genes for the red- and green-sensitive opsins were also identified in this way and, as expected, were found to be on the X chromosome. The red and green genes are highly similar, sharing 98% of their DNA sequence.

Initially, many investigators expected that people with color vision defects would display the usual array of deletions and missense and nonsense mutations seen in other disorders. But further study revealed some surprises. It was found that the red and green opsin genes are located directly adjacent to one another on the distal long arm of the X chromosome and that normal individuals have one copy of the red gene but could have from one to several copies of the green gene. The multiple green genes are 99.9% identical in DNA sequence, and the presence of multiple copies of these genes has no effect on color perception. However, when there are *no* green genes, deuteranopia is produced. Individuals lacking the single red gene have protanopia. The unique aspect of these deletions is that they are the result of **unequal crossover** during meiosis (Fig. 5-17). Unlike ordinary crossover, in which equal segments of chromosomes are exchanged (see Chapter 2), unequal crossover results in a loss of chromosome material on one homolog and a gain of material on the other. Unequal crossover seems to be facilitated by the high similarity in DNA sequence among the red and green genes: it is relatively easy for the cellular machinery to make a "mistake" in deciding where the crossover should occur. Thus, a female with one red gene and two green genes could produce one gamete containing a red gene with one green gene and another gamete containing a red gene with three green genes. Unequal crossover could also result in gametes with no copies of a gene, producing protanopia or deuteranopia.

Unequal crossover also explains protanomalous and deuteranomalous color vision. Here, crossover takes place *within* the red or green genes (see Fig. 5-17), resulting in new chromosomes with hybrid genes (e.g., a portion of

Continued

FIG. 5-17 Normal individuals (A) have one red gene and one to several green genes. Unequal crossover causes normal variation in the number of green genes (B). Unequal crossover can produce a green dichromat with no green genes (deuteranopia). Unequal crossover occurring *within* the red and green genes (D) can produce a red dichromat (protanopia) or a green anomalous trichromat (deuteranomaly). Crossovers within the red gene and green genes (E) can also produce red anomalous trichromats (protanomaly). The degree of red and green color perception depends on where the crossover occurs within the genes.
(Modified from Nathans J, Merbs SL, Sung C, et al. [1989] Sci. Am. 260:42-49.)

the red gene fused with a portion of the green gene). The relative proportion of red and green components of these **fusion genes** determines the extent and nature of the red-green anomaly.

Since the opsin genes have DNA sequence similarity and perform similar functions, they are members of a gene family, much like the globin genes (see Chapter 3). This suggests that they evolved from a single ancestral gene that, through time, duplicated and diverged to encode different but related proteins. Evidence for this process is provided by comparing these genes in humans and other species. Because the X-linked red and green opsin genes share the greatest degree of DNA sequence similarity, we would ex-

pect that these two genes would be the result of the most recent duplication. Indeed, humans share all four of their opsin genes with apes and Old World monkeys, but the less closely related New World monkeys have only a single opsin gene on their X chromosomes. It is thus likely that the red-green duplication occurred sometime after the split of the New and Old World monkeys, which took place about 30 to 40 million years ago. Similar comparisons date the split of the X-linked and autosomal cone opsin genes to approximately 500 million years ago. And finally, comparisons with the fruit fly, *Drosophila melanogaster*, indicate that the split between the rod and cone visual pigment genes may have occurred as much as 1 billion years ago.

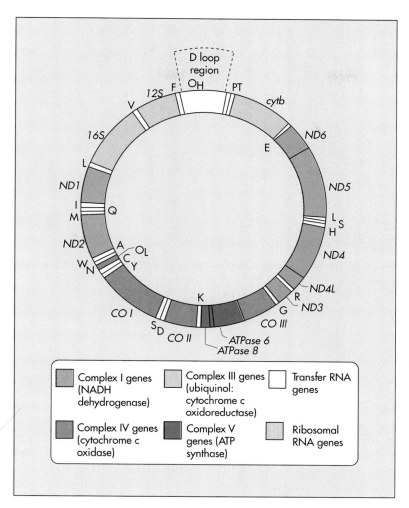

FIG. 5-18   The circular mitochondrial DNA genome. Locations of protein-coding genes (NADH dehydrogenase, cytochrome c oxidase, cytochrome c oxidoreductase, and ATP synthase) are shown, as are the locations of the two ribosomal RNA genes and 22 transfer RNA genes (designated by single letters). The replication origins of the heavy (O_H) and light (O_L) chains and the noncoding D loop (also known as the control region) are also shown. (Modified from Wallace DC [1992] *Science* 256:628-632.)

Each human cell contains several hundred or more mitochondria in its cytoplasm. Through the complex process of oxidative phosphorylation, these organelles produce adenosine triphosphate (ATP), the energy source essential for cellular metabolism. Mitochondria are thus critically important for cell survival.

The mitochondria have their own DNA molecules, occurring in several copies per organelle and consisting of 16,569 base pairs arranged on a double-stranded circular molecule (Fig. 5-18). The mitochondrial genome encodes two ribosomal RNAs, 22 transfer RNAs, and 13 polypeptides involved in oxidative phosphorylation (another 90 or so nuclear DNA genes also encode polypeptides that are transported into the mitochondria to participate in oxidative phosphorylation). Transcrip-

tion of mitochondrial DNA (mtDNA) takes place in the mitochondrion, independently of the nucleus. Unlike nuclear DNA, mtDNA contains no introns. Because it is located in the cytoplasm, mtDNA is inherited exclusively through the maternal line (Fig. 5-19). Males inherit their mtDNA from their mothers, but they cannot pass it to their offspring because sperm cells contain only a few mtDNA molecules that do not enter the egg. The mutation rate of mtDNA is about 10 times higher than that of nuclear DNA. This is caused by a lack of DNA repair mechanisms in the mtDNA and possibly also by damage from free oxygen radicals released during the oxidative phosphorylation process.

Since each cell contains a *population* of mtDNA molecules, a single cell can harbor some molecules that

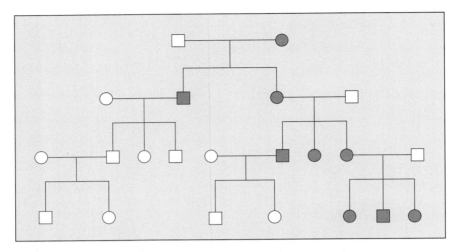

FIG. 5-19 A pedigree showing the inheritance of a disease caused by a mitochondrial DNA mutation. Only females can transmit the disease mutation to their offspring.

have an mtDNA mutation and other molecules that do not. This heterogeneity in DNA composition, termed **heteroplasmy**, is an important cause of variable expression in mitochondrial diseases. The larger the proportion of mutant mtDNA molecules, the more severe the expression of the disease. The proportion of mutant mtDNA molecules may change through **replicative segregation** as cells divide and as mitochondria proliferate. Changes in the proportion of mutant alleles can occur through chance variation (identical in concept to genetic drift, discussed in Chapter 3) or because of a selective advantage (e.g., deletions produce a shorter mitochondrial DNA molecule that can replicate more quickly than a full-length molecule).

Each tissue type requires a certain amount of mitochondrially produced ATP for normal function. Although some variation in ATP levels may be tolerated, there is typically a threshold level below which cells begin to degenerate and die. Organ systems with large ATP requirements and high thresholds tend to be the ones most seriously affected by mitochondrial diseases. For example, the central nervous system consumes about 20% of the body's ATP production and is thus often affected by mtDNA mutations.

Like the globin disorders, mitochondrial disorders can be classified according to the type of mutation that causes them. Missense mutations in protein-coding mtDNA genes cause one of the best-known mtDNA diseases, Leber hereditary optic neuropathy (LHON). This disease is characterized by rapid loss of vision in the central visual field as a result of optic nerve death. Vision loss typically begins in the third decade of life and is usually irreversible. Heteroplasmy is rare in LHON, so expression tends to be relatively uniform and

pedigrees for this disorder usually display a clear pattern of mitochondrial inheritance.

Single-base mutations in a tRNA gene can result in myoclonic epilepsy with ragged-red fiber disease (MERRF), a disorder characterized by epilepsy, dementia, ataxia (uncoordinated muscle movement), and myopathy (muscle disease). MERRF is heteroplasmic and thus highly variable in its expression. Another example of a mitochondrial disease caused by a single-base tRNA mutation is mitochondrial encephalomyopathy and strokelike episodes (MELAS). Like MERFF, MELAS is heteroplasmic and highly variable in expression. **www**

The final class of mtDNA mutations consists of duplications and deletions. These can produce Kearns-Sayre disease (muscle weakness, cerebellar damage, and heart failure), Pearson syndrome (infantile pancreatic insufficiency, pancytopenia, and lactic acidosis), and chronic progressive external ophthalmoplegia (CPEO).

Mitochondrial mutations are also involved in some common human diseases. A mitochondrial deletion causes a form of deafness, and the MELAS mutation is seen in 1% to 2% of individuals with non–insulin dependent diabetes mellitus. An mtDNA mutation is seen in up to 5% of patients with Alzheimer disease, but it is not yet clear whether this mutation plays a causal role. It has also been suggested that mtDNA mutations, which accumulate through the life of the individual as a result of free radical formation, could contribute to the aging process.

▼ **The mitochondria, which produce ATP, have their own unique DNA. Mitochondrial DNA is maternally inherited and has a high mutation rate. Several mitochondrial diseases have been identified.** ▲

STUDY QUESTIONS

1. Females have been observed with five X chromosomes in each somatic cell. How many Barr bodies would such females have?

2. Explain why 8% to 10% of female carriers of the DMD gene have muscle weakness.

3. For X-linked recessive disorders, the ratio of affected males to affected females in populations increases as the disease frequency decreases. Explain this in terms of gene and genotype frequencies.

4. Fig. 5-20 shows the inheritance of hemophilia A in a family. What is the risk that the male in generation IV is affected with hemophilia A? What is the risk that the female in this generation is a heterozygous carrier? What is the risk that she is affected with the disorder?

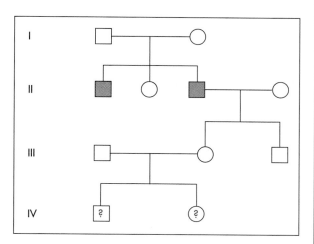

FIG. 5-20 Pedigree for study question 4.

5. Pedigrees for autosomal dominant and X-linked dominant diseases are sometimes difficult to distinguish. Name as many features as you can that would help to tell them apart.

6. How would you distinguish mitochondrial inheritance from other modes of inheritance?

7. A man with Becker muscular dystrophy marries a phenotypically normal female. On average, what proportion of their male offspring will be affected, and what proportion of their female offspring will be affected with this disorder?

8. A female carrier of a Duchenne muscular dystrophy mutation marries a phenotypically normal man. On average, what proportion of their male offspring will be affected, and what proportion of their female offspring will be affected with the disorder?

9. A boy and his brother both have hemophilia A. What is the probability that the boys' aunt (the mother's sister) is a heterozygous *carrier* of the disease gene?

SUGGESTED READINGS

Brown RH (1997) Dystrophin-associated proteins and the muscular dystrophies. Ann. Rev. Med. 48:457-466

Cahill MR, Colvin BT (1997) Haemophilia. Postgrad. Med. J. 73:201-206

Deeb SS, Motulsky AG (1996) Molecular genetics of color vision. Behav. Genet. 26:195-207

Emery AEH (1993) Duchenne Muscular Dystrophy. Oxford University Press, Oxford

Grossman LI, Shoubridge EA (1996) Mitochondrial genetics and human disease. BioEssays 18:983-991

Hoyer LW (1994) Hemophilia A. N. Eng. J. Med. 330:38-47

Lahn BT, Page DC (1997) Functional coherence of the human Y chromosome. Science 278:675-680

Latham KE (1996) X chromosome imprinting and inactivation in the early mammalian embryo. Trends Genet. 12:134-138

Lee JT, Jaenisch R (1997) The (epi)genetic control of mammalian X-chromosome inactivation. Curr. Opin. Genet. Dev. 7:274-280

Straub V, Campbell KP (1997) Muscular dystrophies and the dystrophin-glycoprotein complex. Curr. Opin. Neurol. 10:168-175

Suomalainen A (1997) Mitochondrial DNA and disease. Ann. Med. 29:235-246

Wallace DC (1997) Mitochondrial DNA in aging and disease. Sci. Amer. 277:40-47

Warren ST (1997) Trinucleotide repetition and fragile X syndrome. Hosp. Pract. 32:73-98

6

Clinical Cytogenetics:
The Chromosomal Basis of Human Disease

The previous two chapters have dealt with single-gene diseases. We turn now to diseases caused by chromosome alterations that are sufficiently large to be observable under a microscope. Such alterations are termed **chromosome abnormalities**. The study of chromosomes and their abnormalities is called **cytogenetics**.

Chromosome abnormalities are responsible for a significant proportion of genetic diseases, occurring in approximately 1/150 live births. They are the leading known cause of both mental retardation and pregnancy loss. Chromosome abnormalities are seen in 50% and 20% of first- and second-trimester spontaneous abortions, respectively. Thus, they are an important cause of morbidity and mortality.

As in other areas of medical genetics, advances in molecular genetics have contributed many new insights in the field of cytogenetics. For example, molecular techniques have permitted the identification of chromosome abnormalities, such as deletions, that affect very small regions. In some cases, specific genes responsible for cytogenetic syndromes are being pinpointed. Thus, the distinction between "chromosome abnormalities" and "single-gene diseases" is becoming somewhat blurred. In addition, the ability to identify DNA polymorphisms in parents and offspring has enabled researchers to specify whether an abnormal chromosome is derived from the mother or father. This has increased our understanding of the biological basis of meiotic errors and chromosome abnormalities.

In this chapter we discuss abnormalities of chromosome number and structure. The chromosomal and genetic basis of sex determination will be reviewed. The role of chromosome alterations in cancer will be examined, and several diseases caused by chromosomal instability will be discussed. Emphasis will be given to the new contributions of molecular genetics to cytogenetics.

CYTOGENETIC TECHNOLOGY AND NOMENCLATURE

Although it was possible to visualize chromosomes under microscopes as early as the mid-1800s, it was quite difficult to observe individual chromosomes. It was thus hard to count the number of chromosomes in a cell or to examine structural abnormalities. Beginning in the 1950s, several techniques were developed that improved our ability to observe chromosomes. These included (1) the use of spindle poisons, such as colchicine and colcemid, that arrest dividing somatic cells in metaphase, when chromosomes are maximally condensed and easiest to see; (2) the use of a hypotonic (low salt) solution, which causes swelling of cells, rupture of the nucleus, and better separation of individual chromosomes; and (3) the use of staining materials that are absorbed differentially by different parts of chromosomes, thus producing the characteristic bands that help to identify individual chromosomes.

▼ Our ability to study chromosomes has been improved by the visualization of chromosomes in metaphase, by hypotonic solutions that cause nuclear swelling, and by staining techniques that bring out chromosome bands. ▲

Chromosomes are analyzed by collecting a living tissue (usually blood), culturing the tissue for the appropriate amount of time (usually 48 to 72 hours for peripheral lymphocytes), adding colcemid to produce metaphase arrest, harvesting the cells, placing the cell sediment on a slide, rupturing the cell nucleus with a hypotonic saline solution, staining with a designated nuclear stain, and photographing the metaphase "spreads" of chromosomes on the slide. The chromosome images are then cut out from the photograph, and the 22 pairs of autosomes are arranged according to

FIG. 6-1   A banded karyotype of a normal female. The banded metaphase chromosomes are arranged from largest to smallest in size.

length, with the sex chromosomes in the right-hand corner. This ordered display of chromosomes is termed a **karyotype** (Fig. 6-1). Currently, computerized image analyzers are usually used to display chromosomes.

After sorting by size, chromosomes are further classified according to the position of the centromere. When the centromere occurs near the middle of the chromosome, the chromosome is said to be **metacentric** (Fig. 6-2). An **acrocentric** chromosome has its centromere near the tip, and **submetacentric** chromosomes have centromeres somewhere between the middle and the tip. The tip of each chromosome is termed the **telomere**. The short arm of a chromosome is labeled *p* (for *petite*), and the long arm is labeled *q*. In metacentric chromosomes, where the arms are of roughly equal length, the p and q arms are designated by convention.

▼ A karyotype is a display of chromosomes ordered according to length. Depending on the position of the centromere, a chromosome may be acrocentric, submetacentric, or metacentric. ▲

FIG. 6-2   Metacentric, submetacentric, and acrocentric chromosomes. Note the stalks and satellites present on the short arms of the acrocentric chromosomes.

A normal female karyotype is designated 46,XX; a normal male karyotype is designated 46,XY. The nomenclature for various chromosome abnormalities is summarized in Table 6-1 and will be indicated for each condition discussed in the chapter.

TABLE 6-1 Standard Nomenclature for Chromosome Karyotypes

Karyotype	Description
46,XY	Normal male chromosome constitution
47,XX,+21	Female with trisomy 21, Down syndrome
47,XY,+21/46,XY	Male who is a mosaic of trisomy 21 cells and normal cells
46,XY,del(4)(p14)	Male with distal deletion of the short arm of chromosome 4 band designated 14
46,XX,dup(5p)	Female with a duplication of the short arm of chromosome 5
45,XY,−13,−14,t(13q;14q)	A male with a balanced Robertsonian translocation of chromosomes 13 and 14; karyotype shows that one normal 13 and one normal 14 are missing
46,XY,t(11;22)(q23;q22)	A male with a balanced reciprocal translocation between chromosomes 11 and 22; the break points are at 11q23 and 22q22
46,XX,inv(3)(p21;q13)	An inversion on chromosome 3 that extends from p21 to q13; because it includes the centromere, this is a pericentric inversion
46,X,r(X)	A female with one normal X chromosome and one ring X chromosome
46,X,i(Xq)	A female with one normal X chromosome and an isochromosome of the long arm of the X chromosome

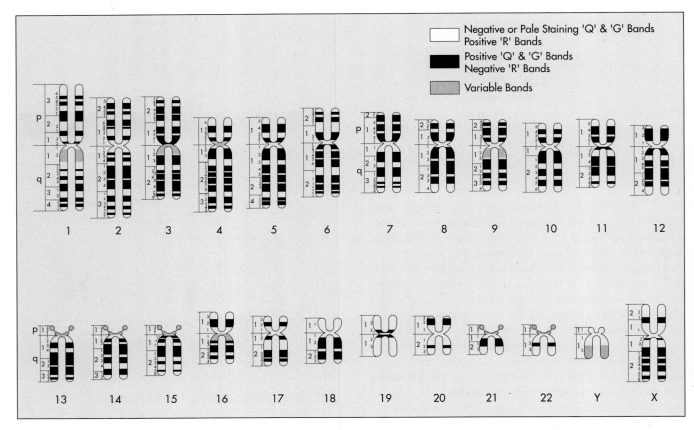

FIG. 6-3 A schematic representation of the banding pattern of a G-banded karyotype. 300 bands are represented in this ideogram. The short and long arms of the chromosomes are designated, and the segments are numbered according to the standard nomenclature adopted at the Paris conference, 1971. In this illustration, both sister chromatids are shown for each chromosome.

Chromosome Banding

Early karyotypes were useful in counting the number of chromosomes, but structural abnormalities, such as chromosomal deletions, were often undetectable. Staining techniques were developed in the 1970s to produce the chromosome bands characteristic of modern karyotypes. Chromosome banding helps greatly in the detection of deletions, duplications, and other structural abnormalities, and it facilitates the correct identification of individual chromosomes. The major bands on each chromosome are numbered (Fig. 6-3). Thus, 14q32 refers to the second band in the third region of the long arm of chromosome 14. Sub-bands are designated by decimal points following the band (e.g., 14q32.3 is the third sub-band of band 2).

Several chromosome-banding techniques are used in cytogenetics laboratories. **Quinacrine** banding (Q-banding) was the first staining method used to produce specific banding patterns. This method requires a fluorescence microscope and is no longer as widely used as **Giemsa banding** (G-banding). To produce G bands, a Giemsa stain is applied after the chromosomal proteins are partially digested by trypsin. **Reverse banding** (R-banding) requires heat treatment and reverses the usual white and black pattern that is seen in G-bands and Q-bands. This method is particularly helpful in staining the distal ends of chromosomes. Other staining techniques include **C-banding** and **NOR** (nucleolar organizing region) **stains**. These latter methods specifically stain certain portions of the chromosome. C-banding stains the **constitutive heterochromatin**, which usually lies near centromeres, and NOR staining highlights the satellites and stalks of acrocentric chromosomes (see Fig. 6-2).

High-resolution banding involves the staining of chromosomes during prophase or early metaphase (prometaphase), before they reach maximal condensation. Because prophase and prometaphase chromosomes are more extended than metaphase chromosomes, the number of bands observable for all chromosomes increases from about 300 to 450 (as in Fig. 6-3) to as many as 800. This allows the detection of less obvious abnormalities usually not seen with conventional banding. High-resolution banding is rather tedious and time consuming, so it is usually used when the clinician is looking for a specific, subtle chromosomal abnormality. An example would be the deletion of the 15q11-13 bands seen in the Prader-Willi syndrome. **WWW**

▼ Chromosome bands help to identify individual chromosomes and structural abnormalities in chromosomes. Banding techniques include quinacrine, Giemsa, reverse, C, and NOR banding. High-resolution banding, using prophase or prometaphase chromosomes, increases the number of observable bands. ▲

Fluorescence In Situ Hybridization and Comparative Genomic Hybridization

Fluorescence in situ hybridization (**FISH**) is a recently developed technique in which a labeled chromosome-specific DNA segment (probe) is hybridized with metaphase, prophase, or interphase chromosomes and then visualized under a fluorescence microscope. A common use of FISH is to determine whether a portion of a chromosome is deleted in a patient. In a normal individual, a probe will hybridize in two places, reflecting the presence of two homologous chromosomes in a somatic cell nucleus. If a probe from the chromosome segment in question hybridizes to only one of the patient's chromosomes, then the patient is likely to have the deletion on one chromosome. Excess chromosome material can also be detected using FISH. In this case, the probe will hybridize in three places instead of two. Combinations of FISH probes can also be used to detect chromosome rearrangements such as translocations (see later discussion).

Fig. 6-4 illustrates a FISH result for a child who is missing a small piece of the short arm of chromosome 17. Although a centromere probe hybridizes to both copies of chromosome 17, a probe corresponding to a specific region of 17p hybridizes to only one chromosome. This demonstrates the deletion that causes the Smith-Magenis syndrome (see Table 6-3). **WWW**

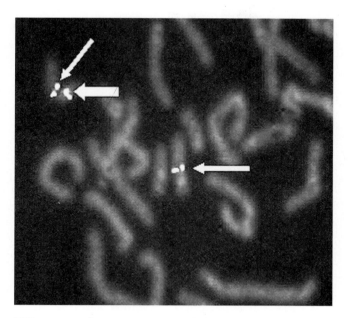

FIG. 6-4   A fluorescence in situ hybridization (FISH) result. The larger arrows point to a centromere-hybridizing probe for chromosome 17, and the smaller arrow points to a probe that hybridizes to 17p. The latter probe reveals only one spot in this individual, who has a deletion of 17p, producing the Smith-Magenis syndrome.

(Courtesy Dr. Arthur Brothman, University of Utah Health Sciences Center.)

▼ Fluorescence in situ hybridization (FISH) is a technique in which a labeled probe is hybridized to metaphase, prophase, or interphase chromosomes. FISH can be used to test for missing or additional chromosomal material as well as chromosome rearrangements. ▲

The FISH technique has been extended by using multiple probes, each labeled with a different color, so that several of the most common numerical abnormalities can be tested simultaneously in the same cell (e.g., abnormal numbers of chromosomes 13, 18, 21, X and Y) (see Color Plate 4 following p. 116). In addition, new techniques such as **spectral karyotyping** utilize varying combinations of five different fluorescent probes in conjunction with special cameras and image-processing software so that each chromosome is uniquely colored ("painted") for ready identification (see Color Plate 5 following p. 116). Such images are especially useful in identifying chromosome rearrangements (see Color Plate 6 following p. 116).

Losses or duplications of specific chromosome regions can be detected by a technique known as **comparative genomic hybridization**, or **CGH** (Fig. 6-5). DNA taken from a test source (e.g., tumor cells) is labeled with a substance that exhibits one color (e.g., green) under a fluorescence microscope; DNA taken from normal control cells is labeled with a second color (e.g., red). Both sets of DNA are then hybridized to normal metaphase chromosomes. If any chromosome region is duplicated in the tumor cell, then this region of the metaphase chromosome will hybridize with excess quantities of the green-labeled DNA. This region will exhibit a green color under the microscope. Conversely, if a region is deleted in the tumor cell, then the corresponding region of the metaphase chromosome will hybridize with excess red-labeled DNA, and the region will exhibit a red color under the microscope. CGH is especially useful in scanning for deletions and duplications of chromosome material in cancer cells, where detection of such alterations may help to predict the severity of the cancer.

▼ The FISH technique can be extended with multiple colors to detect several possible alterations of chromosome number simultaneously. Multiple probes can be used to paint each chromosome with a unique color, facilitating the detection of structural rearrangements. The comparative genomic hybridization (CGH) technique, in which differentially labeled DNA from test and control sources is hybridized to normal metaphase chromosomes, allows the detection of chromosome duplications and deletions. ▲

ABNORMALITIES OF CHROMOSOME NUMBER
Polyploidy

A cell that contains a multiple of 23 chromosomes in its nucleus is said to be **euploid** (Greek, *eu* = "good," *ploid* = "set"). Thus, haploid gametes and diploid somatic cells are euploid. **Polyploidy**, the presence of a complete set of extra chromosomes in a cell, is seen commonly in plants and often improves their agricultural value. Polyploidy also occurs in humans, although much less frequently. The polyploid conditions that have been observed in humans are **triploidy** (69 chromosomes in the nucleus of each cell) and **tetraploidy** (92 chromosomes in each cell nucleus). The karyotypes for these two conditions would be designated 69,XXX and 92,XXXX, respectively (assuming that all of the sex chromosomes were X; other combinations of the X and Y chromosomes may be seen). Because the number of chromosomes present in each of these conditions is a multiple of 23, the cells are euploid in each case. However, the additional chromosomes encode a large amount of surplus gene product, causing multiple anomalies such as defects of the heart and central nervous system. Triploidy and tetraploidy are both lethal. www

Triploidy is seen among only about 1/10,000 live births, but it accounts for an estimated 15% of the chromosome abnormalities occurring at conception. Thus, the vast majority of triploid conceptions are sponta-

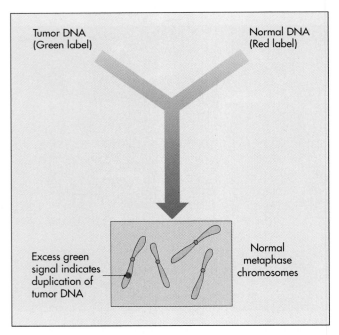

FIG. 6-5 The comparative genomic hybridization (CGH) technique. Green-labeled test DNA (from a tumor sample in this case) and red-labeled reference DNA (from normal cells) are both hybridized to normal metaphase chromosomes. The ratio of green to red signal on the hybridized metaphase chromosomes indicates the location of duplications (excess green) and deletions (excess red) in the tumor chromosomes.

Tumor DNA (Green label)

Normal DNA (Red label)

Excess green signal indicates duplication of tumor DNA

Normal metaphase chromosomes

neously aborted. The most common cause of triploidy is the fertilization of an egg by two sperm (**dispermy**). The resulting zygote then receives 23 chromosomes from the egg and 23 chromosomes from each of the two sperm cells. Triploidy can also be caused by the fusion of an ovum and a polar body, each containing 23 chromosomes, and subsequent fertilization by a sperm cell. **Meiotic failure**, in which a diploid sperm or egg cell is produced, can also produce a triploid zygote.

Tetraploidy is much rarer than triploidy, both at conception and among live births. It has been recorded among only a few live births, and these infants have survived for only short periods. Tetraploidy can be caused by a mitotic failure in the early embryo, in which all of the duplicated chromosomes migrate to one of the two daughter cells. It can also result from the fusion of two diploid zygotes.

▼ Cells that have a multiple of 23 chromosomes are said to be euploid. Triploidy (69 chromosomes) and tetraploidy (92 chromosomes) are polyploid conditions found in humans. Most polyploid conceptions are spontaneously aborted, and all are incompatible with long-term survival. ▲

Autosomal Aneuploidy

Cells that do not contain a multiple of 23 chromosomes are termed **aneuploid**. These cells contain missing or additional chromosomes. Usually only one chromosome is affected, but it is possible for more than one chromosome to be missing or duplicated. Aneuploidies of the autosomes are among the most clinically important of the chromosome abnormalities. They consist primarily of **monosomy** (the presence of only one copy of a chromosome in an otherwise diploid cell) and **trisomy** (three copies of a chromosome). Autosomal monosomies are nearly always incompatible with survival to term, so only a small number of them have been observed among live-born individuals. In contrast, some trisomies are seen with appreciable frequencies among live births. The fact that trisomies produce less severe consequences than monosomies illustrates an important principle: *the body can tolerate excess genetic material more readily than it can tolerate a deficit of genetic material.*

The most common cause of aneuploidy is **nondisjunction**, the failure of chromosomes to disjoin normally during meiosis (Fig. 6-6). Nondisjunction can occur during meiosis I or meiosis II. The resulting gamete either lacks a chromosome or has two copies

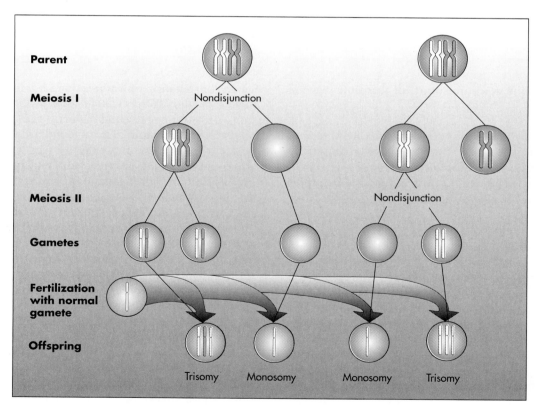

FIG. 6-6 In meiotic nondisjunction, two chromosome homologs migrate to the same daughter cell instead of disjoining normally and migrating to different daughter cells. This produces monosomic and trisomic offspring.

FIG. 6-7 **A,** An infant with Down syndrome, illustrating typical features of this disorder: upslanting palpebral fissures, redundant skin of the inner eyelid (epicanthic fold), protruding tongue, and low nasal bridge. **B,** Same girl as in **A** 7 years later. Note that the typical features are present but less obviously expressed.

of it, producing a monosomic or trisomic zygote, respectively.

▼ Aneuploid conditions consist primarily of monosomies and trisomies. They are usually caused by nondisjunction. Autosomal monosomies are virtually always lethal, while some autosomal trisomies are compatible with survival. ▲

Trisomy 21

Trisomy 21 (47,XY,+21 or 47,XX,+21)* is seen in approximately 1/800 live births, making it the most common aneuploid condition compatible with survival to term. This trisomy produces Down syndrome, a phenotype originally described by John Langdon Down in 1866. Nearly 100 years elapsed between Down's description of this syndrome and the discovery (in 1959) that it is caused by the presence of an extra 21st chromosome.

Although there is considerable variation in the appearance of individuals with Down syndrome, they pre-

sent a constellation of features that help the clinician to make a diagnosis. The facial features include a low nasal root, upslanting palpebral fissures, measurably small and sometimes overfolded ears, and a flattened maxillary and malar region, giving the face a characteristic appearance (Fig. 6-7). Some of these features led to the use of the term "mongolism" in earlier literature, but this term is inappropriate. The cheeks are round, and the corners of the mouth are sometimes downturned. The neck is short, and the skin is redundant at the nape of the neck, especially in newborns. The occiput is flat, and the hands and feet tend to be rather broad and short. Approximately 50% of individuals with Down syndrome have a deep flexion crease across their palms (termed a simian crease). Decreased muscle tone (hypotonia) is a highly consistent feature that is helpful in making a diagnosis. **WWW**

Several medically significant problems occur with increased frequency among infants and children with Down syndrome. About 3% of these infants will develop an obstruction of the duodenum or atresia (closure or absence) of the esophagus, duodenum, or anus. Respiratory infections are quite common, and the risk of developing leukemia is 15 to 20 times higher in

---

*For brevity, the remainder of the karyotype designations for abnormalities not involving the sex chromosomes will indicate an affected male.

FIG. 6-7, cont'd **C,** A karyotype of a male with trisomy 21.

Down syndrome patients than in the general population. The most significant medical problem is that approximately 40% are born with structural heart defects. The most common of these is an AV (atrioventricular) canal, a defect in which the inter-atrial and inter-ventricular septa fail to fuse normally during fetal development. The result is blood flow from the left side of the heart to the right side and then to the pulmonary vasculature, producing pulmonary hypertension. Ventricular septal defects (VSDs) are also common among babies with Down syndrome. Moderate to severe mental retardation (IQ ranging from 25 to 60) is seen in most individuals with Down syndrome. This syndrome alone accounts for 10% of all cases of mental retardation in the United States. www

Several other medical problems occur in infants and young children with Down syndrome. Conductive and sometimes neural hearing loss, hypothyroidism, and various eye abnormalities are the most important and

frequent. Clinical Commentary 6-1 outlines a plan for routine medical care in infants and children with Down syndrome.

Because of the medical problems seen in children with Down syndrome, their survival rates are significantly decreased. Congenital heart defects are the most important single cause of decreased survival. In the early 1960s, only about half of children with this disorder survived until age 5. As a result of improvements in corrective surgery, antibiotic treatment, and management of leukemia, the survival rates have increased considerably in the past 30 years. Currently, it is estimated that approximately 75% to 80% of children with Down syndrome survive to age 10. There is strong evidence that enriched environments can produce significant improvements in intellectual function.

Males with Down syndrome are nearly always sterile; only two cases have been reported in which a male with Down syndrome has reproduced. Some females with

CLINICAL COMMENTARY 6-1
ANTICIPATORY GUIDANCE IN CHILDREN WITH DOWN SYNDROME

In recent years, an approach termed "anticipatory guidance" has evolved in the care and treatment of individuals with genetic syndromes and chronic diseases. After a thorough study of the disease in question (including an extensive literature review), basic guidelines are established for the screening, evaluation, and care of patients. If followed by the primary care practitioner or the specialist, these guidelines should help to prevent further disability or illness. We will illustrate the anticipatory guidance approach with current guidelines for the care of children with Down syndrome.

- Evaluation of heart defects. As mentioned in the text, AV canals are the most common congenital heart defect seen in newborns with Down syndrome. Surgical correction of this condition is appropriate if it is detected before 1 year of age (after this time, pulmonary hypertension has been present too long for surgery to be successful). Accordingly, it is now recommended that an *echocardiogram* be performed during the newborn period.
- Because Down syndrome patients often have strabismus (deviation of the eye from its normal visual axis) and other eye problems, they should be examined regularly by their physician. In asymptomatic children, an *ophthalmological examination* before the age of 4 years is recommended to evaluate visual acuity.
- Hypothyroidism is common, especially during adolescence. Thus, *thyroid hormone levels* should be measured annually.
- Sensorineural and conductive hearing loss are both seen in children with Down syndrome. The routine follow-up should include a *hearing test* at 6 to 8 months of age and as needed afterward.
- Instability of the first and second vertebrae has led to spinal cord injuries in some older Down syndrome patients. It is thus suggested that *imaging studies* be carried out in children with neurological symptoms or in those planning to participate in athletic activities.
- It is appropriate to refer children with Down syndrome to preschool programs to provide intervention for developmental disabilities.

Similar series of guidelines have been developed for children with trisomy 18 and Turner syndrome. In principle, the anticipatory guidance approach can be applied to any genetic disease for which there is sufficient knowledge.

this condition can reproduce, although approximately 40% fail to ovulate. Since reproduction is so uncommon, nearly all cases of trisomy 21 can be regarded as new mutations. The risk for a female with Down syndrome to produce a gamete with two copies of chromo-

some 21 (which would then produce a trisomic zygote) is 50%. However, since approximately 75% of trisomy 21 conceptions are spontaneously aborted, the Down syndrome female's risk of producing affected live-born offspring is considerably lower than 50%.

Approximately 95% of Down syndrome cases are caused by nondisjunction, with most of the remainder being caused by chromosome translocations (see later discussion). Based on comparisons of chromosome morphology in the affected offspring and their parents, it was long thought that about 80% of chromosome 21 nondisjunctions occur in the mother. A more accurate assessment is now made possible by comparing microsatellite polymorphisms on chromosome 21 in parents and offspring. This approach shows that the extra chromosome is contributed by the mother in 90% to 95% of trisomy 21 cases. About 75% of these maternal nondisjunctions occur during meiosis I, with the remainder occurring during meiosis II. As discussed in greater detail later, there is a strong correlation between maternal age and the risk of producing a child with Down syndrome.

Mosaicism is seen in approximately 1% to 3% of trisomy 21 live births. These individuals have some normal somatic cells and some cells with trisomy 21. This type of mosaicism in a male would be designated 47,XY,+21/46,XY. Mosaicism often results in a milder clinical expression of Down syndrome. The most common cause of mosaicism for a trisomy is a trisomic conception followed by loss of the extra chromosome in some cells during mitosis in the embryo.

Depending on the timing and manner in which the mosaicism originated, some individuals may be **tissue-specific mosaics**. As the term suggests, this type of mosaicism is confined only to certain tissues. This can complicate diagnosis, since karyotypes are usually made from a limited number of tissue types (usually circulating lymphocytes derived from a blood sample, or, less commonly, fibroblasts derived from a skin biopsy). Mosaicism affecting primarily the germ line of a parent can lead to multiple recurrences of Down syndrome in the offspring. This factor helps to account for the fact that the recurrence risk for Down syndrome among mothers under the age of 30 is about 1% (i.e., ten times higher than the population risk for this age group).

Because of the prevalence and clinical importance of Down syndrome, considerable effort has been devoted to defining the critical portion of chromosome 21 responsible for this disorder. This region has been narrowed to 21q22, a portion of the distal long arm. Persons with a trisomy of *only* this part of the chromosome will develop Down syndrome. Molecular approaches, such as cloning and sequencing, are being used to identify specific genes in this region that are responsible for the Down syndrome phenotype. For example, a strong candidate for mental retardation in

COLOR PLATE 1 Automated DNA sequencing. **A,** Gel image produced by an automated DNA sequencer. Each lane (labeled 1 to 19) represents a separate DNA sequence. Fluorescent labels that emit different colors on the gel image distinguish between bases. This permits the identity and order of bases in a strand of DNA to be determined. **B,** Analyzed data from a single DNA template sequenced on an automated DNA sequencer. Peaks of different colors represent the identity and relative location of different nucleotides in the DNA sequence. For example, the peak on the upper left is blue and identifies the position of a cytosine. The next peak is red, indicating the presence of a thymine. This "base-calling" continues until the end of the DNA template is reached (typically a few hundred base pairs).

COLOR PLATE 2 An African woman with oculocutaneous albinism. Note her light-colored hair and skin. She is looking away from the camera because her eyes are more sensitive to bright light than are those of individuals with normally pigmented retinas.
(Courtesy Dr. Phil Fischer, University of Utah Health Sciences Center.)

A

 B

COLOR PLATE 3 Fundus photos of ocular albinism. **A,** Fundus photograph of a female heterozygous carrier for X-linked ocular albinism. The pigmented and nonpigmented patches demonstrate mosaicism of the X chromosome as a result of random X inactivation. **B,** Fundus photograph of the heterozygous carrier's affected son, showing a distinct lack of melanin pigment.
(**A** and **B,** Courtesy Dr. Don Creel, University of Utah Health Sciences Center.)

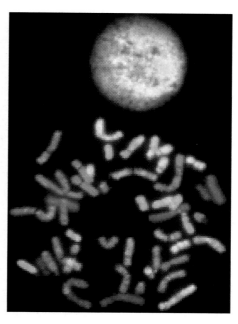

COLOR PLATE 4 Fluorescence in situ hybridization (FISH) technique using different-colored probes (multicolor FISH) that identify the X (green) and Y (red) chromosomes in a male. Multicolor FISH can also be used to label each chromosome with a different color.
(Courtesy Dr. Art Brothman, University of Utah Health Sciences Center.)

COLOR PLATE 5 Spectral karyotype. Each pair of metaphase chromosomes is colored differently. In the nucleus of a cell in interphase *(top)*, chromosome-specific coloring illuminates a tangled web of chromatin fibers.
(Courtesy Dr. Art Brothman, University of Utah Health Sciences Center.)

COLOR PLATE 6 Spectral karyotype. The power of spectral karyotyping is demonstrated by the identification of a rearrangement between chromosomes 2 and 22. Note that a portion of chromosome 2 (brown) has exchanged places with a portion of chromosome 22 (yellow).
(Courtesy Dr. Art Brothman, University of Utah Health Sciences Center.)

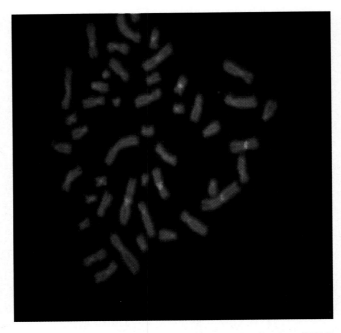

COLOR PLATE 7 Fluorescence in situ hybridization (FISH) analysis of the elastin locus. This region is commonly deleted in patients with Williams syndrome. A control signal (green) is used to identify the pericentromeric region of chromosome 7 (note that there are two signals). The elastin locus is identified by a red signal. Only a single red signal is observed, indicating that the elastin locus is absent from the chromosome 7 with only a green signal.
(Courtesy Dr. Art Brothman, University of Utah Health Sciences Center.)

COLOR PLATE 8 An example of a fiber FISH analysis, in which a chromatin fiber is extended to show the locations of three probes that are located within a 50-kb region. This technique permits the ordering of DNA sequences or loci that are very close to one another.
(Courtesy Aurelia Meloni-Ehrig, University of Utah Health Sciences Center.)

Down syndrome is *DYRK*, a kinase gene located in the critical region. Over-expression of this gene in the mouse causes learning and memory defects. Another gene located in the critical region, *APP*, encodes the amyloid beta precursor protein. A triple copy of *APP* is likely to account for the occurrence of Alzheimer-like dementia in nearly all Down syndrome patients by age 35 to 40. Mutations of *APP* cause a small percentage of Alzheimer disease cases (see Chapter 12), and Down syndrome individuals with partial trisomies that do not include the *APP* gene do not develop Alzheimer-like dementia.

▼ Trisomy 21, which causes Down syndrome, is the most common autosomal aneuploidy seen among live births. The most significant problems include mental retardation, GI tract obstruction, congenital heart defects, respiratory infections, and leukemia. The extra 21st chromosome is contributed by the mother in approximately 90% of cases. Mosaicism is seen in 1% to 3% of Down syndrome cases, and it usually accompanies a milder phenotype. Specific genes contributing to the Down syndrome phenotype are now being identified. ▲

Trisomy 18 (47,XY,+18)

This trisomy, also known as Edwards syndrome, is the second most common autosomal trisomy, with a prevalence of about 1/6,000 live births. It is, however, much more common at conception and is the most common chromosome abnormality among stillborns with congenital malformations. The Edwards syndrome phenotype is as discernable as Down syndrome, but because it is less common, it is less likely to be recognized clinically. Trisomy 18 patients have prenatal growth deficiency (weight that is low for the gestational age), characteristic facial features, and a distinctive hand ab-

normality that often allows the clinician to make the initial diagnosis (Fig. 6-8). Minor anomalies of diagnostic importance include small ears with unraveled helices, a small mouth that is often hard to open, a short sternum, and rather short big toes. Most babies with trisomy 18 have major malformations. Congenital heart defects, particularly ventricular septal defects, are the most common. Other medically significant congenital malformations include omphalocele (protrusion of the bowel into the umbilical cord), diaphragmatic hernia, and, occasionally, spina bifida. **www**

Recent studies have indicated that about 50% of children with trisomy 18 die in the first month, and only about 10% are still alive at 12 months of age. A combination of factors, including aspiration pneumonia, predisposition to infections and apnea, and (most importantly) congenital heart defects, account for the high mortality rate.

Those with trisomy 18 who have survived infancy have a marked developmental disability. The degree of delay is much more significant than in Down syndrome, and most children are not able to walk. However, children with trisomy 18 do progress somewhat in their milestones, and older infants learn some communication skills.

More than 95% of individuals with Edwards syndrome have complete trisomy 18. A small percentage have mosaicism. As in trisomy 21, there is a significant maternal age effect. Molecular analyses indicate that, as in trisomy 21, approximately 90% of trisomy 18 cases are the result of a maternally contributed extra chromosome.

Trisomy 13 (47,XY,+13)

This condition, also termed Patau syndrome, is seen in about 1/10,000 births. The malformation pattern is

FIG. 6-8 An infant with trisomy 18 (Edwards syndrome), exhibiting characteristic facial features, short sternum, overlapping fingers with clenched fists, and a left-sided clubfoot.

A

B

FIG. 6-9 **A,** A newborn male with full trisomy 13 (Patau syndrome). This baby has a cleft palate, atrial septal defect, inguinal hernia, and postaxial polydactyly of the left hand. **B,** An individual with full trisomy 13 at age 7 years (survival beyond the first year is uncommon). He has significant visual and auditory impairments.

(**B,** Courtesy Susan Barg.)

quite distinctive and usually permits clinical recognition. It consists primarily of oral-facial clefts, microphthalmia (small, abnormally formed eyes), and postaxial polydactyly (Fig. 6-9). Malformations of the central nervous system are seen frequently, and cutis aplasia (a scalp defect on the posterior occiput) may also be seen.

The survival rate is very similar to that of trisomy 18, with 90% of live-born cases dying during the first year of life. As in trisomy 18, the children who survive infancy have significant developmental retardation, with skills seldom progressing beyond those of a child of 2 years. However, as in trisomy 18, children with trisomy 13 do progress somewhat in their development and are often able to communicate with their families.

About 80% of cases of Patau syndrome have full trisomy 13. Most of the remaining cases have trisomy of the long arm of chromosome 13 due to a translocation (see later discussion). As in trisomies 18 and 21, the risk of bearing a child with this condition increases with advanced maternal age. It is estimated that 95% or more of trisomy 13 and 18 conceptions are spontaneously lost during pregnancy. **www**

▼ Trisomies of the 13th and 18th chromosomes are sometimes compatible with survival to term, although 95% or more of affected fetuses are spontaneously aborted. These trisomies are much less common at birth than trisomy 21, and they produce a much more seriously affected phenotype, with 90% mortality during the first year of life. As in trisomy 21, there is a maternal age effect, and the mother contributes the extra chromosome in approximately 90% of cases. ▲

Trisomies, Nondisjunction, and Maternal Age

The prevalence of Down syndrome among mothers of different ages is shown in Fig. 6-10. Among mothers under the age of 30, the risk is less than 1/1,000. It increases to approximately 1/400 among women at age 35, to approximately 1/100 at age 40, and to 1/50 or more after age 45. Most other trisomies, including those in which the fetus does not survive to term, also increase in prevalence as maternal age increases. This risk is one of the primary indications for prenatal diagnosis among women over age 35 (see Chapter 13).

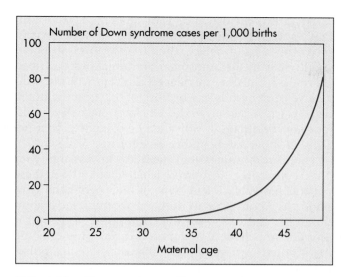

FIG. 6-10 The prevalence of Down syndrome among live births in relation to age of the mother. The prevalence increases with maternal age and becomes especially notable after the age of 35.
(Data from Hook EB, Chambers GM [1977] Birth Defects: Original Articles Series, 23[3A]:123-141.)

Several hypotheses have been advanced to account for this increase, including the idea that older women are less likely to spontaneously abort a trisomic pregnancy. Direct studies of the frequency of chromosome abnormalities in sperm and egg cells indicate that the pattern is instead due to an increase in nondisjunction among older mothers. Recall that all of a female's oocytes are formed during her embryonic development. They remain suspended in prophase I until they are shed during ovulation. Thus, an ovum produced by a 45-year-old woman is itself about 45 years old. This long period of suspension in prophase I may impair normal disjunction. However, the precise nature of this mechanism is not understood.

Many factors have been examined to determine whether they may affect the frequency of nondisjunction in women. These include hormone levels, cigarette smoking, autoimmune thyroid disease, alcohol consumption, and radiation (the latter does increase nondisjunction when administered in very large doses to experimental animals). None of these has shown consistent correlations with nondisjunction in humans, however, and maternal age remains the only known correlated factor.

Although maternal age is strongly correlated with the risk of Down syndrome, it should be pointed out that approximately three fourths of Down syndrome children are born to mothers under the age of 35. This is because the great majority of children (>90%) are borne by women in this age group.

Numerous studies, including direct analysis of sperm cells, have tested the hypothesis of a paternal age effect for trisomies. The consensus is that such an effect, if it exists at all, is minor. This may reflect the fact that spermatocytes, unlike oocytes, are generated throughout the life of the male.

▼ Nearly all autosomal trisomies increase with maternal age as a result of nondisjunction among older mothers. There is little evidence for a paternal age effect on nondisjunction in males. ▲

Sex Chromosome Aneuploidy

Among live births, about 1/400 males and 1/650 females have some form of sex chromosome aneuploidy. Primarily because of X inactivation, the consequences of this class of aneuploidy are less severe than those of autosomal aneuploidy. With the exception of a complete absence of an X chromosome, all of the sex chromosome aneuploidies are compatible with survival in at least some cases.

Monosomy of the X Chromosome (Turner Syndrome)

The phenotype associated with a single X chromosome (45,X) was originally recognized by Henry Turner in 1938. Individuals with Turner syndrome are female and usually have a characteristic phenotype. The findings include the variable presence of (1) proportionate short stature, (2) sexual infantilism and ovarian dysgenesis, and (3) a pattern of major and minor malformations. The physical features may include a triangle-shaped face; posteriorly rotated external ears; and a broad, "webbed" neck (Fig. 6-11). In addition, the chest is broad and shield-like in shape. Lymphedema of the hands and feet is observable at birth. Many patients with Turner syndrome have congenital heart defects, most commonly obstructive lesions of the left side of the heart (bicuspid aortic valve in 50% of patients and coarctation [narrowing] of the aorta in 15% to 20%). Severe obstructions should be surgically repaired. About 50% of individuals with Turner syndrome have structural kidney defects, but they usually do not cause medical problems. There is typically some diminution in spatial perceptual ability, but females with Turner syndrome are not mentally retarded. **www**

Girls with Turner syndrome exhibit proportionate short stature and do not undergo an adolescent growth spurt. Growth hormone administration produces increased height in these girls. Gonadal dysgenesis (lack of ovaries) is commonly seen in Turner syndrome. Instead of ovaries, most females with Turner syndrome have streaks of connective tissue. Lacking normal ovaries, they do not usually develop secondary sexual characteristics, and most women with this condition are

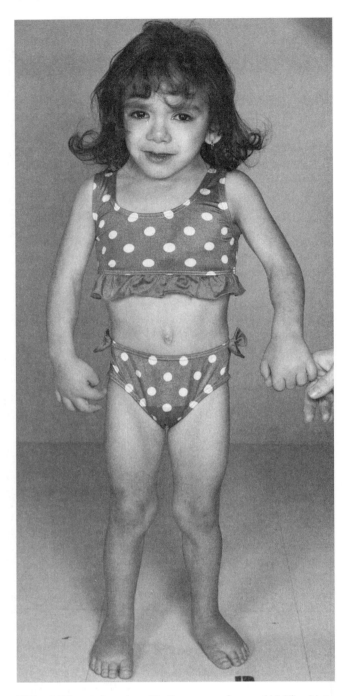

FIG. 6-11 A female with Turner syndrome (45,X). Note the characteristically broad, "webbed" neck. Stature is reduced, and swelling (i.e., lymphedema) is seen in the ankles and wrists.

infertile (about 5% to 10% have sufficient ovarian development to undergo menarche, and a small number have borne children). Teenagers with Turner syndrome are typically treated with estrogen to promote the development of secondary sexual characteristics. The dose is then continued at a reduced level to maintain these characteristics.

Frequently the diagnosis is made in the newborn infant, especially if there is a striking neck webbing coupled with a heart defect. The facial features are more subtle than in the autosomal abnormalities described previously, but the experienced clinician will often diagnose Turner syndrome because of one or more of the listed clues. If Turner syndrome is not diagnosed in infancy or childhood, it will often be diagnosed later because of short stature and/or amenorrhea.

The chromosome abnormalities in females with Turner syndrome are quite variable. About 50% of these patients have a 45,X karyotype in their peripheral lymphocytes. About 30% to 40% are mosaics, most commonly 45,X/46,XX and less commonly 45,X/46,XY. Mosaics who have Y chromosomes in some cells are predisposed to developing malignancies (gonadoblastomas) in their gonadal streaks. About 10% to 20% of patients with Turner syndrome have structural X chromosome abnormalities involving a deletion of some or all of the short arm. This variation in chromosome abnormality helps to explain the considerable phenotypic variation seen in this syndrome.

Molecular studies have shown that approximately 80% of monosomy X cases are caused by meiotic error in the father (i.e., the offspring receives an X chromosome from the mother but no sex chromosome from the father). The prevalence of the 45,X karyotype is low compared to those of other sex chromosome abnormalities, with only about 1/2,500 to 1/5,000 live-born females having the disorder. The 45,X karyotype is very common among conceptions, however, accounting for 15% to 20% of the chromosome abnormalities seen among spontaneous abortions. Thus, the great majority (>99%) of 45,X conceptions are lost prenatally. Among those that do survive to term, many are chromosomal mosaics, with mosaicism of the placenta alone (**confined placental mosaicism**) being especially common. It is likely that the presence of some normal cells in mosaic fetuses contributes to survival.

Molecular analysis has pinpointed specific genes involved in the Turner syndrome phenotype. For example, mutations in the *SHOX* gene, which encodes a transcription factor, produce short stature. This gene is located on the distal tip of the X and Y short arms (in the pseudoautosomal region) (see Clinical Commentary 6-2). Thus, it is normally present in two copies in both males and females. In females with Turner syndrome, however, this gene would be present in only one active copy, and the resulting haploinsufficiency is likely to contribute to short stature.

It was recently reported that females with Turner syndrome who receive the X chromosome from their father have higher verbal IQ scores and better social cognition than those who receive the X chromosome from their mother. This difference implies the presence of a genomic imprinting effect on a specific region of the X chromosome. Interestingly, a study of partial deletions of the X chromosome shows that the imprinted region escapes X inactivation. Because normal females inherit active copies of this region from both parents, while males inherit a copy only from their mothers (the existence of a Y homolog is not yet known), this finding could have important implications for general male-female differences in social cognition and verbal intelligence.

▼ Turner syndrome is most commonly caused by a 45,X karyotype. While common at conception, this disorder is relatively rare among live births, reflecting a very high rate of spontaneous abortion. Mosaicism, including confined placental mosaicism, appears to increase the probability of survival to term. Several specific genes that contribute to the Turner syndrome phenotype have been identified. ▲

Klinefelter Syndrome

Like the Down and Turner syndromes, the syndrome associated with a 47,XXY karyotype was described long before the underlying chromosomal abnormality was understood. Described in 1942 by Harry Klinefelter, the syndrome that bears his name is seen in approximately 1/1,000 male births. Although Klinefelter syndrome is a common cause of primary hypogonadism in the male, the phenotype is less striking than those of the syndromes described thus far. Males with Klinefelter syndrome tend to be taller than average, with disproportionately long arms and legs (Fig. 6-12). Clinical examination of postpubertal patients reveals small testes (<10 ml), and most males with Klinefelter syndrome are sterile as a result of atrophy of the seminiferous tubules. Gynecomastia (breast development) is seen in approximately one third of affected males and leads to an increased risk of breast cancer. The risk can be reduced by mastectomy (breast removal). In addition, there is a predisposition for learning disabilities and sub-average intelligence. Although males with Klinefelter syndrome are not usually mentally retarded, the IQ is on average 10 to 15 points below that of the affected individual's siblings. Because of the subtlety of this disorder, many patients with Klinefelter syndrome are not diagnosed until after puberty, and the condition is sometimes first ascertained in fertility clinics. **www**

The extra X chromosome is derived maternally in about 50% of Klinefelter cases, and the syndrome increases in incidence with advanced maternal age. Mosaicism is seen in about 15% of patients. Despite the relatively mild phenotypic features of this disorder, it is estimated that at least half of 47,XXY conceptions are spontaneously aborted.

Individuals with the 48,XXXY and 49,XXXXY karyotypes have also been reported. Because they have a Y chromosome, they still have a male phenotype, but the

FIG. 6-12 A male with Klinefelter syndrome (47,XXY). Stature is increased, gynecomastia may be present, and body shape may be somewhat feminine.
(From McKusick VA [1960] J. Chron. Dis. 12:1-202.)

degree of mental deficiency and physical abnormality increases with each additional X chromosome.

Testosterone therapy may enhance secondary sex characteristics in postpubertal males with Klinefelter syndrome. There is some evidence that this treatment also improves general well-being, but this has not been clearly substantiated.

▼ Klinefelter syndrome (47,XXY) males are taller than average, may have a reduction in IQ, and are usually sterile. Testosterone therapy and mastectomy for gynecomastia are sometimes recommended. ▲

Trisomy X

The 47,XXX karyotype occurs in approximately 1/1,000 females and usually has benign consequences. Overt physical abnormalities are rarely seen, but these females sometimes suffer from sterility, menstrual irregularity, or mild mental retardation. As in Klinefelter syndrome, females with the 47,XXX karyotype are often first ascertained in fertility clinics. The great majority of cases are the result of nondisjunction in the mother, and, as in other trisomies, the incidence increases among older mothers.

Females have also been seen with four, five, or even more X chromosomes. Each additional X chromosome is accompanied by increased mental retardation and physical abnormality.

47,XYY Syndrome

The final sex chromosome aneuploidy to be discussed is the 47,XYY karyotype. Males with this karyotype tend to be taller than average, and they have a 10 to 15 point reduction in average IQ. This condition, which causes few physical problems, achieved great notoriety when its incidence in male prison populations was discovered to be as high as 1/30, compared with 1/1,000 in the general male population. This led to the suggestion that this karyotype might confer a predisposition to violent, criminal behavior. Several dozen studies have addressed this issue, and they have shown that XYY males are not inclined to commit violent crimes. There is, however, evidence of minor behavioral disorders, such as hyperactivity, attention deficit disorder, and learning disabilities.

▼ **The 47,XXX and 47,XYY karyotypes are seen in about 1/1,000 females and males, respectively. Each involves a slight degree of reduction in IQ but few physical problems.** ▲

CHROMOSOME ABNORMALITIES AND PREGNANCY LOSS

For a long time it was difficult to detect the early stages of pregnancy with certainty. Thus, it was possible for a woman to become pregnant but lose the embryo before knowing of the pregnancy. Sensitive urinary assays of chorionic gonadotropin levels, which show an increase when the embryo implants in the uterine wall, have allowed researchers to pinpoint accurately the occurrence of pregnancy at this early stage. Follow-up of women in whom implantation was verified in this way has shown that about one third of pregnancies are lost after implantation (the number lost before implantation is unknown). Thus, spontaneous pregnancy loss is common in the human.

As mentioned earlier, chromosome abnormalities are the leading known cause of pregnancy loss. It is estimated that a *minimum* of 10% to 15% of conceptions have a chromosome abnormality. At least 95% of these chromosomally abnormal conceptions are lost before term. Karyotype studies of miscarriages indicate that about 50% of the chromosome abnormalities are trisomies, 20% are monosomies, 15% are triploids, and the remainder consist of tetraploids and structural abnormalities. Some chromosome abnormalities that are common at conception seldom or never survive to term. For example, trisomy 16 is thought to be the most common trisomy at conception, but it is never seen in live births.

It is possible to study chromosome abnormalities directly in sperm and egg cells. Oocytes are typically obtained from unused material in in vitro fertilization studies. Karyotypes obtained from these cells indicate that 20% to 25% of oocytes have missing or extra chromosomes (this may be an underestimate because the oocyte's chromosomes are difficult to visualize and count). Human sperm cells can be studied after fusing them with hamster oocytes so that their DNA begins mitosis and condenses, allowing easier visualization. The frequency of aneuploidy in these sperm cells is about 3% to 4%. Structural abnormalities (see later discussion) are seen in about 5% of sperm cells and about 1% of oocytes (it is noteworthy that structural abnormalities increase with advanced paternal age). Undoubtedly this high rate of chromosome abnormality contributes importantly to later pregnancy loss.

These approaches, while informative, may involve some biases. For example, mothers in whom *in vitro* fertilization is performed are not a representative sample of the population. In addition, their oocytes have been stimulated artificially, and only those oocytes that could not be fertilized by sperm cells are studied. Thus, the oocytes themselves may not be a representative sample. The sperm cells studied in human-hamster hybrids represent only those that are capable of penetrating the hamster oocyte and again may not be a representative sample.

Recently, FISH has been used to detect missing or extra chromosomes in human sperm cells. This approach can evaluate thousands of cells fairly rapidly, giving it an important advantage over the human-hamster technique. In general, the results of the FISH studies have yielded results similar to those of the human-hamster studies. These studies have also confirmed a tendency for elevated frequencies of nondisjunction of the sex chromosomes and chromosome 21 in sperm cells.

▼ **Pregnancy loss is common in the human, with approximately one third of pregnancies lost spontaneously after implantation. Chromosome abnormalities, which have been studied in sperm cells, egg cells, and in miscarriages and stillbirths, are an important cause of pregnancy loss.** ▲

ABNORMALITIES OF CHROMOSOME STRUCTURE

In addition to the loss or gain of whole chromosomes, parts of chromosomes can be lost or duplicated as gametes are formed, and the arrangement of portions of chromosomes can be altered. Structural chromosome abnormalities may be **unbalanced** (the rearrangement causes a gain or loss of chromosomal material) or **balanced** (the rearrangement does not produce a loss or gain of chromosome material). Unlike aneuploidy and polyploidy, balanced structural abnormalities often do not produce serious health consequences. Nevertheless, abnormalities of chromosome structure, especially those that are unbalanced, can produce serious disease in individuals or their offspring.

CLINICAL COMMENTARY 6-2

XX MALES, XY FEMALES, AND THE GENETIC BASIS OF SEX DETERMINATION

During normal meiosis in the male, crossover occurs between the tip of the short arm of the Y chromosome and the tip of the short arm of the X chromosome. These regions of the X and Y chromosomes contain highly similar DNA sequences. Because this crossover resembles the behavior of autosomes during meiosis, the distal portion of the Y chromosome is known as the **pseudoautosomal** region (Fig. 6-13). It spans approximately 2.5 Mb. Just centromeric of the pseudoautosomal region lies a gene known as *SRY* (sex-determining region on the Y). This gene, which is expressed in embryonic development, encodes a product that interacts with other genes to initiate the development of the undifferentiated embryo into a male (e.g., Sertoli cell differentiation, secretion of Mullerian inhibiting substance, etc.). As mentioned in Chapter 2, the *SRY* gene product is a member of the HMG family of DNA-bending transcription factors. By bending DNA, the protein is thought to promote DNA-DNA interactions that trigger events in the developmental cascade leading to male differentiation. When the *SRY* gene is inserted experimentally into a female mouse embryo, a male mouse is produced. Mutations of *SRY* can produce individuals with an XY karyotype but a female phenotype. Thus, there is very good evidence that the *SRY* gene is the initiator of male sexual differentiation in the embryo. Mutations in another member of this gene family, *SOX9*, can produce sex reversal (XY females) and campomelic dysplasia (malformations of bone and cartilage). WWW

Approximately 1/20,000 males presents with a condition similar to Klinefelter syndrome, but chromosome evaluation shows that they have a normal *female* karyotype (46, XX). It was demonstrated that these XX males have an X chromosome that includes the *SRY* gene. This is explained as a result of a faulty crossover between the X and Y chromosomes during male meiosis, such that the *SRY* gene, instead of remaining on the Y chromosome, is transferred to the X chromosome (see Fig. 6-13). The offspring who inherits this X chromosome from his father consequently has a male phenotype. Conversely, it should

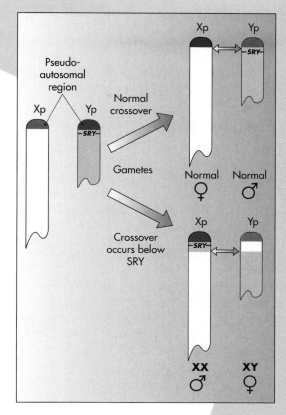

FIG. 6-13 The distal short arms of the X and Y chromosomes exchange material during meiosis in the male. The region of the Y chromosome in which this crossover occurs is called the pseudoautosomal region. The *SRY* gene, which triggers the process leading to male gonadal differentiation, is located just outside the pseudoautosomal region. Occasionally, the crossover occurs on the centromeric side of the *SRY* gene, causing it to lie on an X chromosome instead of the Y chromosome. An offspring receiving this X chromosome will be an XX male, and an offspring receiving the Y chromosome will be an XY female.

be apparent that an offspring who inherits a Y chromosome that lacks the *SRY* gene would be an XY female. These females have gonadal streaks rather than ovaries and have poorly developed secondary sexual characteristics.

Alterations of chromosome structure can occur when homologous chromosomes line up improperly during meiosis (e.g., unequal crossover, as described in Chapter 5). In addition, **chromosome breakage** can occur during meiosis or mitosis. Mechanisms exist to repair these breaks, and generally the break is repaired perfectly with no damage to the daughter cell. Sometimes, however, the breaks remain, or they heal in a fashion that alters the structure of the chromosome. The likelihood of chromosome breakage may be increased in the presence of certain harmful agents, called **clastogens**. Clastogens identified in experimental systems include ionizing radiation, some viral infections, and some chemicals. However, none of these agents has conclusively been shown to cause chromosome breakage in humans.

Translocations

A **translocation** is the interchange of genetic material between nonhomologous chromosomes. Balanced translocations represent one of the most common chromosomal aberrations in humans, with a prevalence of at least 1/500 individuals (Table 6-2). There are two basic types of translocations, termed **reciprocal** and **Robertsonian**.

Reciprocal Translocations

These translocations happen when breaks occur in two different chromosomes and the material is mutually exchanged. The resulting chromosomes are called **derivative chromosomes**. The carrier of a reciprocal translocation is usually normal because he or she has a normal complement of genetic material. However, the carrier's offspring can be normal, can carry the translocation, or can have duplications or deletions of genetic material.

An example of a reciprocal translocation between chromosomes 3 and 6 is shown in Fig. 6-14. The distal half of the short arm of chromosome 6 is translocated to the short arm of chromosome 3, and a small piece of chromosome 3 is translocated to the short arm of chromosome 6. This karyotype is 46,XX,t(3p;6p). The offspring of this woman received the derivative chromosome 3 [der(3)] and the normal 6; thus, the child has a **partial trisomy** of the distal portion of chromosome 6 (i.e., 6p trisomy). This is a well-established but rather uncommon chromosomal syndrome.

FIG. 6-14 A, The parent has a reciprocal balanced translocation involving the short arms of chromosomes 6 and 3. The distal short arm of the 6 has been translocated to the very distal tip of the 3. A small piece of chromosome 3 is attached to the derivative 6. This individual had a child whose chromosomes are depicted in **B.** The child received the derivative chromosome 3 (with part of the 6 short arm attached) and the normal 6. The child received a normal 3 and a normal 6 from the other parent. Thus, the child has a partial trisomy of the 6 short arm and presumably a small deletion of the 3 short arm (see text).

TABLE 6-2 Prevalence of Chromosomal Abnormalities Among Newborns

Abnormality	Prevalence at birth
Autosomal Syndromes	
Trisomy 21	1/800
Trisomy 18	1/6,000
Trisomy 13	1/10,000
Unbalanced rearrangements	1/17,000
Balanced rearrangements	
Robertsonian translocations	1/1,000
Reciprocal translocations	1/11,000
Sex Chromosome Abnormalities	
47,XXY	1/1,000 Male births
47,XYY	1/1,000 Male births
45,X*	1/5,000 Female births
47,XXX	1/1,000 Female births
All Chromosomal Abnormalities	
Autosomal disorders and unbalanced rearrangements	1/230
Balanced rearrangements	1/500[†]

*Note that the 45,X karyotype accounts for about half of cases of Turner syndrome.

[†]This figure is based primarily on older studies of unbanded chromosomes. More recent studies, using banded preparations (Jacobs PA et al. [1992]), show that the prevalence of balanced structural abnormalities is approximately 1/200.

▼ Reciprocal translocations are caused by two breaks on different chromosomes, with a subsequent exchange of material. While carriers of balanced reciprocal translocations usually have normal phenotypes, their offspring may have a partial trisomy or a partial monosomy and an abnormal phenotype. ▲

Robertsonian Translocations

In this type of translocation, the short arms of two non-homologous chromosomes are lost and the long arms fuse at the centromere, forming a single chromosome (Fig. 6-15). This type of translocation is confined to chromosomes 13 to 15, 21, and 22 because the short arms of these acrocentric chromosomes are very small and contain no essential genetic material. When a Robertsonian translocation takes place, the short arms are usually lost during subsequent cell divisions. Since the carriers of Robertsonian translocations lose no essential genetic material, they are phenotypically normal but have only 45 chromosomes in each cell. Their offspring, however, may inherit a missing or extra long arm of an acrocentric chromosome.

A common Robertsonian translocation involves the fusion of the long arms of chromosomes 21 and 14. The karyotype of a male carrier of this translocation would be 45,XY,−14,−21,+t(14q21q), with −14 and −21 showing that the carrier lacks one normal 14 and one normal 21. During meiosis, the translocation chromosome must still pair with its homologs (Fig. 6-16). The figure illustrates the ways in which these chromosomes may segregate in the gametes formed by the translocation carrier. If **alternate segregation** occurs, then the offspring are either chromosomally normal or have a balanced translocation with a normal phenotype. If either of the **adjacent segregation** patterns occur, then the gametes are unbalanced and the offspring may have trisomy 14, monosomy 14, monosomy 21, or trisomy 21 (note that these trisomies and monosomies are genetically the same as trisomies and monosomies produced by nondisjunction because only the long arms of these chromosomes contain genetically significant material). Fetuses with the former three possibilities do not survive to term, while the last translocation results in an infant with three copies of the long arm of chromosome 21 and a Down syndrome phenotype. Robertsonian translocations are responsible for approximately 5% of Down syndrome cases.

It is expected that the three types of conceptions compatible with survival would occur in equal frequencies. Thus, one third would be completely normal, one third would carry the translocation but be phenotypically normal, and one third would have Down syndrome. In part because of prenatal loss, the actual proportion of live-born offspring with Down syndrome is less than one third (about 10% to 15% for mothers carrying the translocation, and only 1% to 2% for fathers who carry it). This recurrence risk, however, is greater than the risk for parents of a child who has the nondisjunction type of Down syndrome, which is 1% for mothers younger than age 30. This difference in recurrence risks demonstrates why it is critical to order a chromosome study whenever a condition such as Down syndrome is suspected.

▼ Robertsonian translocations occur when the long arms of two acrocentric chromosomes fuse at the centromere. The carrier of a Robertsonian translocation can produce conceptions with monosomy or trisomy. ▲

Deletions

A **deletion** is caused by a chromosome break and subsequent loss of genetic material. A single break leading to a loss that includes the chromosome's tip is called

FIG. 6-15 In a Robertsonian translocation, shown here, the long arms of two acrocentric chromosomes (13 and 14) fuse, forming a single chromosome.

FIG. 6-16 The possible segregation patterns for the gametes formed by a carrier of a Robertsonian translocation. Alternate segregation (quadrant A alone, or quadrant B with quadrant C) produces either a normal chromosome constitution or a translocation carrier with a normal phenotype. Adjacent segregation (quadrant A with C, or quadrant A with B) produces unbalanced gametes and will result in conceptions with trisomy 14, trisomy 21, monosomy 14, or monosomy 21.

a **terminal deletion**. When two breaks occur and the material between the breaks is lost, an **interstitial deletion** occurs. For example, a chromosome segment with normal DNA might be symbolized ABCDEFG. An interstitial deletion could produce the sequence ABEFG, while a terminal deletion could produce ABCDE.

Usually, a gamete containing a chromosome with a deletion unites with a normal gamete to form a zygote. The zygote then has one normal chromosome and a homolog with the deletion. Microscopically visible de-letions generally involve multiple genes, and the consequences of losing this much genetic material from even one member of the chromosome pair can be severe.

After the three autosomal aneuploidies described earlier, the autosomal deletion syndromes are the most common group of clinically significant chromosome abnormalities. A well-known example of a chromosome deletion syndrome is the *cri-du-chat* syndrome. This term (French, "cry of the cat") describes the distinctive cry of the child. This cry usually becomes less obvious as the child ages, making a clinical diagnosis more difficult after 2 years of age. *Cri-du-chat* syndrome is caused by a deletion of the distal short arm of chromosome 5 (karyotype 46,XY,del[5p]). Seen in approximately one in 50,000 live births, it is also characterized by mental retardation (average IQ about 35), microcephaly (small head), and a characteristic but not dis-

FIG. 6-17 A child with Wolf-Hirschhorn syndrome (46,XY,del[4p]). Note the wide-spaced eyes and repaired cleft lip.

FIG. 6-18 RFLP loss of heterozygosity demonstrates a microdeletion in tumor cells. Autoradiograms for three RFLPs on the tip of the short arm of chromosome 11 are shown. In each autoradiogram, the lane labeled "L" contains DNA taken from a patient's lymphocytes, while the lane labeled "T" contains DNA taken from the patient's malignant astrocytoma. Because a tiny part of 11p was deleted in the tumor cells, the tumor DNA is homozygous for the HRAS and TH RFLPs, whereas the lymphocyte DNA is heterozygous for these markers. The FSHB marker lies outside the region of the deletion and is thus heterozygous in both the tumor and the lymphocyte DNA.

(Courtesy Dr. Dan Fults, University of Utah Health Sciences Center.)

tinctive facial appearance. Survival to adulthood has been observed but is not common.

Wolf-Hirschhorn syndrome (Fig. 6-17), caused by a deletion of the distal short arm of chromosome 4, is another well-characterized deletion syndrome. Other well-known deletions include those of 18p, 18q, and 13q. With the exception of the 18p deletion syndrome, each of these disorders is relatively distinctive, and the diagnosis can often be made before obtaining the karyotype. The features of the 18p deletion syndrome are more subtle, and usually children with this condition are recognized when chromosome analysis is performed for evaluation of developmental disability. **www**

▼ **Microscopically observable chromosome deletions, which may be either terminal or interstitial, usually affect a fairly large number of genes and produce recognizable syndromes.** ▲

Microdeletion Syndromes

The deletions described thus far all involve relatively large segments of chromosomes. Each of these was described before chromosome banding techniques were developed. With the advent of high-resolution banding,

it has become possible to identify microscopically a large number of deletions that were previously too small for detection. In addition, advances in molecular genetics, particularly the FISH technique and the development of large numbers of easily identified polymorphisms, have permitted the detection of deletions often too small to be observed microscopically (i.e., <5 Mb). Such deletions can be detected by showing that a series of RFLPs or other polymorphisms in a defined chromosome region all produce single, relatively faint bands, indicating that one copy of this region of the chromosome is missing (Fig. 6-18).

Prader-Willi syndrome, a disorder discussed in Chapter 4, is a good example of a **microdeletion syndrome.** Although this condition was described in the 1950s,* it was not until 1981 that advanced banding techniques detected a small deletion of chromosome bands 15q11-q13 in about 50% of these patients. By using molecular techniques, deletions that were too small to be detected cytogenetically were also discovered. In total, about

---

*Although Prader is commonly credited with the first complete description of Prader-Willi syndrome in 1956, John Langdon Down (of Down syndrome fame) published a fairly complete description of the disorder in 1887.

70% of Prader-Willi cases are caused by microdeletions of 15q. Because of imprinting, the inheritance of a microdeletion of the paternal chromosome 15 material produces Prader-Willi syndrome, while a microdeletion of the maternally derived chromosome 15 produces the phenotypically and genetically distinct Angelman syndrome (see Chapter 4).

High-resolution banding and molecular genetic techniques have often led to a more precise specification of the critical chromosome region that must be deleted to cause a given syndrome. Wolf-Hirschhorn syndrome, for instance, can be produced by the deletion of only a very small telomeric segment of 4p. In some instances, specific genes responsible for chromosome abnormality syndromes can be pinpointed. For example, individuals with a deletion of 11p may present with a series of features including <u>W</u>ilms tumor (a kidney tumor), <u>a</u>niridia (absence of the iris), <u>g</u>enitourinary abnormalities,* and mental <u>r</u>etardation (sometimes termed the WAGR syndrome). The genes responsible for the kidney tumor and for aniridia have now each been identified and cloned. Because the WAGR syndrome involves the deletion of a

---

*Because individuals with the WAGR syndrome also have gonadoblastomas (gonadal tumors), some authorities feel that the "G" should stand for gonadoblastoma rather than genitourinary abnormality.

series of adjacent genes, it is sometimes referred to as an example of a **contiguous gene syndrome.** In addition to microdeletions, microduplications can also produce contiguous gene syndromes. **WWW**

Williams syndrome, which is characterized by mental retardation, supravalvular aortic stenosis (SVAS), multiple peripheral pulmonary arterial stenoses, characteristic facial features, dental malformations, and hypercalcemia, is another example of a microdeletion syndrome (Fig. 6-19; see Color Plate 7 following p. 116). A series of molecular analyses have identified some of the individual genes responsible for the Williams syndrome phenotype. The *elastin* gene, for example, is located in the Williams syndrome critical region and is expressed in blood vessels. Elastin is an important component of the aortic wall (microfibrils, which were discussed in Chapter 4 in the context of Marfan syndrome, are another component). Mutations or deletions of *elastin* alone result in isolated SVAS without the other features of Williams syndrome. Larger deletions, encompassing additional genes, produce the complete Williams syndrome phenotype. A second gene in the critical region, *LIMK1*, encodes a brain-expressed kinase that is likely to be involved in the visual-spatial cognition defects observed in Williams syndrome patients. This is supported by the observation of patients with partial deletions of

A

B

FIG. 6-19 **A,** A girl with Williams syndrome, illustrating typical facial features: broad forehead, short palpebral fissures, low nasal bridge, anteverted nostrils, long filtrum, full cheeks, and relatively large mouth with full lips. **B,** An angiogram illustrating supravalvular aortic stenosis (narrowing of the ascending aorta).

(Courtesy Dr. Mark Keating, University of Utah Health Sciences Center)

the critical region affecting only the *elastin* and *LIMK1* genes. These individuals have SVAS and visual-spatial cognitive deficiency but none of the other features of Williams syndrome. WWW

Some of the microdeletion syndromes, such as Prader-Willi and Williams syndromes, often manifest deletions of a fairly consistent portion of a chromosome. Recent studies show that this is caused by the presence of multiple repeated sequences (such as *Alu* elements [Chapter 2]) at the deletion boundaries. It appears that these repeated sequences promote unequal crossing over (see Chapter 5), which then produces duplications and deletions of the region bounded by the repeat elements.

Several additional examples of microdeletions are given in Table 6-3. Many of these conditions, including the Prader-Willi, Miller-Dieker, Williams, and velocardio-facial syndromes (Clinical Commentary 6-3), are now diagnosed using the FISH technique.

▼ Microdeletions are a subtype of chromosome deletion that can be observed only in banded chromosomes or, in some cases, using molecular genetic approaches. Because these abnormalities generally involve the deletion of a series of adjacent genes, they are also sometimes called contiguous gene syndromes. ▲

Uniparental Disomy

As just mentioned, about 70% of Prader-Willi cases are caused by microdeletions. Most of the remainder have **uniparental disomy** (di = two), a condition in which one parent has contributed two copies of a chromosome and the other parent has contributed no copies. If the parent has contributed two copies of one homolog, the condition is termed **isodisomy.** If the parent

has contributed one copy of each homolog, it is termed **heterodisomy.** This phenomenon, only recently discovered in humans, can arise in a number of ways. For example, a trisomic conception can lose one of the extra chromosomes, resulting in an embryo that has two copies of the chromosome contributed by one parent. Disomy can also arise from a monosomic conception followed by mitotic nondisjunction, producing cells with two copies of the monosomic chromosome. Uniparental disomy, although fairly rare, has been observed in several conditions besides Prader-Willi and Angelman syndromes. These include cystic fibrosis (see Chapter 4) and the Beckwith-Wiedemann syndrome (see Chapters 4 and 14).

Duplications

A partial trisomy, or a **duplication**, of genetic material may be seen in the offspring of individuals who carry a reciprocal translocation. Duplications can also be caused by unequal crossover during meiosis, as described for the X-linked color vision loci (see Chapter 5) and Charcot-Marie-Tooth disease (see Chapter 3). Duplications tend to produce less serious consequences than deletions, again illustrating the principle that a loss of genetic material is more serious than is an excess of genetic material.

▼ Duplications can arise from unequal crossover or can occur among the offspring of reciprocal translocation carriers. Duplications generally produce less serious consequences than deletions. ▲

Ring Chromosomes

Deletions sometimes occur at both tips of a chromosome. The remaining chromosome ends can then

TABLE 6-3 Microdeletion Syndromes

Syndrome	Clinical features	Chromosomal deletion
Prader-Willi	Mental retardation, short stature, obesity, hypotonia, characteristic facies, small feet	15q11-13
Langer-Giedion	Characteristic facies, sparse hair, exostosis, variable mental retardation	8q24
Miller-Dieker	Lissencephaly, characteristic facies	17p13.3
DiGeorge anomaly/velo-cardio-facial	DiGeorge anomaly/characteristic facies, cleft palate, heart defect	22q11
Smith-Magenis	Mental retardation, hyperactivity, dysmorphic features, self-destructive behavior	17p11.2
Williams	Developmental disability, characteristic facies, supravalvular aortic stenosis	7q1
Aniridia/Wilms tumor	Mental retardation, aniridia, predisposition to Wilms tumor, genital defects	11p13

CLINICAL COMMENTARY 6-3
THE DIGEORGE ANOMALY,
THE VELO-CARDIO-FACIAL SYNDROME,
AND MICRODELETIONS OF CHROMOSOME 22

The DiGeorge anomaly consists of a pattern of structural or functional defects of the thymus, hypoparathyroidism (reduced parathyroid function), secondary hypocalcemia (decreased serum calcium), and conotruncal heart defects. This pattern is a malformation complex probably caused by an alteration of the embryonic migration of neural crest cells to the developing structures of the neck. In the 1980s it was learned that some children with the DiGeorge anomaly had a deletion of part of the long arm of chromosome 22, often related to an unbalanced translocation between this and another chromosome. This led to the hypothesis that genes on chromosome 22 were responsible for the DiGeorge anomaly. WWW

Independent of this work, a condition called the velo-cardio-facial (VCF) or Shprintzen syndrome was described in the late 1970s. This autosomal dominant syndrome involves palate (velum) abnormalities (including clefts), a characteristic facial appearance, and, in some cases, heart disease. In addition, these patients have learning disabilities and developmental delay. Later it was discovered that some individuals with VCF have dysfunctional T-cells (these cells mature in the thymus), and some have all features of the DiGeorge anomaly. This suggested that the DiGeorge anomaly was somehow related to VCF.

The resemblance between the DiGeorge anomaly and VCF led to the hypothesis that both conditions were caused by abnormalities on chromosome 22. High-resolution chromosome studies, including FISH, of patients with the DiGeorge anomaly and patients with VCF revealed small deletions of chromosome 22 in both groups. This analysis also helped to narrow the critical region that causes both conditions. Approximately 90% of infants with the DiGeorge anomaly have a microdeletion of the 22q11.2 region, and about 70% of VCF patients have the same microdeletion. In addition, 15% of individuals with isolated conotruncal defects exhibit this deletion. It is now postulated that alterations of a gene or genes in this region can produce a variable phenotype ranging from the DiGeorge anomaly to the full VCF syndrome. It is possible that the VCF syndrome is a contiguous gene syndrome, and the gene or genes causing the DiGeorge anomaly are a subset of those that cause VCF.

This example illustrates how cytogenetic studies can demonstrate potential biological relationships between genetic syndromes. Further studies are under way to identify the individual genes that cause the DiGeorge anomaly and VCF.

fuse, forming a **ring chromosome** (Fig. 6-20). The karyotype of a female with a ring X chromosome would be 46,X,r(X). If the ring chromosome includes a centromere, it can often proceed through cell division, but its structure can create difficulties. Ring chromosomes are often lost, resulting in monosomy for the chromosome in at least some cells (i.e., mosaicism for the ring chromosome may be seen). Ring chromosomes have been described in at least one case in each of the human autosomes.

Inversions

An **inversion** is the result of two breaks on a chromosome followed by the reinsertion of the missing fragment at its original site but in inverted order. Thus, a chromosome symbolized as ABCDEFG might become ABEDCFG after an inversion. When the inversion includes the centromere, it is called a **pericentric inversion**. Inversions not involving the centromere are termed **paracentric inversions**.

Like reciprocal translocations, inversions are a balanced structural rearrangement. Consequently, they seldom produce disease in the inversion carrier (recall from Chapter 5, though, that an inversion that interrupts the factor VIII gene produces severe hemophilia A). Inversions can interfere with meiosis, however, producing

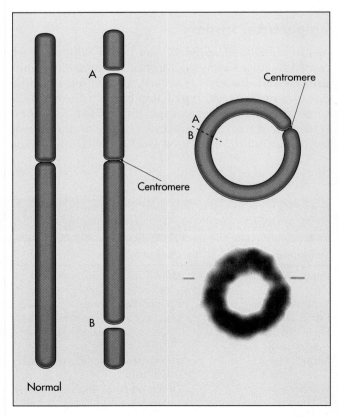

FIG. 6-20 Both tips of a chromosome can be lost, leaving sticky ends that attach to one another, forming a ring chromosome. A chromosome 12 ring is shown here.

chromosome abnormalities in the offspring of inversion carriers. Because chromosomes must line up in perfect order during prophase I, a chromosome with an inversion must form a loop to line up with its normal homolog (Fig. 6-21). Crossing over within this loop can result in duplications or deletions in the chromosomes of daughter cells. Thus, the offspring of individuals who carry inversions often have chromosome deletions or duplications. It is estimated that about one in 1,000 people carries an inversion and is therefore at risk for producing gametes with duplications or deletions.

Fig. 6-21 gives an example of a pericentric inversion that has occurred on chromosome 8 (46,XX,inv[8]). About 5% of the offspring of those who carry this inversion will receive a deletion or duplication of the distal portion of 8q. This combination results in the relatively well-described recombinant 8 syndrome. **WWW**

▼ Chromosome inversions are a relatively common structural abnormality and may be either pericentric (including the centromere) or paracentric (not including the centromere). Parents with inversions are usually normal in phenotype but can produce offspring with deletions or duplications. ▲

Isochromosomes

Sometimes a chromosome divides along the axis perpendicular to its usual axis of division (Fig. 6-22). The result is an **isochromosome**, a chromosome that has two copies of one arm and no copies of the other. Because the genetic material is substantially altered, isochromosomes of most autosomes are lethal. Most isochromosomes observed in live births involve the X chromosome, and babies with isochromosome Xq

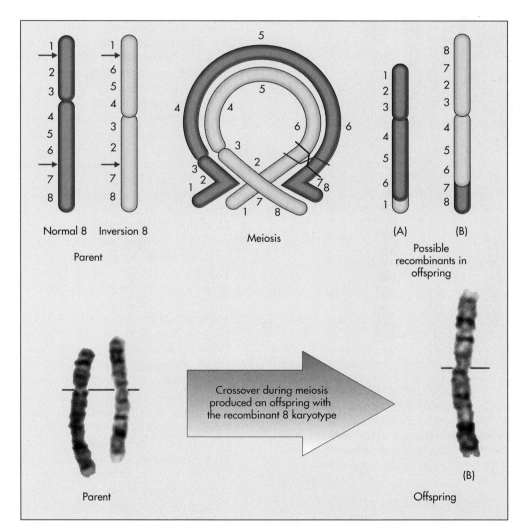

FIG. 6-21   A pericentric inversion in chromosome 8 causes the formation of a loop during the alignment of homologous chromosomes in meiosis. Crossing over in this loop can produce duplications or deletions of chromosome material in the resulting gamete. The offspring in the lower panel received one of the recombinant 8 chromosomes from this parent.

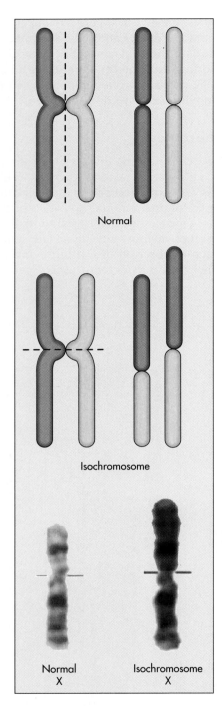

FIG. 6-22 An isochromosome is formed when a chromosome divides along an axis perpendicular to its usual axis of division. This produces one chromosome with only the short arms and another with only the long arms. A normal X chromosome is compared with an isochromosome of Xq.

(46,X,i[Xq]) usually have features of Turner syndrome. Isochromosome 18q, producing an extra copy of the long arm of chromosome 18, has been observed in infants with Edwards syndrome. Although most isochromosomes appear to be formed by faulty division, they

can also be created by Robertsonian translocations of homologous acrocentric chromosomes.

CHROMOSOME ABNORMALITIES AND CLINICAL PHENOTYPES

As we have seen, most autosomal aberrations induce consistent patterns of multiple malformations, minor anomalies, and phenotypic variations with variable degrees of developmental retardation. Although the individual features are usually nonspecific (e.g., simian creases can be seen in both Down syndrome and trisomy 18), the general pattern of features is usually distinctive enough to permit a clinical diagnosis. This is especially true of the well-known chromosome syndromes: Down syndrome, Edwards syndrome, Patau syndrome, and Turner syndrome. However, there is considerable phenotypic variability even within these syndromes. No one patient has every feature; most congenital malformations (e.g., heart defects) are seen in only some affected individuals. This phenotypic variability, and the attendant potential for misdiagnosis, underscores the need to order a karyotype whenever clinical features suggest a chromosome abnormality.

Usually, the biological basis for this phenotypic variability is unknown, although mechanisms such as mosaicism, which leads to milder expression, are being uncovered. The basis of variable expression of chromosome syndromes will be better understood as the individual genes involved in these abnormalities are identified and characterized.

In spite of the variability of chromosome syndromes, it is possible to make several generalizations:

1. Most chromosome abnormalities (especially those involving autosomes) are associated with developmental delay in children and mental retardation in older individuals. This reflects the fact that a large number of our genes, perhaps 30,000 or more, participate in the development of the central nervous system. Thus, a chromosome abnormality, which typically may affect hundreds or thousands of genes, is very likely to involve genes affecting nervous system development.

2. Most chromosome syndromes involve alterations of facial morphogenesis that produce characteristic facial features. For this reason the patient often resembles other individuals with the same disorder more than members of his or her own family. Usually the facial features and minor anomalies of the head and neck are the best aids to diagnosis (see Chapter 14).

3. Growth delay (short stature and/or poor weight gain in infancy) is commonly seen in autosomal syndromes.

4. Congenital malformations, especially congenital heart defects, occur with increased frequency in most autosomal chromosome disorders. These defects occur in specific patterns. For example, while AV canals and ventricular septal defects are common in children with Down syndrome, other congenital heart defects, such

as aortic coarctation or hypoplastic (underdeveloped) left ventricle, are seldom seen in these children but may be seen in those with Turner syndrome. The most common clinical indications for a chromosome analysis are the newborn with multiple congenital malformations or a child with developmental retardation. A summary of clinical situations in which a chromosome evaluation should be considered is given in Box 6-1.

Chromosome abnormalities typically result in developmental delay, mental retardation, characteristic facial features, and various types of congenital malformations. Despite some overlap of phenotypic features, many chromosome abnormalities can be recognized by clinical examination.

CANCER CYTOGENETICS

Most chromosome abnormality syndromes are caused by errors that occur in the meiotic process leading to gamete formation. Chromosome rearrangements in somatic cells are responsible for a number of important cancers in humans. The first of these to be recognized was a chromosome alteration seen consistently in patients with chronic myelogenous leukemia (CML). Initially, it was suggested that the chromosome alteration was a deletion of the long arm of either chromosome 21 or 22. With the subsequent development of chromosome banding techniques, the abnormality was identified as a reciprocal translocation between chromosomes 9 and 22. The **Philadelphia chromosome**, as this translocation is commonly known, consists of a translocation of most of chromosome 22 onto the long arm of chromosome 9. A small distal portion of 9q in turn is translocated to chromosome 22. The net effect is a smaller chromosome 22, which explains why the Philadelphia chromosome was thought to be a deletion. This translocation (Fig. 6-23) is seen in most cases of CML. **www**

Much has been learned about the effects of this translocation by isolating the genes that are located near the translocation **breakpoints** (i.e., the locations on the chromosomes at which the breaks occur preceding translocation). A proto-oncogene called *abl* is moved from its normal position on 9q to 22q. This alters the *abl* gene product, causing it to exhibit increased tyrosine kinase activity. This appears to bring about malignancy in hematopoietic cells (i.e., cells that form blood cells such as lymphocytes). In fact, the introduction of this altered gene into the bone marrow of normal mice causes them to develop malignancies, including CML.

A second example of a translocation that produces cancer is given by Burkitt lymphoma, a childhood jaw tumor that is quite common in equatorial Africa but rare elsewhere. In this case a reciprocal translocation involving chromosomes 8 and 14 moves the *myc* proto-oncogene from 8q24 to 14q32, near the immunoglobulin heavy chain loci (see Chapter 9). There is good evidence that transcription regulation sequences near

FIG. 6-23 A reciprocal translocation between chromosome 22 and the long arm of chromosome 9 (the "Philadelphia" chromosome). The occurrence of this translocation in hematopoietic cells can produce chronic myelogenous leukemia.

the immunoglobulin genes then activate *myc*, causing malignancies to form.

More than 100 different rearrangements involving nearly every chromosome have been observed in over 40 different types of cancer. Some of these are summarized in Table 6-4. In some cases, identification of the chromosome rearrangement leads to more accurate prognosis and therapy. Hence, the cytogenetic evaluation of bone marrow cells from leukemia patients is a routine part of diagnosis. Furthermore, identification and characterization of the genes that are altered in translocation syndromes is leading to a better understanding of carcinogenesis in general.

▼ Balanced translocations in somatic cells can sometimes cause malignancies by interrupting or altering genes or their regulatory sequences. ▲

CHROMOSOME INSTABILITY SYNDROMES

Several autosomal recessive disease conditions exhibit an increased incidence of chromosome breaks under specific laboratory conditions. These conditions, which are termed **chromosome instability syndromes**, include ataxia-telangiectasia, Bloom syndrome, Fanconi anemia, and xeroderma pigmentosum (see Chapter 2). Among Fanconi anemia patients, the frequency of breaks can be increased further when the chromosomes are exposed to certain alkylating agents. Patients with Bloom syndrome also have a high incidence of somatic cell sister chromatid exchange (exchange of chromosome material between sister chromatids; see Chapter 2). Each of these

TABLE 6-4 Specific Cytogenetic Changes Observed in Selected Leukemias and Solid Tumors

Condition	Most common chromosome aberration
Leukemias	
Chronic myelogenous leukemia	t(9;22)(q34;q11)
Acute myeloblastic leukemia	t(8;21)(q22;q22)
Acute promyelocytic leukemia	t(15;17)(q22;q11-12)
Acute non-lymphocytic leukemia	+8,−7,−5,del(5q),del(20q)
Solid Tumors	
Burkitt lymphoma	t(8;14)(q24;q32)
Ewing sarcoma	t(11;22)(q24;q12)
Meningioma	Monosomy 22
Retinoblastoma	del(13)(q14)
Wilms tumor	del(11)(p13)

syndromes is associated with a significant increase in cancer risk. All are thought to be the result of faulty DNA replication or repair, as discussed in Chapter 2.

▼ The chromosome instability syndromes all involve increased frequencies of chromosome breakage and an increased risk of malignancy. All are associated with defects in DNA replication or repair. ▲

STUDY QUESTIONS

1. Distinguish among haploidy, diploidy, polyploidy, euploidy, and aneuploidy.
2. Explain the uses and relative advantages of FISH, spectral karyotyping, and comparative genomic hybridization (CGH).
3. Describe three ways in which triploidy could arise.
4. Studies of karyotypes obtained by prenatal diagnosis at 10 weeks' gestation (chorionic villus sampling; see Chapter 13) reveal prevalence rates of chromosome abnormalities that differ from those obtained in karyotypes at 16 weeks' gestation (amniocentesis; see Chapter 13). Explain this.
5. Even though conditions like Down syndrome and Edwards syndrome can usually be diagnosed accurately by clinical examination alone, a karyotype is always recommended. Why?
6. Rank the following in terms of the risk for producing a child with Down syndrome:
   45-year-old female with no previous family history of Down syndrome
   25-year-old female who has had one previous child with Down syndrome
   25-year-old male carrier of a 21/14 Robertsonian translocation
   25-year-old female carrier of a 21/14 Robertsonian translocation
7. Females with the 49,XXXXX karyotype have been reported. Explain how this karyotype could occur.
8. A male with hemophilia A and a normal female produce a child with Turner syndrome (45,X). The child has normal factor VIII activity. In which parent did the meiotic error occur?
9. A cytogenetics laboratory reports a karyotype of 46,XY,del(8p) for one patient and a karyotype of 46,XY,dup(8p) for another patient. Based on this information alone, which patient is expected to be more severely affected?
10. Why do translocations in somatic cells sometimes lead to cancer?

SUGGESTED READINGS

Ashkenas J (1996) Williams syndrome starts making sense. Am. J. Hum. Genet. 59:756-761

Baty BJ, Blackburn BL, Carey JC (1994a) Natural history of trisomy 18 and trisomy 13. I. Growth, physical assessment, medical histories, survival, and recurrence risk. Am. J. Med. Genet. 49:175-188

Baty BJ, Jorde LB, Blackburn BL, Carey JC (1994b) Natural history of trisomy 18 and trisomy 13: II. Psychomotor development. Am. J. Med. Genet. 49:189-194

Carey JC (1992) Health supervision and anticipatory guidance for children with genetic disorders (including specific recommendations for trisomy 21, trisomy 18, and neurofibromatosis I). Pediatr. Clin. N. Am. 39:25-53

Cooper CS (1996) Translocations in solid tumors. Curr. Opin. Genet. Dev. 6:71-75

Ekong R, Wolfe J (1998) Advances in fluorescence in situ hybridization. Curr. Opin. Biotechnol. 9:19-24

Epstein CJ (1995) Down syndrome (trisomy 21). In: Scriver CR, Beaudet AL, Sly WS, Valle D (eds) The Metabolic Basis of Inherited Disease. Vol. 1. McGraw-Hill, New York, pp 749-794

Fisher JM, Harvey JF, Morton NE, Jacobs PA (1995) Trisomy 18: studies of the parent and cell division of origin and the effect of aberrant recombination on nondisjunction. Am. J. Hum. Genet. 56:669-675

Forozan F, Karhu R, Kononen J, Kallioniemi A, Kallioniemi O (1997) Genomic screening by comparative genomic hybridization. Trends Genet. 13:405-409

Guttenbach M, Engel W, Schmid M (1997) Analysis of structural and numerical chromosome abnormalities in sperm of normal men and carriers of constitutional chromosome aberrations: a review. Hum. Genet. 100:1-21

Hassold T, Hunt PA, Sherman S (1993) Trisomy in humans: incidence, origin and etiology. Curr. Opin. Genet. Dev. 3:398-403

Hassold TJ (1998) Nondisjunction in the human male. Curr. Top. Dev. Biol. 37:383-406

Heiskanen M, Peltonen L, Palotie A (1996) Visual mapping by high resolution FISH. Trends Genet. 12:379-382

Heng HHQ, Spyropoulos B, Moens PB (1997) FISH technology in chromosome and genome research. BioEssays 19:75-84

Hernandez D, Fisher EMC (1996) Down syndrome genetics: unravelling a multifactorial disorder. Hum. Molec. Genet. 5:1411-1416

Jacobs PA, Browne C, Gregson N, Joyce C, White H (1992) Estimates of the frequency of chromosome abnormalities detectable in unselected newborns using moderate levels of banding. J. Med. Genet. 29:103-108

Lahn BT, Page DC (1997) Functional coherence of the human Y chromosome. Science 278:675-680

Leana-Cox J, Pangkanon S, Eanet KR, Curtin MS, Wulfsberg EA (1996) Familial DiGeorge/Velocardiofacial syndrome with dele-

tions of chromosome area 22q11.2: report of five families with a review of the literature. Am. J. Med. Genet. 65:309-316

Ledbetter DH, Ballabio A (1995) Molecular cytogenetics of contiguous gene syndromes: mechanisms and consequences of gene dosage imbalance. In: Scriver CR, Beaudet AL, Sly WS, Valle D (eds) The Metabolic and Molecular Bases of Inherited Disease. Vol. 1. McGraw-Hill, New York, pp 811-839

Ledbetter DH, Engel E (1995) Uniparental disomy in humans: development of an imprinting map and its implications for prenatal diagnosis. Hum. Molec. Genet. 4:1757-1764

Lenhoff HM, Wang PP, Greenberg F, Bellugi U (1997) Williams syndrome and the brain. Sci. Am. 277(6):68-77

Lichter P (1997) Multicolor FISHing: what's the catch? Trends Genet. 13:475-479

MacDonald M, Hassold T, Harvey J, Wang LH, Morton NE, Jacobs P (1994) The origin of 47,XXY and 47,XXX aneuploidy: heterogeneous mechanisms and role of aberrant recombination. Hum. Molec. Genet. 3:1365-1371

Madan K (1995) Paracentric inversions: a review. Hum. Genet. 96:503-515

Robinson A, de la Chapelle A (1997) Sex chromosome abnormalities. In: Rimoin DL, Connor JM, Pyeritz RE (eds) Emery and Rimoin's Principles and Practice of Medical Genetics. Vol. 1. Churchill Livingstone, New York, pp 973-997

Saenger P (1996) Turner's syndrome. N. Eng. J. Med. 335:1749-1754

Sandberg A (1994) Cancer cytogenetics for clinicians. CA Cancer J. Clin. 44:136-159

Schafer AJ, Goodfellow PN (1996) Sex determination in humans. BioEssays 18:955-963

Schrock E, du Manoir S, Veldman T, Schoell B, Weinberg J, Ferguson-Smith MA, Ning Y, et al. (1996) Multicolor spectral karyotyping of human chromosomes. Science 273:494-497

Speicher MR, Ballard SG, Ward DC (1996) Karyotyping human chromosomes by combinatorial multi-fluor FISH. Nature Genet. 12:368-375

Spinner NB, Emanuel BS (1997) Deletions and other structural abnormalities of the autosomes. In: Rimoin DL, Connor JM, Pyeritz RE (eds) Emery and Rimoin's Principles and Practice of Medical Genetics. Vol. 1. Churchill Livingstone, New York, pp 999-1025

Therman E (1993) Human Chromosomes: Structure, Behavior, Effects. Springer-Verlag, New York

Witkin HA, Mednick SA, Schulsinger F, et al. (1976) Criminality in XYY and XXY men. Science 193:547-555

Yoon PW, Freeman SB, Sherman SL, Taft LF, Gu Y, Pettay D, Flanders WD, et al. (1996) Advanced maternal age and the risk of Down syndrome characterized by the meiotic stage of the chromosomal error: a population-based study. Am. J. Hum. Genet. 58:628-633

7

Biochemical Genetics: Disorders of Metabolism

Each of us is composed of a large number of complex molecules that are hierarchically arranged in space to form cells, tissues, organs, and ultimately a complete human being. These molecules are constructed from individual elements that may be synthesized endogenously and/or obtained from our environment. Once created, these molecules are not static. In fact, they are perpetually being synthesized, degraded, excreted, and sometimes recycled in a tightly choreographed metabolic dance.

Each metabolic process consists of a sequence of catalytic steps mediated by enzymes encoded by our genes. Usually, these genes are replicated with high fidelity, and enzymatic systems continue to work effectively from generation to generation. Occasionally, mutations reduce the efficiency of encoded enzymes to a level at which normal metabolism cannot occur. Such variants of metabolism were recognized by Sir Archibald Garrod at the turn of the century, based partly on his studies of alkaptonuria. Garrod recognized that these variants illustrated our "chemical individualities" and called these disorders "inborn errors of metabolism," thus setting the cornerstone for contemporary biochemical genetics.

Alkaptonuria (AKU) is a rare disorder in which homogentisic acid (HGA), an intermediate metabolite in phenylalanine and tyrosine metabolism (Fig. 7-1), is excreted in large quantities in urine, causing it to darken upon standing. Hence it was classically referred to as "black urine disease." Additionally, an oxidation product of HGA is directly deposited in connective tissues, resulting in abnormal pigmentation and debilitating arthritis.

Garrod proposed in 1902 that AKU was caused by a deficiency of the enzyme that normally splits the aromatic ring of HGA. Fifty years later, it was established that AKU is produced by a failure to synthesize homogentisate 1,2 dioxygenase (HGO). However, it was not until 1996 that the gene for AKU was cloned, based on homology to a gene encoding an HGO enzyme that was isolated from a fungus species. The coding region of *HGO* comprises 14 exons distributed over 60 kb of DNA. One of two missense mutations identified in *HGO* encodes a protein that shows no HGO activity when expressed in vitro. This indicates that AKU is caused by a loss-of-function mutation, confirming the hypothesis put forth by Garrod nearly a century ago.

> ▼ Almost all biochemical processes of human metabolism are catalyzed by enzymes. Variation of enzymatic activities among humans is common, and a minority of these variants cause disease. These concepts were introduced by Archibald Garrod and exemplified by his studies of alkaptonuria. ▲

VARIANTS OF METABOLISM
Prevalence of Metabolic Disease

More than 350 different inborn errors of metabolism have been described to date, and most of these are rare. Taken together, however, metabolic disorders account for a substantial percentage of the morbidity and mortality directly attributable to genetic disease (Table 7-1). Moreover, we are beginning to understand that different alleles can alter one's risk for many common diseases. For example, polymorphisms in the gene encoding angiotensinogen have been associated with heightened risks for hypertension and pre-eclampsia.*

The diagnosis of a metabolic disorder can be challenging (see Clinical Commentary 7-1); thus, the morbidity

---

*Pre-eclampsia is a disorder of pregnancy characterized by hypertension, excess excretion of protein in the urine, and excess fluid accumulation.

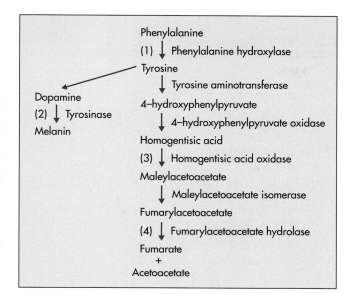

Phenylalanine
(1) ↓ Phenylalanine hydroxylase
Tyrosine
↓ Tyrosine aminotransferase
4–hydroxyphenylpyruvate
↓ 4–hydroxyphenylpyruvate oxidase
Homogentisic acid
(3) ↓ Homogentisic acid oxidase
Maleylacetoacetate
↓ Maleylacetoacetate isomerase
Fumarylacetoacetate
(4) ↓ Fumarylacetoacetate hydrolase
Fumarate
+
Acetoacetate

Dopamine
(2) ↓ Tyrosinase
Melanin

FIG. 7-1 Major pathway of phenylalanine metabolism. Different enzymatic defects in this pathway cause (1) classical PKU, (2) tyrosinase-negative oculocutaneous albinism, (3) alkaptonuria, and (4) tyrosinemias.

associated with metabolic defects is probably underestimated. In the 1970s many children were diagnosed with an often fatal acute metabolic encephalopathy called Reye syndrome. In the following decades, we learned that some children diagnosed with an encephalopathy indistinguishable from Reye syndrome had a urea cycle defect that produced hyperammonemia (increased levels of circulating ammonia) and death. Recognition of Reye syndrome as a **phenocopy** of a urea cycle defect is important because, in addition to supportive care,* the urea cycle defects are directly treatable. Similarly, on postmortem examination, some children who have died from sudden infant death syndrome (SIDS) have been found to have a defect of fatty acid metabolism. These are also treatable disorders, and life-threatening episodes can be avoided with appropriate care.

▼ Although individual metabolic disorders are rare, their overall direct and indirect contribution to morbidity and mortality is substantial. ▲

Inheritance of Metabolic Defects

Most metabolic disorders are inherited in an autosomal recessive pattern; only individuals having two mutant alleles are affected. Although a mutant allele produces reduced or no enzyme activity, it usually does not alter

*Supportive care is care that supports the elementary functions of the body, such as maintenance of fluid balance, oxygenation, and blood pressure, but is not aimed at treating the disease process directly.

the health of a heterozygous carrier. Since many of the genes encoding disease-related enzymes have been cloned and their mutations characterized, carrier testing and prenatal diagnosis for many metabolic disorders is available. However, testing samples of dried blood for elevated levels of metabolites in the newborn period (e.g., for phenylketonuria and galactosemia; see Chapter 13) remains the most commonly used population-based screening test for metabolic disorders. Unfortunately, most deaths caused by inborn errors of metabolism are due to enzyme variants that are not included in newborn screening programs. As the technology for rapid and efficient DNA testing of mutant alleles progresses, population-based screening for additional disorders is likely to be incorporated.

▼ Most inborn errors of metabolism are inherited in an autosomal recessive pattern. The carrier state is usually not associated with morbidity. Carrier and diagnostic testing are becoming widely available for many disorders. ▲

Types of Metabolic Processes

Metabolic disorders have been classified in many different ways, including: (1) the pathological effects of the pathway blocked (e.g., absence of end product, accumulation of substrate); (2) different functional classes of proteins (e.g., receptors, hormones); (3) associated co-factors (e.g., metals, vitamins); and (4) pathways affected (e.g., glycolysis, citric acid cycle). Each of these has advantages and disadvantages, and none of them encompasses all metabolic disorders. However, the classification that most completely integrates our knowledge of cell biology, physiology, and pathology with metabolic disorders categorizes defects of metabolism by the types of processes that are disturbed.

DEFECTS OF METABOLIC PROCESSES

Almost all biochemical reactions in the human body are controlled by enzymes, which act as **catalysts**. The catalytic properties of enzymes typically increase reaction rates by more than a millionfold. These reactions mediate the synthesis, transfer, utilization, and degradation of biomolecules to build and maintain the internal structures of cells, tissues, and organs. Biomolecules can be categorized into four primary groups: nucleic acids, proteins, carbohydrates, and lipids. The major metabolic pathways that metabolize these molecules include glycolysis, citric acid cycle, pentose phosphate shunt, gluconeogenesis, glycogen and fatty acid synthesis/storage, degradative pathways, energy production, and transport systems. We will discuss how defects in each of these metabolic pathways can cause human disease.

TABLE 7-1 Disorders of Metabolism

Name	Prevalence	Mutant gene product	Chromosomal location
Carbohydrate Disorders			
Classical galactosemia	1/35,000 to 1/60,000	Galactose-1-phosphate uridyl transferase	9p13
Hereditary fructose intolerance	Rare	Fructose 1,6-bisphosphate aldolase	9q13-q32
Fructosuria	~1/100,000	Fructokinase	2p23
Hypolactasia (adult)	Common	Lactase	2q21
Diabetes mellitus (type I)	1/400 (Caucasians)	Unknown	Polygenic
Diabetes mellitus (type II)	1/20	Unknown	Polygenic
Maturity onset diabetes of youth (MODY)	~1/400	Glucokinase (60%)	7p13
Amino Acid Disorders			
Phenylketonuria	1/10,000	Phenylalanine hydroxylase	12q24
Tyrosinemia (type 1)	1/100,000	Fumarylacetoacetate hydrolase	15q23-25
Maple syrup urine disease	1/180,000	Branched-chain α-ketoacid decarboxylase (multiple subunits)	Multiple loci
Alkaptonuria	1/250,000	Homogentisic acid oxidase	3q2
Homocystinuria	1/340,000	Cystathionine β-synthase	21q2
Oculocutaneous albinism	1/35,000	Tyrosinase	11q
Cystinosis	1/100,000	Unknown	17p
Cystinuria	1/7,000	SLC3A1 (type I)	2p
Lipid Disorders			
MCAD	1/20,000	Medium-chain acyl-CoA dehydrogenase	1p31
LCAD	Rare	Long-chain acyl-CoA dehydrogenase	2q34-q35
SCAD	Rare	Short-chain acyl-CoA dehydrogenase	12q22qter
Organic Acid Disorders			
Methylmalonic acidemia	1/20,000	Methylmalonyl-CoA mutase	6p
Propionic acidemia	Rare	Propionyl-CoA carboxylase	13q32; 3q
Urea Cycle Defects			
Ornithine transcarbamylase deficiency	1/70,000 to 1/100,000	Ornithine carbamyl transferase	Xp21
Carbamyl phosphate synthetase deficiency	1/70,000 to 1/100,000	Carbamyl phosphate synthetase I	2p
Argininosuccinic acid synthetase deficiency	1/70,000 to 1/100,000	Argininosuccinic acid synthetase	9q34
Energy Production Defects			
Cytochrome C oxidase deficiency	Rare	Cytochrome oxidase peptides	Multiple loci
Pyruvate carboxylase deficiency	Rare	Pyruvate carboxylase	11q
Pyruvate dehydrogenase complex (E_1) deficiency	Rare	Pyruvate decarboxylase, $E_1\alpha$	Xp22
NADH-CoQ reductase deficiency	Rare	Multiple nuclear genes	Multiple loci
Heavy Metal Transport Defects			
Wilson disease	1/50,000	ATP7B	13q14
Menkes disease	1/250,000	ATPase7A	Xq13
Hemochromatosis	1/200 to 1/500 (Europeans)	HFE	6p21

Carbohydrate Metabolism

Because of the many different applications that they serve in all organisms, carbohydrates are the most abundant organic substance on Earth. Carbohydrates function as substrates for energy production and storage, intermediates of metabolic pathways, and the structural framework of DNA and RNA. Consequently, carbohydrates account for a major portion of the human diet and are metabolized into three principal monosaccharides: glucose, galactose, and fructose. Galactose and fructose are converted to glucose before glycolysis. The failure to effectively utilize these sugars accounts for the majority of the inborn errors of human carbohydrate metabolism.

Galactosemia

The most common monogenic disorder of carbohydrate metabolism, transferase deficiency galactosemia (classical galactosemia) affects 1/55,000 newborns. It is caused by mutations in the gene encoding galactose-1-phosphate uridyl transferase (Fig. 7-2; *GAL-1-P uridyl transferase*). This gene is composed of 11 exons distributed across 4 kb of DNA, and approximately 70% of galactosemia-causing alleles contain a single missense mutation in exon 6. As a result of diminished GAL-1-P uridyl transferase activity, affected individuals cannot effectively convert galactose to glucose; consequently, galactose is alternatively metabolized to galactitol and galactonate (see Fig. 7-2). Although galactose and its metabolites accumulate in many tissues, the pathophysiology of classical galactosemia is not well understood.

The most common clinical signs of classical galactosemia include failure to thrive, hepatic insufficiency, cataracts (opacification of the lens of the eye) and developmental delay.* Long-term disabilities include poor growth, mental retardation, and ovarian failure in females. Newborn screening for galactosemia is widespread and commonly performed by measuring plasma GAL-1-P uridyl transferase activity from a dried drop of blood. Early identification affords prompt treatment, which consists largely of eliminating dietary galactose. This substantially reduces the morbidity associated with the acute effects of elevated levels of galactose metabolites. However, prospective dietary therapy has no effect on the prevalence of central nervous system disease or ovarian dysfunction in patients with classical galactosemia.

Galactosemia can also be caused by mutations in the genes encoding galactokinase and uridine diphosphate galactose-4-epimerase (UDP-galactose-4-epimerase; see Fig. 7-2). Deficiency of galactokinase is associated with the formation of cataracts but does not cause growth

---

*Developmental delay is the delayed attainment of age-appropriate motor, speech, and/or cognitive milestones; the outcomes of developmental delay range from normal to profound mental retardation.

FIG. 7-2 Major pathways of galactose metabolism. The most common enzymatic abnormality producing galactosemia is a defect of GAL-1-P uridyl transferase. Defects of galactokinase or UDP-galactose 4 epimerase are much less common causes of galactosemia.

failure, mental retardation, or hepatic disease. Dietary restriction of galactose is also the treatment for galactokinase deficiency. Deficiency of UDP-galactose-4-epimerase can be limited to red blood cells and leukocytes, causing no ill effects, or it can be systemic and result in symptoms similar to those of classical galactosemia. Treatment is aimed at reducing the dietary intake of galactose, but not as severely as in patients with classical galactosemia. This is because some galactose must be provided to produce UDP-galactose for the synthesis of some complex carbohydrates.

▼ Galactosemia is one of the most common inherited disorders of carbohydrate metabolism. Newborn screening for galactosemia is widespread. Early identification affords prompt treatment, which consists largely of eliminating dietary galactose. If untreated, children with galactosemia develop liver disease, poor growth, and mental retardation. Mutations in *GAL-1-P uridyl transferase* are the most common cause of galactosemia. ▲

Fructose

Three autosomal recessive defects of fructose metabolism have been described. The most common is a deficiency of fructokinase (Fig. 7-3), which results in asymptomatic fructosuria (presence of fructose in the urine). The molecular basis of fructokinase deficiency remains unknown.

In contrast, hereditary fructose intolerance (HFI) results in poor feeding, failure to thrive, hepatic and renal insufficiency, and death. HFI is caused by a deficiency of fructose 1,6 bisphosphate aldolase in the liver, kidney cortex, and small intestine. Infants and adults with HFI are asymptomatic unless they ingest fructose or sucrose (a sugar composed of fructose and glucose). Infants who

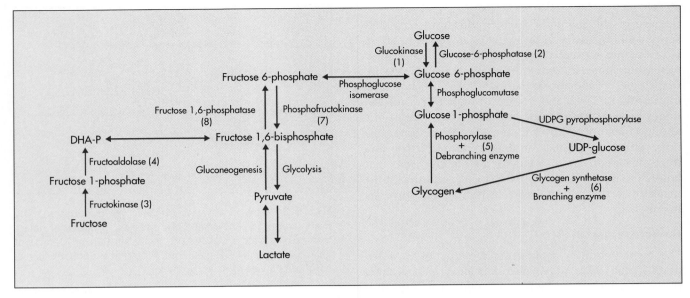

FIG. 7-3 Summary of glucose, fructose, and glycogen metabolism. Enzymatic defects in this pathway cause (1) hyperglycemia, (2) Von Gierke disease, (3) fructosuria, (4) hereditary fructose intolerance, (5) Cori disease, (6) Anderson disease, (7) Tarui disease, and (8) FDPase deficiency.

are breast-fed become symptomatic after weaning, when fruits and vegetables are added to their diet. Affected infants may survive into childhood because they avoid foods they consider noxious, thereby self-limiting their intake of fructose. The prevalence of HFI may be as high as 1/20,000, and, since the cloning of the gene encoding fructose-1 phosphate aldolase, differences in the geographic distribution of mutant alleles have been found.

Deficiency of hepatic fructose 1,6-biphosphatase (FDPase) causes impaired gluconeogenesis, hypoglycemia (reduced level of circulating glucose), and severe metabolic acidemia (serum pH less than 7.4) shortly after birth. If patients are adequately supported beyond childhood, growth and development appear to be normal. Although the gene encoding FDPase has been cloned, no mutations have yet been identified.

▼ **Asymptomatic deficiency of fructokinase is the most common defect of fructose metabolism. Hereditary fructose intolerance is less prevalent but associated with much more severe problems.** ▲

Glucose

Abnormalities of glucose metabolism are the most common errors of carbohydrate metabolism. However, the causes of these disorders are heterogeneous and include both environmental and genetic factors. Historically, disorders associated with elevated levels of plasma glucose (hyperglycemia) have been classified into three

categories: diabetes mellitus types 1 and 2 (DM type 1 and DM type 2) and maturity-onset diabetes of youth (MODY). DM type 1 is associated with reduced or absent levels of plasma insulin and usually presents in childhood. DM type 2 is characterized by insulin resistance and adult onset. A more detailed discussion of DM types 1 and 2 can be found in Chapter 12.

Substantial advances in our understanding of the pathophysiology of common diabetes have been achieved by identifying mutations that cause rare forms of hyperglycemia. Mutations in the insulin receptor gene have been associated with a disorder characterized by insulin resistance and acanthosis nigricans (hypertrophic skin with a corrugated appearance). These mutations may decrease the number of insulin receptors on a cell's surface or may decrease the insulin-binding activity level or insulin-stimulated tyrosine kinase activity level. Mutations in mitochondrial DNA and in the genes encoding insulin and glucokinase have also been associated with hyperglycemic disorders.

▼ **Studies of rare, monogenic forms of diabetes (abnormal glucose metabolism) define the pathways that may be disturbed in the more common form(s) of diabetes mellitus.** ▲

Lactose

The ability to metabolize lactose (a sugar composed of glucose and galactose) is dependent, in part, on the activity of an intestinal brush-border enzyme called lactase. In most mammals lactase activity diminishes after

TABLE 7-2   Glycogen Storage Disorders

Type	Defect	Major affected tissues
Ia (Von Gierke)	Glucose-6-phosphatase	Liver, kidney, intestine
Ib	Microsomal glucose 6-phosphate transport	Liver, kidney, intestine, neutrophils
Ic	Microsomal pyrophosphate transport	Liver, kidney, intestine
Id	Microsomal glucose transport	Liver
II (Pompe)	Lysosomal acid α-glucosidase	Muscle
IIIa (Cori)	Glycogen debranching enzyme	Liver, muscle
IIIb	Glycogen debranching enzyme	Liver
IV (Anderson)	Branching enzyme	Liver, muscle
V (McArdle)	Muscle phosphorylase	Muscle
VI (Hers)	Liver phosphorylase	Liver
VII (Tarui)	Muscle phosphofructokinase	Muscle

infants are weaned from maternal milk. However, the persistence of intestinal lactase activity is a common polymorphism in human populations, with a frequency ranging from 5% to 90%. The geographic distribution of persistent lactase activity is concordant with areas of high milk intake such as Northwestern Europe and certain parts of Africa. The persistent ability for adults to use dairy products as a source of Vitamin D may have had a selective advantage in these populations.

Restricted lactase activity is common in most tropical and subtropical countries. Individuals with restricted lactase activity may experience nausea, bloating, and diarrhea after ingesting lactose. Thus, in many regions where reduced lactase activity is prevalent, the lactose in dairy products is often partially metabolized (e.g., by lactobacilli in the preparation of yogurt) before consumption. The role of lactase restriction as a cause of abdominal pain and symptoms of irritable bowel syndrome is controversial.

Lactase activity is determined by at least two common alleles, with persistent lactase activity (*LAC*P*) dominant to restricted lactase activity (*LAC*R*). The gene encoding lactase on chromosome 2 has been cloned, although differences between *LAC*P* and *LAC*R* have not been found. Thus, differences between alleles may reflect pre- or post-translational modification. Mutations that abolish lactase activity cause congenital lactase deficiency and produce severe diarrhea and malnutrition in infancy. Such mutations are very rare.

Glycogen

Carbohydrates are most commonly stored as glycogen in humans. Consequently, enzyme deficiencies that lead to impaired synthesis or degradation of glycogen are also considered disorders of carbohydrate metabolism. Defects of each of the proteins involved in glycogen metabolism have been identified (Table 7-2). These cause different forms of glycogen storage disorders and are classified numerically according to the chronological order in which their enzymatic basis was described. The two organs most severely affected by glycogen storage disorders are the liver and skeletal muscle. Glycogen storage disorders that affect the liver typically cause hepatomegaly (enlarged liver) and hypoglycemia (low plasma glucose level). Glycogen storage disorders that affect skeletal muscle cause exercise intolerance, progressive weakness, and cramping. Some glycogen storage disorders can also affect cardiac muscle, causing cardiomyopathy and early death.

▼ **Each disorder of carbohydrate metabolism is uncommon, yet taken together these defects account for substantial morbidity. Early intervention can prevent severe disabilities and/or early death.** ▲

Amino Acid Metabolism

Proteins play the most diverse roles of the major biomolecules (e.g., providing mechanical support, coordinating immune responses, and generating motion). Indeed, nearly all known enzymes are proteins. The fundamental structural units of proteins are amino acids. Some amino acids can be synthesized endogenously (non-essential), while others must be obtained from the environment (essential). Many defects of the metabolism of amino acids have been described.

Hyperphenylalaninemias

Defects in the metabolism of phenylalanine (an essential amino acid) cause the hyperphenylalaninemias, some of the most widely studied of all metabolic defects. The hyperphenylalaninemias are disorders caused by mutations of the loci encoding components of the phenylalanine hydroxylation pathway (see Fig. 7-1). Elevated levels of plasma phenylalanine disrupt essential cellular processes in the brain such as myelination and protein synthesis, eventually producing severe mental retardation. Most cases of hyperphenylalaninemia are caused by mutations of *phenylalanine hydroxylase* (*PAH*) and produce classical phenylketonuria (PKU). More than 100 mutations have been identified in *PAH*, including substitutions, insertions, and deletions. The prevalence of hyperphenylalaninemia varies widely among ethnic groups, with PKU ranging from 1/10,000 in Caucasians to 1/90,000 in Africans. Less commonly, hyperphenylalaninemia is caused by defects in the synthesis of tetrahydrobiopterin, a co-factor necessary for the hydroxylation of phenylalanine, or by a deficiency of dihydropteridine reductase.

Treatment of most hyperphenylalaninemias is aimed at restoring normal blood phenylalanine levels by restricting dietary intake of phenylalanine-containing foods (Box 7-1). However, phenylalanine is an essential amino acid, and adequate supplies are necessary for normal growth and development. A complete lack of phenyl-

alanine is fatal. Thus, a fine balance must be maintained between providing enough protein and phenylalanine for normal growth and preventing the serum phenylalanine level from rising too high. Most children with PKU are maintained on a phenylalanine-restricted diet until they are teenagers, although some studies indicate that individuals benefit from lifelong treatment.

Hyperphenylalaninemia in a pregnant woman can cause an **embryopathy,** consisting of poor growth, congenital malformations, microcephaly, and mental retardation in the fetus (regardless of the fetus' genotype). Thus, it is important that women with PKU receive appropriate pregnancy counseling. Optimally, they should be following a low-phenylalanine diet at conception and throughout gestation. **WWW**

▼ Hyperphenylalaninemias are the most common defects of amino acid metabolism. Classical PKU is caused by mutations in phenylalanine hydroxy-

---

BOX 7-1
DIETARY MANAGEMENT OF INBORN ERRORS OF METABOLISM

The most important component of therapy for many inborn errors of metabolism is manipulation of the diet. This commonly includes restriction of substrates that are toxic such as carbohydrates (e.g., in galactosemia, diabetes mellitus), fats (e.g., in MCAD deficiency), and amino acids (e.g., in PKU, MSUD, urea cycle defects); avoidance of fasting; replacing deficient co-factors (e.g., B vitamins, carnitine); and/or utilizing alternative pathways of catabolism to eliminate toxic substances. Since many metabolic disorders are diagnosed in infants whose nutritional requirements change quickly (sometimes weekly), it is imperative to provide them with diets that provide adequate calories and nutrients for normal growth and development. Thus, the responsibility for maintaining a special diet begins with the parents of an affected child and shifts to the child when he or she is capable of managing independently. For most individuals with metabolic diseases, the use of a special diet is lifelong. This results in many unique challenges that are often unforeseen by families and care providers alike. Consequently, it is important that support and guidance be provided by clinical dietitians, gastroenterologists, psychologists, genetic counselors, and biochemical geneticists.

For example, newborns with PKU are fed a low-phenylalanine diet to prevent the effects of hyperphenylalaninemia on the brain. Breast milk contains too much phenylalanine (see Table 7-2) to be used as the only source of nutrients. Therefore, many infants are fed an expensive low-phenylalanine formula that is available only by prescription, a so-called medical food.* Small quantities of breast milk can be mixed with the formula, although the breast milk must be pumped and carefully titrated to avoid giving the infant

too much phenylalanine. Serum phenylalanine levels are measured frequently, and adjustments must be made to the diet to compensate for an infant's growth and varying individual tolerances for phenylalanine. These interventions may disrupt maternal-infant bonding and distort a family's social dynamics.

As a child with PKU grows older, low-protein food substitutes are introduced to supplement the formula (e.g., low-protein breads, pasta, etc.). To put this in perspective, consider that a 10-year-old child with PKU can eat 300 to 500 mg of phenylalanine per day. Thus, 3 or 4 slices of regular bread would meet a child's nutritional needs and dietary phenylalanine limit, because of the relatively high protein content of grains. Low-protein foods make the diet more substantive and varied. Indeed, 7 slices of low-protein bread contain the phenylalanine equivalent of 1 piece of regular bread. Yet, many of these foods have a taste, texture, and/or appearance that differs distinctively from foods containing normal amounts of protein.

The intake of many fruits, fats, and carbohydrates is less restricted (Table 7-3). However, phenylalanine is found unexpectedly in many food items (e.g., gelatin, beer). In fact, the Food and Drug Administration (FDA) requires manufacturers to label products containing aspartame (a

---
*U.S. Public law 100-290 defines a medical food as a food which is formulated to be consumed or administered enterally under the supervision of a physician and which is intended for the specific dietary management of a disease or condition for which distinctive nutritional requirements, based on recognized scientific principles, are established by medical evaluation.

lase. Hyperphenylalaninemias are treated by restricting dietary intake of phenylalanine-containing foods. ▲

Tyrosinemia

The amino acid tyrosine is the starting point of the synthetic pathways leading to catecholamines, thyroid hormones, and melanin pigments, and it is incorporated into many proteins. Elevated levels of serum tyrosine can be acquired (e.g., severe hepatocellular dysfunction) or may be the result of an inborn error of catabolism, of which there are several. Hereditary tyrosinemia type 1 (HT1) is the most common and is caused by a deficiency of fumarylacetoacetate hydrolase (FAH), which catalyzes the last step in tyrosine catabolism (see Fig. 7-1). Accumulation of FAH's substrate, fumarylacetoacetate, and its precursor, maleylacetoacetate, is thought to be mutagenic and toxic to the liver. Consequently, HT1 is characterized by renal tubular dysfunction, acute

episodes of peripheral neuropathy, progressive liver disease leading to cirrhosis, and a high risk of developing liver cancer (hepatocellular carcinoma). Management of HT1 includes supportive care, dietary restriction of phenylalanine and tyrosine, and liver transplantation. Liver transplantation can be curative.

More recently, administration of 2-(nitro-4-trifluoro-methylbenzoyl)-1,3-cyclohexanedione (NTBC), an inhibitor of an enzyme upstream of FAH (4-hydroxyphenylpyruvate dioxygenase), has produced marked improvement in children with HT1. Unfortunately, long-term use of NTBC does not prevent the development of liver cancer in a mouse model of HT1. A novel therapeutic approach involves using gene therapy (see Chapter 14) to create a substantial population of FAH+ hepatocytes in the HT1 mouse. Long-term stable expression of *FAH* was achieved by effectively repopulating the liver with FAH+ hepatocytes. Because some FAH- hepatocytes remain in these livers, it is unclear whether the risk

---

phenylalanine-containing sweetener) with a warning for individuals with PKU.

Teenagers with PKU sometimes have difficulty socializing with their peers because their dietary restrictions limit food choices at restaurants, sporting events, parties, etc. Adults with PKU must consume more medical food than they did during childhood due to their size and protein requirements (Fig. 7-4). Women with PKU must be on a severely restricted low-phenylalanine diet during pregnancy because hyperphenylalaninemia is a known teratogen (see text).

Inborn errors of metabolism are chronic diseases that are often treated by substantially modifying the diet. This may require considerable changes in lifestyle, precipitating financial and emotional hardships of which health care providers need to be aware.

TABLE 7-3   Phenylalanine Content of Some Common Foods

Food	Measure	Phenylalanine (mg)
Turkey, light meat	1 cup (1/2 cup)	1662
Tuna, water-packed	1 cup (1/2 cup)	1534
Baked beans	1 cup (1/2 cup)	726
Lowfat milk, 2%	1 cup	393
Soy milk	1 ounce	46
Breast milk	1 ounce	14
Broccoli (raw)	3 tablespoons (1 cup)	28
Potato (baked)	2 tablespoons (1 cup)	14
Watermelon	1/2 cup (1 cup)	12
Grapefruit (fresh)	1/4 fruit (1/2 fruit)	13
Beer	6 ounces (12 ounces)	11
Gelatin dessert	1/2 cup	36

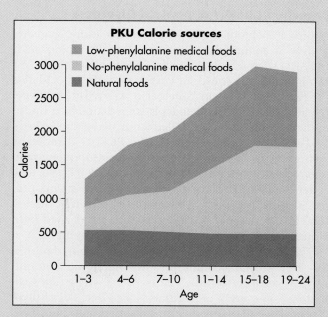

FIG. 7-4 Graph of the sources of calories of individuals with PKU at different ages. The amount of no-protein medical foods and low-protein medical foods eaten increases with age as the need for energy and protein increases.

(Courtesy Kathleen Huntington and Diane Waggoner, University of Oregon Health Sciences.)

of hepatocellular carcinoma is reduced. Gene therapy for HT1 has yet to be attempted in humans.

FAH has been cloned, and mutations have been identified in many families. A splice-site mutation is quite common in French-Canadians, and its high frequency is likely the result of founder effect (see Chapter 3). This mutation results in an in-frame deletion of an exon, which removes a series of critically important amino acids from FAH. Missense and nonsense mutations of *FAH* have also been found in families with HT1.

Tyrosinemia type 2 (oculocutaneous tyrosinemia) is caused by a deficiency of tyrosine aminotransferase. It is characterized by corneal erosions, thickening of the skin on the palms and the soles, and variable mental retardation. Tyrosinemia type 3 is associated with reduced activity of 4-hydroxyphenylpyruvate dioxygenase and neurological dysfunction, although only a few affected individuals have been reported.

▼ **Deficiency of fumarylacetoacetate hydrolase (FAH) is the most common cause of hereditary tyrosinemia type 1 (HT1). Accumulation of the substrates of FAH leads to neurological, kidney, and liver dysfunction. Although liver transplantation has been the cornerstone of treatment for HT1, the use of drugs that block the production of FAH substrates appears promising. ▲**

Branched-Chain Amino Acid Disorders

Approximately 40% of the pre-formed amino acids required by mammals are branched-chain amino acids (BCAAs) such as valine, leucine, and isoleucine. BCAAs can be used as a source of energy through an oxidative pathway that uses an α-ketoacid as an intermediate. Decarboxylation of α-ketoacids is mediated by a multimeric enzyme complex called branched-chain α-ketoacid decarboxylase (BCKAD). The BCKAD complex is composed of at least three catalytic components and two regulatory enzymes, which are encoded by six loci. A deficiency of any one of these five components produces a disorder known as maple syrup urine disease (MSUD), so named because the urine of affected individuals has an odor reminiscent of maple syrup.

The prevalence of MSUD in the general population is low, but MSUD is common in the Mennonite community of Lancaster county, Pennsylvania, where approximately 1 in every 7 individuals is a carrier. All of these carriers have the same disease-causing mutation of *E1α*, one of the loci encoding a catalytic component of BCKAD, and all are descendants of a couple who emigrated from Europe in the eighteenth century. This is another example of founder effect in a small, relatively isolated population (see Chapter 3).

Untreated patients with MSUD accumulate BCAAs and their associated ketoacids, leading to progressive neurodegeneration and death in the first few months of life. Treatment of MSUD consists of dietary restriction of BCAAs to the minimum required for normal growth. Despite treatment, episodic deterioration is common, and supportive care is required during these crises. Because increasing BCKAD levels by only a few percent can alter the course of disease substantially, gene therapy for MSUD is currently being investigated.

▼ **Maple syrup urine disease (MSUD) is caused by defects in branched-chain α-ketoacid decarboxylase. Accumulation of branched-chain amino acids (BCAAs) causes progressive neurodegeneration and death. Treatment of MSUD consists of restricting dietary intake of BCAAs to a minimal level. ▲**

Early detection of amino acid defects coupled with prompt intervention can prevent severe physical impairment and/or death. Moderate increases of enzyme activity can dramatically alter the course of some aminoacidopathies, making them good candidates for the use of somatic gene therapy.

Lipid Metabolism

Lipids (Greek, *lipos* or fat) are a heterogeneous group of biomolecules that are insoluble in water and highly soluble in organic solvents (e.g., chloroform). They provide the backbone for phospholipids and sphingolipids, which are components of all biological membranes. Lipids are also constituents of hormones; they act as intracellular messengers and serve as an energy substrate. Elevated serum lipid levels (hyperlipidemia) are common and result from defective lipid transport mechanisms. Errors of fatty acid (hydrocarbon chains with a terminal carboxylate group) metabolism are much less frequent. Characterizing errors of fatty acid oxidation has been a powerful approach for understanding the biochemical basis of lipid catabolism.

During fasting and prolonged aerobic exercise, fatty acids are mobilized from adipose tissue and become a major substrate for energy production in the liver, skeletal muscle, and cardiac muscle. Major steps in this pathway include the uptake and activation of fatty acids by cells, transport across the outer and inner mitochondrial membranes, and entry into the (β-oxidation spiral in the mitochondrial matrix (Fig. 7-5). Defects in each of these steps have been described in humans.

MCAD Deficiency

The most common inborn error of fatty acid metabolism results from a deficiency of medium-chain acyl-CoA dehydrogenase (MCAD). MCAD deficiency is characterized by episodic hypoglycemia, which is often provoked by fasting (Clinical Commentary 7-1). Commonly, a child with MCAD deficiency presents with vomiting and lethargy after a period of diminished oral

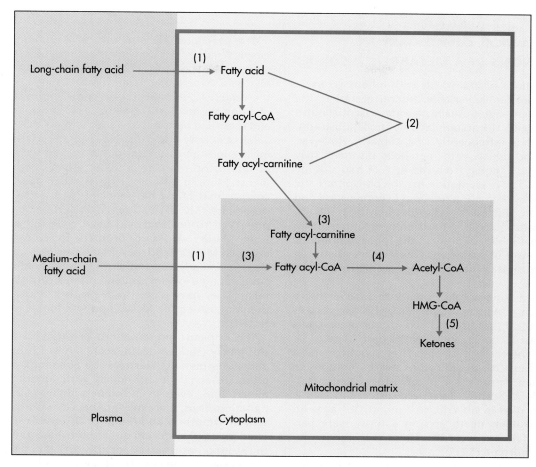

FIG. 7-5 Summary of fatty acid metabolism: fatty acid (1) entry into a cell, (2) activation and transesterification, (3) mitochondrial uptake, (4) oxidation via β-oxidation, and (5) formation of ketone bodies. Note that medium-chain fatty acids can traverse the mitochondrial membrane without carnitine-mediated transport.

intake due to a minor illness (e.g., upper respiratory illness, gastroenteritis). Fasting results in the accumulation of fatty acid intermediates, a failure to produce ketones in sufficient quantities to meet tissue demands, and the exhaustion of glucose supplies. Cerebral edema and encephalopathy result from the indirect and direct effects of fatty acid intermediates in the central nervous system. Death often follows unless a usable energy source such as glucose is provided promptly. Between these episodes, children with MCAD deficiency often have normal examinations. Treatment consists of providing supportive care during periods of nutritional stress, an adequate source of calories, and the avoidance of fasting.

To date, most of the reported MCAD patients are of Northwestern European origin, and 90% of their alleles have an A to G missense mutation that results in the substitution of glutamate for lysine. Additional substitution, insertion, and deletion mutations have been identified but are much less common. The molecular characterization of MCAD has made it possible to offer direct DNA testing as a reliable and inexpensive diagnostic tool. Furthermore, since MCAD deficiency appears to meet the criteria established for newborn screening (see Chapter 13), this test may be added to those already performed on all newborns in the United States (e.g., PKU testing).

LCHAD and SCAD Deficiency

Deficiencies of long-chain acyl-CoA dehydrogenase (LCAD) and long-chain 3-hydroxyacyl-CoA dehydrogenase (LCHAD) have been reported. LCAD-deficient patients may present with fasting-induced coma, hepatomegaly, cardiomyopathy, and hypotonia. They are initially treated similarly to individuals with MCAD deficiency. LCHAD deficiency can cause hepatic disease, cardiomyopathy, muscle weakness, and a peripheral neuropathy. Its clinical and biochemical characteristics clearly differentiate it from other fatty acid oxidation disorders. Short-chain acyl-CoA dehydrogenase (SCAD) deficiency has been described in only a few individuals, and its presentation is highly variable.

CLINICAL COMMENTARY 7-1
THE DIAGNOSIS OF A METABOLIC DISORDER

The presentations of individuals with inborn errors of metabolism are highly variable. During gestation, the maternal-placental unit usually provides essential nutrients and prevents the accumulation of toxic substrates. Thus, a fetus is infrequently symptomatic. However, after birth, individuals with metabolic disorders may present at ages ranging from the first 24 hours of life to adulthood. The presentation may be precipitous and characterized by dramatic alterations in homeostasis and even death. In contrast, the disorder may be insidious, with only subtle changes in function over long periods. For most metabolic disorders, the pre-symptomatic period and onset of symptoms is somewhere between these two extremes. The following case illustrates this point.

Anthony is a 9-month-old Hispanic male who comes to an emergency room accompanied by his parents. His parents complain that he has been irritable and vomiting for the last 36 hours, and over the past 12 hours he has become increasingly sleepy. They sought medical attention because it was difficult to awaken Anthony to breastfeed him. Anthony's medical history is unremarkable. He has a healthy 8-year-old sister and had a brother who died in his crib at 7 months of age. An investigation of his death and an autopsy were performed. The findings were consistent with sudden infant death syndrome (SIDS).

Anthony is hospitalized and noted to be hypoglycemic (low serum glucose level), slightly acidemic (serum pH <7.4), and hyperammonemic (elevated plasma ammonia). Intravenous infusion of glucose transiently improves his level of alertness, but he becomes comatose and dies 5 days later. An autopsy reveals marked cerebral edema (swelling of the brain) and fatty infiltration of the liver consistent with a diagnosis of Reye syndrome. Anthony's mother is concerned that the boys' deaths are related to each other, especially since she is pregnant again. She is counseled that the causes of death are unrelated and neither disorder is likely to recur in her family.

One year later her 6-month-old daughter, Maria, is hospitalized for the third time because of lethargy and weakness. Laboratory studies reveal moderate hypoglycemia, hyperammonemia, and ketonuria (ketones in the urine). Additional studies, including measurement of urine organic acids,* serum amino acids, and free and esterified plasma carnitines, suggest that Maria has a defect of fatty acid oxidation. Therapy is initiated with intravenous glucose, oral carnitine, and the restriction of fats to no more than 20% of her caloric requirements. More specific biochemical and molecular studies confirm that Maria has medium-chain acyl-CoA dehydrogenase (MCAD) deficiency. Molecular studies from preserved tissues that had been collected at autopsy from Maria's deceased brothers indicate that they also had MCAD deficiency. Maria's asymptomatic older sister is similarly affected. Both girls are healthy 2 years later, eating a low-fat diet and using a carnitine supplement. They have a new baby brother who underwent prenatal testing for MCAD and was found to be unaffected.

The disparate presentations of MCAD deficiency in this family (sudden death, acute illness, chronic illness, and asymptomatic) illustrate the phenotypic variability often observed in individuals with inborn errors of metabolism, even in individuals sharing an identical mutation. Thus, there may not be a disease-specific pattern of symptoms and findings. Often it is the heightened index of suspicion of care providers that leads to the testing necessary to identify a metabolic disorder. Supportive therapy can be lifesaving and should be initiated before making a diagnosis. Nevertheless, it is imperative that prudent attempts be made to make a specific diagnosis, as it may have important implications for the family (e.g., prenatal testing, presymptomatic therapy). The treatment of MCAD deficiency is completely effective at preventing early death from the toxic effects of accumulated fatty acid intermediates.

*Organic acids are carbon-based acids that are products of intermediate metabolism and normally do not accumulate in plasma or urine beyond the buffering capacities of these fluids.

▼ The clinical presentation of children with defects of lipid metabolism varies from slow deterioration to sudden death. MCAD deficiency is the most common of these disorders, and a direct DNA test has made widespread screening possible. Deficiencies in long-chain and short-chain acyl-CoA dehydrogenase have also been reported. ▲

Degradative Pathways

Most biomolecules are dynamic, perpetually being recycled as part of the normal metabolic state of a cell. Existing molecules are degraded into their constituents to produce substrates for building new molecules. Furthermore, the by-products of energy production, substrate conversions, and anabolism need to be processed and eliminated. Errors in these degradative pathways result in the accumulation of metabolites that would otherwise have been recycled or eliminated.

Lysosomal Storage Disorders

The lysosomal storage disorders are the prototypic inborn errors of metabolism: disease is a result of the

TABLE 7-4   Mucopolysaccharidoses*

Name	Mutant enzyme	Clinical features
Hurler/Scheie	α-L-Iduronidase	Coarse face, hepatosplenomegaly, corneal clouding, dysostosis multiplex,[†] mental retardation
Hunter	Iduronate sulfatase	Coarse face, hepatosplenomegaly, dysostosis multiplex
Sanfilippo A	Heparan-N-sulfamidase	Behavioral problems, dysostosis multiplex, mental retardation
Sanfilippo B	α-N-Acetylglucosaminidase	Behavioral problems, dysostosis multiplex, mental retardation
Sanfilippo C	Acetyl-CoA: α-glucosaminide N-acetyltransferase	Behavioral problems, dysostosis multiplex, mental retardation
Sanfilippo D	N-Acetylglucosamine-6-sulfatase	Behavioral problems, dysostosis multiplex, mental retardation
Morquio A	N-Acetylgalactosamine-6-sulfatase	Short stature, bony dysplasia, hearing loss
Morquio B	β-Galactosidase	Short stature, bony dysplasia, hearing loss
Maroteaux-Lamy	Aryl sulfatase B	Short stature, corneal clouding, cardiac valvular disease, dysostosis multiplex
Sly	β-Glucuronidase	Coarse face, hepatosplenomegaly, corneal clouding, dysostosis multiplex

*Hunter syndrome is an X-linked recessive disorder, while the remaining MPS disorders are autosomal recessive.
[†]Dysostosis multiplex is a distinctive pattern of bony changes including a thickened skull, anterior thickening of the ribs, vertebral abnormalities, and shortened and thickened long bones.

accumulation of substrate. Enzymes within lysosomes catalyze the stepwise degradation of sphingolipids, glycosaminoglycans (mucopolysaccharides), glycoproteins, and glycolipids. Accumulation ("storage") of undegraded molecules results in cell, tissue, and organ dysfunction. Most of the lysosomal disorders are caused by enzyme deficiencies, although some are caused by the inability to activate an enzyme or to transport an enzyme to a sub-cellular compartment where it can function properly. Many of the lysosomal storage disorders are found with uncommonly high prevalence in different ethnic populations as a result of founder effect, genetic drift, and possibly natural selection (see Chapter 3).

The mucopolysaccharidoses (MPS disorders) are a heterogeneous group of disorders caused by a reduced ability to degrade one or more glycosaminoglycans (e.g., dermatan sulfate, heparan sulfate, keratan sulfate, and chondroitin sulfate). These glycosaminoglycans are degradation products of proteoglycans found in the extracellular matrix. Ten different enzyme deficiencies cause six different MPS disorders, which share many clinical features (Table 7-4), but these disorders can be distinguished from each other by clinical, biochemical, and molecular analyses. Assays that measure enzyme activity in fibroblasts, leukocytes, or serum are available for each MPS disorder, and prenatal testing following amniocentesis or chorionic villus sampling (see Chapter 13) is possible. Except for the X-linked recessive Hunter syndrome, all of the MPS disorders are inherited in an autosomal recessive fashion.

All MPS disorders are characterized by chronic and progressive multisystem deterioration, which causes hearing, vision, joint, and cardiovascular dysfunction

(Fig. 7-6). Hurler, severe Hunter, and Sanfilippo syndromes are characterized by mental retardation, while normal cognition is observed in other MPS disorders.

Deficiency of iduronidase (MPS I) is the prototypic MPS disorder. It produces a spectrum of phenotypes that have been traditionally delimited into three groups: Hurler, Hurler-Scheie, and Scheie syndromes, which manifest severe, moderate, and mild disease respectively. MPS I disorders cannot be distinguished from each other by biochemical analysis; therefore, assignment of the MPS I phenotype is usually made using clinical criteria. The *iduronidase* gene has been cloned, and eventually genotype-phenotype correlations may lead to earlier and more accurate classification.

Hunter syndrome (MPS II) is caused by a deficiency of iduronate sulfatase. It is separated into mild and severe phenotypes based on clinical assessment. The onset of disease usually occurs between 2 and 4 years of age. Affected children develop coarse facial features, short stature, skeletal deformities, joint stiffness, and mental retardation. The gene for iduronate sulfatase is composed of 9 exons spanning 24 kb. Twenty percent of all identified mutations are large deletions, and most of the remainder are missense and nonsense mutations. **WWW**

▼ Defects of glycosaminoglycan degradation cause a heterogeneous group of disorders called mucopolysaccharidoses (MPS disorder). All MPS disorders are characterized by progressive multisystem deterioration causing hearing, vision, joint, and cardiovascular dysfunction. These disorders can be distinguished from each other by clinical, biochemical, and molecular studies. ▲

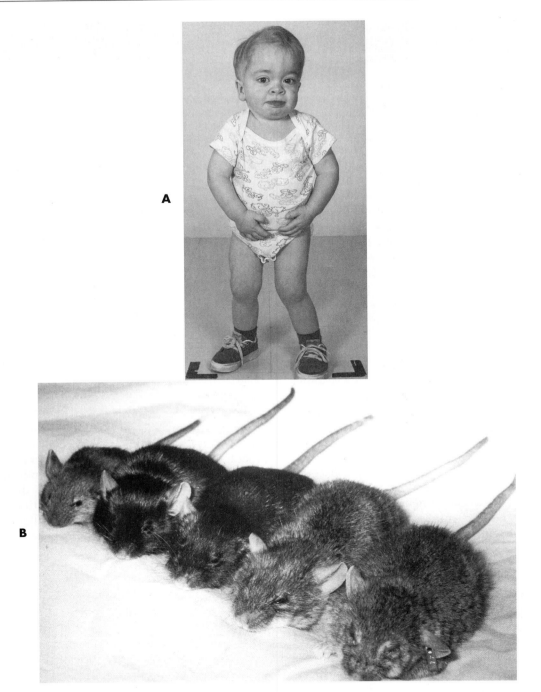

FIG. 7-6   A, A boy with a mutation in *α-L-iduronidase,* which causes Hurler syndrome. Note his coarse facial features, crouched stance, thickened digits, and protuberant abdomen. **B,** Transgenic mice with a targeted disruption of *α-L-iduronidase.* Progressive coarsening of face is apparent as 8-week-old mice *(left)* grow to become 52-week-old mice *(right).* (Courtesy Dr. Lorne Clark, University of British Columbia).

Defects in the degradation of sphingolipids (sphingolipidoses) result in their gradual accumulation, which leads to multiorgan dysfunction (Table 7-5). Deficiency of the lysosomal enzyme, acid β-glucosidase, causes accumulation of glucosylceramide and Gaucher disease. It is characterized by visceromegaly (enlarged visceral organs), multiorgan failure, and debilitating skeletal disease. There are three subtypes of Gaucher disease, and these can be distinguished by their clinical features. Type 1 is most common and does not involve

TABLE 7-5 Lysosomal Storage Disorders*

Name	Mutant enzyme	Clinical features
Tay-Sachs	β-Hexosaminidase (A isoenzyme)	Hypotonia, spasticity, seizures, blindness
Gaucher (type 1; non-neuropathic)	β-Glucosidase	Splenomegaly, hepatomegaly, bone marrow infiltration, brain usually spared
Niemann-Pick, type 1A	Sphingomyelinase	Hepatomegaly, corneal opacities, brain deterioration
Fabry	α-Glucosidase	Paresthesia of the hands and feet, corneal dystrophy, hypertension, renal failure, cardiomyopathy
GM1 gangliosidosis (infantile)	β-Galactosidase	Organomegaly, dysostosis multiplex,[†] cardiac failure
Krabbe	β-Galactosidase (galactosylceramide-specific)	Hypertonicity, blindness, deafness, seizures, atrophy of the brain
Metachromatic leukodystrophy (late-infantile)	Aryl sulfatase A	Ataxia, weakness, blindness, brain atrophy
Sandhoff	β-Hexosaminidase (total)	Optic atrophy, spasticity, seizures
Schindler	α-N-Acetylgalactosaminidase	Seizures, optic atrophy, retardation
Multiple sulfatase deficiency	Aryl sulfatases A, B, C	Retardation, coarse facial features, weakness, hepatosplenomegaly, dysostosis multiplex

*Of the lysosomal storage disorders included in this table, Fabry syndrome is X-linked recessive and the remainder are autosomal recessive.
[†]Dysostosis multiplex is a distinctive pattern of bony changes including a thickened skull, anterior thickening of the ribs, vertebral abnormalities, and shortened and thickened long bones.

the central nervous system. Type 2 is the most severe, often leading to death within the first 2 years of life. Type 3 Gaucher disease is intermediate between the other two forms.

Gaucher disease is rare, although the frequency of disease-causing alleles is more than 0.03 in Ashkenazi Jews. The most common allele is produced by an A to G mutation that results in a single amino acid substitution. DNA screening for the five most common Gaucher alleles detects 97% of all mutations found in this population.

Enzymes that function in lysosomes are targeted and transported into the lysosomal space by specific pathways. Targeting is mediated by receptors that bind mannose-6-phosphate recognition markers attached to the enzyme (i.e., a posttranslational modification). The synthesis of these recognition markers is deficient in I-cell disease (mucolipidosis II), so named because the cytoplasm of fibroblasts from affected individuals were found by light microscopy to contain inclusions. These inclusions represent partially degraded oligosaccharides, lipids, and glycosaminoglycans. As a consequence of recognition marker deficiency, newly synthesized lysosomal enzymes are secreted into the extracellular space instead of being correctly targeted to lysosomes. Individuals with I-cell disease have coarse facial features, skeletal abnormalities, hepatomegaly, corneal opacities, mental retardation, and early death. There is no specific treatment for I-cell disease.

Some of the lysosomal storage disorders may be amenable to treatment by exogenously supplied enzyme or restoration of endogenous enzyme activity by bone marrow transplantation or gene therapy. Children with Hurler syndrome who underwent bone marrow transplantation 2 to 7 years ago have demonstrated less mental deterioration than was expected. It remains to be seen whether these positive results will persist over an extended period. WWW

▼ Many different lysosomal enzymes catalyze the degradation of sphingolipids, glycosaminoglycans, glycoproteins, and glycolipids. Deficiency of a lysosomal enzyme causes accumulation of substrate, visceromegaly, organ dysfunction, and early death if untreated. Genes encoding many of the lysosomal enzymes have been cloned, and treatment with gene therapy is being tested. ▲

Urea Cycle Disorders

The primary role of the urea cycle is to prevent the accumulation of nitrogenous wastes by incorporating nitrogen into urea, which is subsequently excreted by the kidney. Additionally, the urea cycle is responsible for the de novo synthesis of arginine. The urea cycle consists of five major biochemical reactions (Fig. 7-7); defects in each of these steps have been described in humans.

Deficiencies of carbamyl phosphate synthetase (CPS), ornithine transcarbamylase (OTC), argininosuccinic acid

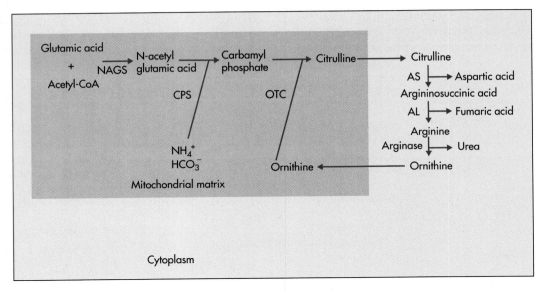

FIG. 7-7 Schematic diagram of the urea cycle. *AL,* Argininosuccinase; *AS,* argininosuccinic acid synthetase; *CPS,* carbamyl phosphate synthetase; *NAGS,* N-acetylglutamate synthetase; *OTC,* ornithine transcarbamylase.

synthetase (ASA), and argininosuccinase (AS) result in the accumulation of urea precursors such as ammonium and glutamine. Consequently, the clinical presentations of individuals with CPS, OTC, ASA, and AS deficiencies are similar, producing progressive lethargy and coma and closely resembling the clinical presentation of Reye syndrome. Affected individuals may present in the neonatal period or anytime thereafter, and there is wide intrafamilial and interfamilial variability in severity. In contrast, arginase deficiency causes a progressive spastic quadriplegia and mental retardation. Differentiation among these disorders is based on biochemical testing.

Each of these disorders, except OTC deficiency, is inherited in an autosomal recessive pattern. Although OTC deficiency is X-linked, women can be symptomatic carriers depending, in part, on the proportion of hepatocytes in which the normal allele is inactivated. The goal of therapy for each disorder is to provide sufficient calories and protein for normal growth and development while preventing hyperammonemia.

OTC deficiency is the most prevalent of the urea cycle disorders and thus has been intensively studied. The *OTC* gene contains 10 exons spanning approximately 85 kb and is located just proximal to *dystrophin* on Xp. A variety of exon deletions and missense mutations have been described. In addition, mutations that affect RNA processing have been observed.

▼ **The urea cycle consists of five major biochemical reactions that convert nitrogenous waste products to urea, which is subsequently excreted by the** **kidney. Enzymatic defects in this pathway lead to the accumulation of urea precursors, progressive neurlogical impairment, and death if untreated. The genes for most of these disorders have been cloned, including the most common observed defect, X-linked ornithine transcarbamylase (OTC) deficiency. ▲**

Energy Production

Energy for cellular activities can be produced from many different substrates such as glucose, ketones, amino acids, and fatty acids. Catabolism of these substrates requires their stepwise cleavage into smaller molecules (via processes such as the citric acid cycle or β-oxidation) followed by passage of hydrogen ions through the oxidative phosphorylation (OXPHOS) system. Alternatively, some substrates may be processed anaerobically.

The OXPHOS system consists of five multiprotein complexes that transfer electrons to oxygen. These complexes are composed of more than 100 polypeptides and are located in the inner mitochondrial membrane. Thirteen of these polypeptides are encoded by the mitochondrial genome (see Fig. 5-18), and the remainder are encoded by nuclear genes. Thus, assembly and function of the OXPHOS system require ongoing signaling and transport between the nucleus and mitochondrion. OXPHOS regulation is mediated by a wide variety of factors, including oxygen supply, hormone levels, and metabolite-induced transcription control.

More than 20 disorders characterized by OXPHOS defects are caused by substitutions, insertions, or deletions in the mitochondrial genome and are maternally inherited (see Chapter 5). However, nuclear genes that can cause mtDNA deletions or depletion of mtDNA have been isolated, and these disorders are inherited in an autosomal recessive pattern. Mutations in genes affecting the OXPHOS system produce very complex phenotypes as a consequence of the varying metabolic requirements of different tissues and systems at different developmental stages.

Electron transfer flavoprotein (ETF) and ETF-ubiquinone oxidoreductase (ETF-QO) are nuclear encoded proteins through which electrons can enter the OXPHOS system. Inherited defects in either of these proteins cause glutaric acidemia type II, which is characterized by hypotonia, hepatomegaly, hypoketotic or nonketotic hypoglycemia, and metabolic acidemia. Most affected individuals present in the neonatal period or shortly thereafter, and despite aggressive therapy, affected children often die within months.

In most tissues, the metabolism of pyruvate proceeds though pyruvate dehydrogenase, the citric acid cycle, and the OXPHOS system. However, in tissues with high glycolytic activity and a reduced or absent OXPHOS capacity, the end-products of metabolism are pyruvate and lactic acid (see Fig. 7-4). Lactate is produced by the reduction of pyruvate, and the bulk of circulating lactate is usually absorbed by the liver and converted to glucose. Defects in the pathways of pyruvate metabolism produce lactic acidemia. The most common of such disorders is a deficiency of the pyruvate dehydrogenase (PDH) complex. It may be caused by mutations in the genes encoding one of five components of the PDH complex: E_1, E_2, E_3, X-lipoate, or PDH phosphatase. These disorders are characterized by varying degrees of lactic acidemia, developmental delay, and abnormalities of the central nervous system. It has been suggested that the facial features of some children with PDH deficiency resemble those of children with fetal alcohol syndrome (see Clinical Commentary 14-6). It has also been proposed that acetaldehyde from the circulation of mothers with alcoholism inhibits PDH in the fetus, creating a phenocopy of PDH deficiency. **www**

▼ The phenotype produced by defects of energy metabolism is complex because of the varying oxidative demands of different tissues and organs. Once the condition is diagnosed, the goal of treatment is to utilize alternative pathways of energy production. ▲

Transport Systems

The efficient movement of molecules between compartments (e.g., organelles, cells, and the environment) and hence across a barrier, often requires a macromolecule that connects the compartments and mediates transport

through the barrier. Abnormalities of these transport systems have myriad effects, depending on whether altered barrier integrity or the accumulation of substrate has a greater impact on normal physiology.

Cystine is the disulfide derivative of the amino acid cysteine. Abnormal cystine transport can produce two diseases, cystinuria and cystinosis. Both disorders are inherited in an autosomal recessive fashion.

Abnormal cystine transport between cells and the extracellular environment causes cystinuria, one of the most common inherited disorders of metabolism. Although cystinuria produces substantial morbidity, early death is uncommon. Cystinuria is a genetically heterogeneous disorder caused by a defect of dibasic amino acid transport affecting the epithelial cells of the gastrointestinal tract and renal tubules. As a result, cystine, lysine, arginine, and ornithine are excreted in urine in quantities higher than normal. Cystine is the most insoluble of amino acids; therefore, elevated urinary cystine predisposes to the formation of renal calculi (kidney stones). Complications of chronic nephrolithiasis (presence of kidney stones) include infection, hypertension, and renal failure. Treatment of cystinuria is directed at reducing cystine production and excretion, altering the solubility of cystine, and converting cystine to a more soluble compound. This is accomplished by reducing methionine intake (cystine is produced from methionine), maintaining a well hydrated state, alkalinizing the urine, and using chelating agents such as penicillamine.

Based on amino acid excretion studies, cystinuria has been divided into 3 phenotypes. Type I cystinuria has been associated with missense, nonsense, and deletion mutations in a gene termed *soluble carrier family 3, member 1 amino acid transporter* (*SLC3A1*) on chromosome 2p. In vitro studies of mutant SLC3A1 protein have demonstrated a marked reduction in transport activity, providing direct evidence for the role of SLC3A1 in type I cystinuria. Types II and III cystinuria have been mapped to a locus on chromosome 19q13, but the gene has not yet been cloned.

Cystinosis is a rare disorder caused by a diminished ability to transport cystine across the lysosomal membrane. This produces an accumulation of cystine crystals in the lysosomes of most tissues. Affected individuals are normal at birth but develop electrolyte disturbances, corneal crystals, rickets, and poor growth by the age of 1 year. Renal glomerular damage is severe enough to necessitate dialysis or transplantation within the first decade of life. Transplanted kidneys function normally, but chronic complications such as diabetes mellitus, pancreatic insufficiency, hypogonadism, myopathy, and blindness occur. Until recently, treatment was largely supportive, including renal transplantation. However, cysteine-depleting agents such as cysteamine have proven successful in slowing renal deterioration and improving growth. A novel gene encoding an integral membrane protein was recently found to be mutated in individuals with cystinosis.

▼ The phenotype of transport defects is partly contingent on the degree of barrier disruption as well as the compartments through which normal traffic is compromised. Abnormal cystine transport between cells and the extracellular environment causes cystinuria, renal disease, and hypertension. Cystinosis is produced by a defect of cystine transport between cytoplasm and lysosome, leading to severe chronic disabilities and, if untreated, death. ▲

Many of the enzymes controlling metabolic processes require additional factors (**co-factors**) to function properly and efficiently. These co-factors are commonly trace elements such as ions of heavy metals (metals that are more dense than those in the first two groups of the periodic table). There are at least 12 trace elements that are essential to humans. For example, a zinc ion acts as a co-factor in carbonic anhydrase, placing a hydroxide ion next to carbon dioxide to facilitate the formation of bicarbonate. Although an adequate supply of trace elements is critical for normal metabolism, excessive amounts of circulating and/or stored heavy metals are highly toxic. Accordingly, a complex series of transport and storage proteins precisely control heavy metal homeostasis. Abnormalities of these proteins cause progressive dysfunction of various organs, often leading to premature death if untreated. Human disorders that disrupt the normal homeostasis of copper (Wilson disease, Menkes disease, occipital horn syndrome), iron (hereditary hemochromatosis; see Clinical Commentary 7-2), and zinc (hereditary acrodermatitis enteropathica) have been described.

Defective biliary excretion of copper and reduced incorporation of copper into ceruloplasmin (the most abundant copper protein in plasma) cause the progressive liver disease and neurological abnormalities seen in Wilson disease (WND). This autosomal recessive disorder was first described by Kinnear Wilson in 1912 and was called hepatolenticular degeneration because of end-stage destruction of the liver and brain. It remained unknown until the 1940s that these findings were due to the accumulation of copper. Further progress in understanding the defect underlying WND did not occur until the 1990s.

Patients with WND usually present with acute or chronic liver disease in childhood. If untreated, the liver disease is progressive, resulting in liver insufficiency, cirrhosis, and failure. Adults commonly develop neurological symptoms such as dysarthria (the inability to correctly articulate words) and diminished coordination. Accumulation of copper can also cause arthropathy (inflammation of the joints), cardiomyopathy (abnormal

function of the heart muscle), kidney damage, and hypoparathyroidism (diminished secretion of or response to parathormone). Deposition of copper in Descemet's membrane (at the limbus of the cornea) produces a characteristic finding in the eye (the Kayser-Fleischer ring), which is observed in 95% of WND patients and 100% of WND patients with neurological symptoms.

Biochemical testing can be used to confirm the diagnosis of WND. Findings include decreased serum ceruloplasmin, increased serum non-ceruloplasmin copper, increased urinary copper excretion, and increased deposition of copper in the liver. The most sensitive indicator of WND is the reduced incorporation of isotopes of copper into cells cultured in vitro. Treatment of WND consists of reducing the load of accumulated copper using chelating agents such as penicillamine and ammonium tetrathiomolybdate.

Menkes disease (MND) is an X-linked recessive disorder described in 1962 by John Menkes, who studied five male siblings, all of whom died before 3 years of age. MND is characterized by mental retardation, seizures, hypothermia, twisted and hypopigmented hair (pili torti), loose skin, arterial rupture, and death in early childhood. In MND patients copper can be absorbed by the gastrointestinal epithelium but cannot be exported from these cells. Consequently, when the intestinal cells slough, the trapped copper is excreted from the body. The lack of available copper leads to impaired enzyme function. Thus, in contrast to Wilson disease, in which excess copper causes disease, Menkes disease results from a lack of copper. Copper is a required co-factor in tyrosinase, lysyl oxidase, superoxide dismutase, cytochrome c oxidase, and dopamine beta-hydroxylase, explaining the major clinical features of MND. For example, lysyl oxidase is required for cross-linking collagen and elastin; therefore, ineffectual cross-linking leads to weakened vascular walls and laxity of the skin.

Treatment of MND consists of restoring copper levels in the body to normal. Since copper cannot be absorbed via the gastrointestinal tract in MND patients, it must be administered by an alternative route such as subcutaneous injections. Patients treated this way have demonstrated some clinical improvement. However, none of the abnormalities is completely corrected or prevented. Based on studies in an animal model of MND, the brindled mouse, it has been proposed that treatment for MND would be most effective if it were started in mid-gestation. Consequently, prenatal therapy is being investigated.

In 1993 the gene causing MND, *ATPase7A*, was cloned. It encodes an ATPase with six tandem copies of a heavy-metal-binding sequence homologous to previously identified bacterial proteins that confer resistance to toxic heavy metals. The high sequence conservation between human and bacterial binding sequences

CLINICAL COMMENTARY 7-2
HEREDITARY HEMOCHROMATOSIS

Hereditary hemochromatosis (HH) is an autosomal recessive disorder of iron metabolism in which excessive iron accumulates in a variety of organs such as the liver, kidney, heart, joints, and pancreas. It was described by von Recklinghausen, the same physician who described NF1, in 1889. Approximately 1/8 Northern Europeans is a carrier for HH, and 1/200 to 1/400 individuals is a homozygote. Thus, it is one of the most common genetic disorders observed in Caucasians. The prevalence of HH is substantially lower in Asian and African populations.

HH exhibits delayed age of onset, with a presymptomatic period of 40 years or more in males. Women commonly develop symptoms 20 years or so later than men because accumulation of iron in women is tempered by iron losses during menstruation, gestation, and lactation. The most common symptom of HH is fatigue, although the clinical presentation of patients with HH can vary considerably. Additional findings include joint pain, diminished libido, diabetes, increased skin pigmentation, cardiomyopathy, liver enlargement, and cirrhosis. Abnormal serum iron parameters can identify most men at risk for iron overload, but many pre-menopausal women may not be detected. The most sensitive diagnostic test for HH is a liver biopsy accompanied by histochemical staining for hemosiderin (a form of stored iron) (Fig. 7-8).

Treatment of HH consists of reducing the accumulated iron. This is accomplished by serial phlebotomy or the use of an iron-chelating agent such as deferoxamine. Depending on the quantity of iron stored, a return to a normal level of iron may take a few years. However, iron reduction prevents further liver damage, cures the cardiomyopathy, returns skin pigmentation to normal, and may improve the diabetes. Individuals who have not developed irreversible liver damage have a nearly normal life expectancy. Thus, there is a clear benefit to presymptomatic testing and early reduction of stored iron.

As early as the 1970s, an increased frequency of the HLA-A3 allele in HH patients indicated that an HH gene might be located near the major histocompatibility locus (MHC) on chromosome 6p. Subsequent linkage studies confirmed this hypothesis in the late 1970s, but it was not until 1996 that the HH gene was cloned. The HH gene is a widely expressed HLA Class I–like gene, designated *HFE*. A single missense mutation that results in the substitution of a tyrosine for cysteine in a putative β_2-microglobulin–binding domain is found on the majority of HH chromosomes. A single ancestral haplotype predominates in Caucasians, suggesting there was a selective advantage conferred by having at least one copy of the HH gene. Since iron deficiency affects one third of the world's population and is significantly less common in HH heterozygotes, it is likely that this explains the higher frequency of HH in many populations.

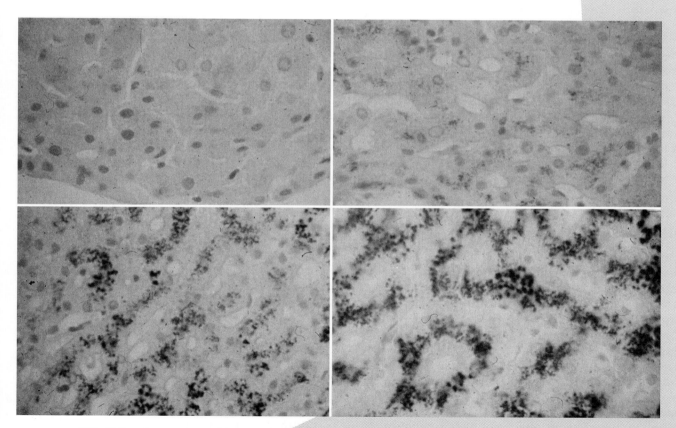

FIG. 7-8   Comparison of hemosiderin stain of normal liver *(upper left)* with hemosiderin stain of livers from individuals affected with hemochromatosis *(upper right, lower right,* and *lower left)*. Note the varying degree of increased deposition of hemosiderin livers of HH homozygotes. This damages the liver, impairs its function, and can lead to cirrhosis and liver cancer.

indicated that *ATPase7A* had an important role in regulating heavy-metal ion transport. *ATPase7A* was expressed in a variety of tissues but not the liver, suggesting that a similar gene that is expressed in the liver might cause WND. Portions of the *ATPase7A* gene were used as a probe to test for the presence of a similar gene on chromosome 13 (the known location of a WND gene, revealed by linkage analysis). This strategy led to the cloning of the gene for WND *(ATPase7B)* in 1993. The protein product is highly homologous (76% amino acid homology) to *ATPase7A*. In contrast to *ATPase7A*, *ATP7B* is expressed predominantly in the liver, kidney, and placenta, the major sites of involvement in WND based on clinical and biochemical data.

A variety of missense, nonsense, and splice site mutations in *ATPase7A* have been found in MND patients. Approximately 15% to 20% of the mutations in *ATPase7A* are large deletions. Several mutations in *ATPase7A* have been associated with another disorder called the occipital horn syndrome (OHS), which is characterized by mild mental retardation, bladder and ureteric diverticula (cul-de-sac-like herniations through the wall), skin and joint laxity, and ossified occipital (the most posterior bone of the calvarium) horns. More than 40 different mutations (mostly missense and small deletions) have been identified that alter the expression of *ATP7B* in patients with WND. **www**

▼ Wilson disease (WND) is an autosomal recessive disorder characterized by progressive liver disease and neurological abnormalities. Menkes disease (MND) is an X-linked recessive disorder characterized by mental retardation, seizures, and death in early childhood. Accumulation of excess copper causes disease in WND, while MND results from a lack of copper and impaired enzyme function. WND and MND are caused by mutations in the highly homologous genes, *ATP7B* and *ATP7A*, respectively. ▲

PHARMACOGENETICS

We often consider errors of metabolism only as deficiencies of enzymes required for metabolism of nutrients and endogenously synthesized molecules. However, many of the drinks and foods that we ingest each day (e.g., coffee) contain thousands of complex compounds that must be processed. Some of these compounds never leave the gastrointestinal tract, but most undergo biotransformation to a variety of products that are utilized immediately, stored, or excreted. Pharmaceuticals are exogenously synthesized compounds that are administered to achieve a specific effect on the human body. Humans vary substantially in terms of their metabolism of these exogenously synthesized compounds. The study of the genetic modification of human responses to pharmacological agents is called **pharmacogenetics**.

The effects of variation of drug metabolizing enzymes can be found in all ethnic groups and in a variety of pharmaceuticals. A deficiency of glucose-6-phosphate dehydrogenase (G6PD) causes increased sensitivity to the anti-malarial drug, primaquine, producing an acute hemolytic anemia. The slow metabolism of isoniazid (a drug commonly used to treat tuberculosis) is caused by a hepatic acetylation polymorphism. Reduced activity of plasma cholinesterases can produce an abnormal prolongation of the effects of succinylcholine (a neuromuscular relaxant). In each of these examples, the exposure of an individual having a common enzyme polymorphism to a specific chemical produces an unanticipated pharmacological effect.

More recently, polymorphisms in enzymes that produce a much broader effect on the body's response to many different pharmaceuticals have been described. An example of such an enzyme is debrisoquine hydroxylase, CYP2D6, an isozyme of the microsomal cytochrome P450 monooxygenase system. The cytochrome P450 superfamily includes genes that encode many different membrane-bound hemoproteins. These enzymes are responsible for the biotransformation of compounds with widely divergent structures. At least nine polymorphisms of CYP2D6 affect the metabolism of more than 30 different pharmaceuticals, including β-adrenergic receptor antagonists, neuroleptics, and tricyclic antidepressants. The gene encoding CYP2D6 is located in a cluster of CYP2D genes in a contiguous 45-kb region of chromosome 22. Each cluster contains between two and four genes composed of nine exons, yet only *CYP2D6* is expressed, as the others appear to be pseudogenes. Frequencies of *CYP2D6* polymorphisms differ widely among ethnic groups.

Although polymorphisms that alter drug metabolism warrant further investigation, the primary issue is whether these variants affect the clinical management of patients. This point is somewhat controversial among many scientists and physicians; consequently, only general guidelines for determining the clinical relevance of a variant that alters drug metabolism, not specific recommendations, are available as of yet. A pharmacogenetic variant may be important if (1) the drug is widely used in clinical practice, (2) the drug's therapeutic and toxic effects are difficult to assess and titrate clinically, and (3) the fate of the active agent is largely dependent on the variant pathway. To date, there is no estimate of how many drug/polymorphism combinations meet these criteria, although most pharmaceuticals are effective and well tolerated in many people.

▼ Each individual's response to natural and synthetic chemicals is partly determined by polymorphisms in genes controlling drug-metabolizing pathways. Most responses produce only minor variations from normal, while others precipitate dramatic deviations. ▲

STUDY QUESTIONS

1. Garrod found alkaptonuria to be more common in the offspring of consanguineous matings. Explain this finding. In general, what is the association between the coefficient of relationship and the prevalence of an inborn error of metabolism?

2. If many metabolic reactions can proceed in the absence of an enzyme, explain how diminished or absent enzyme activity can produce disease.

3. Despite the low prevalence of most metabolic disorders, why is it important to understand the pathogenesis of inborn errors of metabolism?

4. Describe 3 types of metabolic processes and give examples of disorders disturbing each of them.

5. A 1-week-old neonate is diagnosed with galactosemia, yet enzymatic activity of GAL-1-P uridyl transferase is normal. Interpret these results and explain how mutations of different genes can produce a similar phenotype.

6. The prevalence of PKU varies from 1/10,000 to more than 1/100,000. Explain how prevalence rates of inborn errors of metabolism can vary so widely among different ethnic groups.

7. An 18-year-old woman comes to your office for prenatal counseling. She had a younger brother who died from a defect of mitochondrial fatty acid oxidation when he was a few months old. What is her risk of having an affected child? Explain your answer.

8. An 8-year-old girl develops hyperammonemia and is critically ill. Biochemical testing performed on a liver biopsy confirms that she has OTC deficiency. Which genetic test would you order next? Why?

9. Disorders of the OXPHOS system are commonly associated with elevated blood lactic acid levels. Explain this finding.

10. Polymorphisms that affect drug metabolism presumably have been maintained by selection because they offer heterozygotes a slight advantage. Provide an example of how these polymorphisms may have been advantageous to a group of hunter-gatherers 10,000 years ago.

SUGGESTED READINGS

Beutler E (1997) Gaucher disease. Curr. Opin. Hematol. 4:19-23

Bulaj ZJ, Griffen LM, Jorde LB, Edwards CE, Kushner JP (1996) Clinical and biochemical abnormalities in people heterozygous for hemochromatosis. N. Eng. J. Med. 335:1799-1805

Bull PC, Cox DW (1994) Wilson disease and Menkes disease: new handles on heavy-metal transport. Trends Genet. 10:246-252

Feder JN, Gnirke A, Thomas W, Tsuchihashi Z, et al (1996) A novel MHC class-I-like gene is mutated in patients with hereditary hemochromatosis. Nat. Genet. 13:399-408

Fernández-Cañón JM, Granadino B, Beltrán-Valero de Bernabé D, et al (1996) The molecular basis of alkaptonuria. Nat. Genet. 14:19-24

Iafolla AK, Thompson RJ, Roe CR (1994) Medium-chain acyl-CoA dehydrogenase deficiency: clinical course in 120 affected children. J. Peds. 124:409-415

Leonard CO, Nuttall KL (1997) Testing for inborn errors of metabolism in the acutely ill newborn. Ann. Clin. Lab. Sci. 27:34-40

Overturf K, Al-Dhalimy M, Tanguay R, et al (1996) Hepatocytes corrected by gene therapy are selected in vivo in a murine model of hereditary tyrosinemia type 1. Nat. Genet. 12:266-273

Petry KG, Reichardt JKV (1998) The fundamental importance of human galactose metabolism: lessons from genetics and biochemistry. Trends Genet. 14:98-102

Schweitzer S, Shin Y, Jakobs C, Bradehl J (1993) Long term outcome in 134 patients with galactosemia. Eur. J. Ped. 152:36-43

Scriver CR, Eisensmith RC, Woo SLC, Kaufman S (1994) The hyperphenylalaninemias of man and mouse. Annu. Rev. Genet. 28:141-165

Scriver CR, Beaudet AL, Sly WS, Valle D (eds) (1996) The Metabolic and Molecular Bases of Inherited Disease, 1996, McGraw-Hill, New York

8

Gene Mapping and Cloning

The mapping of genes to specific locations on chromosomes is a central focus of medical genetics. Dramatic advances in molecular genetic technology, coupled with important developments in the statistical analysis of genetic data, have greatly increased the rate at which genes are being mapped (Fig. 8-1). Currently, more than 6,000 genes have been assigned to chromosome locations. While this is an admirable rate of progress, this number represents only a small fraction of the estimated 50,000 to 100,000 genes that exist within the human genome. Clearly, a great deal of work remains to be done. One goal of the Human Genome Project (see Box 8-3) is to map all of our genes to specific chromosome locations. As this work progresses, our understanding of the biological basis of genetic disease will surely progress as well.

Gene mapping is an important step in the understanding, diagnosis, and eventual treatment of a genetic disease. When a disease gene's location is pinpointed, it is often possible to provide a more accurate prognosis for individuals at risk for a genetic disease. Locating a disease gene is usually the first step in cloning the gene. Once a gene is cloned, its DNA sequence and protein product can be studied. This can contribute to our understanding of the actual cause of the disease. Furthermore, it may open the way to the manufacture of a normal gene product through recombinant DNA techniques, permitting more effective treatment of many genetic diseases. Gene therapy, the insertion of normal genes into the bodies of individuals affected with a genetic disease, also becomes a possibility. Thus, gene mapping contributes directly to many of the primary goals of medical genetics.

In this chapter we will discuss the approaches commonly used in gene mapping and cloning. Two major types of gene mapping can be distinguished. In **genetic**

mapping, the frequency of meiotic crossovers between loci is used to estimate inter-locus distances. **Physical mapping** involves the use of cytogenetic and molecular techniques to determine the actual physical locations of genes on chromosomes. In addition to discussing mapping procedures, we will see how these techniques lead to more accurate prediction of disease risk in families and how they lead to the isolation and cloning of disease genes.

GENETIC MAPPING
Linkage Analysis

One of Gregor Mendel's laws, the principle of independent assortment, states that an individual's genes will be transmitted to the next generation independently of one another (see Chapter 4). Mendel was not aware that genes are located on chromosomes and that genes located near one another on the same chromosome are transmitted together, not independently. Thus, Mendel's principle of independent assortment holds true for most pairs of loci, but not those that occupy the same region of a chromosome. Such loci are said to be **linked.**

Fig. 8-2 depicts two loci, A and B, that are located close together on the same chromosome. A third locus, C, is located on another chromosome. In the individual in our example, each of these loci has two alleles, designated 1 and 2. A and B are linked, so A_1 and B_1 are inherited together. Because A and C are on different chromosomes and thus unlinked, their alleles do follow the principle of independent assortment. Hence, if the process of meiosis places A_1 in a gamete, the probability that C_1 will be found in the same gamete is 50%.

Recall from Chapter 2 that homologous chromosomes sometimes exchange portions of their DNA during prophase I ("crossing over," or "crossover"). The average chromosome will experience one to three cross-

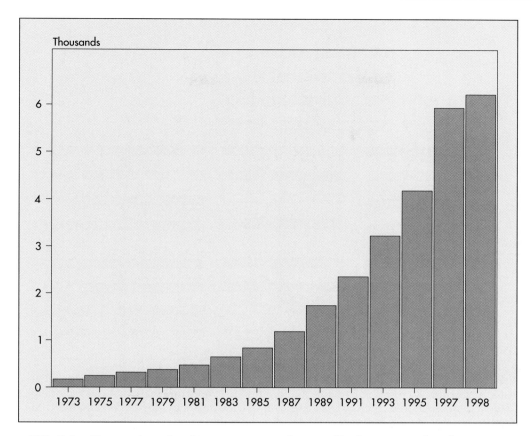

Thousands

FIG. 8-1 The number of coding genes mapped to specific chromosome locations. (From Guyer MS, Collins FS [1995] Proc. Natl. Acad. Sci. USA 92:10841-10848; and the Online Genome Data Base [March 1998].)

A_1 B_1

A_2 B_2

C_1

C_2

FIG. 8-2 Loci A and B are linked on the same chromosome, so alleles A_1 and B_1 are usually inherited together. Locus C is on a different chromosome, so it is not linked to A and B, and its alleles are transmitted independently of the alleles of A and B.

over events during meiosis. As a result of crossover, new combinations of alleles can be formed on a chromosome. Consider the linked loci, A and B, discussed previously. Alleles A_1 and B_1 are located together on one chromosome, and alleles A_2 and B_2 are located on the homologous chromosome. The combination of alleles on each chromosome is termed a **haplotype** (from

"haploid genotype"). The two haplotypes of this individual are denoted as A_1B_1/A_2B_2. As Fig. 8-3, A shows, A_1B_1 is found in one gamete and A_2B_2 is found in the other gamete in the absence of crossover. But when there is a crossover, new allele combinations, A_1B_2 and A_2B_1, are found in each gamete (Fig. 8-3, B). The process of forming such new arrangements of alleles is called **recombination.** Crossover does not *necessarily* lead to recombination, however, because a **double crossover** can occur between two loci, resulting in no recombination (Fig. 8-3, C).

As Fig. 8-4 shows, crossovers are more likely to occur between loci that are situated far apart on a chromosome than between loci that are situated close together. Thus, the distance between two loci can be inferred by estimating how frequently recombinations occur in families (this is called the **recombination frequency).** If, in a large series of meioses studied in families, the alleles of A and B undergo recombination 5% of the time, then the recombination frequency for A and B would be 5%.

The genetic distance between two loci is measured in **centiMorgans (cM),** in honor of T.H. Morgan, who discovered the process of crossing over in 1910. One cM is

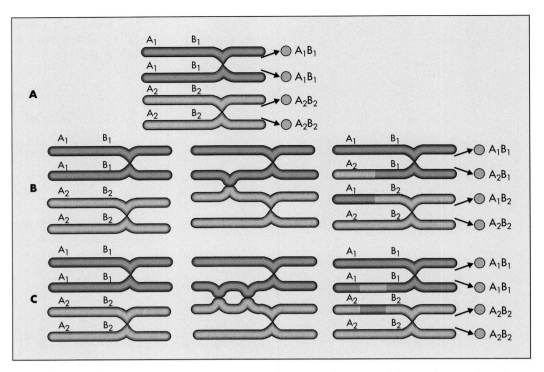

FIG. 8-3 The genetic results of crossover. **A,** No crossover: A_1 and B_1 remain together after meiosis. **B,** A crossover between A and B results in a recombination: A_1 and B_2 are inherited together on a chromosome, and A_2 and B_1 are inherited together on another chromosome. **C,** A double crossover between A and B results in no recombination of alleles. (Modified from McCance KL, Huether SE [1998] Pathophysiology. Ed. 3. Mosby, St. Louis.)

approximately equal to a recombination frequency of 1%. The relationship between recombination frequency and cM is approximate because double crossovers produce no recombination. The recombination frequency thus underestimates map distance, especially as the recombination frequency increases above 5% to 10%. Mapping functions have been devised to correct for this underestimate.

Loci that are on the same chromosome are said to be **syntenic** (meaning "same thread"). If two syntenic loci are 50 cM apart, they are considered to be unlinked. This is because their recombination frequency is just as large as it would be if they were on different chromosomes.

▼ **Crossovers between loci on the same chromosome can produce recombination. Loci on the same chromosome that experience recombination less than 50% of the time are said to be linked. The distance between loci can be expressed in centiMorgans (cM); 1 cM represents a recombination frequency of approximately 1%.** ▲

Recombination frequencies can be estimated by observing the transmission of genes in pedigrees. Fig. 8-5, *A* is an example of a pedigree in which neurofibroma-

tosis type 1 (*NF1*) is being transmitted. The members of this pedigree have also been typed for a two-allele RFLP termed *1F10*, which, like the *NF1* gene, is located on chromosome 17. The *1F10* genotypes are shown below each individual in the pedigree. Examination of generations 1 and 2 allows us to determine that, *under the hypothesis of linkage between NF1 and 1F10*, the *NF1* gene must be on the same chromosome as allele 1 of the *1F10* locus in this family because individual I-2, who is homozygous for allele 2, is unaffected with the disease. Only the affected father (I-1), who is a heterozygote for the *1F10* locus, could have transmitted a chromosome containing both the disease allele and *1F10* allele 1 to the daughter (II-2). The arrangement of these alleles on each chromosome is referred to as **linkage phase.** Knowing the linkage phase, individual II-2's haplotypes would then be *N1/n2*, where *N* indicates the allele causing NF1, *n* indicates the normal allele, and *1* and *2* are the two *1F10* alleles. This woman's husband (individual II-1) is unaffected with the disease and is a homozygote for allele 2 at *1F10*. He must have the haplotypes *n2/n2*. If *NF1* and *1F10* loci are linked, the children of this union who are affected with NF1 should usually have *IF10* allele *1*, while those who are unaffected should have allele *2*. In seven of eight children in generation III,

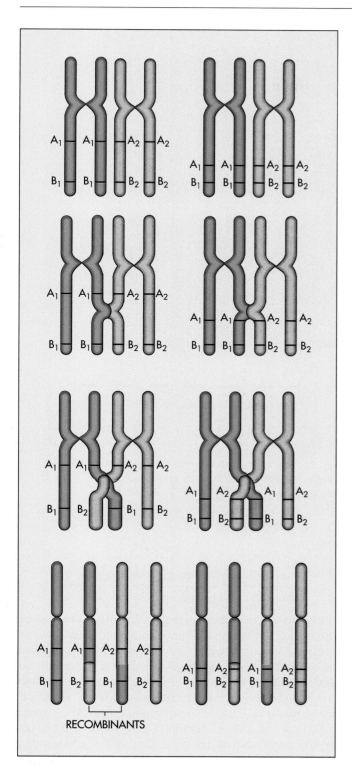

FIG. 8-4 Crossover is more likely between loci that are far apart on chromosomes *(left)* than those that are close together *(right)*.

we find this to be true. In one case a recombination occurred (individual III-6). This gives a recombination frequency of $^1/_8$, or 12.5%, supporting the hypothesis of linkage between the *NF1* and *1F10* loci. A recombination frequency of 50% would support the hypothesis that the two loci are not linked.

In actual practice a much larger sample of families would be used to ensure statistical accuracy of this result (if this were done, it would show that *1F10* and *NF1* are in fact much more closely linked than indicated by this example, with a recombination frequency less than 1%).

▼ Estimates of recombination frequencies are obtained by observing the transmission of alleles in families. Determination of the linkage phase (i.e., the chromosome on which each allele is located) is an important part of this procedure. ▲

Polymorphisms such as *1F10*, which can be used to follow a disease gene through a family, are termed **markers** (i.e., they can "mark" the chromosome on which a disease allele is located). Since linked markers can be typed in an individual of any age (even in a fetus), they are very useful for the early diagnosis of genetic disease (see Chapter 13). It is important to emphasize that a marker locus simply designates which chromosome is being transmitted; it usually has nothing to do with the actual *causation* of the genetic disease.

In general, 1 cM corresponds to approximately 1 million bp (1 Mb) of DNA. However, this is only a very approximate relationship, since several factors are known to influence crossover rates. First, crossovers are roughly 1.5 times more common in female meiosis (oogenesis) than in male meiosis (spermatogenesis). Also, crossovers tend to be more common near the telomeres of chromosomes than near the centromeres. Finally, some chromosome regions exhibit substantially elevated crossover rates. These regions are termed **recombination hot spots.** It is not yet known what causes recombination hot spots in humans, although specific DNA sequences, possibly including *Alu* sequences (see Chapter 2), are thought to be especially prone to crossover.

▼ Although there is a correlation between centi-Morgans and actual physical distances between loci, this relationship is complicated by gender differences in recombination, higher recombination frequencies near telomeres, and the existence of recombination hot spots. ▲

LOD Scores: Determining the Significance of Linkage Results

As in any statistical study, we must be careful to ensure that the results obtained in a linkage study are not due simply to chance. For example, consider a two-allele

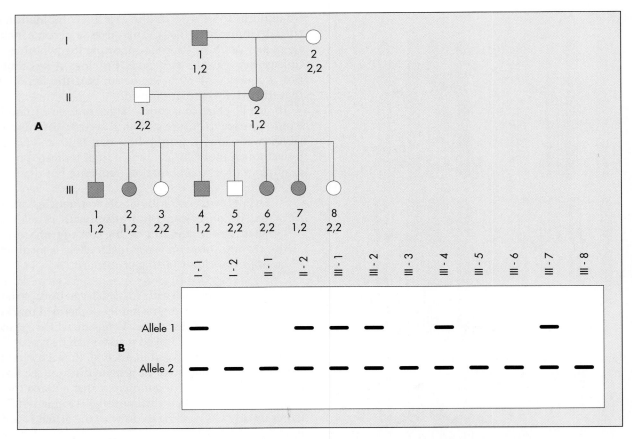

FIG. 8-5 **A,** An NF1 pedigree in which each member has been typed for the *1F10* polymorphism. Genotypes for this two-allele marker locus are shown below each individual in the pedigree. Affected pedigree members are indicated by a shaded symbol. **B,** An autoradiogram for the *1F10* polymorphism in this family.

marker locus that has been typed in a pedigree. It is possible *by chance* for all affected offspring to inherit one allele and for all unaffected offspring to inherit the other allele even if the marker is not linked to the disease gene. This misleading result becomes less likely as we increase the number of subjects in our linkage study (just as the chance of a strong deviation from a 50/50 heads-tails ratio becomes smaller as we toss a coin many times).

How do we determine whether a linkage result is likely to be due to chance alone? In linkage analysis a standard method is used. We begin by comparing the **likelihood** (a likelihood is similar in concept to a probability) that two loci are linked at a given recombination frequency (denoted θ) versus the likelihood that the two loci are not linked (recombination frequency = 50%, or θ = 0.5). Suppose we wish to test the hypothesis that two loci are linked at a recombination frequency of θ = 0.1 versus the hypothesis that they are not linked. We use our pedigree data to form a **likelihood ratio:**

$$\frac{\text{likelihood of observing pedigree data if } \theta = 0.1}{\text{likelihood of observing pedigree data if } \theta = 0.5}$$

If our pedigree data indicate that θ is more likely to be 0.1 than 0.5, then the likelihood ratio (or "odds") will be greater than 1. If, however, the pedigree data argue against linkage of the two loci, then the denominator will be greater than the numerator, and the ratio will be less than 1.0. For convenience, the common logarithm* of the ratio is usually taken; this "logarithm of the odds" is termed a **LOD score.** Conventionally, a LOD score of 3.0 is accepted as evidence of linkage; a score of 3.0 indicates that the likelihood in favor of linkage is 1,000 times greater than the likelihood against linkage. Conversely, a LOD score less than –2.0 (odds of 100 to 1 *against* linkage) is considered to be evidence that two loci are not linked. Box 8-1 provides details on the calculation of LOD scores.

---

*Recall that the common logarithm of a number is the power to which 10 is raised to obtain the number. Thus, the common logarithm of 100 is 2, the common logarithm of 1,000 is 3, and so on.

BOX 8-1
THE ESTIMATION OF LOD SCORES IN LINKAGE ANALYSIS

A simple example will help to illustrate the concepts of likelihood ratios and LOD scores. Consider the pedigree in Fig. 8-6, which illustrates another family in which NF1 is being transmitted. The family has been typed for the *1F10* marker, as in Fig. 8-5. The male in generation 2 had to receive the *1F10-1* allele from his mother, since she can transmit only this marker allele. Thus, his *1F10-2* allele had to come from his father, on the same chromosome as the *NF1* disease gene (under the hypothesis of linkage). This allows us to establish linkage phase in this pedigree: the affected male in generation 2 must have the haplotypes *N2/n1*. He marries an unaffected woman who is a homozygote for the *1F10-2* allele. Thus, the hypothesis of close linkage ($\theta = 0.0$) predicts that each child in generation 3 who receives allele 2 from his or her father must also receive the *NF1* disease allele. Under the hypothesis of linkage, the father can transmit only two possible combinations: either the chromosome having the disease gene and *1F10-2* (*N2*) or the other chromosome, which has the normal gene and *1F10-1* (*n1*). The probability of each of these events is 1/2. Thus, if $\theta = 0.0$, the probability of observing five children with the genotypes shown in Fig. 8-6 is $(1/2)^5$, or 1/32 (i.e., the multiplication rule is applied to obtain the probability of all five of these events occurring together). This is the numerator of the likelihood ratio.

Now consider the likelihood of observing these genotypes if *1F10* and *NF1* were *not* linked ($\theta = 0.5$). Under this hypothesis, there is *independent assortment* of alleles at *1F10* and *NF1*. The father can transmit any of four combinations, *N1*, *N2*, *n1*, and *n2*, with equal probability (1/4). The probability of observing five children with the observed genotypes is then $(1/4)^5 = 1/1024$. This likelihood is the denominator of the likelihood ratio. The likelihood ratio is then 1/32:1/1024 = 32. Thus, the data in this pedigree tell us that *linkage*, at $\theta = 0.0$, is 32 times more likely than *non-linkage*. If we take the common logarithm of 32, we find that the LOD score is 1.5, which is still far short of the value of 3.0 usually accepted as evidence of linkage. To prove linkage, then, we would need to examine data from additional families. LOD scores obtained from individual families can be added together to obtain an overall score (note that adding LOD scores is the same as multiplying the odds of linkage in each family together and then taking the logarithm of the result; this is another example of the use of the multiplication rule to assess the probability of co-occurrence).

Suppose that a recombination had occurred in the meiosis producing the fifth child, III-5, in generation 3 (i.e., she would retain the same marker genotype but be affected with the disease rather than unaffected). This event is impossible under the hypothesis that $\theta = 0.0$, so the numerator of the likelihood ratio becomes zero, and the LOD score for $\theta = 0.0$ is -∞. It is possible, however, that the marker and disease loci are still linked, but at a recombination frequency greater than zero. Let us test the hypoth-

FIG. 8-6 An NF1 pedigree in which each member has been typed for the *1F10* polymorphism. The marker genotypes are shown below each individual in the pedigree.

esis that θ is equal to 0.1. This hypothesis predicts that the disease allele, *N*, will be transmitted along with marker allele 2 90% of the time and with marker allele 1 10% of the time (i.e., when a recombination has occurred). By the same reasoning, the normal allele, *n*, will be transmitted with marker allele 1 90% of the time and with marker allele 2 10% of the time. As in our previous example, the father can transmit either the normal allele or the disease allele with equal probability (0.5) to each child. Thus, the probability of inheriting the disease allele with marker allele 2 (*N2*) is $0.5 \times 0.90 = 0.45$, and the probability of inheriting the disease allele with marker allele 1 (*N1*) is $0.5 \times 0.1 = 0.05$. The probability of inheriting the normal allele with marker 1 (*n1*) is $0.5 \times 0.9 = 0.45$, and the probability of inheriting the normal allele with marker 2 (*n2*) is $0.5 \times 0.1 = 0.05$. In either case, then, the probability of receiving a nonrecombination (*N2* or *n1*) is 0.45, and the probability of receiving a recombination (*N1* or *n2*) is 0.05. We know that four of the children in generation 3 are nonrecombinants, and each of these events has a probability of 0.45. We know that one individual is a recombinant, and the probability of this event is 0.05. Then the probability of four nonrecombinations and one recombination occurring together in generation 3 is obtained by applying the multiplication rule: $0.45^4 \times 0.05$. This becomes the numerator for our LOD score calculation. As before, the denominator (the likelihood that $\theta = 0.5$) is given by the quantity $(1/4)^5$. The LOD score for $\theta = 0.1$, then, is given by $\log_{10}[(0.45^4 \times 0.05)/(1/4)^5] = 0.32$.

To test the hypothesis that $\theta = 0.2$, the approach just outlined is used again, with $\theta = 0.2$ instead of $\theta = 0.1$. This yields a LOD score of 0.42. It makes sense that the LOD score for $\theta = 0.2$ is higher than that of $\theta = 0.1$ because we know that one of five children (0.2) in generation 3 is a

Continued

BOX 8-1—cont'd

THE ESTIMATION OF LOD SCORES IN LINKAGE ANALYSIS—cont'd

recombinant. Applying this formula to a series of possible θ values (0, 0.1, 0.2, 0.3, 0.4, and 0.5) shows that 0.2 yields the highest LOD score, as we would expect.

θ	0	0.1	0.2	0.3	0.4	0.5
LOD	-∞	0.32	0.42	0.36	0.22	0.0

Sometimes the linkage phase in a pedigree is not known. For example, if the grandparents in Fig. 8-6 had not been typed, we would not know the linkage phase of the father in generation 2. It is equally likely that his haplotypes are *N2/n1* or *N1/n2* (i.e., each combination has a probability of 1/2). Thus, we need to take both possibilities into account. If he has the *N2/n1* haplotypes, then the first four children are nonrecombinants, each with probability $(1-\theta)/2$, while the fifth child is a recombinant, with probability $\theta/2$ (using the same reasoning outlined previously). Under the hypothesis that $\theta = 0.1$, the overall probability that the father has haplotypes *N2/n1* *and* that the five children have the observed genotypes is $1/2(0.45^4 \times 0.05) = 0.001$. We now need to take the alternative phase into account (i.e., the father having haplotypes *N1/n2*). Here, the first four children would each be recombinants (with probability $\theta/2$), and only the fifth child would be a nonrecombinant (with probability $(1-\theta)/2$). The probability that the father has the *N1/n2* haplotypes *and* that the children have the observed genotypes is $1/2(0.45 \times 0.05^4) = 0.000001$. This probability is considerably smaller than the probability of the previous phase, which makes sense when we consider that, under the hypothesis of linkage at $\theta = 0.1$, four of five recombinants is unlikely. We can now consider the probability of *either* linkage phase in the father by adding the two probabilities together: $1/2(0.45^4 \times 0.05) + 1/2(0.45 \times 0.05^4)$. This becomes the numerator for the LOD score calculation. As before, the denominator (i.e., the probability that $\theta = 0.5$) is simply $(1/2)^5 = 1/1024$. Then, the total LOD score for unknown linkage phase at $\theta = 0.1$ is $\log_{10} [(1/2[0.45^4 \times 0.05] + 1/2[0.45 \times 0.05^4])/(1/1024)] = 0.02$. As before, we can estimate LOD scores for each recombination frequency:

θ	0	0.1	0.2	0.3	0.4	0.5
LOD	-∞	0.02	0.12	0.09	0.03	0.0

Notice that each LOD score is lower than the corresponding score when linkage phase is known. This follows from the fact that a known linkage phase contributes useful information to allow more accurate estimation of the actual genotypes of the offspring.

FIG. 8-7 **The LOD score (logarithm of the odds; y axis) is plotted against the recombination frequency (x axis) to determine the most likely recombination frequency for a pair of loci.**

LOD scores are often graphed against the θ values, as shown in Fig. 8-7. The highest LOD score on the graph is the **maximum likelihood estimate** of θ. That is, it is the *most likely* distance between the two loci being analyzed.

In practice, the analysis of human linkage data is not as simple as in these examples. Penetrance of the disease gene may be incomplete, recombination frequencies differ between the sexes, and the mode of inheritance of the disease may be unclear. Consequently, linkage data are analyzed using one of several available computer software packages such as LIPED or MLINK (hyperlinks to these sites are provided on our Web page). Many of these packages also allow one to carry out **multipoint mapping,** an approach in which the map locations of several markers are estimated simultaneously. **WWW**

▼ The statistical odds that two loci are a given number of cM apart can be calculated by measuring the ratio of two likelihoods: the likelihood of linkage at a given recombination frequency divided by the likelihood of no linkage. The logarithm of this odds ratio is a LOD score. LOD scores >3.0 are taken as evidence of linkage, and LOD scores <−2.0 are taken as evidence that two loci are not linked. ▲

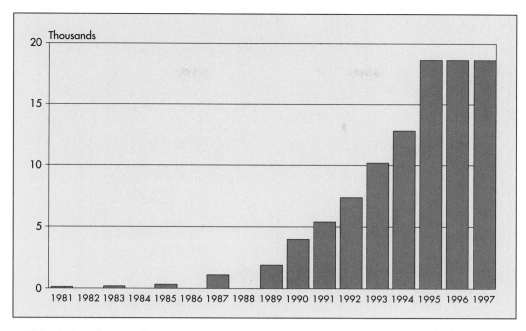

FIG. 8-8 The number of known polymorphic marker loci, showing a rapid rate of increase during the past decade.
(From Guyer MS, Collins FS [1995] Proc. Natl. Acad. Sci. USA 92:10841-10848; and the Online Genome Data Base [March 1998].)

Linkage Analysis and the Human Gene Map

Suppose that we are studying a disease gene in a series of pedigrees, and we wish to map it to a specific chromosome location. Typically we would type the members of our pedigree for marker loci distributed along each chromosome, testing for linkage between the disease gene and each marker. Most of these tests would yield negative LOD scores, indicating no linkage between the marker and the disease gene. Eventually this exercise will reveal linkage between a marker and the disease gene. Because of the large size of the human genome, one may have to type dozens, or even hundreds, of markers before finding linkage. Many important diseases have been localized using this approach, including cystic fibrosis, Huntington disease, Marfan syndrome, and NF1.

A little more than a decade ago, linkage analyses had little chance of success because there were only a few dozen useful polymorphic markers in the entire human genome. Thus, it was unlikely that a disease gene would be located near enough to a marker to yield a significant linkage result. This situation has changed dramatically over the past decade, as thousands of new polymorphic markers (RFLPs, VNTRs, and microsatellite polymorphisms; see Chapter 3) have been generated (Fig. 8-8). With efficient genotyping technologies and large numbers of markers, it is now commonplace to map a disease gene with only a few weeks or months of laboratory and statistical analysis.

To be useful for gene mapping, marker loci should have several properties. First, they should be codominant (i.e., homozygotes should be distinguishable from heterozygotes). This makes it easier to determine linkage phase. RFLPs, VNTRs, and microsatellite polymorphisms fulfill this criterion, while some of the older types of markers, such as the ABO and Rh blood groups, do not. Second, marker loci should be numerous, so that close linkage to the disease gene is likely. As Fig. 8-8 shows, this requirement has been fulfilled. Our chromosomes are rapidly becoming saturated with markers (Fig. 8-9). Finally, marker loci are most useful when they are highly polymorphic (i.e., when the locus has many different alleles in the population). A high degree of polymorphism ensures that most parents will be heterozygous for the marker locus, making it easier to establish linkage phase in families. Microsatellite repeat polymorphisms typically have many alleles and are easy to assay; they are thus especially well suited to gene mapping.

An example will illustrate this last point. Consider the pedigree in Fig. 8-10, *A*. The affected man is a homozygote for a two-allele RFLP that is closely linked to the disease locus (recall that most RFLPs are caused by the presence or absence of a restriction site and thus have only two alleles in a population). His wife is a heterozygote. Their affected daughter is homozygous for the marker allele. Based on these genotypes, it is impossible to determine linkage phase in this generation, so we cannot predict which children will be affected with the disorder and which will not. The mating in generation 1 is called an **uninformative mating.** In contrast, a microsatellite

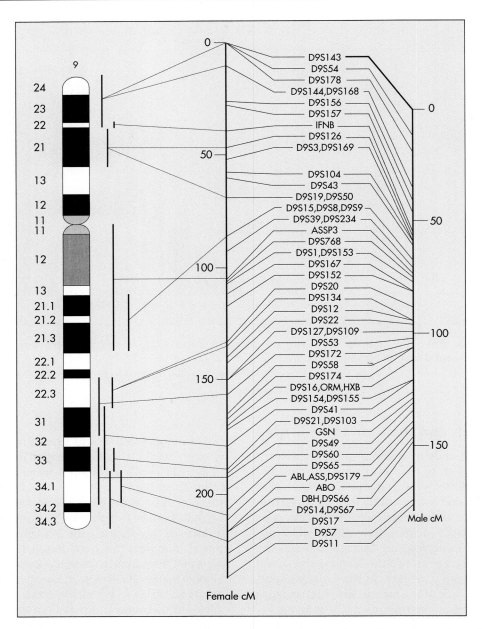

FIG. 8-9 A genetic map of chromosome 9, showing the locations of a large number of polymorphic markers. Because recombination rates are usually higher in female meiosis, the distances between markers (in cM) are larger for females than for males.
(From Atwood J, Chiano M, Collins A, et al. [1994] Genomics 19:203-214.)

repeat polymorphism with six alleles has been typed in the same family (Fig. 8-10, *B*). Because the mother in generation 1 has two alleles that differ from those of the affected father, it is now possible to determine that the affected daughter in generation 2 has inherited the disease gene on the single chromosome that contains marker allele 1. Since she married a man who has alleles 4 and 5, we can predict that each offspring who receives allele 1 from her will be affected, while each one who re-

ceives allele 2 will be normal. Exceptions will be due to recombination. This example demonstrates the value of highly polymorphic markers both for linkage analysis and diagnosing genetic disease (see Chapter 13).

▼ To be useful in gene mapping, linked markers should be codominant, numerous, and highly polymorphic. A high degree of polymorphism increases the probability that matings will be informative. ▲

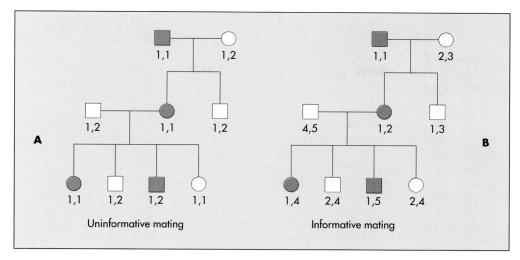

FIG. 8-10 An autosomal dominant disease gene is segregating in this family. **A,** A closely linked two-allele RFLP has been typed for each member of the family, but linkage phase cannot be determined (uninformative mating). **B,** A closely linked six-allele microsatellite polymorphism has been typed for each family member, and linkage phase can now be determined (informative mating).

Sometimes, a linkage analysis will produce a total LOD score close to zero. This could mean simply that the families are uninformative (a LOD score of zero indicates that the likelihoods of linkage and non-linkage are approximately equal). However, a total LOD score of zero can also result when one subset of families has positive LOD scores (indicating linkage) while another subset has negative LOD scores (arguing against linkage). This result would provide evidence of locus heterogeneity for the disease in question (see Chapter 4). For example, osteogenesis imperfecta type I can be caused by mutations on either chromosome 7 or chromosome 17 (see Chapter 4). A study of families with this disease could show linkage to markers on chromosome 17 in some families and linkage to chromosome 7 in others. Linkage analysis has helped to define locus heterogeneity in a large number of diseases, including retinitis pigmentosa, a major cause of blindness (Clinical Commentary 8-1).

Linkage Disequilibrium, the Nonrandom Association of Alleles at Linked Loci

Within families, one allele of a marker locus will be transmitted along with the disease allele if the marker and disease loci are linked. For example, allele 1 of a linked two-allele marker could co-occur with the Huntington disease (HD) allele in a family. This association is part of the definition of linkage. However, if one examines a series of families for linkage between HD and the marker locus, allele 1 will co-occur with the disease in some families, while allele 2 of the marker will co-occur with the disease

in others. This reflects two things. First, disease-causing mutations may have occurred multiple times, sometimes on a chromosome carrying marker allele 1 and other times on a chromosome carrying marker allele 2. Second, even if the disease is the result of only one original mutation, crossovers occurring through time will eventually result in recombination of the marker and disease alleles. A disease allele and a linked marker allele will thus be associated *within* families, but not necessarily *between* families. If we study a large collection of families and find that there is no preferential association between the disease gene and a specific allele at a linked marker locus, the two loci are said to be in **linkage equilibrium.**

Sometimes, however, we do observe the preferential association of a specific marker allele and the disease allele in a population. By this we mean that the chromosome haplotype consisting of one marker allele and the disease allele is found more often than we would expect based on the frequencies of the two alleles in the population. Suppose, for example, that the disease allele has a frequency of 0.01 in the population and the frequencies of the two alleles (labeled 1 and 2) of the marker are 0.4 and 0.6, respectively. Assuming independence between the two loci (i.e., linkage equilibrium), the multiplication rule would predict that the population frequency of the haplotype containing the disease allele and marker allele 1 would be $0.01 \times 0.4 = 0.004$. By collecting family information, we can directly count the haplotypes in the population. If we find that the actual frequency of this haplotype is 0.009 instead of the predicted 0.004, then the assumption of independence has been violated, indicating preferential

CLINICAL COMMENTARY 8-1

RETINITIS PIGMENTOSA, A GENETIC DISORDER CHARACTERIZED BY LOCUS HETEROGENEITY www

Retinitis pigmentosa (RP) describes a collection of inherited retinal defects that together are the most common inherited cause of human blindness, affecting 1/3,000 to 1/4,000 individuals. The first clinical signs of RP are seen as the rod photoreceptor cells begin to die, causing night blindness. With the death of rod cells, other tissue begins to degenerate as well. Cone cells die, and the vessels that supply blood to the retinal membranes begin to attenuate. This leads to a reduction in daytime vision. Patients develop tunnel vision, and most are legally blind by age 60. The name "retinitis pigmentosa" comes from the pigments that are deposited on the retinal surface as pathological changes accumulate (Fig. 8-11). RP is neither preventable nor curable, but its progress can be slowed somewhat by dietary supplementation with vitamin A.

RP is known to be inherited in different families in autosomal dominant, autosomal recessive, and X-linked

FIG. 8-11 A fundus photograph illustrating clumps of pigment deposits and retinal blood vessel attenuation in retinitis pigmentosa.

(Courtesy Dr. Don Creel, University of Utah Health Sciences Center.)

recessive fashion. This disease is an excellent example of locus heterogeneity: linkage analyses have identified more than 20 chromosome regions containing loci that can cause RP. Specific disease-causing genes have been identified in eight of these regions. An early linkage analysis mapped an autosomal dominant form of RP to the long arm of chromosome 3. This was a significant finding because the gene encoding rhodopsin (a retinal visual pigment) had also been mapped to this region. Because of its role in the phototransduction cascade, rhodopsin was a reasonable candidate gene (see text) for RP. Linkage analysis was performed using a polymorphism located within the rhodopsin gene, and a LOD score of 20 was obtained for a recombination frequency of zero in a large Irish pedigree. Subsequently, approximately 100 different mutations in the rhodopsin gene have been shown to cause RP, confirming the role of this locus in causing the disease. Rhodopsin mutations are estimated to account for about 10% of RP cases.

RP-causing mutations have been identified in three other genes that encode rod phototransduction proteins: the α subunit of the rod cGMP cation-gated channel protein and the α and β subunits of rod cGMP photodiesterase. In addition, RP-causing mutations are seen in two genes that encode proteins necessary for maintenance of the structure of the outer segment discs of photoreceptors, the peripherin protein and rod outer segment membrane protein 1. Mutations in the gene that encodes myosin VIIa cause Usher syndrome type 1, a disease that includes both RP and severe congenital deafness. Finally, mutations in the Stargardt disease gene have recently been shown to cause RP in some individuals. Mutations in this photoreceptor transporter gene can also lead to age-related macular degeneration, another common cause of vision loss in the elderly.

Although considerable progress has been made in identifying specific genes involved in RP, it is estimated that the genes discovered thus far account for only about 25% of RP cases. It is sobering to consider that more than 70 loci have been identified in photoreceptor defects in the fruit fly, *Drosophila*. Undoubtedly, continued linkage and cloning analyses will lead to a more complete identification and understanding of genes underlying the pathogenesis of RP.

association of marker allele 1 with the disease allele. This association of alleles at linked loci is termed **linkage disequilibrium.**

Fig. 8-12 illustrates how linkage disequilibrium can come about. Imagine two markers linked to the myotonic dystrophy locus on chromosome 19. Marker *B* is closely linked, at less than 1 cM away. Marker *A* is less closely linked, at about 5 cM away. Since each of these marker loci has two alleles (denoted 1 and 2), there

are four possible combinations of marker alleles at the two loci, as shown in Fig. 8-12. When a new myotonic dystrophy mutation first occurs in a population, it can be found on only one chromosome, in this case the one with the A_1B_2 marker combination. As the disease mutation is passed through multiple generations, crossovers will occur between it and the two markers. Because the disease locus is more closely linked to marker *B* than marker *A*, fewer crossovers will occur between

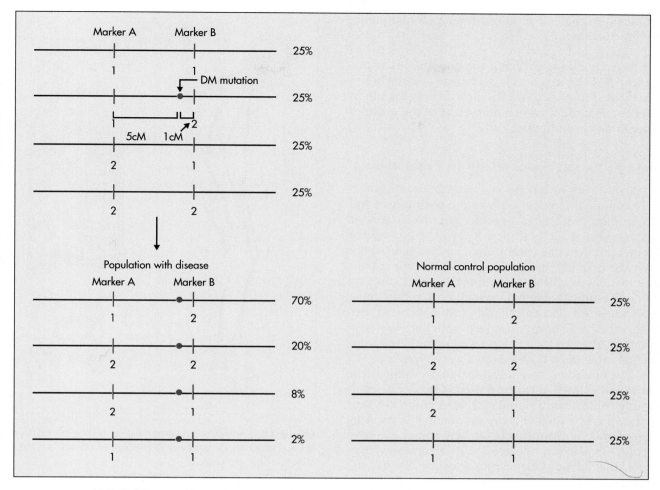

FIG. 8-12 Linkage disequilibrium between the myotonic dystrophy *(DM)* locus and two linked loci, *A* and *B*. The *DM* mutation first arises on the chromosome with the A_1B_2 haplotype. After a number of generations have passed, most chromosomes carrying the *DM* mutation still have the A_1B_2 haplotype, but, as a result of recombination, the *DM* mutation is also found on other haplotypes. Because the A_1B_2 haplotype is seen in 70% of *DM* chromosomes but only 25% of normal chromosomes, there is linkage disequilibrium between *DM* and loci *A* and *B*. Since locus *B* is closer to *DM*, it has greater linkage disequilibrium with *DM* than does locus *A*.

the disease mutation and marker *B*. As a result, the disease mutation is found on a B_2 chromosome 90% of the time, while it is found on an A_1 chromosome 72% of the time. The degree of linkage disequilibrium is stronger between marker *B* and the disease allele than between marker *A* and the disease allele. Notice also that *both* the A_1 and B_2 alleles are still positively associated with the disease allele, since each allele has a much lower frequency (50%) in the population of individuals lacking the disease allele (Fig. 8-12). If enough generations elapse, recombination would eventually eliminate the allelic associations completely, and the loci would be in linkage equilibrium.

Because linkage disequilibrium is a function of the distance between loci, it can be used to help infer the order of genes on chromosomes. Linkage disequilibrium

provides an advantage over linkage analysis in that it reflects the action of recombinations that have occurred during dozens or hundreds of past generations. Linkage analysis, in contrast, is limited to the recombinations that can be directly observed in only the past several generations. Consequently, there are seldom enough recombinants in a series of families to map a gene to a region smaller than one or several cM using linkage analysis, whereas linkage disequilibrium analysis can sometimes map a gene to an interval of 0.1 cM or less. However, linkage disequilibrium can be influenced by evolutionary forces, such as natural selection or genetic drift, that have acted during the history of a population. For example, some loci in the major histocompatibility complex on chromosome 6 (see Chapter 9) are in disequilibrium, presumably because certain allelic combinations confer a selective advantage for immunity to some diseases.

▼ Linkage disequilibrium is the nonrandom association of alleles at linked loci. Linkage disequilibrium between loci diminishes through time as a result of recombination. It can be used to infer the order of genes on chromosomes. ▲

Linkage Versus Association in Populations

The phenomena of linkage and association are sometimes confused. Linkage refers to the positions of loci on chromosomes. When two loci are linked, specific combinations of alleles at these loci will be transmitted together (on the same chromosome) *within families.* But as the HD example cited previously showed, the specific combinations of alleles transmitted together can vary from one family to another. **Association,** on the other hand, refers to a statistical relationship between two traits (which may or may not be genetic) *in the general population.* The two traits occur together in the same individual more often than expected by chance.

As just discussed, two linked loci may exhibit allelic association in the population if there is linkage disequilibrium. In this case a population association can lead to mapping of a disease gene. An example is given by idiopathic hemochromatosis, an autosomal recessive disorder discussed in Chapter 7. One association study showed that 78% of hemochromatosis patients had the *A3* allele of the *HLA-A* locus (see Chapter 9 for further discussion of the HLA system), whereas only 27% of unaffected subjects (controls) had this allele. This strong statistical association prompted linkage analyses using HLA polymorphisms and led to the mapping of the hemochromatosis gene to a region of several cM on chromosome 6. The large size of this region made it very difficult to pinpoint a specific gene. Linkage disequilibrium analysis was subsequently used to narrow the region to approximately 250 kb, prompting the ready identification of an HLA-like gene *(HFE)* in which a single mutation is responsible for approximately 85% of hemochromatosis chromosomes. www

The association between the hemochromatosis gene and the linked *HLA-A* locus is likely the result of a recent hemochromatosis-causing mutation having occurred on a chromosome containing the *HLA-A3* allele. Population associations can also be due to a causal relationship between an allele and a disease condition. An example of such an association involves ankylosing spondylitis, a disease that primarily affects the sacroiliac joint (Fig. 8-13). Inflammation of the ligaments leads to their ossification and eventually to fusion of the joints (ankylosis). The *HLAB27* allele is found in about 90% of U.S. Caucasians who have ankylosing spondylitis but in only 5% to 10% of the general U.S. Caucasian population. Since the population incidence of ankylosing

FIG. 8-13 Ankylosing spondylitis, caused by ossification of discs, joints, and ligaments in the spinal column. Note the characteristic posture.
(Modified from Mourad LA [1991] Orthopedic Disorders. Mosby, St. Louis.)

spondylitis is quite low (<1%), most people who have the *HLAB27* allele do not develop ankylosing spondylitis. However, those who have the *HLAB27* allele are about 90 times more likely to develop the disease than are those who do not have the *B27* allele (i.e., 9% of the *HLA-B27* individuals shown in Table 8-1 have ankylosing spondylitis, while only about 0.1% of those without *HLA-B27* have the disease). Because of this strong association, a test for *HLA-B27* is sometimes included as part of the diagnosis of ankylosing spondylitis. It is important to emphasize that the genetic and environmental factors causing ankylosing spondylitis remain unclear and that the observed population *association* between *HLA-B27* and this disorder does not necessarily imply genetic *linkage.* Because ankylosing spondylitis is thought to be an autoimmune disorder, the association may reflect the fact that the HLA system is a key element in the body's immune response (see Chapter 9).

A population association is also seen between the *HLA-DR3* and *HLA-DR4* alleles and type 1 diabetes (see Chapter 12). Since autoimmunity appears to be a factor in the etiology of type 1 diabetes, there may well be a causative relationship between the *HLA-DR3/DR4*

TABLE 8-1   Association of Ankylosing Spondylitis and the HLA-B27 Allele in a Hypothetical Population.*

HLA-B27	Ankylosing spondylitis	
	Present	Absent
Present	90	1000
Absent	10	9000

*This table shows that individuals with ankylosing spondylitis are much more likely to have the HLA-B27 allele than are normal controls.

alleles and increased susceptibility to this form of diabetes.

Association studies should be interpreted cautiously because many things can produce spurious associations between a disease and a potential risk factor. An example is ethnic stratification in a population: certain diseases are more frequent in certain ethnic groups, and allele frequencies may also differ among these groups because of their evolutionary histories. Thus, if one compares disease cases and controls without proper matching for ethnicity, a false association, due simply to ethnic differences in the two groups, could be found. For example, type 2 diabetes (see Chapter 12) has been studied extensively among the Pima Native American population, where the disease is much more common than among Caucasians. It was observed that the absence of haplotype Gm3;5,13,14 of human immunoglobulin G (abbreviated here as Gm3) was strongly associated with type 2 diabetes among the Pima. This suggested initially that the absence of Gm3 might be involved in the causation of type 2 diabetes. However, further analysis revealed that the proportion of Caucasian ancestry varied substantially among members of the Pima population and that the Gm3 frequency *also* varied with the degree of Caucasian ancestry: Gm3 is absent in Pima individuals with no Caucasian ancestry but increases to 65% among Caucasians. Since type 2 diabetes is much less common among Caucasians, the apparent association between type 2 diabetes and the absence of Gm3 was most likely a consequence of the level of Caucasian mixture. Once the degree of Caucasian ancestry in the study subjects was taken into account, there was no evidence of an association.

Other factors that may produce false associations include imprecise definition of the disease state, inadequate sample sizes, and improper matching of cases and controls for variables such as age and gender. The inability to replicate an association in multiple study populations is a good indication that the association may be invalid. An example is given by an association reported, but not replicated, between alcoholism and a polymorphism near the dopamine D2 receptor locus (discussed further in Chapter 12).

▼ Population associations refer to the nonrandom co-occurrence of factors at the population level. Associations are distinguished from linkage, which refers to the positions of loci on chromosomes. Linkage disequilibrium is a special case of association in which there is nonrandom association of specific alleles at linked loci. ▲

PHYSICAL MAPPING AND CLONING

Linkage analysis allows us to determine the relative distances between loci, but it does not assign specific locations to markers or disease genes. Physical mapping, which involves a variety of methods, accomplishes this goal, and considerable progress has been made in developing high-resolution physical mapping approaches.

Chromosome Morphology

A simple and direct way of mapping disease genes is to show that the disease is consistently associated with a cytogenetic abnormality, such as a duplication, deletion, or other variation in the appearance of a chromosome. Such abnormalities may have no clinical consequences themselves (thus serving as a marker), or they may cause the disease. Because these approaches are historically the oldest of the physical mapping approaches, we will discuss them first.

Heteromorphisms

A **heteromorphism** is a variation in the appearance of a chromosome. Conceptually, heteromorphisms are similar to polymorphisms: they are natural variations that occur among individuals in populations. The difference is that polymorphisms are not detectable microscopically, while heteromorphisms are.

A well-known example of a heteromorphism is an "uncoiled" (and thus elongated) region of chromosome 1, a rare feature that is transmitted regularly in families. In the 1960s a researcher named R.P. Donahue was practicing cytogenetic analysis on his own chromosomes and found that he had this heteromorphism. He studied other members of his family and found that the heteromorphism was transmitted through his family as a Mendelian trait. He then typed his family members for several blood groups. He found that the heteromorphism was perfectly associated in his family with allele *A* of the Duffy blood group. Linkage analysis of the "uncoiler" locus and the Duffy locus showed that they were closely linked, leading to the first assignment of a gene to a specific autosome.

It should be emphasized that heteromorphisms, like marker loci, do not *cause* a genetic variant or disease, but they may be associated with it within a family, thus indicating the gene's location. Although such heteromorphisms can be useful in mapping genes, they are not very common and thus have been useful in only a few instances.

Deletions

Karyotypes of patients with a genetic disease will occasionally reveal deletions of a specific region of a chromosome. This provides a strong hint that the locus causing the disease may lie within the deleted region. The extent of a deletion may vary in several patients with the same disease. Deletions are compared in many patients to define the region that is deleted in all patients, thereby narrowing the location of the disease gene (Fig. 8-14). Deletion mapping has been used, for example, in locating the genes responsible for retinoblastoma (see Chapters 4 and 11), Prader-Willi and Angelman syndromes (see Chapter 4), and Wilms tumor, a childhood kidney tumor that can be caused by mutations on chromosome 11. As opposed to the heteromorphisms just discussed, deletions of genetic material are the direct cause of the genetic disease.

Note that these deletions affect only one member of the homologous pair of chromosomes, making the patient heterozygous for the deletion. If a region large enough to be microscopically observable were missing in both chromosomes, it would usually produce a lethal condition.

Translocations

As discussed in Chapter 6, balanced chromosome translocations often have no effect on a translocation carrier because the individual still has a complete copy of his or her genetic material. However, when a translocation happens to interrupt a gene, it can produce genetic disease. For example, linkage analysis had mapped the *NF1* gene approximately to the long arm of chromosome 17. A more refined location was obtained when two patients were identified, one with a balanced translocation between chromosomes 17 and 22, and the other with a balanced translocation between chromosomes 17 and 1. The breakpoints of these translocations on chromosome 17 were located very close to one another in the same region implicated by linkage analysis. They provided a physical starting point for experiments that subsequently led to cloning of the *NF1* gene.

A similar example is provided by translocations observed between the X chromosome and autosomes in females affected with Duchenne muscular dystrophy (DMD). Because this is a lethal X-linked recessive disorder, affected homozygous females are rare. The translocation breakpoint on the X chromosome was in the same location (Xp21) in several affected females, suggesting that the translocation interrupted the *DMD* gene. This proved to be the case, and these translocations aided considerably in mapping and cloning the *DMD* gene. (Although these females also carried a normal X chromosome, the normal X was preferentially inactivated, leaving only the interrupted X as the active chromosome.)

FIG. 8-14 Localization of a disease gene through deletion mapping. A series of overlapping deletions is studied in which each deletion produces the disease phenotype. The region of overlap of all deletions defines the approximate location of the disease gene.

Dosage Mapping Using Deletions and Duplications

When a deletion occurs on a chromosome, it stands to reason that the protein products encoded by genes in the deleted region would be present in only half the normal quantity. This is the basis of a simple approach known as **dosage mapping.** For example, it was observed that a 50% reduction in the level of the enzyme adenylate kinase was consistently associated with a deletion on chromosome 9, mapping the adenylate kinase gene to this chromosome region. Dosage mapping was also used to map the gene for red cell acid phosphatase to chromosome 2.

Similarly, a duplication of chromosome material should be associated with an increase in gene product levels. Because three genes are present instead of two,

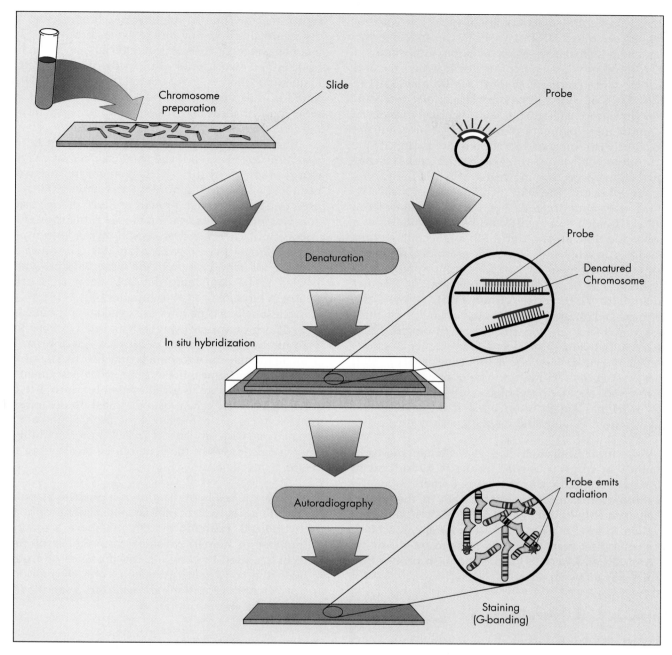

FIG. 8-15   Mapping a DNA segment to a chromosome location through in situ hybridization.

the increase should be approximately 50% above normal. This form of dosage mapping was used to assign the gene encoding superoxide dismutase-1 (SOD-1) to the long arm of chromosome 21.

▼ A gene can be physically mapped to a chromosome region by associating cytogenetically observable variations (heteromorphisms, translocations, deletions, duplications) with gene expression (including the presence of a genetic disease). ▲

In Situ Hybridization

In situ hybridization, illustrated in Fig. 8-15, is a direct and intuitively simple approach to mapping DNA segments. Suppose that we have a segment of DNA, taken from a polymorphic marker or disease gene whose location we wish to know. This DNA can be cloned into a probe using the recombinant DNA methods outlined in Chapter 2. The probe is labeled with a radioactive substance, such as tritium. The probe is then exposed to a slide containing metaphase chromosomes whose DNA has been denatured in place *(in situ)*. The labeled probe undergoes complementary base pairing with the denatured DNA of a specific chromosome segment. Because the probe emits radiation, its position on a chromosome can be pinpointed by placing x-ray film over the slide (autoradiography; see Chapter 3). The probe DNA often hybridizes nonspecifically with random chromosomal segments, so it is usually necessary to repeat the experiment many times to pinpoint the most likely chromosomal location of the probe DNA.

In situ hybridization using radioactive probes is usually a slow process, and the degree of resolution (2 to 5 Mb) is rather low. The FISH technique (see Chapter 6), which uses fluorescent probes instead of radioactive probes, is much faster and offers better resolution of a probe's location, often within 1 Mb for metaphase chromosomes. By using interphase chromosomes, which are less condensed than metaphase chromosomes, FISH resolution can be increased to 25 to 250 kb. Another variation of FISH, termed **fiber FISH,** involves the chemical and physical manipulation of interphase chromosomes to loosen and stretch the chromatin fibers such that individual DNA loops (see Chapter 2) can be visualized (see Color Plate 8 following p. 116). With fiber FISH, probes within a few kb of one another may be resolved. Because of its high resolution and ease of use, FISH has largely supplanted radioactive in situ hybridization as a physical mapping technique.

> ▼ In situ hybridization is a physical mapping technique in which a labeled probe is hybridized to fixed metaphase chromosomes to determine the chromosomal location of the DNA in the probe. Fluorescence in situ hybridization (FISH) can be applied to interphase chromosomes and can achieve much better resolution than radioactive in situ hybridization. Fiber FISH can distinguish probes that are only a few kb apart. ▲

Somatic Cell Hybridization

Another method of gene localization exploits the somewhat surprising fact that somatic cells from different species, when grown in the same culture in the presence of agents such as polyethylene glycol or Sendai virus, will sometimes fuse together to form hybrid cells (**somatic cell hybridization;** Fig. 8-16). When mouse and human cells are grown together in this way, the resulting hybrid cells contain 86 chromosomes: the 46 human chromosomes together with the 40 mouse chromosomes. The cells are exposed to selective media such as HAT (hypoxanthine, aminopterin, and thymidine) to eliminate those that did not fuse. The hybrid cells are then allowed to replicate. These cells will begin to lose some of their human chromosomes as they undergo mitosis. Eventually cells remain that have a full set of mouse chromosomes but only one or a few human chromosomes. The cells are karyotyped to determine which human chromo-

somes remain (human and mouse chromosomes are distinguishable from one another on the basis of size and banding patterns). These sets of cells can then be studied to determine which ones consistently contain the gene in question (Table 8-2). For example, if the gene is always found in cells that contain human chromosome 1 but never found in those that do not, we would conclude that the gene must be located on this chromosome.

Presence of the gene in the hybrid cell can be detected in several ways. If the gene encodes an enzyme that is produced by the cell, then an enzyme assay can be used. Protein electrophoresis (see Chapter 3) may be used to detect a human protein product and to distinguish it from the equivalent mouse protein product. These approaches, however, require that a known protein product can be detected. More often, investigators now test for hybridization of the fused cell lines with a labeled probe containing the DNA of interest using Southern blotting or PCR techniques (Fig. 8-17).

Occasionally a gene can be assigned to a specific *segment* of a chromosome using somatic cell hybridization. Translocations infrequently occur such that only part of a single human chromosome is attached to one of the mouse chromosomes. If the gene or DNA segment of interest is detectable in a cell containing such a translocation, then the gene must be located on the translocated segment of the human chromosome. Similarly, if a gene is consistently absent in cell lines containing a known deletion, then the gene can be localized to the region that is deleted.

> ▼ Somatic cell hybridization is a physical mapping technique in which human and rodent cells are hybridized, resulting in cells that have a reduced number of human chromosomes. Panels of such cells are used to correlate the presence of a gene with the consistent presence of one chromosome (or when translocations are available, a specific segment of a chromosome). ▲

Radiation Hybrid Mapping

This powerful and widely used technique, illustrated in Fig. 8-18, typically begins with a somatic cell hybrid that contains a single human chromosome. The cells are then irradiated with x-rays or γ-rays to induce multiple double-strand breaks in the chromosomes. This radiation kills the cells, so they must be fused with rodent cells to survive. This is accomplished using approaches similar to those described for somatic cell hybridization. Some of the resulting cells, termed **radiation hybrids,** contain small fragments of human chromosomes fused with rodent chromosomes. The presence of human chromosomes can be detected by screening for *Alu* sequences, which occur every few kb in human chromosomes but are not found in rodent chromosomes. Because radiation breaks the human chromo-

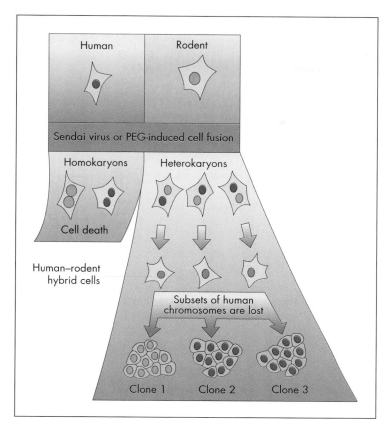

FIG. 8-16   Gene mapping by somatic cell hybridization. The human and rodent cells that fused are selected using a medium such as HAT. The hybrid cells preferentially lose human chromosomes, resulting in clones that each have only a few human chromosomes. Each clone is examined to determine whether the gene is present, thus assigning the gene to a specific chromosome.

TABLE 8-2   Somatic Cell Hybridization Panel

Clone	DNA segment	1	2	3	4	5	6	7	8	9	10	11	12	13	14	15	16	17	18	19	20	21	22	X	Y
1	+	−	−	−	+	−	+	+	+	+	−	+	+	−	−	+	−	+	−	+	−	−	−	+	−
2	−	+	+	+	−	+	−	+	−	−	+	−	−	−	+	+	+	−	−	+	+	+	+	−	−
3	+	−	−	−	+	+	+	+	+	+	−	−	−	+	−	+	−	+	−	+	+	−	+	−	−
4	+	+	−	+	−	−	−	+	−	+	−	+	+	−	−	−	+	−	+	−	−	+	−	−	−
5	−	−	+	+	+	+	+	−	−	−	+	−	−	+	−	+	−	+	−	−	+	+	−	+	+
6	−	+	−	+	−	−	+	−	−	−	+	+	−	+	+	−	+	−	+	−	−	−	+	+	−
7	+	−	+	−	+	−	+	+	+	+	−	+	−	−	−	+	+	−	+	−	+	+	−	+	−
8	−	−	+	+	+	−	−	+	−	−	+	+	+	−	+	−	+	+	−	+	+	−	−	−	−

Note that the DNA segment being tested shows a positive hybridization signal to clones 1, 3, 4, and 7. Each of these clones contains chromosome 9, while clones 2, 5, 6, and 8 do not contain this chromosome. This pattern localizes the DNA segment to chromosome 9.

somes at random intervals, loci that are located closer to one another will be found more often on the same chromosome fragment. Techniques such as PCR can be used to determine which radiation hybrids contain specific combinations of human loci (i.e., locus-specific PCR primers would be used to amplify the locus if it is present in the cell). Then statistical techniques are used to assess how often each pair of loci is found on the same chromosome fragment, providing an estimate of the relative distances between loci. Increased levels of radiation can be used to generate smaller fragments, thereby increasing the resolution of the technique.

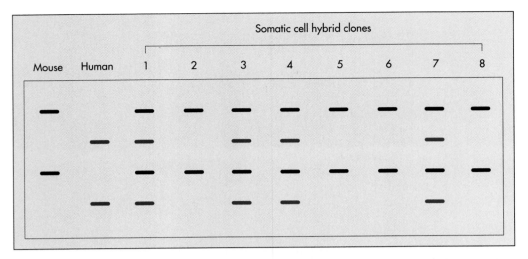

FIG. 8-17 A Southern blot used in a somatic cell hybridization gene mapping experiment (compare with panel shown in Table 8-2). Human and mouse bands differ in size because the two species have different recognition sequences. The human gene probe hybridizes only to the hybrid cells 1, 3, 4, and 7, showing that the probe hybridizes only when chromosome 9 is present.

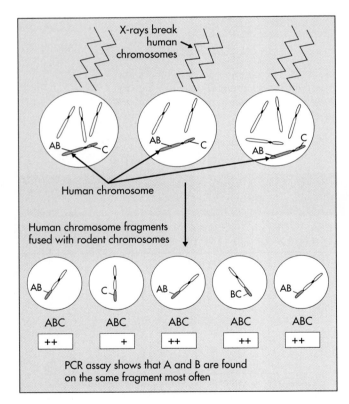

FIG. 8-18 Radiation hybrid mapping. A cell line containing a human chromosome is irradiated to produce chromosome breaks. These human chromosome fragments are fused with rodent chromosomes so that they will survive. The presence of human chromosome material in rodent cells can be detected by the presence of *Alu* sequences. Closely linked loci, such as *A* and *B*, will frequently be found on the same chromosome fragment, while loosely linked loci, such as *A* and *C*, will infrequently be found on the same chromosome fragment.

Closing in on the Gene: Positional Cloning

Sometimes the gene product responsible for a genetic disease is known before the gene itself is identified. This was the case, for example, with the β-globin polypeptide and sickle cell disease. Then one can deduce the DNA sequence from the amino acid sequence of the polypeptide; this DNA sequence can be used to make a probe in order to locate the disease gene using the techniques just described. This type of approach, in which the gene product and its function are used to pinpoint the gene, is an example of **functional cloning.**

More often, however, we have only a linkage result that has localized the disease gene to a region that may be 1 Mb or larger. Such a region can easily contain several dozen genes, interspersed with non-coding DNA. A common approach is to begin with a linked marker and then canvas the region around the marker to locate and clone the disease gene itself. This process, previously known as "reverse genetics," is now usually referred to as **positional cloning.**

Suppose that we know the approximate location of a polymorphic marker that is tightly linked (less than 1 cM, or approximately 1 Mb) to the disease gene we wish to isolate. An approach commonly used to proceed toward the gene is called **chromosome walking.** DNA from the marker can be used as a probe to pick out partially overlapping segments of DNA from a genomic library (Box 8-2). The overlap can be determined by using PCR to show that a portion of the probe and the DNA segment taken from the library can both be amplified by the same primers (Fig. 8-19). Once identified, the overlapping DNA segment itself is used as a probe to pick out another DNA segment from the genomic

FIG. 8-19 A probe was tested against eight clones taken from a human YAC library. The probe hybridized with two of the clones (lanes 6 and 7), indicating overlap between the DNA in the probe and the DNA in each of the two YAC clones.

BOX 8-2
PROBES AND LIBRARIES: THEIR CONSTRUCTION AND USE IN GENE MAPPING

Probes and libraries play central roles in gene mapping and cloning. A DNA library is much like an ordinary library, except that the library is composed of pieces of DNA rather than books. There are several types of DNA libraries. The most general is termed a **genomic library** and consists of fragments of DNA that are the result of a restriction digest of whole genomic DNA. The DNA is partially digested, so that some recognition sites are cleaved while others are not. This produces fragments that will overlap with one another. These fragments are then cloned into vectors such as phage, cosmids, or yeast artificial chromosomes using the recombinant DNA techniques discussed in Chapter 3. A genomic library contains all of the human genome: introns, exons, enhancers, promoters, and the vast stretches of noncoding DNA that separate genes.

A **cDNA library** is much more limited (and thus often easier to search), containing only the DNA corresponding to exons. It is obtained by purifying mRNA from a specific tissue, such as liver or skeletal muscle, and then exposing the mRNA to an enzyme called **reverse transcriptase.** This enzyme copies the mRNA into the appropriate complementary DNA (hence cDNA) sequence. DNA polymerase can then be used to convert this single-stranded DNA to double-stranded DNA, after which it is cloned into phage or other vectors, as in the genomic library. The steps involved in making genomic and cDNA libraries are summarized in Fig. 8-20.

Yet another type of DNA library is the **chromosome-specific library.** Chromosomes are sorted using a method called **flow cytometry,** which separates chromosomes according to the proportion of AT base pairs in each one. The result is a library consisting mostly of DNA from only one chromosome. For example, after the gene for Huntington disease was mapped to a region on the short arm of chromosome 4, a library specific for this chromosome was used to refine the location of the gene.

DNA libraries are often used in making new polymorphic markers. For example, microsatellite polymorphisms can be obtained from DNA libraries by constructing a probe that contains multiple repeated DNA sequences (e.g., multiple CA repeats). Then the DNA library is "screened" with this probe to find fragments in the library that hybridize with the probe. These fragments can be tested in a series of individuals to see whether they are polymorphic. The polymorphism can then be mapped to a specific location by using physical mapping techniques such as in situ hybridization (see text).

Probes are also highly useful in isolating specific disease genes. In this context, they can be made in several different ways. If the defective protein (or part of it) has been identified, the protein's amino acid sequence can be used to deduce part of the DNA sequence of the gene. Generally, a short DNA sequence, only 20 to 30 bp in length, is sufficiently unique so that it will hybridize only to the complementary DNA in the disease gene. These sequences can be synthesized in a laboratory instrument to make oligonucleotide probes (see Chapter 3). Because of the degeneracy of the DNA code, more than one triplet codon may specify an amino acid. For this reason, different possible combinations of base pairs must be tried. These combinations of oligonucleotide probes are mixed together, and the mixture is then used to probe a DNA library (e.g., a cDNA library). When one of the oligonucleotide probes in the mixture

Continued

BOX 8-2—cont'd

PROBES AND LIBRARIES: THEIR CONSTRUCTION AND USE IN GENE MAPPING—cont'd

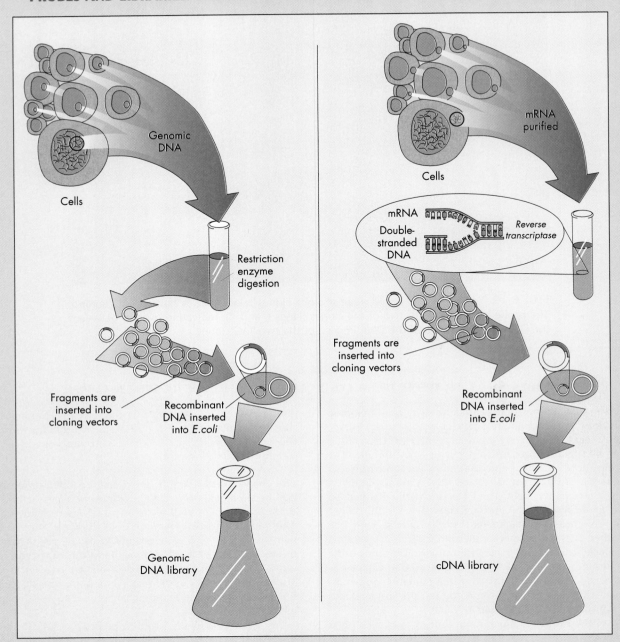

FIG. 8-20 **The creation of human DNA libraries.** *Left,* A total genomic library is created using a partial restriction digest of human DNA and then cloning the fragments into vectors such as phage, cosmids, or YACs. *Right,* A cDNA library is created by purifying mRNA from a tissue and exposing it to reverse transcriptase to create cDNA sequences. These are cloned into vectors.

hybridizes with a fragment in the library, a portion of the desired gene has been identified. This fragment can be mapped using the physical techniques mentioned in the text.

Often the investigator has no knowledge of the sequence of the gene product. In this case it is sometimes possible to isolate the gene by purifying mRNA produced by specialized cell types. For example, reticulocytes (immature red blood cells) produce mostly globin polypeptides. mRNA

taken from these cells can be converted to cDNA using reverse transcriptase, as discussed previously, and then used as a probe to find additional fragments of the gene in a DNA library. It is sometimes easier to obtain mRNA from an experimental animal, such as a pig or rodent. Because of sequence similarity between these animals and humans, the animal-derived probe will usually hybridize appropriately with segments of a human DNA library.

library with which *it* partially overlaps. In this way, one uses partially overlapping DNA segments to "walk" along the chromosome until the disease gene itself is reached. Since we are sometimes uncertain whether the disease gene is on one side of the marker or the other, chromosome walking may proceed in both directions away from the marker (a bidirectional walk).

The determination of overlap among DNA segments has been greatly facilitated by the creation and mapping of tens of thousands of **sequence tagged sites (STSs).** STSs are sequences of a few hundred bp whose chromosome location is known. They are flanked by known PCR primers, so that any laboratory can use PCR to amplify them for analysis. They thus create physical "signposts" of known sequence throughout the genome whose mutual occurrence on different DNA segments indicates overlap between the segments (Fig. 8-21). STSs are localized to specific chromosome locations using techniques such as radiation hybrid mapping. www

The DNA segments used in a chromosome walk may be cloned into vectors such as plasmids, cosmids, or yeast artificial chromosomes (YACs), as discussed in Chapter 3. Plasmids accommodate the smallest DNA inserts, while YACs accommodate the largest ones, 200 to 2000 kb. Nearly all of the human genome has now been cloned into YACs. While very useful, YACs sometimes combine DNA from completely different genomic regions in the same clone (known as chimerism). Obviously, this can complicate a chromosome walk. Other cloning vectors are more stable but accept smaller inserts: **bacterial artificial chromosomes (BACs)** and **bacteriophage P1 artificial chromosomes (PACs)** both accept inserts of 50 to 200 kb. They are often used in combination with YACs in positional cloning experiments. Fig. 8-22 depicts a map of overlapping YACs and

cosmids in the adenomatous polyposis coli region (a form of colon cancer; see Chapter 11). These maps of contiguous DNA segments are termed **contig maps.**

The process of chromosome walking can be further illustrated with an analogy. Imagine that we have been placed somewhere in the state of California and that our ultimate destination is Los Angeles. We do not

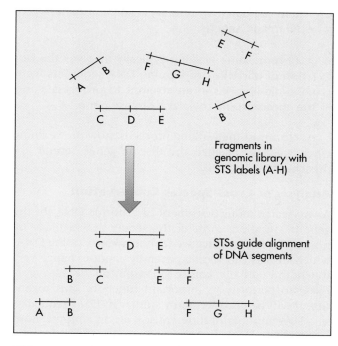

FIG. 8-21 The use of STSs to indicate overlap between DNA segments in a chromosome walk. Overlap is indicated when PCR primers for a specific STS amplify DNA from different DNA segments taken from a genomic library.

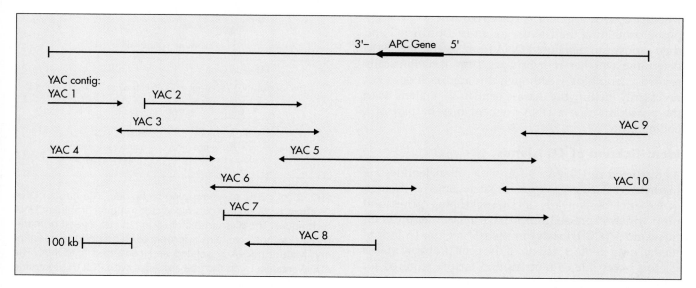

FIG. 8-22 An example of a YAC contig map used in "walking" along chromosome 5 in the region of the adenomatous polyposis coli (APC) gene.

know in which direction Los Angeles lies, nor do we know exactly how far away it is. We are given a map of the county in which we are currently located, and we have access to a library of highway maps of each county of California. These maps are not labeled, but, like most highway maps, there is a small region of overlap between maps of adjacent counties. We then use the first map we were given to search the library for maps that overlap in either direction. Finding such maps, we then use them to search the library again, ultimately progressing to Los Angeles.

▼ Chromosome walking typically involves the isolation of partially overlapping DNA segments from genomic libraries in an attempt to progress along the chromosome toward a disease gene. ▲

As chromosome walking proceeds, how do we know when we have reached the disease gene? Several approaches may be used.

Analysis of Cross-Species Conservation

As we search along a segment of genomic DNA for the gene in question, most of the sequence will likely be noncoding DNA, which we wish to avoid. Coding DNA, which we wish to locate, generally cannot change very much through the course of evolution because it is likely to perform an important function. This means that it will be **conserved,** or similar in DNA sequence, in a large number of different species. In contrast, noncoding DNA is likely to change rapidly and differ substantially among species. Thus, if the sequence we are currently considering in our chromosome walk consists of coding DNA, it is more likely to hybridize (i.e., undergo complementary base pairing) with the DNA of many other species. A nonconserved sequence is less likely to show cross-species hybridization. To test whether a DNA segment is conserved across species, a probe containing the DNA segment is constructed and then exposed to denatured DNA from several species to determine whether it hybridizes (this is whimsically termed a "zoo blot"). Although this approach does not necessarily identify the disease gene itself, it alerts us to the possibility that a DNA segment may be part of a coding gene.

Identification of CG Islands

As discussed in Chapter 3, most CG dinucleotides are methylated. However, approximately 60% of human genes, including nearly all housekeeping genes and most widely expressed genes, have *unmethylated* CG dinucleotides **(CG islands)** in their 5′ region. (A lack of methylation in the 5′ region of the gene probably makes it more accessible to transcription factors required for active expression.) The identification of a series of CG islands can often pinpoint a coding gene.

Exon Identification Techniques

Several approaches are now used to identify exons in a genomic DNA sequence. In one approach, termed **exon trapping,** the presence of an exon or exons in a DNA sequence is detected by inserting the sequence into a plasmid vector that is allowed to undergo transcriptional processing in yeast or mammalian cells (Fig. 8-23). Normal mRNA processing takes place, and all sequences except the exons are spliced out. If the DNA sequence in question contains exons, a larger fragment will be produced after mRNA processing; if the DNA sequence does not contain exons, a smaller fragment will be produced.

Another commonly used exon detection technique is termed **direct cDNA selection.** Here, the genomic DNA sequence under scrutiny is inserted into a YAC. The

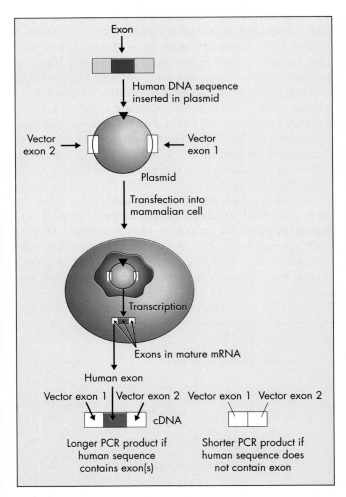

FIG. 8-23   The exon trapping technique. The human DNA segment is placed in a plasmid vector using recombinant DNA techniques. The plasmid vector is cloned into a yeast or mammalian cell that contains appropriate transcriptional machinery. Mature mRNA is isolated and converted to cDNA. The cDNA sequence can then be amplified with PCR to determine its length. If the human DNA segment contains an exon or exons, the resulting fragment will be longer than if it does not.

YACs are then hybridized to cDNA clones taken from a complete human cDNA library. If the DNA sequence in the YAC contains exons, they should undergo complementary base pairing with sequences in the cDNA library (since cDNA is made only from coding DNA; see Box 8-2). If the DNA sequence does not contain exons, it should not hybridize effectively. After several repeated cycles of hybridization, the cDNA clones corresponding to exons in the DNA sequence will be greatly enriched, permitting their identification. A weakness of this approach is that it may miss genes that are poorly represented in the cDNA library because they are expressed only rarely.

Further Linkage Analysis

As chromosome walking proceeds, polymorphisms within the overlapping segments can be analyzed as new markers for the disease gene. These markers are then used in new linkage analyses in families. If we find that the recombination frequency has increased between our new markers and the disease gene, then we are likely to be moving away from the disease gene rather than toward it. Because recombination in genomic regions smaller than 1 Mb is rare, additional linkage analysis is often of limited usefulness. Linkage disequilibrium analysis, which sometimes permits resolution at a finer scale, may also be used in this way.

Computer Analysis of DNA Sequence

Computer analysis, sometimes termed *in silico* research, has become an effective and popular approach for identifying genes. Sophisticated computer algorithms, such as GRAIL, can test a DNA sequence for patterns that signal a coding gene (e.g., transcription initiation sites, stop codons, intron-exon boundaries). This approach was used, for example, to help identify and characterize one of the adult polycystic kidney disease genes (*PKD1*; see Chapter 4). In addition, these algorithms can often recognize patterns typical of genes that encode specific classes of proteins (e.g., transcription factors, transmembrane proteins).

Computerized databases of known DNA sequences also play an important role in gene identification. When studying a specific region of DNA to find a gene, it is common to search for similarity between DNA sequences from the region and DNA sequences in the database. The sequences in the database may derive from genes with known function or tissue-specific expression patterns. Suppose, for example, that we have used linkage analysis to identify a region containing a gene that causes a developmental disorder such as a limb malformation. As we proceed with chromosome walking, we would look for similarity between a DNA sequence from this region and a plausible sequence from the database (e.g., sequence from a gene that encodes a protein involved in bone development, such as a fibroblast

growth factor). Because genes that encode similar protein products usually have similar DNA sequences, a match between the sequence from our region and a sequence in the database could be a vital clue that this particular DNA sequence is actually part of the gene that causes the limb malformation.

A computerized database commonly used in these searches consists of small DNA sequences known as **expressed sequence tags (ESTs).** ESTs are obtained by sequencing several hundred bp from both ends of cDNA clones taken from a cDNA library (see Box 8-2). Because these clones consist of DNA that is complementary to mRNA, the ESTs represent *expressed* portions of genes. Often, they are expressed only in certain tissues at certain points in time. ESTs can be mapped to specific chromosome locations using previously discussed physical mapping techniques, such as radiation hybrid mapping or FISH. Then the investigator can search for sequence similarity between DNA sequences in a region of interest and ESTs known to be located in the same region (and possibly known to be expressed in a tissue that would be consistent with the disease in question). This strategy was used, for example, to identify one of the genes known to cause Alzheimer disease (see Chapter 12). The identification of ESTs has proceeded rapidly, with more than one million ESTs now available in computerized databases. **WWW**

The similarity search need not be confined to human genes. Often, sequence similarity is observed with genes of known function in other organisms, such as mouse or even yeast or bacteria. Because genes with important protein products tend to be highly conserved throughout evolution, the identification of a human homolog in another organism can provide important information about the gene's function in the human. For example, many of the genes involved in cell cycle regulation are quite similar in yeast and human (e.g., portions of the *NF1* gene and the yeast *IRA2* gene). Indeed, approximately one third of human disease-causing genes identified to date have homologs in yeast. These genes and their products can easily be manipulated in experimental organisms, so their well-understood functions in these organisms can provide useful inferences about their functions in humans. A number of important human disease genes have been identified because homologous candidate genes had been identified in other organisms (e.g., the mouse "small eye" gene and aniridia, the mouse "splotch" gene and Waardenburg syndrome, the *Drosophila* and mouse "patched" genes and basal cell nevus syndrome, the mouse "pink eye" gene and oculocutaneous albinism type 2).

Screen for Mutations in the Sequence

Once a portion of coding DNA has been isolated, it can be examined for mutations using techniques such as SSCP, DGGE, and direct DNA sequencing (see Chapter

3). If a DNA sequence represents the disease gene, then mutations should be found in individuals with the disease, but they should not be found in unaffected individuals. To help to distinguish disease-causing mutations from polymorphisms that vary naturally among individuals, it is particularly useful to compare the DNA of patients whose disease is caused by a *new mutation* with the DNA of their unaffected parents. While a harmless polymorphism will be seen in both the affected offspring and the unaffected parents, a mutation re-sponsible for the disease in the offspring will not be seen in the parents. This approach is especially useful in identifying mutations in highly penetrant autosomal dominant diseases such as NF1.

Another type of mutation that can be tested is a submicroscopic deletion (i.e., a deletion too small to be observable under a microscope). Small deletions can be detected using Southern blotting techniques (see Chapter 3). A deletion will produce a smaller-than-normal restriction fragment, which migrates more quickly

FIG. 8-24   An example of a Northern blot, showing the hybridization of a cDNA probe from the *EVI2A* gene (a gene embedded within an intron of the *NF1* gene) with mRNA from adrenal gland, brain, and fibroblasts. This result indicates that *EVI2A* is expressed in the brain at a much higher level than in the other two tissues.
(Courtesy Dr. Richard Cawthon, University of Utah Health Sciences Center.)

through a gel. Somewhat larger deletions can be detected through **pulsed field gel electrophoresis,** a variation on the Southern blotting technique in which restriction digests are done with enzymes that, because their recognition sequences are rare, cleave the DNA infrequently. This produces restriction fragments that can be tens or hundreds of kb in length. These fragments are too large to be distinguished from one another using standard gel electrophoresis, but they will migrate differentially according to size when the electrical current is pulsed in alternating directions across the gel.

Test for Gene Expression

To help verify that a gene is responsible for a given disease, one can test various tissues to determine the ones in which the gene is expressed (i.e., transcribed into mRNA). This can be done by purifying mRNA from the tissue, placing it on a blot, and hybridizing it with a probe made from the gene. This technique, known as **Northern blotting** (Fig. 8-24), is conceptually similar to Southern blotting except that mRNA, rather than DNA, is being probed. If the gene in question causes the disease, the mRNA may be expressed in tissues known to be affected by the disease (the same reasoning is applied to the analysis of ESTs obtained from tissue-specific cDNA libraries). For example, one would expect the phenylalanine hydroxylase gene (in which mutations can cause PKU) to be expressed in the liver, where this enzyme is known to be synthesized.

A more direct gene expression test involves inserting the normal version of the DNA sequence into a defective cell from an affected individual (or animal model), using recombinant DNA techniques. If the normal sequence corrects the defect, then it is very likely to represent the disease gene of interest. This approach has been used, for example, to prove that mutations in the CFTR gene can cause cystic fibrosis.

Many things can complicate the positional cloning procedure. For example, the isolation of overlapping DNA sequences can become very difficult when long sequences of repetitive DNA are encountered. As a result, this process can be very laborious and time-consuming. The Huntington disease gene, for example, was localized to chromosome 4p by linkage analysis in 1983, but 10 years of hard work by a large group of dedicated researchers elapsed before the disease gene itself was cloned. Four years of positional cloning were required to isolate the cystic fibrosis gene. The positional cloning process has been accelerated as better cloning techniques and vectors have been devised (e.g., BACs, PACs, and YACs, which can carry much larger inserts than cosmids). The development of physical mapping landmarks (STSs) as part of the Human Genome Project has also increased the speed and efficiency of positional cloning.

▼ **During the course of chromosome walking, one needs to determine whether the DNA segment cur-** rently under consideration is part of a disease gene. Tests used for this purpose include cross-species hybridization, identification of unmethylated CG islands, exon trapping, direct cDNA selection, further linkage analysis using polymorphisms in the newly isolated DNA segment as markers, computer analysis of DNA sequence, mutation screening in affected individuals, and tests of gene expression. ▲

Candidate Genes

The gene hunting process can be expedited considerably when a **candidate gene** is available. As the name implies, this is a gene whose known protein product makes it a likely candidate for the disease in question. For example, the various collagen genes were considered to be reasonable candidates for Marfan syndrome because collagen is an important component of connective tissue. However, linkage analysis using collagen gene markers in Marfan syndrome families consistently yielded negative results. Another candidate gene emerged when the *fibrillin-1* gene was identified on chromosome 15. Fibrillin, as discussed in Chapter 4, is also a connective tissue component. Linkage analysis had localized the Marfan syndrome gene to chromosome 15, so *fibrillin-1* became an even stronger candidate. Analysis of *fibrillin-1* mutations showed that they were consistently associated with Marfan syndrome, confirming these mutations as a cause of the disease. This combination of linkage analysis to identify the region containing a gene followed by a search of the region for plausible candidate genes is sometimes called the **positional candidate** approach.

Another example of candidate gene analysis is provided by hyperkalemic periodic paralysis, an autosomal dominant muscle disorder characterized by transient episodes of weakness or paralysis. The electrophysiological abnormalities observed in this disorder suggested that a defect in a voltage-gated sodium channel could be involved. A sodium channel gene on chromosome 17 thus presented itself as a likely candidate, and a polymorphism in this gene showed perfect linkage with the disease phenotype in large families. Subsequent analyses verified the pathogenic role of the sodium channel gene by detecting mutations in affected individuals.

▼ **Candidate genes are those whose characteristics (such as protein product) suggest that they may be responsible for a genetic disease. The analysis of candidate genes in a region known to contain the disease-causing gene is termed the "positional candidate approach."** ▲

Using the techniques described in this chapter, a large number of important disease genes have now been mapped, and many of them have also been cloned. Some examples are given in Table 8-3.

TABLE 8-3 Examples of Disease Genes That Have Been Mapped and Cloned

Disease	Chromosome location	Gene product
α-1-Antitrypsin deficiency	14q	Serine protease inhibitor
α-Thalassemia	16p	α-Globin component of hemoglobin
β-Thalassemia	11p	β-Globin component of hemoglobin
Achondroplasia	4p	Fibroblast growth factor receptor 3
Adult polycystic kidney disease	16p	Polycystin-1 membrane protein
	4p	Polycystin-2 membrane protein
Albinism, oculocutaneous (type 1)	11q	Tyrosinase
Albinism, oculocutaneous (type 2)	15q	Tyrosine transporter
Alzheimer disease*	14q	Presenilin 1
	1q	Presenilin 2
	19q	Apolipoprotein E
	21q	β-Amyloid precursor protein
Amyotrophic lateral sclerosis	21q	Superoxide dismutase 1
Angelman syndrome	15q	Ubiquitin-protein ligase E3A
Ataxia telangiectasia	11q	Cell cycle control protein
Beckwith-Wiedemann syndrome	11p	Insulin-like growth factor II
Bloom syndrome	15q	RecQ helicase
Breast cancer (familial)	17q	BRCA1 tumor suppressor
	13q	BRCA2 tumor suppressor
Charcot-Marie-Tooth disease (type 1B)*	1q	Myelin protein zero
(type 1A)	17p	Peripheral myelin protein 22
(CMTX1)	Xq	Connexin-32 gap junction protein
Cystic fibrosis	7q	Cystic fibrosis transmembrane regulator (CFTR)
Deafness (nonsyndromic)	13q	Connexin-26 gap junction protein
	5q	Actin polymerization regulator
	11q	Myosin VIIA
Diabetes (MODY1)	20q	Hepatocyte nuclear factor-4α
(MODY2)	7p	Glucokinase
(MODY3)	12q	Hepatocyte nuclear factor-1α
Duchenne/Becker muscular dystrophy	Xp	Dystrophin
Familial polyposis coli	5q	APC tumor suppressor
Fragile X syndrome	Xq	FMR1 RNA-binding protein
Friedreich ataxia	9q	Frataxin mitochondrial protein
Hemochromatosis	6p	HLA-like protein
Hemophilia A	Xq	Clotting factor VIII
Hemophilia B	Xq	Clotting factor IX
Hereditary nonpolyposis colorectal cancer	3p	MLH1 DNA mismatch repair protein
	2p	MSH2 DNA mismatch repair protein
	2q	PMSL1 DNA mismatch repair protein
	7p	PMSL2 DNA mismatch repair protein
Hirschsprung disease (type 1)*	10q	RET tyrosine kinase proto-oncogene
(type 2)	13q	Endothelin receptor type B
Huntington disease	4p	Huntingtin
Hypercholesterolemia (familial)	19p	LDL receptor
Long QT syndrome (LQT3)*	3p	SCN5A cardiac sodium channel
(LQT2)	7q	HERG cardiac potassium channel
(LQT1)	11p	KVLQT1 cardiac potassium channel α subunit
(LQT5)	21q	KCNE1 cardiac potassium channel β subunit
Marfan syndrome	15q	Fibrillin-1
Melanoma (familial)*	9p	Cyclin-dependent kinase inhibitor tumor suppressor
	12q	Cyclin-dependent kinase 4
Myotonic dystrophy	19q	Protein kinase
Myoclonus epilepsy (Unverricht-Lundborg)	21q	Cystatin B cysteine protease inhibitor
Neurofibromatosis type 1	17q	Neurofibromin tumor suppressor
Neurofibromatosis type 2	22q	Merlin (schwannomin) tumor suppressor

TABLE 8-3	Examples of Disease Genes That Have Been Mapped and Cloned—cont'd	

Disease	Chromosome location	Gene product
Phenylketonuria	12q	Phenylalanine hydroxylase
Retinitis pigmentosa*	3q	Rhodopsin
	6p	TULP1 tubby-like protein
	1p	Retina-specific ABC transporter
	6p	Peripherin
	11q	Rod outer segment membrane protein
	4p	Retinal rod photoreceptor cGMP phosphodiesterase, β subunit
	5q	Retinal rod photoreceptor cGMP phosphodiesterase, α subunit
	4p	Retinal rod cGMPgated channel, α subunit
	11q	Myosin VIIA
Retinoblastoma	13q	pRb tumor suppressor
Sickle-cell disease	11p	β-globin component of hemoglobin
Tay-Sachs disease	15q	Hexosaminidase A
Tuberous sclerosis (type 1)*	9q	Hamartin tumor suppressor
(type 2)	16p	Tuberin tumor suppressor
Waardenburg syndrome (types 1 and 3)*	2q	PAX3 transcription factor
(type 2)	3p	MITF leucine zipper protein
(type 4)	14q	Endothelin 3 or endothelin B receptor
Wilms tumor*	11p	WT1 zinc finger protein tumor suppressor
Wilson disease	13q	Copper transporting ATPase
von Willebrand disease	12q	von Willebrand clotting factor

*Additional disease-causing loci have been mapped and/or possibly cloned.

BOX 8-3
THE HUMAN GENOME PROJECT

The Human Genome Project is one of the most widely publicized and ambitious undertakings in the history of biomedical research. Initiated in October 1990, this 15-year project has three major goals: (1) a genetic marker map, (2) a physical map, and (3) the complete three billion bp sequence of the human genome.

Considerable progress has been made in achieving these goals. The marker map was completed several years ago and currently includes nearly 20,000 polymorphisms distributed throughout the genome. These include RFLPs, VNTRs, and microsatellite polymorphisms. On average, a useful polymorphism can be found at intervals of less than 1 cM. Thus, a closely linked marker can be found for virtually any disease gene. Recently, a project was initiated to amass a collection of approximately 100,000 **single nucleotide polymorphisms** (SNPs) distributed throughout the genome. SNPs are single-base variants that individually are less polymorphic than a microsatellite or VNTR polymorphism. However, they have a lower mutation rate than these polymorphisms, and they are especially amenable to computerized automated processing (e.g., DNA chips; see Chapter 3). They will thus add even further to the usefulness of the human genetic map.

The second goal, a physical map of known STSs distributed at 100 kb intervals throughout the genome, is nearly complete, with more than 44,000 STSs catalogued as of early 1998. These physical signposts are invaluable in positional cloning experiments, where they can be used to place a series of DNA sequences (e.g., those inserted in YACs, BACs, PACs, or cosmids) in relative order.

The final goal, the complete genome sequence, is in many ways the most challenging of all. Starting from a chromosome-specific library, sequencing centers typically obtain the sequences of thousands of small inserts of 1000 bp or less. These must then be arranged in order to assemble the sequence of a chromosome. This is a formidable task because of potential gaps, difficulties with repetitive sequences, and so forth. Much effort is still being devoted to the development of methods that will minimize the time and expense required for this project. To be useful, a high degree of accuracy must be attained; the currently accepted error rate is 1 in every 10,000 bp. Sequencing the genomes of several smaller, genetically simpler organisms (e.g., bacteria [E. coli] and yeast [S. cerevisiae]) has helped to optimize the methods being used for the much larger human genome. In addition, homology between the genes of these organisms and the human have helped us to understand the nature of a number of human disease genes.

Currently, about 3% of the human genome has been sequenced. This figure is expected to increase rapidly as

BOX 8-3—cont'd

THE HUMAN GENOME PROJECT—cont'd

methods are optimized, and researchers are optimistic that the sequencing project will be completed before the projected end of the Human Genome Project in 2005.

Completion of this project will provide many benefits. Already, gene mapping projects can often be completed in a matter of weeks because of dense and freely available marker maps. Positional cloning, once the bane of genetics laboratories, is now much more feasible because of the existing physical map. The amount of time required to identify genes via positional cloning continues to decrease, and the number of disease genes pinpointed this way is growing each year. The cloning of disease genes yields many important benefits: improved genetic diagnosis, the potential for manufacture of gene products by recombinant DNA techniques, and improved treatment through more specific drugs or gene therapy (see Chapter 13).

The complete genome sequence is likely to yield predictable—and unpredictable—results and benefits. Having a complete sequence in hand will greatly speed the identification of all human genes. It will provide the ultimate genetic "blueprint" of the human. It is also quite possible that the vast expanses of non-coding DNA will surprise us with previously unknown insights about our biology and our origins.

It is a mistake to think of the completion of the human genome sequence as the end of an era of research. The genome sequence, while of immense value, is still nothing more than a long string of nucleotides. The challenge will be to use this vast pool of information to identify genes, understand their regulation and expression, and characterize the many complex interactions among genes and environment that ultimately give rise to phenotypes. The human genome sequence thus represents the beginning, rather than the end, of an era of fruitful and exciting biological research.

STUDY QUESTIONS

1. In Fig. 8-25, a pedigree for an autosomal dominant disease, each family member has been typed for a four-allele microsatellite marker, as shown in the autoradiogram below the pedigree. Determine the linkage phase for the disease and marker locus in the affected male in generation 2. Based on the meioses that produced the offspring in generation 3, what is the recombination frequency for the marker and the disease locus?

FIG. 8-25 Pedigree for Study Question 1.

STUDY QUESTIONS—cont'd

2. In the Huntington disease pedigree in Fig. 8-26, the family has been typed for two two-allele markers, A and B. The genotypes for each marker are shown below each family member; the genotype for marker A is shown above the genotype for marker B. Under the hypothesis that θ = 0.0, what is the LOD score for linkage between each marker locus and the Huntington disease locus?

FIG. 8-26   Pedigree for Study Question 2.

3. Interpret the following table of LOD scores and recombination frequencies (θ):

θ	0.0	0.05	0.1	0.2	0.3	0.4	0.5
LOD	-∞	1.7	3.5	2.8	2.2	1.1	0.0

4. Two pedigrees for an autosomal dominant disease are shown in Fig. 8-27. The families have been typed for a six-allele microsatellite polymorphism. Based on the data in these families, what is the re-combination frequency between the marker locus and the disease locus? What is the LOD score for linkage between the marker and disease loci under the hypothesis that θ = 0.0?

FIG. 8-27   Pedigrees for Study Question 4.

5. Consider the pedigree in Fig. 8-28, in which an autosomal recessive gene is being transmitted and each family member has been typed for a five-allele microsatellite polymorphism. Carrier status in each individual has been established by an independent enzymatic assay. What is the recombination frequency between the microsatellite polymorphism and the disease locus?

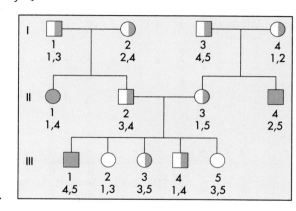

FIG. 8-28   Pedigree for Study Question 5.

6. An autosomal dominant disease is being transmitted in the pedigree in Fig. 8-29. A two-allele marker has been typed for each family member. What is the recombination frequency for the marker and the disease locus? What is the LOD score for a recombination frequency of 0.0? What is the LOD score for a recombination frequency of 0.1?

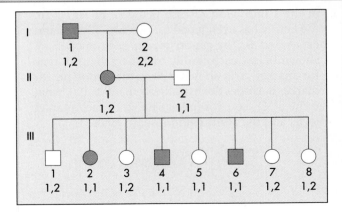

FIG. 8-29   Pedigree for Study Question 6.

7. The family shown in the pedigree in Fig. 8-30 has been presented for genetic diagnosis. The disease in question is autosomal dominant. The family members have been typed for a closely linked two-allele marker locus. What can you tell the family about the risks for their offspring?

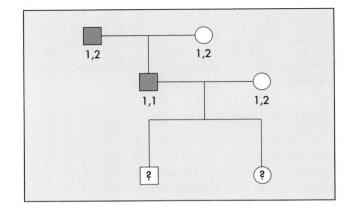

FIG. 8-30   Pedigree for Study Question 7.

8. Distinguish the differences among the concepts of synteny, linkage, linkage disequilibrium, and association.
9. A recent study showed no linkage disequilibrium between neurofibromatosis type 1 and a very closely linked marker locus. Explain this, keeping in mind that the neurofibromatosis type 1 gene has a high rate of new mutations.

10. The somatic cell hybridization panel in Fig. 8-31 indicates the clones that yielded a positive hybridization signal for a cDNA segment. Based on this information, on which chromosome is the cDNA segment likely to reside?

Clone	DNA segment	1	2	3	4	5	6	7	8	9	10	11	12	13	14	15	16	17	18	19	20	21	22	X	Y
1	−	−	−	+	−	−	−	+	−	+	−	+	+	−	+	+	+	−	−	+	−	−	−	+	−
2	−	−	+	+	−	−	−	+	−	−	+	−	−	−	+	−	+	−	−	+	−	+	−	+	−
3	+	−	+	+	−	+	−	+	−	+	−	+	+	+	−	+	−	+	−	+	−	−	+	−	−
4	−	+	−	+	−	−	−	+	−	−	−	+	+	−	+	−	+	−	+	+	+	+	−	−	−
5	−	−	+	+	+	−	+	−	−	−	+	−	−	+	−	−	+	−	+	+	+	−	+	+	−
6	+	−	+	+	−	+	−	+	+	+	+	+	+	−	−	−	+	−	+	+	−	−	+	+	+

FIG. 8-31   Somatic cell hybridization panel for Study Question 10.

SUGGESTED READINGS

Berson EL (1996) Retinitis pigmentosa: unfolding its mystery. Proc. Natl. Acad. Sci. USA 93:4526-4528

Collins FS (1995) Positional cloning moves from perdition to traditional. Nature Genet. 9:347-350

Collins FS (1997) Sequencing the human genome. Hosp. Practice 32:35-54

Cross SH, Bird AP (1995) CpG islands and genes. Curr. Opin. Genet. Dev. 5:309-314

Dib C, Faure S, Fizames C, Samson D, Drouot N, Vignal A, Millasseau P, et al (1996) A comprehensive genetic map of the human genome based on 5,264 microsatellites. Nature 380:152-154

Dryja TP, Li T (1995) Molecular genetics of retinitis pigmentosa. Hum. Molec. Genet. 4:1739-1743

Foury F (1997) Human genetics diseases: a cross-talk between man and yeast. Gene 195:1-10

Gerhold D, Caskey CT (1996) It's the genes! EST access to human genome content. BioEssays 18:973-981

Guyer MS, Collins FS (1995) How is the Human Genome Project doing, and what have we learned so far? Proc. Natl. Acad. Sci. USA 92:10841-10848

Hudson TJ, Stein LD, Gerety SS, Ma J, Castle AB, Silva J, Slonim DK, et al. (1995) An STS-based map of the human genome. Science 270:1945-1954

Jorde LB (1995) Invited editorial: Linkage disequilibrium as a gene mapping tool. Am. J. Hum. Genet. 56:11-14

Leach RJ, O'Connell P (1995) Mapping of mammalian genomes with radiation (Goss and Harris) hybrids. Adv. Genet. 33:63-99

Marra MA, Hillier L, Waterston RH (1998) Expressed sequence tags—ESTablishing bridges between genomes. Trends Genet. 14:4-7

McKusick VA (1997) Genomics: structural and functional studies of genomes. Genomics 45:244-249

Morton NE (1995) LODs past and present. Genetics 140:7-12

Nelson DL (1995) Positional cloning reaches maturity. Curr. Opin. Genet. Dev. 5:298-303

Ott J (1991) Analysis of Human Genetic Linkage. Johns Hopkins University Press, Baltimore

Rawlings CJ, Searls DB (1997) Computational gene discovery and human disease. Curr. Opin. Genet. Dev. 7:416-423

Rowen L, Mahairas G, Hood L (1997) Sequencing the human genome. Science 278:605-607

Schuler GD, Boguski MS, Stewart EA, Stein LD, Gyapay G, Rice K, White RE, et al. (1996) A gene map of the human genome. Science 274:540-546

Sheffield VC, Nishimura DY, Stone EM (1995) Novel approaches to linkage mapping. Curr. Opin. Genet. Dev. 5:335-341

Wang DG, Fan J-B, Siao C-J, Berno A, Young P, Sapolsky R, Ghandour G, et al. (1998) Large-scale identification, mapping, and genotyping of single-nucleotide polymorphisms in the human genome. Science 280:1077-1082

9

Immunogenetics

Each day, our bodies are confronted with a formidable series of invaders: viruses, bacteria, and many other disease-causing organisms whose goal is to overcome our natural defenses. These defenses, known collectively as the immune system, consist of a diverse collection of trillions of cells. The immune system must be able to cope with a multitude of invading microorganisms, and it must be able to distinguish "self" from "non-self" with a high degree of accuracy.

As one might expect, the genetic basis of the immune system is complex. The study of the genetics of the immune system, known as **immunogenetics,** has benefited enormously from new developments in gene mapping and cloning. Most of the techniques discussed in earlier chapters (e.g., linkage analysis, chromosome walking, DNA sequencing) have been used to study genes responsible for the immune response. Many new genes have been discovered, and their functions and interactions have been studied intensely. This chapter provides a brief review of basic immunology, and it discusses the genes underlying our capacity to defend against a highly diverse array of pathogens. Aspects of autoimmune disease are examined, and some of the major immunodeficiency disorders are discussed.

THE IMMUNE RESPONSE: BASIC CONCEPTS
The Innate Immune System

When a pathogenic microorganism is encountered, the body's first line of defense includes **phagocytes** (a type of cell that engulfs and destroys the microorganism) and the **complement system.** The complement proteins can destroy microbes directly by perforating their cell membranes, and they can also attract phagocytes and other immune system agents to microbes by coating the microbial surface (it is because of this assisting role that

the term "complement" originated). **Natural killer cells,** a specific type of lymphocyte, can respond to certain viral infections and some tumor cells. These various components of the immune system can distinguish foreign bodies in a variety of ways. For example, bacteria are often identified because they produce distinctive peptides beginning with formyl methionine, and many possess distinctive carbohydrate side chains. Viruses are often recognized because some of them produce double-stranded RNA, which is relatively rare in mammals. These elements of the early phase of the immune response, termed the **innate immune system,** recognize only general features of foreign microbes. All multicellular organisms have some type of innate immune response system.

▼ The innate immune system, which includes some phagocytes, natural killer cells, and the complement system, is an early part of the immune response and recognizes general features of invading microorganisms. ▲

The Adaptive Immune System

While the innate immune system may help to hold an infection in check in its early phases, it is often incapable of overcoming the infection. This is the task of a more specialized component of the immune system, the **adaptive immune system.** As its name suggests, this part of the immune system is capable of "adapting" to features of the invading microorganism in order to mount a more specific and more effective immune response. The adaptive immune system is a more recent evolutionary development than the innate immune system and is found only in vertebrates.

Key components of the adaptive immune response include **T lymphocytes** (or **T cells**) and **B lymphocytes** (or **B cells**). These cells are created in the body's primary lymphoid organs (bone marrow for B cells and the thymus for T cells). In the thymus, T cells that can tolerate the body's own peptides are selected, and those that would attack the body's peptides are eliminated. The B and T cells then progress to secondary lymphoid tissues, such as the lymph nodes, spleen, and tonsils, where they encounter disease-causing microorganisms. Mature B lymphocytes secrete circulating **antibodies,** which combat infections. The B lymphocyte component of the immune system is sometimes called the **humoral immune system** because it produces antibodies that circulate in the bloodstream. T lymphocytes help B lymphocytes to respond to infections more effectively, and they can directly kill infected cells. Because some of the T cells destroy infected cells directly, the T-cell component of the immune system is sometimes called the **cellular immune system.** It is estimated that the body contains several trillion B and T cells.

▼ B lymphocytes are a component of the adaptive immune system; they produce circulating antibodies in response to infection. T lymphocytes, another component of the adaptive immune system, interact directly with infected cells to kill these cells, and they aid in the B cell response. ▲

The B Cell Response: Humoral Immune System

A major element of the adaptive immune response begins when specialized types of phagocytes engulf invading microbes and then present peptides derived from these microbes on their cell surfaces. These cells, which include **macrophages** and **dendritic cells,** are termed **antigen presenting cells (APCs).** B cells are also capable of engulfing microbes and presenting foreign peptides on their cell surfaces. The foreign peptide is transported to the surface of the APC by a **class II major histocompatibility complex (MHC)** molecule, which carries the foreign peptide in a specialized groove (Fig. 9-1). This complex, which projects into the extracellular environment, is recognized by another cell, the **helper T lymphocyte.** This cell has a receptor on its surface capable of binding (i.e., forming non-covalent bonds) to the MHC-peptide complex. As shown in Fig. 9-2, other cell-surface proteins, such as the various **cell adhesion molecules** and **costimulatory molecules,** also participate in the binding interaction. Binding the MHC-peptide complex stimulates the helper T lymphocyte to secrete **cytokines,** which are signaling proteins that mediate communication between cells. In particular, these cytokines help to stimulate the subset of B lymphocytes whose cell surface receptors, termed **immunoglobulins,** can bind to the invading microorganism's peptides. The immunoglobulin's capacity to bind a specific foreign peptide (i.e., its **affinity** for the peptide) is determined by its shape and other characteristics.

▼ In the humoral immune response, foreign particles are displayed in conjunction with class II MHC molecules by antigen presenting cells. These displayed molecules are recognized by helper T cells, which then stimulate proliferation of B cells whose immunoglobulins can bind to the foreign pathogen. ▲

It is estimated that, upon initial exposure to a foreign microbe, as few as one in every million B lymphocytes happens to produce immunoglobulins capable of binding to the microbe. This number is too small to fight an infection effectively. Furthermore, the immunoglobulins' binding affinity is likely to be relatively poor. However, once this relatively small population of B lymphocytes is stimulated, they begin an adaptive process in which minor DNA sequence variations are introduced with each mitotic division (somatic hypermutation; see later discussion). These DNA sequence variations in turn produce alterations in the binding characteristics of immunoglobulins (e.g., the shape of the protein). Some of these variant immunoglobulins will possess a higher level of binding affinity for the microorganism. The B cells producing these immunoglobulins are favorably selected because they bind the pathogen for a longer period of time. They thus proliferate rapidly. These B cells then become **plasma cells,** which secrete immunoglobulins into the bloodstream. The secreted immunoglobulins, which are structurally identical to the immunoglobulins that act as receptors on the B cell's surface, are antibodies. It can now be seen how the adaptive immune system gets its name: it involves the initial selection of B cells whose receptors can bind with the pathogen and subsequent fine-tuning of these B cells to achieve higher binding affinity.

▼ During the B cell response to a foreign peptide, the binding affinity of immunoglobulins for the invading pathogen increases. When mature, the B cell becomes an antibody-secreting plasma cell. ▲

After initial stimulation by the disease pathogen, the process of B-cell differentiation and maturation into antibody-producing plasma cells requires about 5 to 7 days for completion. Each plasma cell is capable of secreting approximately 10 million antibody molecules per hour. Antibodies bind to the pathogen's surface **antigens** (from "*anti*body *gen*erating") and may destroy the microorganism directly. More often, the antibody "tags" the pathogen for destruction by other components of the immune system, such as complement proteins and phagocytes.

Another important activity of the humoral immune response is the creation of **memory cells,** a subset of high-affinity-binding B cells that persist in the body after the infection has subsided. These cells, which have already been highly selected for response to the pathogen,

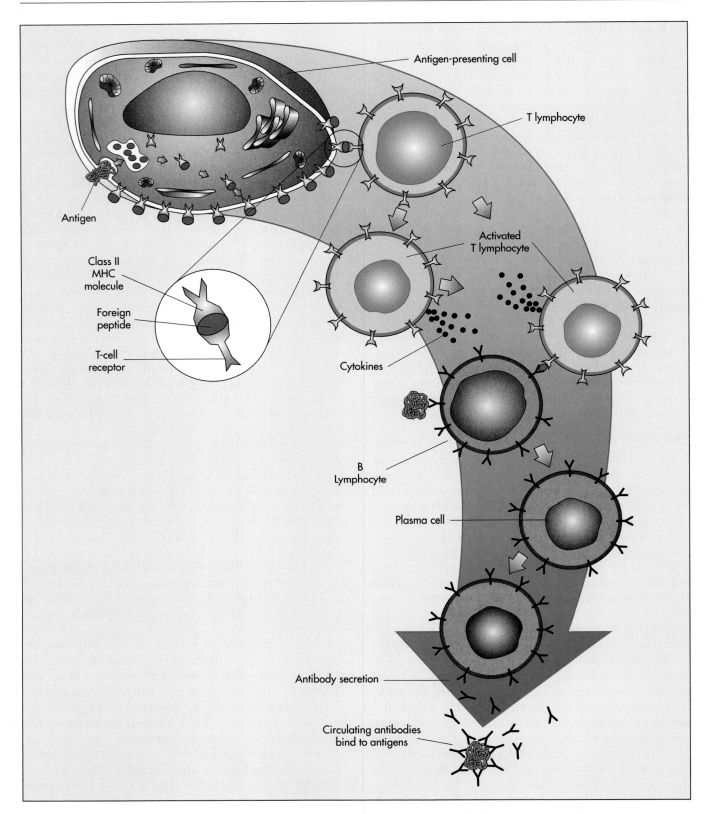

FIG. 9-1 The humoral immune response. Class II MHC molecules in antigen-presenting cells carry foreign peptides to the surface of the cell, where the foreign peptide is recognized by a helper T cell. The T cell secretes cytokines, which stimulate B cells whose immunoglobulins will bind to the foreign peptide. These B cells become plasma cells, which secrete antibodies into the circulation to bind with the microbe, helping to combat the infection. (Modified from Nossal JVN [1993] Sci. Am. 269:53-62.)

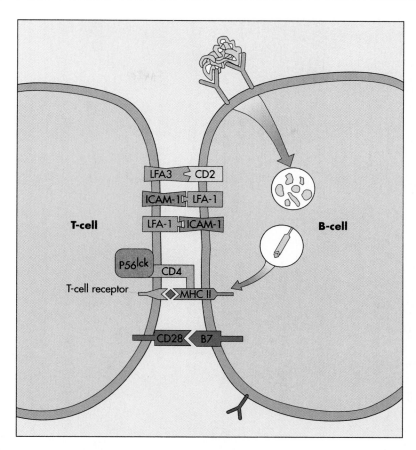

FIG. 9-2   A detailed view of the binding between a helper T cell and a B cell. In addition to the binding of the T-cell receptor to the MHC-peptide complex, a number of other molecules interact with one another, such as the costimulatory B7-CD28 complex.
(Modified from DeFranco AL [1991] Nature 351:603-604.)

provide a more rapid response should the pathogen be encountered again later in the individual's life. Vaccinations are effective because they induce the formation of memory cells that can respond to a specific pathogen.

The Cellular Immune System

Some microorganisms, such as viruses, are very adept at quickly inserting themselves into the body's cells. Here, they are inaccessible to antibodies, which are water-soluble proteins that cannot pass through the cell's lipid membrane. A second component of the adaptive immune system, the cellular immune system, has evolved to combat such infections. A key member of the cellular immune system is the **class I MHC molecule,** which is found on the surfaces of nearly all of the body's cells. In a normal cell the class I MHC molecule binds with small peptides (8 to 10 amino acids in length) derived from the interior of the cell. It migrates to the cell's surface, carrying the peptide with it and displaying it outside the cell. Because this is one of the body's *own* peptides, no immune

response is elicited. In an infected cell, however, the class I MHC molecule binds to small peptides that are derived from the infecting organism. Cell-surface presentation of the *foreign peptide* by the class I MHC molecule alerts the immune system, T cells in particular. Recall that T lymphocytes learn to tolerate "self" peptides while developing in the thymus, but they are highly intolerant of foreign peptides. The MHC-peptide complex binds to receptors on the appropriate T cell's surface, which prompts the T cell to emit a chemical that destroys the infected cell (Fig. 9-3). Because of their ability to destroy cells in this way, these T lymphocytes are termed **cytotoxic T lymphocytes** (or **killer T lymphocytes**).* Each cytotoxic T lymphocyte can destroy one infected cell every 1 to 5 minutes.

---

*They are also known as CD8 T cells because of the presence of CD8 (cluster of differentiation antigen 8) coreceptors on their surfaces (see Fig. 9-3). Helper T cells have CD4 coreceptors on their cell surfaces (see Fig. 9-2) and are thus a type of CD4 T lymphocyte.

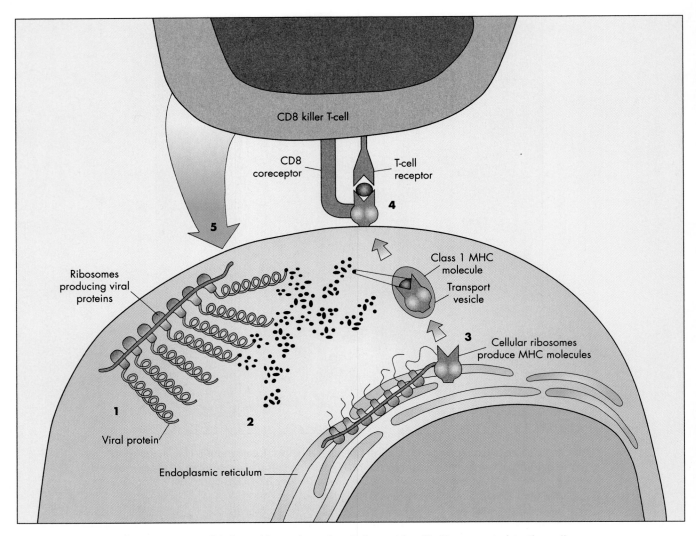

FIG. 9-3 In a cell infected by a virus, the viral peptides *(1, 2)* are carried to the cell surface by class I MHC molecules *(3)*. The T-cell receptor of a CD8 cytotoxic T cell binds to the peptide-MHC complex *(4)*. Recognizing the peptide as foreign, the cytotoxic T cell secretes chemicals that either kill the infected cell directly or induce it to undergo programmed cell death (apoptosis; see Chapter 11) *(5)*.
(Modified from Janeway CA [1993] Sci. Am. 269:73-79.)

▼ The cellular immune system is capable of destroying the body's cells once they are infected. Peptides from the pathogen are displayed on cell surfaces by class I MHC molecules. These are recognized by cytotoxic (killer) T lymphocytes, which destroy the infected cell. ▲

As with B lymphocytes, only a small proportion of the body's T cells will have binding affinity for the infecting pathogen. By secreting cytokines, helper T cells stimulate the proliferation of the cytotoxic T lymphocytes whose receptors can bind to the infected cells. In addition, circulating dendritic cells present the foreign peptides on their cell surfaces and migrate to secondary lymphoid tissues, where most of the T cells reside, helping to alert the appropriate T cells to the infection.

The humoral immune system is specialized to combat extracellular infections, such as circulating bacteria and viruses. The cellular immune system combats intracellular infections, such as parasites and viruses within cells. However, this division of labor is not strict, and there is a great deal of interaction between the two components of the adaptive immune system. Furthermore, components of the innate immune system interact with and help to coordinate components of the adaptive immune system.

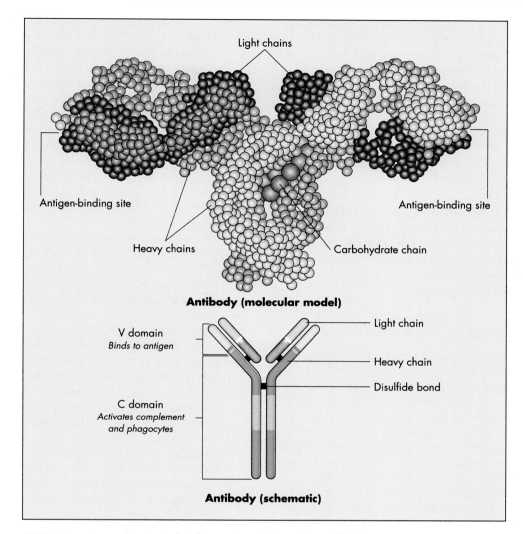

Light chains

Antigen-binding site

Antigen-binding site

Heavy chains

Carbohydrate chain

Antibody (molecular model)

V domain
Binds to antigen

C domain
Activates complement and phagocytes

Light chain

Heavy chain

Disulfide bond

Antibody (schematic)

FIG. 9-4 An antibody molecule consists of two identical light chains and two identical heavy chains. The light chain includes variable, joining, and constant regions; the heavy chain includes these regions as well as a diversity region located between its variable and joining regions. The upper portion of the figure depicts a molecular model of antibody structure.

IMMUNE RESPONSE PROTEINS: GENETIC BASIS OF STRUCTURE AND DIVERSITY
Immunoglobulin Molecules and Genes

As illustrated in Fig. 9-4, each antibody (or immunoglobulin) molecule is composed of four chains: an identical pair of longer **heavy chains** and an identical pair of shorter **light chains.** The chains are linked together by disulfide bonds. There are five different types of heavy chains (termed γ, μ, α, δ, and ϵ) and two types of light chains (κ and λ). The five types of heavy chains determine the major **class** (or **isotype**) to which an immunoglobulin (Ig) molecule belongs: γ, μ, α, δ, and ϵ correspond to the immunoglobulin isotypes IgG, IgM, IgA, IgD, and IgE, respectively. Immature B lymphocytes produce only IgM, but as they mature, a rearrangement

of heavy chain genes called **class switching** occurs. This produces the other four major classes of immunoglobulins, each of which differs in amino acid composition, charge, size, and carbohydrate content. Each class tends to be localized in certain parts of the body, and each tends to respond to a different type of infection. The two types of light chains can be found in association with any of the five types of heavy chains.

The heavy and light chains both contain a **constant** and a **variable** region, which are located at the C-terminal and N-terminal ends of the chains, respectively. The arrangement of genes encoding the constant region determines the major class of the Ig molecule (e.g., IgA, IgE). The variable region is responsible for antigen recognition and binding and thus varies within immunoglobulin classes.

Three distinct gene segments encode the light chains: C for the constant region, V for the variable region, and J for the region joining the constant and variable regions. Four gene segments encode the heavy chains, with C, V, and J coding again for the constant, variable, and joining regions, respectively, and a "diversity" (D) region located between the joining and variable regions. The genes encoding the κ light chain are located on chromosome 2, and those encoding the λ light chain are on chromosome 22. The genes that encode the heavy chains are on chromosome 14.

▼ Immunoglobulin molecules consist of two identical heavy chains and two identical light chains. The heavy chain constant region determines the major class to which an immunoglobulin belongs. The variable regions of the light and heavy chains recognize and bind antigens. ▲

The Genetic Basis of Antibody Diversity

Our bodies face an enormous variety of infectious organisms. Because the immune system cannot "know" in advance what types of microbes it will encounter, the system must contain a huge reservoir of structurally diverse immune cells so that at least a few cells can respond (i.e., bind) to any invading microbe. Indeed, the humoral immune system is capable of generating at least 10 billion structurally distinct antibodies. At one time, it was thought that, since each antibody has a unique amino acid sequence, each must be encoded by a different gene. However, this "one gene—one antibody" hypothesis could not possibly be correct because the human has only 50,000 to 100,000 genes. Further study has shown that several mechanisms are responsible for generating antibody diversity:

1. *Multiple germline immunoglobulin genes.* Molecular genetic studies (cloning and DNA sequencing) have shown that, for each heavy and light chain, an individual has more than 80 different V segments located contiguously in his or her germ line and six different J segments. There are at least 30 D segments in the heavy chain region.

2. *Somatic recombination (VDJ recombination).* As immunoglobulin molecules are formed during B lymphocyte maturation, a specific combination of single V and J segments is selected for the light chain, and another combination of V, J, and D segments is selected for the heavy chain. This is accomplished by deletion of the DNA sequences separating the single V, J, and D segments before they are transcribed into mRNA (Fig. 9-5). The deletion process is carried out in part by **recombinases** (encoded by the *RAG1* and *RAG2* genes) which initiate double-strand DNA breaks at specific DNA sequences that flank the V

and D gene segments. After the deletion of all but one V, D, and J segment, the non-deleted segments are joined by ligases. This "cutting and pasting" process is known as **somatic recombination,** as opposed to the germline recombination that takes place during meiosis. Somatic recombination produces a rather unique result: unlike most other cells of the body, whose DNA composition is identical, mature B lymphocytes *vary* in terms of their rearranged immunoglobulin DNA sequences. Because there are many possible combinations of single V, J, and D segments, somatic recombination can generate a large number of different types of antibody molecules.

3. *Junctional diversity.* As the V, D, and J regions are assembled, slight variations occur in the position at which they are joined, and small numbers of nucleotides may be deleted or inserted at the junctions joining the regions. This creates even more variation in antibody amino acid sequence.

4. *Somatic hypermutation.* After stimulation by a foreign antigen, the B lymphocytes undergo a "secondary differentiation" process characterized by **somatic hypermutation,** as mentioned previously. The mutation rate of the genes encoding the immunoglobulins increases to approximately 10^{-3} per base pair per cell division. This causes minor variation in the DNA sequences encoding immunoglobulins and thus in their peptide-binding characteristics. Somatic hypermutation of the V, D, and J genes, which may be caused by an error-prone DNA polymerase or a lack of accurate DNA repair, produces considerable antibody diversity.

5. *Multiple combinations of heavy and light chains.* Further diversity is created by the random combination of different heavy and light chains in assembling the immunoglobulin molecule.

FIG. 9-5 Somatic recombination in the formation of a heavy chain of an antibody molecule. The functional heavy chain is encoded by only one segment each from the multiple V, D, and J segments.
(Modified from Roitt I, Brostoff J, Male D [1998] Immunology, Ed 5. Mosby, St. Louis.)

Each of these mechanisms contributes to antibody diversity. Considering all of them together, it has been estimated that as many as 10^{10} to 10^{14} distinct antibodies can potentially be produced.

▼ Mechanisms that produce antibody diversity include multiple germline immunoglobulin gene segments, somatic recombination of the immunoglobulin gene segments, junctional diversity, somatic hypermutation, and the potential for multiple combinations of heavy and light chains. ▲

T-Cell Receptors

The T-cell receptors are similar in many ways to the immunoglobulins produced by B cells. Like the immunoglobulins, T-cell receptors must be able to bind to a large variety of peptides from invading organisms. Unlike immunoglobulins, however, T-cell receptors are never secreted from the cell, and T-cell activation requires the presentation of foreign peptide along with an MHC molecule. Approximately 90% of T-cell receptors are heterodimers composed of an α and a β chain, and approximately 10% are heterodimers composed of a γ and a δ chain (Fig. 9-6). The genes encoding the α and δ chains are located on chromosome 14, and those encoding the β and γ chains are located on chromosome 7. A given T cell will have either the α-β receptor or the γ-δ receptor.

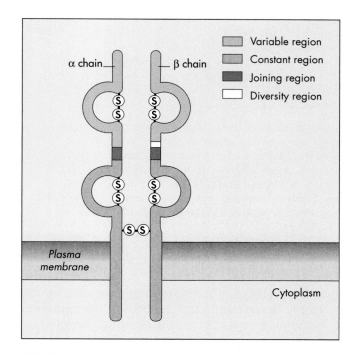

FIG. 9-6 The T-cell receptor, a heterodimer that consists of either an α and a β chain, or a γ and a δ chain.
(Modified from Raven PH, Johnson GB [1992] Biology. Ed 3. Mosby, St. Louis.)

Most of the mechanisms involved in generating immunoglobulin diversity—multiple germ-line gene segments, VDJ somatic recombination, and junctional diversity—are also important in generating T-cell receptor diversity. However, somatic hypermutation does not occur in the genes that encode the T-cell receptors. This is probably a consequence of the requirement that T-cell receptors must be able to tolerate normal "self" peptides and also recognize MHC molecules.

▼ T-cell receptors are similar in function to B-cell receptors (immunoglobulins). Unlike immunoglobulins, however, they can bind to foreign peptide only when it is presented by an MHC molecule. Their diversity is created by the same mechanisms that produce immunoglobulin diversity, with the exception of somatic hypermutation. ▲

THE MAJOR HISTOCOMPATIBILITY COMPLEX
Class I, II, and III Genes

The major histocompatibility complex (or MHC) includes a series of at least 80 genes that lie in a 4-Mb region on the short arm of chromosome 6 (Fig. 9-7). The MHC is commonly classified into three groups: class I, class II, and class III. As previously mentioned, the class I MHC molecule forms a complex with foreign peptides that is recognized by receptors on the surfaces of cytotoxic T lymphocytes. Class I presentation is thus essential for the cytotoxic T cell response; some viruses evade cytotoxic T cell detection by down-regulating the expression of MHC class I genes in the cells they infect.

Class I MHC molecules are composed of a single heavy glycoprotein chain and a single light chain called β2-microglobulin; the latter protein is encoded by a gene on chromosome 15 (Fig. 9-8, *A*). The most important of the class I loci are labeled ***HLA**** *A*, *B*, and *C*. Each of these loci has dozens of alleles, resulting in a high degree of class I MHC variability among individuals. The class I region spans 1.8 Mb and includes at least 20 genes, but the other genes in this region are less polymorphic than the *HLA A*, *B*, and *C* genes and play a lesser role in T-cell receptor recognition. The region also includes several **pseudogenes** (genes that are similar in DNA sequence to coding genes but that have been altered so that they cannot be transcribed or translated).

The class I molecules were first discovered in the 1940s by scientists who were experimenting with tissue grafts in mice. When the class I alleles in donor and recipient mice differed, the grafts were rejected. This is

---

*HLA stands for "human leukocyte antigen," reflecting the fact that these molecules were seen in early studies on leukocyte (white cell) surfaces. However, as mentioned previously, they are found on the surfaces of nearly all cells.

FIG. 9-7 A map of the human MHC. The 4-Mb complex is divided into three regions: classes I, II, and III.

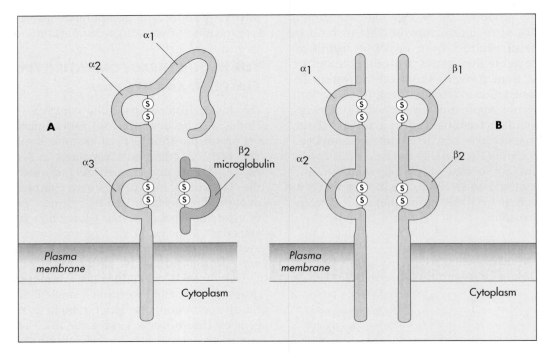

FIG. 9-8 **A,** A class I MHC molecule, showing the structure of the heavy chain, which consists of three extracellular domains (α_1, α_2, and α_3), a membrane-spanning domain, and a cytoplasmic domain. A groove formed by the α_1 and α_2 domains carries peptide for presentation to T-cell receptors. The α_3 domain associates closely with the β_2-microglobulin chain. **B,** A class II MHC molecule, showing the structure of the α and β chains. Each has two globular extracellular domains, a membrane-spanning domain, and a cytoplasmic domain. The α_1 and β_1 domains form a groove into which peptide nestles for presentation to T-cell receptors.
(Modified from Raven PH, Johnson GB [1992] Biology. Ed 3. Mosby, St. Louis.)

the historical basis for the term "major histocompatibility complex." In humans, matching of the donor's and recipient's class I alleles increases the probability of graft or transplant tolerance. Since grafts and transplants are a relatively new phenomenon in human history, the MHC obviously did not evolve to effect transplant rejection. Instead, T cells, when confronted with foreign MHC molecules on donor cells, interpret these as foreign peptides and attack the cells.

▼ The class I MHC molecules are encoded by the highly polymorphic *HLA A, B,* and *C* loci on chromosome 6. In addition to presenting foreign peptides on the surfaces of infected cells, they can also bring about transplant rejection when foreign MHC molecules stimulate cytotoxic T cells. ▲

Whereas the class I MHC molecules are found on the surfaces of nearly all cells and can bind with cytotoxic

T-cell receptors, the class II MHC molecules ordinarily are found only on the surfaces of the immune system's APCs (phagocytes and B lymphocytes). When associated with foreign peptides, they stimulate helper T cell activity after binding to the T cells' receptors, as described previously. The class II molecules are heterodimers consisting of an α and a β chain, each of which is encoded by a different gene located on chromosome 6 (Fig. 9-8, *B*). In addition to the genes encoding major class II systems (*HLA DP, DQ,* and *DR*), the class II region includes genes that encode peptide transporter proteins (*TAP1* and *TAP2*) that help to transport peptides into the endoplasmic reticulum, where they initially form complexes with class I molecules before migration to the cell surface.

▼ Class II MHC molecules are heterodimers encoded by genes on chromosome 6. They present peptides on the surfaces of antigen-presenting cells. These peptides, in conjunction with class II MHC molecules, are bound by receptors on helper T cells. ▲

Like the major class I *MHC* loci, the major class II loci are highly polymorphic, expressing hundreds of different alleles. Indeed, the *MHC* loci are, as a class, the most polymorphic loci known in the human. This high degree of polymorphism is thought to be the result of natural selection for allelic variability. Each *MHC* allele encodes a molecule with slightly different binding properties: some variants will bind peptide from a given pathogen more effectively than will others.* Consequently, an individual who expresses a greater variety of MHC molecules has a better chance of dealing effectively with a variety of infectious organisms. For example, someone who is homozygous for each of the major class I loci (*A, B,* and *C*) will express only three class I MHC molecules, while someone who is heterozygous for each of these loci will express six class I MHC molecules and will be able to cope more successfully with pathogenic diversity. A higher degree of polymorphism in the general population increases the chance that any individual in the population will be heterozygous. In addition, greater MHC polymorphism in a population decreases the chance that an infectious pathogen can spread easily through the population.

In some cases, specific *MHC* alleles are known to produce proteins that are effective against specific pathogens. For example, the *HLA-B53* allele has been shown to have a strong protective effect against severe malaria in the population of Gambia, Africa, and the *HLA-DRB1*1302* allele protects against hepatitis B infection in the same population. These alleles produce MHC molecules that have higher-affinity binding of the infectious agents.

*Because of the relatively limited repertoire of different MHC molecules, peptide binding affinity of MHC molecules is usually much lower than the binding affinity of finely-tuned T-cell receptors.

▼ Like the class I *MHC* genes, class II genes are highly polymorphic. This increases the ability of individuals and populations to respond to a wide variety of pathogens. ▲

It can be seen that both class I and class II MHC molecules guide T-cell receptors (cytotoxic and helper, respectively) to specific cells. The T-cell requirement for MHC presentation is called **MHC restriction.** Not all components of the immune system are MHC restricted. The complement system, for example, does not require direct interaction with MHC molecules. Natural killer cells, a previously discussed component of the innate immune system, are also independent of MHC presentation for their activity and are thus not necessarily MHC restricted. Indeed, natural killer cells can destroy some virus-infected cells and tumor cells that lose their MHC molecules and would otherwise be ignored by the cellular immune system (Clinical Commentary 9-1).

The class III MHC region spans 680 kb and contains at least 36 genes, only some of which are involved in the immune response. Among the most important of these are the genes encoding the complement proteins.

The genes encoding the immunoglobulins, the T-cell receptors, and the class I and class II MHC proteins all share similar DNA sequences and structural features. Thus, they are members of a gene family, like the globin genes, the color vision genes, and the collagen genes described in earlier chapters. Table 9-1 provides a summary of the major genes of the immune system and their chromosome locations.

It is important to emphasize that the class I and class II MHC molecules differ greatly *among* individuals, but each cell within an individual has the same class I and class II molecules (this uniformity is necessary for recognition by T cells). In contrast, after VDJ recombination the T-cell receptors and immunoglobulins differ from cell to cell *within* individuals, allowing the body to respond to a large variety of different infectious agents.

▼ The immunoglobulin, T-cell receptor, and MHC genes are members of a gene family. Whereas immunoglobulins and T-cell receptors vary between cells within an individual, MHC molecules vary between individuals. ▲

MHC-Disease Associations

A number of diseases show significant associations with specific *MHC* alleles: those individuals who have the allele are much more likely to develop the disease than are those who lack it. Some examples, mentioned in earlier chapters, include the *HLA-B27* (i.e., allele 27 of the *HLA-B* locus) association with ankylosing spondylitis and the *HLA-DR3/HLA-DR4* association with type 1 diabetes. An especially strong association is seen

CLINICAL COMMENTARY 9-1

THE IMMUNE RESPONSE AS A MOLECULAR ARMS RACE

The vast majority of the pathogens that assault the human body are destroyed by our immune system. Consequently, there is strong natural selection for pathogens that can evade immune surveillance and destruction. These microorganisms often have high mutation rates, and their numbers are huge. Thus, despite their biological simplicity, viruses and other pathogens have evolved some very clever ways of overcoming the immune response. Our immune systems in turn are constantly creating new ways to deal with pathogenic ingenuity. Three examples of this molecular "arms race" are discussed here.

The cytomegalovirus (CMV) is a common infectious agent that can produce mononucleosis, hemolytic anemia, pneumonitis, congenital infections, and thrombocytopenia (a decrease in the number of platelets). Cells infected with CMV are the targets of cytotoxic T cell destruction. However, some CMV strains (as well as other viruses and tumor cells) can evade T-cell detection by down-regulating the expression of class I molecules. Without viral peptide presentation by class I molecules, the cytotoxic T cells are blind to the presence of CMV, and they do not destroy the infected cell. At this point, the cell would normally become the target of natural killer cells, which attack cells that lack MHC class I molecules on their surfaces. But the CMV has devised a way to outwit natural killer cells, too. The virus encodes a cell-surface protein that resembles class I molecules closely enough so that the natural killer cells mistake the viral protein for a true class I molecule. The viral protein is also sufficiently *different* from a true class I MHC molecule that it does not trigger destruction by the more finely tuned cytotoxic T cell. In this way, the CMV can avoid destruction by both T cells and natural killer cells.

Although a fetus is by no means a pathogen, pregnancy does present an interesting immunological challenge in that placental cells express foreign class I MHC molecules derived from the father. Ordinarily, such cells would be quickly destroyed by the mother's cytotoxic T cells. To avoid this, class I MCH expression is down-regulated in these cells. As with viral down-regulation of class I molecules, this lack of MHC class I expression leaves the placental cells liable to destruction by the mother's natural killer cells. In this case, the cells are saved from destruction by presenting HLA-G molecules on their surface. This relatively nonvariant MHC molecule does not stimulate a T-cell response, which is limited to presentation of HLA A, B, and C molecules. It does inhibit the natural killer cell, which has HLA-G receptors on its surface. The fetus, like the CMV, has thus devised ways of avoiding destruction by both T cells and natural killer cells.

A third example of the molecular arms race is given by one of the most feared infectious agents of modern times, the human immunodeficiency virus (HIV). Some strains of this virus gain entry to helper T cells via a T-cell receptor that normally binds to a cytokine. Once inside the cell, HIV inserts its genetic material into the nucleus and takes advantage of the cell's machinery to replicate itself (HIV is a retrovirus, a type of virus to be discussed further in Chapter 13). Helper T cells, as already discussed, are a critical component of the body's immune system, and their destruction by HIV leads to severe secondary immunodeficiency. Recently, it has been demonstrated that individuals who are homozygous for a 32-bp deletion of the gene that encodes the cytokine receptor *(CMKBR5)* are remarkably resistant to HIV infection. This deletion is especially common in northeastern European populations, where the gene frequency reaches 0.16. Analysis of linkage disequilibrium in the chromosomal region that contains *CMKBR5* indicates that the deletion arose in these populations only a few thousand years ago. Since HIV originated only a few decades ago, the high gene frequency in northeastern Europe must be due to some other selective force or perhaps to genetic drift. Clearly, there would be strong selection in favor of this mutation in populations now heavily exposed to HIV, and the deletion would eventually rise in frequency in these populations. Even now, knowledge of the consequences of this deletion may well help to accelerate the medical arms race against HIV.

---

between *HLA-DR2* and narcolepsy, a disorder characterized by sudden and uncontrollable episodes of sleep. As Table 9-2 shows, most of the HLA-disease associations involve the class II *MHC* genes.

In some cases the association between *MHC* alleles and a disease is caused by linkage disequilibrium. For example, the hemochromatosis locus is closely linked to *HLA-A*, and significant associations occur between *HLA-A3* and the hemochromatosis disease gene (see Chapter 8). There is no known causal link between *HLA-A3* and this disorder, however. More likely, the

association represents a past event in which the primary hemochromatosis mutation arose on a chromosome that had the *HLA-A3* allele.

In other cases a causal association may exist. Some MHC-disease associations may involve **autoimmunity,** a puzzling situation in which the body's immune system attacks its own normal cells. For example, type 1 diabetes is characterized by T-cell infiltration of the pancreas and subsequent T-cell destruction of the insulin-producing β cells. The biological basis of autoimmunity remains poorly understood, but it is signifi-

TABLE 9-1 Chromosome Location and Function of Major Immune Response Genes

Gene system	Chromosome location	Gene product function
Immunoglobulin heavy chain (C, V, D, and J genes)	14q32	Heavy chain is part of antibody molecule, which binds foreign antigens
Immunoglobulin κ light chain (C, V, and J genes)	2p13	Light chain is the second part of antibody molecule
Immunoglobulin λ light chain (C, V, and J genes)	22q11	Light chain is the second part of antibody molecule (either κ or λ may be used)
T-cell receptor α	14q11	One chain of the α-β T-cell receptor, which recognizes antigen with MHC molecule
T-cell receptor β	7q35	The other chain of the α-β T-cell receptor
T-cell receptor γ	7p15	One chain of the γ-δ T-cell receptor
T-cell receptor δ	14q11	The second chain of the γ-δ T-cell receptor
MHC (class I, II, and III); includes TAP1 and TAP2	6p21	Cell-surface molecules that present peptides to T-cell receptors. TAP1 and TAP2 are transporter molecules that process foreign peptides and carry them to the endoplasmic reticulum
β2-microglobulin	15q21-22	Forms second chain of the class I MHC molecule
RAG1, RAG2	11p13	Recombinases that participate in VDJ somatic recombination

TABLE 9-2 Some Examples of MHC-Disease Associations

Disease	MHC (HLA)–associated allele	Approximate relative risk*
Type 1 diabetes	DR3 and DR4	Approximately 5 for DR3 or DR4 alone; 20 to 40 for DR3/DR4 heterozygotes
Ankylosing spondylitis	B27	90
Narcolepsy	DR2	>100
Celiac disease	DR3, DR7	10
Rheumatoid arthritis	DR1, DR4	5
Myasthenia gravis	DR3, DR7	2.5
Multiple sclerosis	DR2	4
Pemphigus vulgaris	DR4	24
Systemic lupus erythematosus	DR2, DR3	1 to 3
Hemochromatosis	A3	20
Malaria	B53	0.59
Graves disease	DR3	5
Psoriasis vulgaris	Cw6	8
Squamous cell cervical carcinoma	DQw3	7

Data from Bell JI, Todd JA, McDevitt HO (1989) The molecular basis of HLA-disease association. Adv. Hum. Genet. 18:1-41; Langdon N et al. (1984) Genetic markers in narcolepsy. Lancet II. 1178-1180; Wank R, Thomssen C (1991) High risk of squamous cell carcinoma of the cervix for women with HLA-DQw3. Nature 352:723-725; Hill AV et al. (1991) Common West African HLA antigens are associated with protection from severe malaria. Nature 352:595-600; Doherty DG, Nepom GT (1997) The human major histocompatibility complex and disease susceptibility. In Rimoin DL, Connor JM, Pyeritz RE (eds) (1997) Emery and Rimoin's Principles and Practice of Medical Genetics. Vol. 1. Churchill Livingstone, New York.

*Relative risk can be interpreted loosely as the odds that an individual who has a risk factor (in this case, an MHC antigen) will develop the disease, compared to an individual who lacks the risk factor. Thus, a relative risk of four for DR2 and multiple sclerosis means that persons with DR2 are four times more likely to develop multiple sclerosis than are those without DR2. A relative risk less than one (as seen for malaria and B53) indicates that the factor is *protective* against the disease.

cant that autoimmunity is often seen when class II molecules are inappropriately expressed on the surfaces of cells *not* involved in the immune response. It is thought that such cells may be interpreted by T cells as viral peptides in association with MHC molecules, triggering an immune response. There is also evidence for such "molecular mimicry" in ankylosing spondylitis, another autoimmune disease. Infections of *HLA-B27*-positive individuals with specific microbes, such as *Klebsiella*, may lead to a **cross-reaction** in which the immune system mistakes some of the body's normal *B27*-bearing cells for the microbe.

Other common MHC-associated diseases that involve autoimmunity include rheumatoid arthritis, systemic lupus erythematosus, and multiple sclerosis. It is estimated that approximately 5% of the population suffers from some type of autoimmune disease.

▼ A significant number of diseases are associated with specific MHC alleles. Some of these associations are the result of linkage disequilibrium, but most are likely to result from causal associations involving autoimmunity. ▲

THE ABO AND RH BLOOD GROUPS

Another component of the immune system involves red-cell surface molecules that can cause an immune reaction during blood transfusions. The ABO and Rh red-cell antigen systems were discussed in Chapter 3 as early examples of polymorphic marker loci. They are also the most important systems determining transfusion compatibility.

The ABO System

There are four major ABO blood types: A, B, AB, and O. The first three groups respectively represent individuals who carry the A, B, and A and B antigens on their erythrocyte surfaces. Those with type O have neither the A nor the B antigen. Individuals who have a given antigen on their erythrocyte surfaces possess antibodies against all other ABO antigens in their bloodstream (these are formed as a result of exposure to antigens that are identical to the A and B antigens but present in various microorganisms). Thus, if a type B individual received type A or AB blood, his or her anti-A antibodies would produce a severe and possibly fatal reaction. Type O individuals, who have neither antigen and both anti-A and anti-B antibodies, would react strongly to blood of the other three types (A, B, and AB). It was once thought that type O persons, because they lack both types of antigens, could be "universal donors" (anyone could accept their blood). Similarly, type AB persons were termed "universal recipients" because they lacked both anti-A and anti-B antibodies. However, when transfusions of whole blood containing large volumes of serum are conducted, the donor's *antibodies* can react with the recipient's erythrocyte *antigens*, and a reaction can result. Hence, complete matching is nearly always done for blood transfusions.

▼ The ABO locus encodes red cell antigens that can cause a transfusion reaction if donors and recipients are not properly matched. ▲

The Rh System

The Rh blood group is encoded by two tightly linked loci, one of which is labeled *D*. The other locus produces Rh systems labeled *C* and *E* through alternative splicing mechanisms. The *D* locus is of primary interest because it is responsible for Rh maternal-fetal incompatibility and the resulting disease, hemolytic disease of the newborn (HDN). Persons with the *DD* or *Dd* genotype have the Rh antigen on their erythrocytes and are termed "Rh-positive." The recessive homozygotes, with genotype *dd*, are "Rh-negative" and do not have the Rh antigen. About 85% of North Americans are Rh-positive, and about 15% are Rh-negative.

Unlike the ABO system, in which antibodies are formed in response to antigens presented by other organisms, anti-Rh antibody production requires a stimulus by the human Rh antigen itself. An Rh-negative person does not begin to produce anti-Rh antibodies unless he or she is exposed to the Rh antigen, usually through a blood transfusion or during pregnancy. Maternal-fetal incompatibility results when an Rh-positive man and an Rh-negative woman produce children. If the man's genotype is *DD*, all of their offspring will be Rh-positive and will have Rh antigens on their erythrocytes. If the man is a heterozygote, with genotype *Dd*, half of their children will be Rh-positive, on average.

There are usually no difficulties with the first Rh-incompatible child because very few of the fetus's red blood cells cross the placental barrier during gestation. When the placenta detaches at birth, a large number of fetal red blood cells typically enter the mother's bloodstream. These cells, carrying the Rh antigens, stimulate production of anti-Rh antibodies by the mother. These antibodies persist in the bloodstream for a long time, and if the next offspring is again Rh-positive, the mother's anti-Rh antibodies enter the fetus's bloodstream and destroy its red blood cells. As this destruction proceeds, the fetus becomes anemic and begins to release many erythroblasts (immature nucleated red cells) into its bloodstream. This phenomenon is responsible for the descriptive term *erythroblastosis fetalis*. The anemia can lead to a spontaneous abortion or stillbirth. Because the maternal antibodies remain in the newborn's circulatory system, destruction of red cells can continue in the neonate. This causes a buildup of bilirubin and a jaundiced appearance shortly after birth. Without replacement transfusions, in which the child receives Rh-negative red cells, the bilirubin is deposited in the brain, producing cerebral damage and usually death. Those infants who do not die may suffer from mental retardation, cerebral palsy, and/or high-frequency deafness.

In North American Caucasians, approximately 13% of all matings are Rh-incompatible. Fortunately, a simple therapy now exists to avoid Rh sensitization of the mother. During and after pregnancy, an Rh-negative mother is given injections of Rh immune globulin, which consists of anti-Rh antibodies. These antibodies destroy the fetal erythrocytes before they stimulate production of maternal anti-Rh antibodies. Since the injected antibodies do not remain in the mother's bloodstream for long, they do not affect subsequent offspring. To avoid sensitization, these injections must be administered with each pregnancy. The Rh-negative mother must also be careful not to receive a transfusion containing Rh-positive blood because this would also stimulate production of anti-Rh antibodies.

> ▼ Maternal-fetal Rh incompatibility (Rh-negative mother and Rh-positive fetus) can produce hemolytic disease of the newborn if the mother's Rh antibodies attack the fetus. Administration of Rh immune globulin prevents this reaction. ▲

A rarer form of maternal-fetal incompatibility can result when a mother with type O blood carries a fetus with type A or B blood. The HDN produced by this combination is usually so mild that it does not require treatment. Interestingly, if the mother is also Rh-negative and the child is Rh-positive, the ABO incompatibility *protects* against the more severe Rh incompatibility. This is because any fetal red blood cells entering the mother's circulatory system are quickly destroyed by her anti-A or anti-B antibodies before she can form anti-Rh antibodies.

IMMUNODEFICIENCY DISEASES

Immunodeficiency disease results when one or more components of the immune system (e.g., T cells, B cells, MHC, complement proteins) are missing or fail to function normally. **Primary immunodeficiency diseases** are caused by abnormalities in cells of the immune system and are usually produced by genetic defects. **Secondary immunodeficiency** occurs when components of the immune system are altered or destroyed by other factors, such as radiation, infection, or drugs. For example, the human immunodeficiency virus, which causes AIDS, attacks the CD4 T lymphocytes, a central component of the immune system. The result is increased susceptibility to a multitude of opportunistic infections rarely seen in healthy individuals.

B-cell immunodeficiency diseases render the patient especially susceptible to recurrent bacterial infections, such as *Streptococcus pneumoniae*. An important example of a B-cell immunodeficiency is X-linked agammaglobulinemia (XLA). Patients with this disorder, the overwhelming majority of whom are males, lack B cells completely and have no IgA, IgE, IgM, or IgD in their serum. Because IgG crosses the placenta during pregnancy, infants with XLA have some B-cell immune response for the first several months of life. However, the IgG supply is soon depleted, and the infants develop recurrent bacterial infections. They were treated with large amounts of gamma-globulin. XLA is caused by mutations in a gene (*BTK*) that encodes a B-cell tyrosine kinase necessary for normal B-cell maturation.

T-cell immunodeficiency diseases directly affect T cells, but they also affect the humoral immune response because B-cell proliferation is largely dependent on helper T cells. Thus, these patients develop severe combined immune deficiency (SCID) and are susceptible to many opportunistic infections, including *Pneumocystis carinii* (a protozoan that commonly infects AIDS patients). Without bone marrow transplants, these patients usually die within the first several years. About half of SCID cases are caused by X-linked recessive mutations in a gene encoding the γ chain of a cytokine receptor (specifically, the interleukin-2 receptor and parts of the receptors for interleukins 4, 7, 11 and 15). Lacking these receptors, T cells cannot receive the signals they need for normal maturation. About 25% of SCID cases are caused by adenosine deaminase (ADA) deficiency, an autosomal recessive disorder of purine metabolism that results in a buildup of metabolites that are toxic to B and T cells. ADA deficiency is sometimes treated by bone marrow transplants, and it is now being treated with gene therapy (see Chapter 13). Other T-cell immunodeficiency disorders are listed in Table 9-3.

Several immune system defects result in lymphocytes that lack MHC molecules on their surfaces. These are collectively termed "bare lymphocyte syndrome." One form of this syndrome is caused by mutations in the *TAP2* gene. The TAP2 protein, as mentioned previously, helps to transport peptides to the endoplasmic reticulum, where they are bound by class I MHC molecules. A defect in the TAP2 protein destabilizes the class I MHC molecules so that they are not expressed on the cell surface. The result is a severe reduction in the number of functional T and B cells. Bare lymphocyte syndrome can also be caused by defects in several different transcription factors that bind to promoters in the class II MHC region. The result is a lack of class II MHC molecules on antigen presenting cells, a deficiency of helper T cells, and a consequent lack of antibody production.

Chronic granulomatous disease (CGD) is a primary immunodeficiency disorder in which phagocytes can ingest bacteria and fungi but are then unable to kill them. This brings about a persistent cellular immune response to the ingested microbes, and granulomas (nodular inflammatory lesions containing macrophages) form, giving the disease its name. These patients develop pneumonia, lymph node infections, and abscesses of the skin, liver, and other sites. The most common cause of CGD is an X-linked gene, but there are also at least three autosomal recessive genes that can cause CGD. The gene that causes X-linked CGD was the first disease gene to be isolated through positional cloning. It encodes a subunit of cytochrome b, a protein

TABLE 9-3   Some examples of primary immunodeficiency diseases

Condition	Mode of inheritance	Brief description
X-linked agammaglobulinemia	XR	Absence of B cells leads to recurrent bacterial infections
Severe combined immune deficiency (SCID) (γ chain cytokine receptor defect or ADA deficiency)	XR, AR	T-cell deficiency leading also to impairment of humoral immune response; fatal unless treated by bone marrow transplants or gene therapy
Zap-70 kinase deficiency	AR	Lack of cytotoxic T cells; defective helper T cells and natural killer cells; impaired antibody response
Jak-3 deficiency	AR	Protein kinase deficiency leading to reduced interleukin-2 expression and T-cell and B-cell deficiency
Purine nucleoside phosphorylase deficiency	AR	Purine metabolism disorder leading to T-cell deficiency
Bare lymphocyte syndrome (BLS)	AR	Deficient MHC class I expression (*TAP2* mutation) leads to T-cell and B-cell deficiency in type 1 BLS; mutations in transcription factors for MHC class II genes lead to a relative lack of helper T cells in type 2 BLS
Complement system defects	Mostly AR	Increased susceptibility to bacterial and other infections
DiGeorge anomaly	AD, sporadic	Congenital malformations include abnormal facial features, congenital heart disease, and thymus abnormality leading to T-cell deficiency
Ataxia telangiectasia	AR	DNA repair defect characterized by unsteady gait (ataxia), telangiectasia (dilated capillaries), and thymus abnormality producing T-cell deficiency
Wiskott-Aldrich syndrome	XR	Abnormal, small platelets, eczema, and abnormal T cells causing susceptibility to opportunistic infections
Chediak-Higashi syndrome	AR	Partial albinism, defective lysosomal assembly, giant cytoplasmic granules, abnormal natural killer cells and neutrophils leading to recurrent bacterial infections
Leukocyte adhesion deficiency	AR	Mutations in integrin receptor gene produce phagocytes that cannot recognize and ingest microorganisms, resulting in severe bacterial infections
Chronic granulomatous disease	XR, AR	Phagocytes ingest microbes but cannot kill them; leads to formation of granulomas and recurrent infections

that the phagocyte requires for a burst of microbe-killing oxygen metabolism.

Multiple defects in the various proteins that make up the complement system have been identified. Most of these are inherited as autosomal recessive disorders, and most result in increased susceptibility to bacterial infections.

Finally, a number of syndromes include immuno-deficiency as one of their features. One example is the DiGeorge anomaly (see Chapter 6), in which a lack of thymic development leads to T-cell deficiency. Wiskott-Aldrich syndrome is an X-linked recessive disorder that involves deficiencies of platelets and B and T cells. It is caused by mutations in a gene (*WAS*) whose protein

product is needed for normal formation of the cellular cytoskeleton. Several syndromes that involve DNA instability are characterized by immunodeficiency (e.g., ataxia telangiectasia, Bloom syndrome, and Fanconi anemia; see Chapter 3).

▼ Primary immunodeficiency diseases involve intrinsic defects of immune response cells (e.g., B cells, T cells, MHC, complement system, or phagocytes) and are usually caused by genetic alterations. Secondary immunodeficiency disorders, of which AIDS is an example, are caused by external factors. Immunodeficiency is also seen in a number of genetic syndromes, including several DNA instability disorders. ▲

STUDY QUESTIONS

1. Compare the functions of class I and class II MHC molecules.

2. MHC molecules and immunoglobulins both display a great deal of diversity, but in different ways. How and why do these types of diversity differ?

3. In what ways are T-cell receptors and immunoglobulins similar? In what ways are they different?

4. If there are 80 V segments, 6 J segments, and 30 D segments that can encode an immunoglobulin heavy chain of one particular class, how many different immunoglobulins can be formed on the basis of somatic recombination alone?

5. When matching donors and recipients for organ transplants, siblings are often desirable donors because they are more likely to be HLA-compatible with the recipient. If we assume no crossing over within the HLA loci, and assuming four distinct HLA haplotypes among the parents, what is the probability that a transplant recipient will be HLA-identical with a sibling donor?

6. What types of matings will produce Rh maternal-fetal incompatibility?

SUGGESTED READINGS

Abbas AK, Murphy KM, Sher A (1996) Functional diversity of helper T lymphocytes. Nature 383:787-793

Doherty DG, Nepom GT (1997) The human major histocompatibility complex and disease susceptibility. In: Rimoin DL, Connor JM, Pyeritz RE (eds) Emery and Rimoin's Principles and Practice of Medical Genetics. Vol. 1. Churchill Livingstone, New York, pp 479-504

Fearon DT (1997) Seeking wisdom in innate immunity. Nature 388:323-324

Fearon DT, Locksley RM (1996) The instructive role of innate immunity in the acquired immune response. Science 272:50-54

Green NS, Lin MM, Scharff MD (1998) Somatic hypermutation of antibody genes: a hot spot warms up. BioEssays 20:227-234

Huston DP (1997) The biology of the immune system. JAMA 278:1804-1814

Medzhitov R, Janeway CA (1997) Innate immunity: the virtues of a nonclonal system of recognition. Cell 91:295-298

Parham P, Ohta T (1996) Population biology of antigen presentation by MHC Class I molecules. Science 272:67-74

Pleogh HL (1998) Viral strategies of immune invasion. Science 280:248-253

Puck JM (1997) Primary immunodeficiency diseases. JAMA 278:1835-1841

Ridgway WM, Fathman CG (1998) The association of MHC with autoimmune diseases: understanding the pathogenesis of autoimmune diseases. Clin. Immunol. Immunopathol. 86:3-10

Roitt I, Brostoff J, Male D (1998) Immunology. Ed 5. Mosby, St. Louis

Smith CIE, Notarangelo LD (1997) Molecular basis for X-linked immunodeficiencies. Adv. Genet. 35:57-115

Strominger JL, Wiley DC (1995) The class I and class II proteins of the human major histocompatibility complex. JAMA 274:1074-1076

Unanue ER (1995) The concept of antigen processing and presentation. JAMA 274:1071-1073

Vyse TJ, Todd JA (1996) Genetic analysis of autoimmune disease. Cell 85:311-318

Weaver DT, Alt FW (1997) V(D)J recombination: from RAGs to stitches. Nature 388:428-429

Willerford DM, Swat W, Alt FW (1996) Developmental regulation of V(D)J recombination and lymphocyte differentiation. Curr. Opin. Genet. Dev. 6:603-609

10

Developmental Genetics

Birth defects are the most common cause of infant* death in the United States. Approximately 100,000 children are born each year with a birth defect, and the prevalence is even higher among miscarriages. Birth defects can be isolated abnormalities, or they can be features of one of more than 2,000 known genetic syndromes. The etiology of most birth defects is unknown; however, it is estimated that a substantial proportion are caused by mutations in genes that control normal development. Thus, the characterization of genes coordinating animal development is revolutionizing our understanding of the molecular basis of human birth defects. This chapter provides a brief review of the genes and proteins that control development and then discusses some of the cardinal developmental processes that, when disturbed, cause birth defects.

DEVELOPMENT: BASIC CONCEPTS

Animal development can be defined as the process by which a fertilized ovum becomes a mature organism capable of reproduction. A single fertilized egg divides and grows to form different cell types, tissues, and organs, all of which are arranged in a species-specific **body plan** (i.e., the arrangement and pattern of body parts). Many of the instructions necessary for normal development are encoded by an animal's genes. Because the genes in each cell of an organism are identical, several questions arise: How do cells with identical genetic constitutions form a complex adult organism composed of many different cells and tissues? What controls the fate of each cell, instructing a cell to become, for example, a brain cell or a liver cell? How do cells organize into discrete tissues? How is the body plan of an organism

determined? Answering such fundamental questions has been a major focus of developmental biology for more than a century. The pace of discovery has accelerated dramatically in the last 10 years, and these discoveries are helping us to understand the causes of human malformations and genetic syndromes.

For ethical and technical reasons, it is difficult to study early developmental events in human embryos. Consequently, a variety of non-human model organisms are used to facilitate the study of development (Table 10-1). This approach is feasible because the major elements (genes and pathways) that control animal development are conserved across a wide range of species and body plans. In addition, many regulatory switches and signaling pathways are used repeatedly during development to control various patterning and differentiation events. This underscores the point that the evolution of species proceeds, in part, by continual tinkering with similar developmental programs to effect changes in an organism's phenotype.

For example, **ectopic expression** (i.e., expression of the gene product in an abnormal location) of the *Drosophila* gene, *eyeless*, results in the formation of a well-formed but misplaced eye. Mice have a homologous gene, *Pax6*,[†] in which mutations can produce abnormally small eyes. When inserted ectopically into *Drosophila*, *Pax6* again produces a misplaced eye. Mutations in the human homolog, *PAX6*, cause defects of the eye such as cataracts and aniridia (absence of the iris). *PAX6*, *Pax6*, and *eyeless* are homologous genes that encode DNA transcription factors (see Chapter 3). Although the ancestors of *Drosophila* and mouse diverged from the lineage leading to humans 500 and 60 million years ago, respectively, the genes and pathways

---

* An infant is an individual who is less than 1 year of age.

[†]It is conventional to capitalize all letters of the names of human genes but only the first letter of the names of mouse genes.

TABLE 10-1   Animal Models of Human Development

Organism	Generation time*	Advantages	Disadvantages
C. elegans (roundworm)	9 days	Fate of every cell known Genome well-characterized Easy to breed and maintain	Alternative body plan compared to vertebrates Targeted mutagenesis not yet possible Tissues cannot be cultured
D. melanogaster (fruit fly)	10 days	Easy to breed Large populations Vast database of mutants	Alternative body plan compared to vertebrates Targeted mutagenesis not yet possible Must be stored live; cannot be frozen
D. rerio (zebrafish)	3 months	Transparent embryo Easy to maintain large populations	Small size of embryo makes manipulation difficult
X. laevis (frog)	12 months	Transparent embryo is large and easy to manipulate	Tetraploid genome makes genetic experiments difficult
G. gallus (chicken)	5 months	Easy to observe and manipulate embryo Development accompanied by growth	Genetic experiments difficult
M. musculus (mouse)	2 months	Easy to breed Large populations Many different strains available Dense genetic maps available Large regions of genome syntenic with human chromosomes	Relatively expensive to maintain Manipulation of embryo is challenging
P. hamadryas (baboon)	60 months	Physiology similar to that of humans Genetic linkage map complete	Very expensive to maintain Small populations Long generation times

*Generation time is defined as the age at which the organism is first capable of reproduction.

involved in development of the eye have been conserved. **WWW**

▼ Approximately 2% to 3% of babies are born with a recognizable birth defect. Some birth defects are caused by mutations in genes encoding elements in pathways that control development. These pathways are highly conserved among animal species. Thus, studies of non-human animal models are invaluable for understanding human development and the causes of birth defects. ▲

A Brief Overview of Major Processes in Embryonic Development

Several major processes are involved in the development of the embryo. These include **axis specification, pattern formation**, and **organogenesis**. As its name suggests, pattern formation describes a series of steps in which differentiated cells are arranged spatially to form tissues and organs. The interactions of these cells are mediated by processes such as **induction**, which occurs when the cells of one embryonic region influence the organization and

differentiation of cells in a second region. Axis specification involves the definition of the major axes of the body: ventral/dorsal and anterior/posterior. Specification of **polarity** (direction) is an important part of this process. As the axes are specified, the formation of organs and limbs (organogenesis) begins. Each of these major processes involves many different proteins that form structures and provide signals to coordinate the development of the embryo. The major types of these proteins, and the genes that encode them, are described next.

▼ Embryonic development involves the processes of pattern formation, axis specification, and organogenesis. Each of these processes is controlled by a series of proteins that provide signals and form structures necessary for normal development of the embryo. ▲

GENETIC MEDIATORS OF DEVELOPMENT: THE MOLECULAR TOOLBOX

The genes required for normal development encode many different products, including signaling molecules

TABLE 10-2   Genes Causing Human Birth Defects

Gene	Type of protein	Syndrome	Birth defects
BOR1	Transcription factor	Branchio-oto-renal	External ear anomalies, hearing loss, kidney defects
EMX2	Transcription factor	Schizencephaly	Clefting of the cerebral cortex
GLI3	Transcription factor	Greig	Premature fusion of the cranial sutures, extra digits
GLI3	Transcription factor	Pallister-Hall	Hypothalamic hamartomas, extra digits
GLI3	Transcription factor	Polydactyly type A	Extra posterior digits
HOXD13	Transcription factor	Synpolydactyly	Extra digits that are often fused with other digits
HOXA13	Transcription factor	Hand-foot-genital	Hypoplasia of the first digits, kidney and genital defects
KIT	Receptor molecule	Piebaldism	Hypopigmented patches of skin
PAX3	Transcription factor	Waardenburg	Hypopigmentation, hearing impairment
MITF	Transcription factor	Waardenburg	Hypopigmentation, hearing impairment
PAX6	Transcription factor	Aniridia	Hypoplasia or aplasia of the irides
PAX2	Transcription factor	—	Kidney and optic nerve defects
RIEG1	Transcription factor	Rieger	Defects of teeth, eyes, and umbilicus
SALL1	Transcription factor	Townes-Brocks	Anal, kidney, limb, and ear defects
SOX9	Transcription factor	Campomelic	Skeletal defects, sex-reversal
SOX10	Transcription factor	Hirschsprung	Bowel hypomotility
SHH	Signaling molecule	Holoprosencephaly	Lack of midline cleavage of the brain
TBX3	Transcription factor	Ulnar-mammary	Posterior upper limb anomalies, breast and genital anomalies
TBX5	Transcription factor	Holt-Oram	Anterior upper limb anomalies, heart defects
TCOF1	Transcription factor	Treacher Collins	Mid-face hypoplasia, small jaw, external ear defects
WT1	Transcription factor	Denys-Drash	Kidney defects, sex reversal

and their receptors, DNA transcription factors, components of the extracellular matrix, enzymes, transport systems, and other proteins. Each of these genetic mediators is expressed in combinations of spatially and temporally overlapping patterns that control different developmental processes. As detailed in this chapter, mutations in the genes mediating development are a common cause of human birth defects (Table 10-2).

Paracrine Signaling Molecules

Interactions between neighboring cells are usually mediated by proteins that can diffuse across small distances to induce a response. These molecules are often called paracrine factors because they are secreted into the space surrounding a cell, unlike hormones, which are secreted into the bloodstream. Closely related paracrine factors have been isolated from a variety of organisms, making it clear that homologous molecules are utilized throughout the animal kingdom. To date, four major families of paracrine signaling molecules have been described: (1) the fibroblast growth factor (FGF) family; (2) the Hedgehog family; (3) the Wingless (Wnt) fam-

ily; and (4) the Transforming Growth Factor β (TGF-β) family. Each of these signaling molecules binds to one or more receptors to effect a response, and mutations in genes encoding these molecules may lead to abnormal communication between cells. Clinical Commentary 10-1 discusses the FGF family and associated receptors; the other three families are described in this section.

The first member of the Hedgehog family was originally isolated in a *Drosophila* mutant that has bristles in an area that is naked in the normal fly (hence it was named *hedgehog*). Vertebrates have several homologs of *hedgehog*, the most widely used of which is termed *Sonic hedgehog* (*Shh*). Among its many roles, Shh participates in axis specification, induction of the neural plate, and patterning of the limbs. One of the receptors of Shh is a transmembrane protein encoded by a gene called *patched*. Binding of Shh to the patched receptor suppresses transcription of genes encoding members of the TGF-β and Wnt families and inhibits cell growth. Mutations in the human homolog, *PATCHED* (*PTC*), cause Gorlin syndrome, a birth defect characterized by rib anomalies, cysts of the jaw, and basal cell carcinomas (a form of skin cancer). Mutations in *PTC* have also

CLINICAL COMMENTARY 10-1
DISORDERS OF FIBROBLAST GROWTH FACTOR RECEPTORS

Fibroblast growth factor receptors (FGFRs) are highly homologous glycoproteins with a common structure consisting of a signal peptide (an amino acid sequence that helps to direct the protein to its proper cellular location), three immunoglobulin-like (Ig-like) domains, a membrane-spanning segment, and an intracellular tyrosine kinase domain (Fig. 10-1). FGFRs are receptors for at least 13 fibroblast growth factors (FGFs) that participate in a wide variety of biological processes, including cell migration, growth, and differentiation. With varying affinities, FGFs bind FGFRs, leading to phosphorylation, and hence activation, of the tyrosine kinase domain.

FGFRs are widely expressed in developing bone, and many common human autosomal dominant disorders of bone growth (i.e., skeletal dysplasias) are caused by mutations in *FGFR* genes. The most prevalent of these disorders is achondroplasia (ACH), which is characterized by disproportionate short stature (i.e., the limbs are disproportionately shorter than the trunk) and macrocephaly (see Chapter 4). Nearly all individuals with ACH have a glycine → arginine substitution in the transmembrane domain of FGFR3 (see Fig. 10-1), resulting in FGFR3 activation. WWW

FGFR3 is normally expressed in resting chondrocytes, where it restrains chondrocyte proliferation and differentiation. In mice, FGFR3-inactivating mutations cause expansion of the zones of proliferating cartilage and increased long bone growth. Thus, overactivation causes further inhibition of chondrocyte growth, producing skeletal defects. The degree of FGFR3 activation, which may vary depending on the domain that is altered, corresponds to the severity of long bone shortening. Lesser degrees of activation result in the milder skeletal abnormalities observed in hypochondroplasia, while markedly increased activation causes a virtually lethal disorder called thanatophoric dysplasia.

Abnormal bone growth is also a feature of a group of disorders characterized by premature fusion (synostosis) of the cranial sutures, misshapen skulls, and various types of limb defects. Collectively, these disorders are called craniosynostosis syndromes. Mutations in *FGFR1*, *FGFR2*, and *FGFR3* cause at least five distinct craniosynostosis disorders (Table 10-3). The same mutation can sometimes cause two or more different craniosynostosis syndromes. For example, a cysteine → tyrosine substitution in FGFR2 can cause either Pfeiffer or Crouzon syndrome. This suggests that additional factors, such as modifying genes, are partly responsible for creating different phenotypes. WWW

FIG. 10-1   Schematic drawing of fibroblast growth factor 3 receptor (FGFR3) protein. Important functional domains of FGFR3 include a signal peptide *(SP)*, three immunoglobulin-like *(Ig)* domains, an acid box *(AB)*, a transmembrane *(TM)* domain, and a split tyrosine kinase *(TK)* domain. The locations of point mutations causing achondroplasia *(A*; gray), hypochondroplasia *(H*; dark blue), and thanatophoric dysplasia *(T*; light blue) are indicated. (Modified from Webster MK, Donoghue DJ [1997] Trends Genet. 13:178-182.)

TABLE 10-3	Craniosynostosis Syndromes Due to Mutations in Fibroblast Growth Factor Receptors	

Gene	Syndrome	Characteristics
FGFR1	Pfeiffer	Broad first digits, hypertelorism
FGFR2	Apert	Fusion of digits, mid-face hypoplasia
	Pfeiffer	Broad first digits, hypertelorism
	Crouzon	Mid-face hypoplasia, ocular proptosis
	Beare-Stevenson	Mid-face hypoplasia, corrugated skin
	Jackson-Weiss	Mid-face hypoplasia, foot anomalies
FGFR3	Crouzon	Mid-face hypoplasia, ocular proptosis, acanthosis nigricans*
	Non-syndromic craniosynostosis	Digital defects, hearing loss

*Acanthosis nigricans is characterized by hyperplastic and hypertrophic skin of varying pigmentation, most often covering the axillae, neck, genitalia, and flexural surfaces.

been found in sporadic basal cell carcinomas. Thus, germline mutations in *PTC* alter the regulation of developing cells to cause birth defects, while somatic mutations in *PTC* can alter the regulation of terminally differentiated cells to cause cancer. **WWW**

The Wnt family of genes is named after the *Drosophila* gene *wingless* and one of its vertebrate homologs, *integrated*. The *wingless* gene establishes polarity during *Drosophila* limb formation, and members of the Wnt family play similar roles in vertebrates. Wnt genes encode secreted glycoproteins that participate in a wide variety of developmental processes, including specification of the dorsal/ventral axis and formation of the brain, muscle, gonads, and kidneys.

The TGF-β supergene family* is composed of at least 30 structurally related genes that encode proteins that form homodimers or heterodimers. Members of the TGF-β supergene family include the TGF-β family itself, the bone morphogenetic protein (BMP) family, the activin family, and the Vg1 family. Although the role of BMPs is not limited to bone development, members of the BMP family were originally isolated because of their ability to induce bone formation.

Mutations in a member of the BMP family, *cartilage-derived morphogenetic protein 1* (*CDMP1*), cause various skeletal abnormalities. Different mutations can produce distinct phenotypes (allelic heterogeneity; see Chapter 4). For example, a nonsense mutation in *CDMP1* causes dominantly inherited brachydactyly (short digits). Individuals homozygous for a 22-bp duplication in *CDMP1* have brachydactyly as well as shortening of the long bones of the limbs (an autosomal recessive disorder called acromesomelic dysplasia). A homozygous missense mutation produces autosomal recessive Grebe chondrodysplasia, characterized by severe shortening of the long bones and digits. The mutant protein is not secreted, and it is thought to inactivate other BMPs by forming heterodimers with them and preventing their secretion. Thus, mutations causing Grebe chondrodysplasia produce a novel type of "dominant negative" effect by inactivating the products of other genes. **WWW**

▼ Paracrine signaling molecules are secreted, diffuse a short distance, and bind to a receptor that effects a response. There are four major families of paracrine signaling molecules: (1) the fibroblast growth factor (FGF) family; (2) the Hedgehog family; (3) the Wingless (Wnt) family; and (4) the Transforming Growth Factor β (TGF-β) family. ▲

DNA Transcription Factors

There are many different ways to regulate the expression of a gene. For example, a gene may not be transcribed,

the transcribed mRNA may not be translated into protein, or the rate of transcription may be altered. As discussed in Chapter 2, genes encoding proteins that turn on (activate) or turn off (repress) other genes are called transcription factors. Transcription factors commonly do not activate or repress only a single target. Often they regulate the transcription of many genes that, in turn, regulate other genes in a cascading effect. Consequently, mutations in transcription factor genes typically have pleiotropic effects.

There are many different families of transcription factors, members of which commonly share specific properties such as a common DNA-binding domain. Members of these different families have pivotal roles in controlling development, and alterations can cause birth defects. Examples include homeobox-containing genes such as the HOX, PAX, EMX, and MSX families; HMG-box containing genes such as the SOX family; and the T-box family.

As described in Chapter 2, the HMG domain of SOX proteins appears to activate transcription indirectly by bending DNA so that other factors can make contact with promoter regions of genes. Several SOX genes act in different developmental pathways. *Sox9* is expressed in the genital ridges of both sexes, but it is up-regulated in males and down-regulated in females prior to differentiation of the gonads. Furthermore, *Sox9* regulates chondrogenesis and the expression of *Col2A1*, a collagen gene (see Chapter 2). As might be predicted from these expression and interaction patterns, mutations in *SOX9* cause a disorder characterized by skeletal defects (campomelic dysplasia) and sex reversal that produces XY females. Mutations in a related gene, *SOX10*, result in a syndrome characterized by Hirschsprung disease (hypomotility of the bowel caused by a reduced number of enteric nerve cells), pigmentary disturbances, and deafness (see Clinical Commentary 10-2). **WWW**

▼ There are many different families of transcription factors, each of which regulates the transcription of specific genes. The same transcription factor is often used in different developmental pathways. Thus, disorders caused by mutations in genes encoding transcription factors are often pleiotropic. ▲

Extracellular Matrix Proteins

Extracellular matrix proteins (EMPs) are secreted macromolecules that serve as scaffolding for all tissues and organs. These molecules include collagens, fibrillins, proteoglycans, and large glycoproteins such as fibronectin, laminin, and tenascin. EMPs are not simply passive structural elements. By separating adjacent groups of cells and forming matrices on which cells may migrate, they are active mediators of development. For example, the proteins encoded by *fibrillin-1* and *elastin*

---

* A supergene family is a group of related gene families.

coordinate microfibril assembly in the extracellular matrix. Mutations in these two genes result in Marfan syndrome (see Chapter 4) and supravalvular aortic stenosis (see Chapter 6), respectively. Both of these diseases are characterized by malformations of the heart and/or large blood vessels. **WWW**

In order to facilitate cell migration, EMPs must transiently adhere to a cell's surface. This is commonly accomplished by two families of cell surface receptors: integrins and glycosyltransferases. Integrins are so named because they integrate the extracellular matrix and the cytoskeleton, allowing them to function in tandem. Attachment of cells and the extracellular matrix can be more permanent as well. Because of an inability of epithelial cells to properly anchor themselves to the basement membrane, the skin of individuals with autosomal recessive junctional epidermolysis bullosa (JEB) spontaneously forms large blisters. JEB is caused by mutations in *LAMC2*, a gene encoding a subunit of laminin. **WWW**

> ▼ Extracellular matrix proteins (EMPs) are secreted macromolecules that serve as a dynamic scaffolding for tissues and organs. They are also active mediators of development. ▲

PATTERN FORMATION

The process by which ordered spatial arrangements of differentiated cells create tissues and organs is called pattern formation. The general pattern of the animal body plan is laid down during embryogenesis. This leads to the formation of semi-autonomous regions of the embryo in which the process of pattern formation is repeated to form organs and appendages. Such regional specification takes place in several steps: (1) definition of the cells of a region, (2) establishment of signaling centers that provide positional information, and (3) differentiation of cells within a region in response to additional cues. For example, cells in the vertebrate upper limb differentiate into many cell types, including cartilage (chondrocytes) and bone cells (osteocytes). However, these cells must also be arranged in a temporal-spatial pattern that creates functional bone. Additional information is required to determine whether a bone becomes an ulna or a humerus. How do particular structures develop in specific places? How do cells acquire information about their relative positions? Answering such questions is an area of intense investigation.

For pattern formation to occur, cells and tissues communicate with each other through many different signaling pathways. It has become clear that these pathways are used repeatedly and are integrated with one another to control specific **cell fates** (i.e., the eventual location and function of the cell). For example, the

Sonic hedgehog protein is involved in patterning of the vertebrate neural tube, somites, and limbs, as well as the way the left is distinguished from the right. Point mutations in the human Shh gene, *SHH*, can cause abnormal midline brain development (holoprosencephaly; Fig. 10-2), severe mental retardation, and early death. (Not all affected individuals have holoprosencephaly, however; some have only minor birth defects such as a single upper central incisor.) Attachment of the SHH protein to cholesterol appears to be necessary for proper patterning of hedgehog signaling. This may partly explain how midline brain defects could be caused by some environmental substances that inhibit embryonic cholesterol biosynthesis and by genetic disorders of cholesterol metabolism (e.g., Smith-Lemli-Opitz syndrome). **WWW**

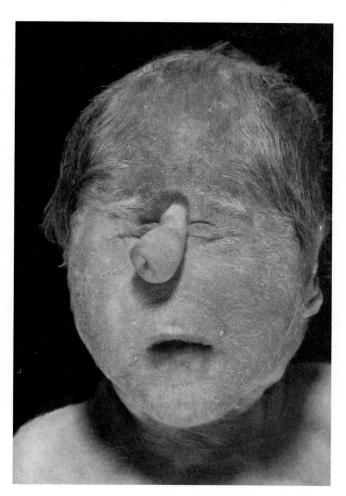

FIG. 10-2 Postmortem photograph of a neonate with holoprosencephaly (failure of the forebrain to completely separate). Note the sloping forehead, reduced midline scalp hair, small and closely spaced palpebral fissures, single nostril (proboscis), and small mouth. Holoprosencephaly can be caused by mutations in *Sonic hedgehog* that produce abnormal formation of the dorsal/ventral axis.

(Courtesy Dr. Edward Klatt, University of Utah Health Sciences Center.)

▼ The process by which ordered spatial arrangements of differentiated cells create tissues and organs is called pattern formation. Regional specification takes place in several steps: (1) definition of the cells of a region, (2) establishment of signaling centers that provide positional information, and (3) differentiation of cells within a region in response to additional cues. ▲

Gastrulation

Gastrulation is the process of cell and tissue movements whereby the cells of the blastula are rearranged so that they have new positions and neighbors. In the human embryo, gastrulation occurs between days 14 and 28 of gestation. In this process, the embryo is transformed into a three-layer (trilaminar) structure composed of three germ layers: ectoderm (outer layer), endoderm (inner layer), and mesoderm (middle layer) (Fig. 10-3). The formation of these layers is a prerequisite for the next phase of development, organogenesis. The major structural feature of mammalian gastrulation is the **primitive streak,** which appears as a thickening of epiblast tissue extending along the anterior-to-posterior axis (see Fig. 10-3). In placental animals such as humans, gastrulation includes the formation of the extra-embryonic tissues, primarily from trophoblastic cells. As might be predicted, the process of gastrulation is dominated by cell migration. Thus, many of the genes expressed during gastrulation encode proteins that facilitate cell movement.

▼ Human gastrulation is characterized by cell and tissue movements that result in the formation of three germ layers: ectoderm, endoderm, and mesoderm. The major structural feature of mammalian gastrulation is the primitive streak. ▲

Neurulation and Ectoderm

Once a trilaminar embryo is formed, the dorsal mesoderm and the overlying ectoderm interact to form the hollow neural tube. This event is called **neurulation** and is mediated by induction. In amphibians, induction of the neural tube and transformation of the flanking mesoderm into an embryo with clear anterior/posterior and dorsal/ventral axes is controlled by a group of cells known as the Spemann-Mangold organizer. A number of proteins are expressed almost exclusively in the organizer. Chordin is a secreted protein that prevents dorsalized mesoderm from being ventralized. Another secreted protein, Noggin, induces neural tissue from dorsal ectoderm and dorsalizes the mesoderm. Understanding the major functions of the organizer and the molecules that mediate these functions is an area of active investigation.

Neurulation is a critical event in development because it initiates organogenesis and divides the ectoderm into three different cell populations: (1) the neural tube, which will eventually form the brain and spinal cord, (2) the epidermis of the skin, and (3) the neural crest cells. In humans, neural tube closure begins at five separate sites, which correspond to the locations of common neural tube defects such as anencephaly (absence of the brain), occipital encephalocele, and lumbar spina bifida (see Chapter 12). Neural crest cells migrate from the neuroepithelium along defined routes to tissues where they differentiate into cell types such as sensory neurons, melanocytes, neurons of the small bowel, and smooth muscle cells (Clinical Commentary 10-2). WWW

▼ Induction is the process by which cells of one embryonic region influence the organization and differentiation of cells in a second embryonic region. Neurulation initiates organogenesis and induces the ectoderm to divide into the neural tube and neural crest cells. Defects of neural tube closure and neural crest migration or differentiation cause birth defects. ▲

Mesoderm and Endoderm

The formation of a layer of mesoderm between the endoderm and ectoderm is one of the major events in gastrulation. Mesoderm can be divided into five components: the notochord; the dorsal, intermediate, and lateral mesoderms; and head **mesenchyme.** * The notochord is a transient midline structure that induces the formation of the neural tube and body axis. Dorsal mesoderm is observed on either side of the notochord. It differentiates into elements that form the axial skeleton, appendicular skeleton, skeletal muscles, and connective tissue of the skin. Intermediate mesoderm forms the kidneys and genitourinary system. Lateral plate mesoderm differentiates into the heart, the connective tissue of viscera, and the connective tissue elements of the amnion and chorion. Finally, the muscles of the eyes and head arise from head mesenchyme.

The primary function of embryonic endoderm is to form the linings of the digestive tract and the respiratory tree. Outgrowths of the intestinal tract form the pancreas, gallbladder, and liver. A bifurcation of the respiratory tree produces the left and right lungs. The endoderm also produces the pharyngeal pouches, which, in conjunction with cells derived from the neural crest, give rise to endodermal-lined structures such as the middle ear, thymus, parathyroids, and thyroids.

---

*Mesenchyme is tissue that forms the connective tissues, blood vessels, and lymphatic vessels.

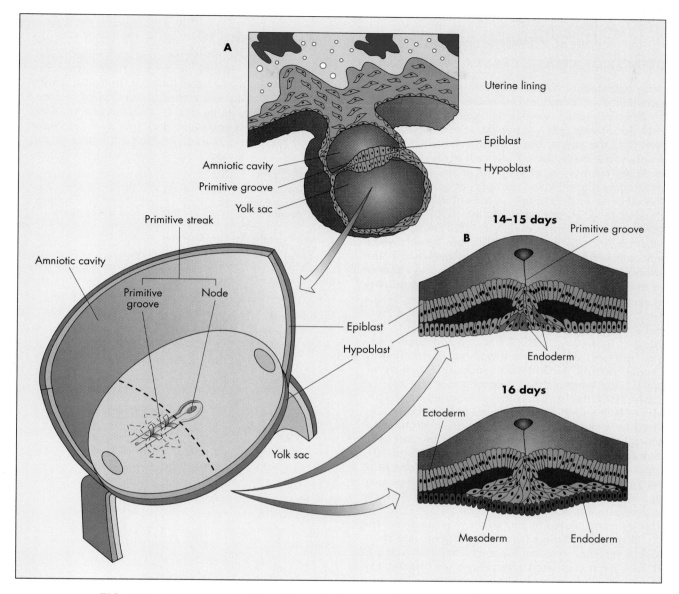

FIG. 10-3 Human gastrulation. **A,** Sagittal section through the midline of an embryo embedded in the uterine lining. **B,** Dorsal surface of an embryo exposed by removing part of the embryonic mesoderm surrounding the amniotic cavity and yolk sac. Arrows denote ingressing epiblast cells. On day 14 to 15, epiblast cells replace hypoblast cells to form endoderm. A day later, migrating epiblast cells are creating a layer of mesoderm.

A process common to endoderm-derived structures is budding and branching. This process appears to be controlled, in part, by fibroblast growth factors (FGFs), bone morphogenetic proteins (BMPs), and their respective receptors. Mutations in *fibroblast growth factor receptor 3 (FGFR3)*, one of four FGF receptors, cause three different skeletal dysplasias (see Clinical Commentary 10-1). The most severe of these, thanatophoric dysplasia, is caused by mutations that activate FGFR3, resulting in shortened long bones, a poorly developed vertebral column, a small thoracic cage, and a relatively large skull. Children with thanatophoric dysplasia may also have pulmonary hypoplasia and brain anomalies, suggesting that FGFR3 plays a role in formation of the lung and brain. **www**

▼ Formation of a layer of mesoderm between endoderm and ectoderm is one of the major events of gastrulation. Mesoderm contributes to the formation of the skeleton, urogenital system, and limbs. Endoderm lines the digestive and respiratory tracts and forms visceral organs and the lungs. ▲

CLINICAL COMMENTARY 10-2
DEFECTS OF NEURAL CREST DEVELOPMENT

During neurulation, neural crest cells migrate from the neuroepithelium along defined routes to tissues where they differentiate into various cell types (Fig. 10-4). One fate of neural crest cells is to populate the small and large bowel (i.e., the enteric tract) with nerve cells to create the enteric nervous system. These cells partly control and coordinate the normal movements of the enteric tract that facilitate digestion and transport of bowel contents. Reduced or absent nerve cells in the enteric tract causes a disorder called Hirschsprung disease (HSCR).

HSCR occurs in approximately 1/5,000 live births and is characterized by hypomotility of the bowel, which leads to severe constipation. It often presents in the newborn period, although it is also found in children and sometimes adults. If untreated, bowel hypomotility can lead to obstruction and gross distention of the bowel. Consequently, HSCR was formerly termed "congenital megacolon." WWW

Most individuals with HSCR have no additional problems. However, HSCR is also a well-recognized feature of some multiple birth defect syndromes such as trisomy 21 and Waardenburg syndrome. For the last few decades HSCR has been considered an example of a disorder that fit a multifactorial model of inheritance (i.e., caused by a combination of genes plus environmental factors; see Chapter 12). However, it has become clear that half of all cases of familial HSCR and 15% to 20% of sporadic cases are caused by mutations in one of at least four different genes. Study of these genes provides us with a window through which we can observe the development of neural crest cells.

HSCR can be caused by mutations that inactivate the RET (REarranged during Transfection) gene, which encodes a receptor tyrosine kinase (other mutations in RET have been associated with cancer; see Chapter 11). Normal signaling through RET appears to be required for neural crest migration into the distal portions of the bowel and for differentiation into nerve cells. The penetrance of RET mutations is higher in males than in females, suggesting that sex-specific modifiers of the phenotype might exist.

Mutations of another cell membrane receptor, *endothelin-B (EDNRB)*, or its ligand, *endothelin-3 (EDN3)*, also cause HSCR. Penetrance appears to vary by sex and genotype. In a large Mennonite community, individuals homozygous for an *EDNRB* mutation were four times more likely to develop HSCR than were heterozygous individuals. In addition to HSCR, some individuals with mutations in either *EDNRB* or *EDN3* have melanocyte abnormalities producing hypopigmented patches of skin and sensorineural hearing loss (normal melanocytes are required for auditory development). This disorder is called the Waardenburg-Shah syndrome. Thus, normal EDNRB and

EDN3 signaling is required for the development of neural crest cells into enteric nerve cells and melanocytes.

More recently, mutations in the *SOX10* transcription factor gene have been found in individuals with Waardenburg-Shah syndrome. Disruption of the homologous mouse gene, *Sox-10,* causes coat spotting and aganglionic megacolon. Although Sox genes are involved in many different biological processes, the role of SOX10 in neural crest cell development remains to be determined.

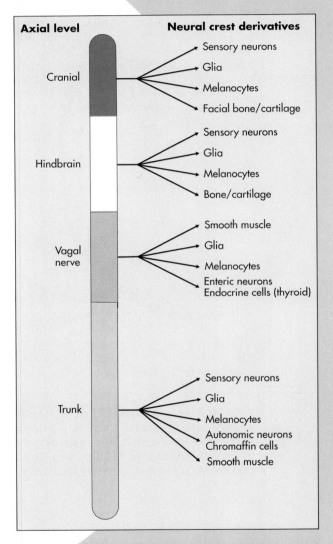

FIG. 10-4 Fates of selected populations of neural crest cells migrating from different levels along the anterior/posterior axis of the developing embryo. Appropriate fate of neural crest derivatives is dependent on normal cell migration and terminal differentiation. Defects of neural crest cells can cause Hirschsprung disease or Waardenburg-Shah syndrome (see text).

Axis Specification

Animal body plans have evolved into a wide variety of symmetries. Some animals, such as the volvox, are completely symmetrical. Other animals exhibit only a dorsal/ventral symmetry (e.g., starfish). To many animals, such as worms, an anterior/posterior axis has been added. All chordates (animals that develop a notochord) have a third axis that is perpendicular to the first two, the left/right axis. Specification and formation of the axes are critical events in development because they determine the orientation of the body plan. The proteins mediating these processes are rapidly being discovered. Many of these mediators have additional roles in patterning of the body plan and tissues.

Formation of the Anterior/Posterior Axis

The anterior/posterior axis of a developing mammalian embryo is defined by the primitive streak. At the anterior end of the primitive streak is a structure called the node. Expression of a gene called *nodal* is required for initiation and maintenance of the primitive streak, and later in gastrulation, its expression is important in forming the left/right axis (Clinical Commentary 10-3).

Patterning along the anterior/posterior axis is controlled by a cluster of genes that encode transcription factors containing an approximately 60–amino acid DNA-binding domain called the **homeodomain**. These genes compose the homeotic gene complex (HOM-C) in *Drosophila*, the organism in which they were first

---

CLINICAL COMMENTARY 10-3
LATERALITY DEFECTS: DISORDERS OF THE LEFT/RIGHT AXIS

Left/right (L/R) asymmetry is common in nature. For example, all animals utilize only L-amino acids and D-sugars. Likewise, all vertebrates have asymmetric structures that are consistently oriented along the L/R axis. For example, looping of the heart tube toward the right, the first observable sign of L/R asymmetry in the embryo, is seen in all chordates. How did L/R asymmetry evolve? How and when is L/R asymmetry established? Substantial progress is being made toward understanding the molecular basis of L/R axis formation so that answers may be obtained for these questions. This is important because disorders of L/R symmetry (i.e., laterality defects) are found in approximately 1/10,000 live births.

The final position of asymmetrically placed vertebrate structures is determined by at least three different mechanisms. Unpaired organs in the chest and abdomen (e.g., the heart and liver) begin their development in the midline and then lateralize to their adult positions. The mirror image of a paired structure may regress, leaving a lateralized, unpaired structure (e.g., some blood vessels). Some organs (e.g., lungs) begin as asymmetric outgrowths from a midline structure. It is unknown whether the molecular basis of laterality determination differs among these mechanisms. Disorders of L/R symmetry may cause randomization (*situs ambiguus*) or L/R reversal of organ position (*situs inversus*) (Fig. 10-5). These defects may by limited to a single organ (e.g., a right-sided heart, or dextrocardia) or may include many organs with L/R asymmetry (e.g., stomach and spleen). WWW

Initially, L/R axis establishment requires a mechanism that generates asymmetry. Studies of chick and frog embryos suggest that this is accomplished by a cascade of signaling molecules beginning with asymmetric expression of *Sonic hedgehog (Shh)* from the notochord. This results in left-sided expression of a member of the TGF-β family called *nodal*, which is responsible for rightward looping of the heart tube. L/R expression of *nodal* is randomized in a naturally occurring mouse mutant that exhibits a form of randomized organ asymmetry called *inversus viscerum*. This phenotype is caused by mutations in a gene that encodes dynein, a component of the motor that drives ciliary movement. Defects of dynein have also been described in humans with immotile cilia and a reversal of L/R asymmetry (Kartagener syndrome).

Mutations in *zinc-finger protein of the cerebellum (ZIC3)*, a member of the Gli transcription factor family located on the X chromosome, have been identified in humans with laterality defects. Affected males exhibit randomization defects, while some carrier females have L/R reversal. In *Drosophila*, some members of the Gli family are known to be regulated by forming a complex with costal2, a motor molecule similar to dynein. Because of these similarities, it has been suggested that ZIC3 and dynein may interact in humans. This could explain how mutations in genes encoding dissimilar proteins both cause human laterality disorders.

Once L/R asymmetry has been established in the early embryo, the left and right sides of individual organs must also be patterned. For example, two related transcription factors, dHAND and eHAND, play roles in patterning the right and left ventricles of the heart. In mice, homozygous mutation of *dHAND* produces animals that fail to form a right ventricle, indicating that dHAND participates in cardiac differentiation.

Abnormalities of L/R axis formation are found more frequently in human conjoined twins than in singletons or dizygotic twins. Most commonly, it is the twin arising

Continued

CLINICAL COMMENTARY 10-3—cont'd
LATERALITY DEFECTS: DISORDERS OF THE LEFT/RIGHT AXIS—cont'd

on the right side that exhibits randomization of the L/R axis information. It has been suggested that ran- domization of the right-sided twin is due to inade- quate signaling from the left-sided embryo. A candi- date for this signaling molecule discovered in frogs is Vg1. This suggests a possible molecular pathway for the formation of birth defects in human conjoined twins. WWW

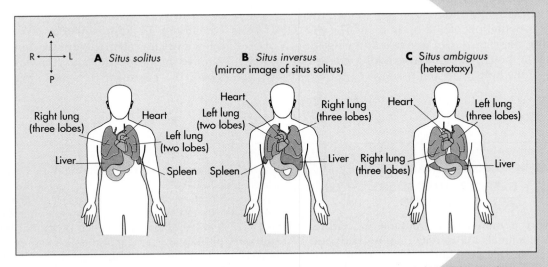

FIG. 10-5 Abnormalities of left/right (L/R) symmetry in humans. **A,** The normal positions of organs arranged along the L/R axis *(situs solitus).* The apex of the heart points toward the left. The right lung is trilobed and the left lung is bilobed. In the abdominal cavity, the spleen and stomach are positioned on the left side and the liver is on the right. The small bowel is looped in a counterclockwise direction. **B,** A complete mirror image of organ arrange- ment along the L/R axis is called *situs inversus.* Individuals with *situs inversus* may not be symptomatic. **C,** Random- ization of the arrangement the heart, lungs, liver, spleen, and stomach along the L/R axis *(situs ambiguus,* or het- erotaxy). *Situs ambiguus* is often associated with congenital heart defects. *Situs inversus* and *situs ambiguus* can be caused by mutations in *ZIC3.*

isolated through mutation identification (a classic example of such a mutation, termed "Antennapedia," disturbs axis patterning so that antennae are replaced by legs). Four copies of HOM-C (Hox A through D) are found in the human and the mouse (Fig. 10-6). There are 39 Hox genes, and each 100-kb gene cluster is located on a different chromosome. Mammalian Hox genes are numbered from 1 to 13, although not each cluster contains 13 genes. Equivalent genes in each complex (e.g., *Hoxa-13, Hoxc-13, Hoxd-13*) are called **paralogs**.

Hox genes are expressed along the dorsal axis from the anterior boundary of the hindbrain to the tail. Within each cluster, 3' Hox genes are expressed earlier than 5' Hox genes (**temporal collinearity**). Also, the 3' Hox genes are expressed anterior to the 5' Hox genes (**spatial collinearity**). Thus, *Hoxa-1* expression occurs earlier and in a more anterior location than does the expression of *Hoxa-2* (see Fig. 10-6). These overlapping domains of Hox gene expression produce combinations of codes that specify the positions of cells and tissues. Collectively these codes identify various regions along the anterior/ posterior axis of the trunk and limbs. To study the role of different Hox genes in mammalian development, it has been common to produce a "knock-out" mouse that lacks a functional copy of the gene of interest (Box 10-1).

▼ The anterior/posterior axis of a developing mam- malian embryo is defined by the primitive streak and patterned by combinations of Hox genes. Col- lectively these combinations identify various re- gions along the anterior/posterior axis of the body and limbs. Disruption of Hox genes produces de- fects in body, limb, and organ patterning. ▲

FIG. 10-6 **A,** Distribution of 39 Hox genes among clusters on four chromosomes in human (HOX) and mouse (Hox). Individual Hox genes are labeled from 1 (3′) to 13 (5′) within each cluster (A/a through D/d). Hox genes sharing the same number but located in different clusters are called paralogs (e.g., *HOXA13* and *HOXD13* are paralogs). Paralogs often exhibit more sequence homology than different Hox genes in the same cluster. Hox genes are expressed from 3′ to 5′ along the anterior/posterior axis of the embryo, and Hox genes located 3′ are expressed earlier than Hox genes located 5′. **B,** Schematic of combinatorial codes of overlapping Hox gene expression domains along the anterior/posterior body axis. Hox codes determine the identity of each segment. Thus, if expression of *Hoxb-4* is eliminated (e.g., in a knockout), the combinatorial code in the third segment is altered from 1+2+3 to 1+2. This results in the transformation of the third segment into another second segment. The transformation of one structure into another is called a homeotic transformation.

BOX 10-1
ANIMAL MODELS IN THE STUDY OF HUMAN DEVELOPMENT

There are significant obstacles to the study of genes that affect human development. Many of these genes are expressed embryonically, and it is difficult (or in some cases ethically undesirable) to analyze human embryos directly. Humans have relatively small family sizes and a long generation length. And human mating patterns are often not conducive to genetic study. For these and other reasons, animal models of human diseases are a useful alternative to the direct study of the disease in humans.

The mouse is commonly used as an animal model of human disease because it is a well-understood and easily manipulated experimental system and because many developmental genes are conserved in most mammalian species. In some cases a naturally occurring mouse model of a human genetic disease may exist (e.g., dog and mouse models for muscular dystrophy), but natural mouse models are relatively uncommon. To overcome this difficulty, human genes can be inserted directly into mouse embryonic stem cells, which are then placed into mouse embryos to create a **transgenic** mouse (Fig. 10-8). The expression of the human gene can then be studied directly in mouse embryos. It is also possible to use **targeted disruption** to alter a specific mouse gene so that it is not expressed. This is termed a **knockout** model. Mice that are heterozygous for the disrupted gene can be bred to produce homozygotes. Many human genetic diseases have been studied using mouse knockouts, including neurofibromatosis type 1, Gaucher disease, Huntington disease, myotonic dystrophy, fragile X syndrome, cystic fibrosis, and subtypes of Alzheimer disease.

These models do not always mimic their human counterparts accurately. Sometimes this reflects differences in the interactions of gene products in the model system and the human. Such differences may account for the fact that a heterozygous mouse knockout of the retinoblastoma homolog (*RB*) develops pituitary tumors instead of retinoblastomas. In some cases the knockout has little detectable effect, possibly reflecting **genetic redundancy**: even though the expression of one gene product is blocked, a "backup" system may compensate for its loss. Thus, the mouse knockout of either *Hoxa-11* or *Hoxd-11* alone has little phenotypic effect, but the simultaneous knockout of both genes produces a severe reduction of length of the radius and ulna. Despite these potential shortcomings, the introduction or disruption of genes in mice and other model systems can be a powerful approach for analyzing human genetic disease.

Formation of the Dorsal/Ventral Axis

Dorsal/ventral patterning of the vertebrate depends on the interaction between dorsalizing and ventralizing signals (Fig. 10-7). As previously mentioned, *noggin* and *chordin* are expressed in the amphibian organizer and encode secreted proteins that are capable of dorsalizing ventral mesoderm and restoring dorsal structures that have been ventralized. In contrast, *Bmp-4* is expressed ventrally and induces ventral fates, patterning the dorsal/ventral axis. Noggin and Chordin bind directly to Bmp-4 to prevent it from activating its receptor. Thus, the organizer promotes dorsalization by repressing a ventralizing signal encoded by *Bmp-4*. This mechanism, in which a signal promotes one process by repressing another competing process, is a common feature of embryonic development.

▼ Dorsal/ventral patterning of the embryo is an active process coordinated by signaling molecules and their antagonists. ▲

Formation of Organs and Appendages

The formation of organs and limbs (organogenesis) occurs after gastrulation. Many of the proteins used during this process are the same ones used earlier in embryonic development. As might be expected, how-

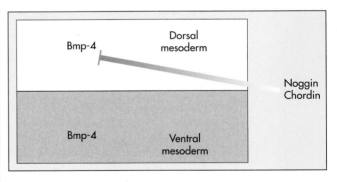

FIG. 10-7 Schematic illustration of signals that dorsalize or ventralize mesoderm in the developing embryo. Noggin and Chordin are secreted from cells in the node and bind to Bmp-4 to prevent it from activating its receptor. Because the ventralizing signal is blocked, mesoderm expressing Chordin and Noggin is dorsalized.

ever, a number of genes that were transcriptionally silent now become active. To date, most of the developmental genes known to cause human birth defects have prominent roles in this phase of development. This could represent an ascertainment bias because mutations in genes that disrupt earlier developmental events may be lethal.

BOX 10-1 ANIMAL MODELS IN THE STUDY OF HUMAN DEVELOPMENT—cont'd

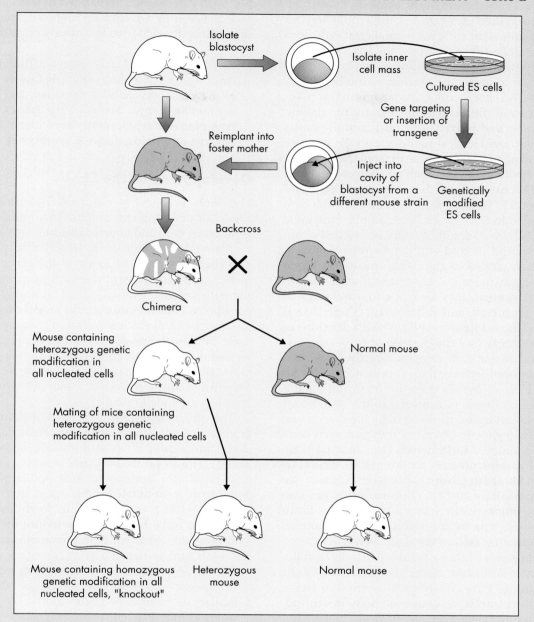

FIG. 10-8 Construction of an animal model. Blastocysts are collected from a pregnant mouse that has a marker that identifies its strain (e.g., light coat color). The inner cell mass is isolated, and embryonic stem (ES) cells are cultured. ES cells can be modified to introduce foreign genes (to create a transgenic animal) or disrupt the normal function of an endogenous gene (to create a knockout animal). Genetically modified ES cells are implanted into blastocysts from a different mouse strain that has a marker recessive to the marker in the modified strain (e.g., dark coat color is recessive to light coat color). Modified blastocysts are injected into a pseudopregnant surrogate mouse. Development of introduced blastocysts results in chimeric animals with two populations of cells (i.e., some cells have the genetic modification and other cells do not). Chimeras can be detected by the presence of two markers in the same mouse (e.g., two different coat colors in the same mouse). Backcrossing of chimeras and mating of heterozygotes can produce mice that are homozygous for a genetic modification (e.g., a knockout), heterozygous for a genetic modification, or normal.

(Modified from Strachan T, Read AP [1996] Human Molecular Genetics. Oxford, Bios Scientific.)

Craniofacial Development

Development of the craniofacial region is directly related to the formation of the underlying central nervous system. In mammalian embryos, neural crest cells from the forebrain and midbrain become the nasal processes, palate, and mesenchyme of the first pharyngeal pouch. This mesenchyme forms the maxilla, mandible, incus, and malleus. The neural crest cells of the anterior hindbrain migrate and differentiate to become the mesenchyme of the second pharyngeal pouch and the stapes and facial cartilage. Cervical neural crest cells produce the mesenchyme of the third, fourth, and sixth pharyngeal arches (in humans the sixth pharyngeal arch degenerates). This mesenchyme becomes the muscles and bones of the neck. The fate of each group of neural crest cells is specified by Hox genes. For example, functional inactivation of *Hoxa-3* results in mice with small or absent thymuses and thyroid and parathyroid glands, as well as malformations of the heart and major blood vessels. Although the number of neural crest cells in these mice is normal, they lack fate information and thus fail to proliferate and differentiate. These defects are similar to those found in children with deletions of chromosome 22q11 (see Chapter 6).

The bones of the skull develop directly from mesenchyme produced by neural crest cells. Complete fusion of these bones usually does not occur until adulthood. Premature fusion (synostosis) of the skull bones (craniosynostosis) causes the head to be misshapen and can impair brain growth. Often, craniosynostosis is associated with additional birth defects (e.g., hearing loss). Many of the craniosynostosis syndromes are caused by mutations in fibroblast growth factor receptor genes (see Clinical Commentary 10-1). Craniosynostosis can also be caused by mutations in *MSX2*, a transcription factor that may play a role in controlling the programmed death of neural crest cells in the skull. **WWW**

Craniosynostosis is also a feature of Greig cephalopolysyndactyly, a disorder caused by mutations of the gene encoding GLI3, a zinc-finger transcription factor. *GLI3* encodes at least seven conserved domains, including DNA-binding, zinc-finger, and microtubular anchor domains. Studies of the *Drosophila* homolog of *GLI3* suggest that this gene may be regulated so that it can have either activator or repressor functions. Mutations causing Greig cephalopolysyndactyly occur in the carboxy-terminal portion of *GLI3*, eliminating both its activator and repressor functions. Mutations in the region between the zinc-finger and the microtubular anchor domains produce a protein in which the amino terminal is cleaved so that it can migrate to the nucleus and repress transcription. Such mutations in *GLI3* cause a disorder called Pallister-Hall syndrome, characterized by hypothalamic hamartomas, visceral anomalies, and posterior polydactyly. Mutations 3′ of the microtubular anchor domain produce a protein retaining both repressor and activator functions and have been described in individuals with isolated posterior polydactyly, a relatively minor birth defect. Thus, mutations in *GLI3* alter the balance between its activator and repressor functions and cause three distinct disorders of varying severity. **WWW**

▼ The majority of craniofacial structures are derived from neural crest cells. The fate of each group of neural crest cells is specified by homeobox-containing genes. Some of the genes controlling craniofacial development have been isolated by analysis of craniosynostosis syndromes. ▲

Development of the Limb

The limb is arguably our best understood classical model of development. Surgical manipulation, ectopic gene expression, and targeted disruption of genes in animal models (see Box 10-1) have led to the isolation and characterization of many of the genes controlling growth and patterning of the limb. Many of the signaling pathways and transcriptional control elements that coordinate limb development in model organisms such as *Drosophila* and chick appear to be conserved in mammals. Because the newborn prevalence of limb defects is second only to that of congenital heart defects, the limb defect phenotypes are well documented. As a result, our knowledge of the molecular basis of human limb defects has expanded rapidly.

The vertebrate limb is composed of elements derived from lateral plate mesoderm (bone, cartilage, and tendons) and somitic mesoderm (muscle, nerve, and vasculature). The signal that initiates induction of forelimbs and hindlimbs appears to arise in the intermediate mesoderm. A candidate for this signal, fibroblast growth factor 8 (FGF8), is expressed in forelimbs and hindlimbs, and FGF8 is sufficient to induce the entire limb bud program. Once initiated, proximal/distal growth of the limb bud is dependent on a region of ectoderm called the apical ectodermal ridge (AER), which extends from anterior to posterior along the dorsal/ventral boundary of the limb bud (Fig. 10-9).

Prior to AER differentiation, two genes, *Radical fringe* (*r-Fng*) and *Wnt-7a*, are expressed in the dorsal ectoderm. In the ventral ectoderm, expression of *r-Fng* and *Wnt-7a* is blocked by Engrailed-1 (En-1), a homeobox-containing transcription factor. The AER forms at the interface of *r-Fng*–expressing and non–*r-Fng*-expressing cells, while expression of *Wnt-7a* instructs the mesoderm to adopt dorsal characteristics. Mesoderm in which *Wnt-7a* expression is blocked becomes ventralized. Thus, the processes of AER formation and dorsal/ventral patterning are interconnected and coordinated by En-1. In the mouse, functional inactivation of *Wnt-7a* results in ventralization of the dorsal surface (i.e., pads on both sides of the foot). Ventralization of the dorsal surface of the limb has been described in humans, but the etiology remains unknown.

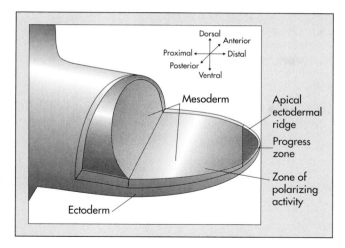

FIG. 10-9 Schematic illustration of a limb bud. The apical ectodermal ridge (AER) extends from anterior to posterior along the dorsal/ventral boundary of the limb bud. Proximal to the AER is a region of rapidly proliferating mesodermal cells called the progress zone (PZ). Located in the posterior mesoderm is an important signaling center called the zone of polarizing activity (ZPA). The signaling pathways of the AER, PZ, and ZPA are interconnected so that pattern formation and growth are partly dependent on their coordinated function.

Mediation of proximal/distal growth by the AER is controlled in part by fibroblast growth factors (e.g., FGF2, FGF4, FGF8) that stimulate proliferation of an underlying population of mesodermal cells in the progress zone (PZ). Maintenance of the AER is dependent on a signal from a posterior portion of the limb bud known as the zone of polarizing activity (ZPA). The signaling molecule of the ZPA is Sonic hedgehog (Shh), which is also responsible for dorsal/ventral patterning of the central nervous system and establishment of the embryonic left/right axis. The ZPA also specifies positional information along the anterior/posterior of the limb bud.

Defects of the anterior and posterior elements of the upper limb occur in the Holt-Oram syndrome (HOS) and ulnar-mammary syndrome (UMS), respectively. HOS is caused by mutations in a gene called *TBX5*, while UMS is caused by mutations in the tightly linked gene, *TBX3*. *TBX3* and *TBX5* are members of a highly conserved family of DNA transcription factors containing a DNA-binding domain called a T-box (see Chapter 2). It appears that *TBX3* and *TBX5* have evolved from a common ancestral gene, and each has acquired specific yet complementary roles in patterning the anterior/posterior axis of the mammalian upper limb. **www**

If the early events of limb bud signaling provide positional information to developing cells, what controls the growth and differentiation of these cells? One important component is the transcription factors encoded by Hox genes. The expression patterns of *Hoxa-9* through *Hoxa-13* define overlapping domains along the proximal/distal axis of the developing limb bud.

Combinations of Hox paralogs preferentially promote growth within different segments of the limb according to their 5' position within a Hox cluster. For example, mice with *Hoxa-11* or *Hoxd-11* mutations have only minor abnormalities, whereas *Hoxa-11/Hoxd-11* double mutants exhibit a marked reduction in the size of the radius and ulna. Similarly, deletion of increasing numbers of Hox-13 paralogs has a cumulative effect on phenotypic abnormalities of the hands or feet. It is presumed that this is because the functions of Hox paralogs are partially redundant.

For this reason, it was suspected that mutations in Hox genes would be unlikely causes of human birth defects. However, Hox mutations have recently been described in individuals with synpolydactyly and hand-foot-genital syndrome. Synpolydactyly is characterized by duplication and fusion of the middle digits of the hands and feet. It is caused by mutations in *HOXD13* that produce an expansion of a polyalanine tract in the amino terminal end of the HOXD13 protein. A similar defect can be reproduced by simultaneous disruption of *Hoxd-13*, *Hoxd-12*, and *Hoxd-11*, suggesting that expansion of the polyalanine tract in *HOXD13* results in the functional inactivation of its 3' neighbors. **www**

▼ **The vertebrate limb is composed of elements derived from lateral plate mesoderm and somitic mesoderm. Growth and patterning are controlled by proteins secreted from specialized collections of cells called the apical ectodermal ridge, the progress zone, and the zone of polarizing activity.** ▲

Organ Formation

Many developmental processes must be coordinated simultaneously to construct the specific arrangement of cells and tissues that compose an organ. As in limb development, the formation of organs involves numerous interactions. These interactions are mediated by secreted signaling molecules that bind to receptors, conduct signals through various interconnected pathways, and stimulate or repress DNA transcription. Use of the same elaborate networks to form different organs allows for genomic economy while maintaining developmental flexibility.

Once a specialized cell within an organ is terminally differentiated, various proteins turn on its molecular machinery so that it may perform its intended function. Often, development of the organ and function of the differentiated cell are interrelated. For example, the endocrine pancreas is largely composed of three different cell types: α, β, and δ. Transcription of insulin in β cells is stimulated by the binding of insulin promoter factor 1 (IPF1) to the insulin promoter region. Mutations in the gene encoding IPF1 prevent pancreatic development, indicating that IPF1 is necessary for the maturation and differentiation of pancreatic precursor cells.

Interactions between mesenchymal and epithelial cells are prominent in the development of cutaneous structures (e.g., hair, sweat glands, breasts), parenchymal organs (e.g., liver, pancreas), lungs, thyroid, kidneys, and teeth. These interactions are dynamic in that expression patterns in the epithelia and mesenchyme change over time and continue to influence one another. For example, during tooth development, the epithelium secretes Bmp-4, which signals the underlying mesenchyme to express a set of transcription factors, including Msx1. The mutual exchange of signals between epithelium and mesenchyme leads to formation of a dental papilla and cusp and finally to terminal differentiation of mesenchyme into tooth-forming odontoblasts. In humans, mutations in *MSX1* disrupt tooth formation and cause loss of the second premolars. Similarly, mutations in the human homolog of the mouse gene, *hairless*, cause loss of all body hair, including that of the scalp, eyebrows, axilla, and pubis.

One of the largest organs in the body is the skeleton. Skeletal formation is dependent on bone-forming cells called osteoblasts. The differentiation of osteoblasts is regulated by an osteoblast-specific transcription factor, Cfba1. Targeted disruption of *Cfba1* produces mice with a complete lack of ossification of the skeleton. Heterozygous mice have widened cranial sutures, shortened digits, and abnormalities of the shoulder girdle. Similar defects are found in individuals with cleidocranial dysplasia, which is caused by mutations in *CFBA1*, the human homolog of mouse *Cfba1*. **www**

▼ **Formation of organs involves reciprocal interactions between epithelium and mesenchyme. This interaction is mediated by secreted signaling molecules that bind to receptors, conduct signals through various interconnected pathways, and stimulate or repress DNA transcription.** ▲

RECOMMENDED READINGS

Anderson DJ (1997) Cellular and molecular biology of neural crest cell lineage determination. Trends Genet. 13:276-280

Anderson E, Beddington R (1997) Pattern formation and developmental mechanisms. Curr. Opin. Genet. Dev. 7:3455-458

Bowers PN, Brueckner M, Yost HJ (1996) The genetics of left-right development and heterotaxia. Semin. Perinatol. 20:577-588

DeMoerlooza L, Dickson C (1997) Skeletal disorders associated with fibroblast growth factor receptor mutations. Curr. Opin. Genet. Dev. 7:378-385

Epstein CJ (1995) The new dysmorphology: application of insights from basic developmental biology to the understanding of human birth defects. Proc. Natl. Acad. Sci. USA 92:8566-8573

Farese RV, Herz J (1998) Cholesterol metabolism and embryogenesis. Trends Genet. 14:115-120

Gilbert SF (1997) Developmental Biology. Sinauer Press, Sunderland

Hammerschmidt M, Brook A, McMahon AP (1997) The world according to hedgehog. Trends Genet. 13:14-21

Hogan BLM (1996) Bone morphogenetic proteins in development. Curr. Opin. Genet. Dev. 6:432-438

Innis JW (1997) Role of HOX genes in human development. Curr. Opin. Pediatr. 9:617-622

Johnson RL, Tabin C (1997) Molecular models for vertebrate limb development. Cell 90:979-990

Mark M, Rijli FM, Chambon P (1997) Homeobox genes in embryogenesis-pathogenesis. Pediatr. Res. 42:421-429

Moon RT, Brown JD, Torres M (1997) WNTs modulate cell fate and behavior during vertebrate development. Trend Genet. 13:157-162

Papaioannou VE, Sliver LM (1998) The T-box gene family. BioEssays 20:9-19

Pevny LH, Lovell-Badge R (1997) *Sox* genes find their feet. Curr. Opin. Genet. Dev. 7:338-344

Shubin N, Tabin C, Carroll S (1997) Fossils, genes, and the evolution of animal limbs. Nature 388:639-648

Shuldiner, AR (1996) Transgenic animals. N. Eng. J. Med. 334:653-655

Webster MK, Donoghue DJ (1997) FGFR activation in skeletal disorders: too much of a good thing. Trends Genet. 13:178-182

Winter RM (1996) Analyzing human developmental abnormalities. BioEssays 18:965-971

Wood WB (1997) Left/right asymmetry in animal development. Annu. Rev. Cell Dev. Biol. 13:53-82

STUDY QUESTIONS

1. Explain how non-human animal models are useful for studying human development and birth defects. Give at least one example.

2. Mutations in fibroblast growth factor receptors (FGFRs) cause at least five different craniosynostosis syndromes. Moreover, the same mutation in FGFR2 causes Pfeiffer syndrome in some families but Crouzon syndrome in other families. How can the same mutation produce two distinct disorders?

3. Disorders caused by mutations in genes encoding transcription factors are often pleiotropic. Explain this finding.

4. Define pattern formation, and give an example of a birth defect caused by disruption of this process.

5. If the control of developmental processes is tightly regulated, how can you explain that mutations in some developmental genes (e.g., *Hox* genes) produce subtle phenotypes?

6. Loss-of-function mutants in mammals are commonly studied by creating a knockout mouse model. Explain why it is impractical to use some organisms (e.g., baboons) to generate knockouts. Can you think of a way to circumvent some of these obstacles?

7. Give an example of a birth defect that can be caused by a defect in a ligand or its receptor.

8. Explain what may be some of the obstacles to using gene therapy to treat birth defects.

11
Cancer Genetics

Present evidence indicates that approximately one in four deaths is now due to cancer and that more than half of the population will be diagnosed with invasive cancer at some point in their lives. Many cancers are increasing in frequency, largely due to the increasing proportion of our population in older age groups. As shown in this chapter, the causes of cancer are a mixture of environmental components and genetic alterations occurring in our tissues. Inherited predisposition plays a role in some families. Dramatic advances in molecular biology and genetics have now clarified the basic molecular elements of cancer and provide a schematic outline of the cellular events leading to cancer. This understanding will be crucially important in the control of cancer, providing the beginnings of a base of knowledge that should lead to significantly improved therapies and possibly prevention.

"Cancer" is a collection of disorders that share the common feature of uncontrolled cell growth. This leads to a mass of cells termed a **neoplasm** (Greek, "new formation"), or **tumor.** The formation of tumors is called **tumorigenesis. Malignant** neoplasms invade nearby tissues and often **metastasize** (spread) to more distant sites in the body. The capacity to invade and metastasize distinguishes malignant from **benign** neoplasms. Tumors are classified according to the tissue type in which they arise. Major types of tumors include those of epithelial tissue **(carcinomas,** the most common tumors), connective tissue **(sarcomas),** lymphatic tissue **(lymphomas),** glial cells of the central nervous system **(gliomas),** and hematopoietic organs **(leukemias).** The cells composing a tumor are usually derived from a single ancestral cell, making them a single clone **(monoclonal).**

Many of the basic biological features of **carcinogenesis** (cancer development) are now understood. Throughout our lives, many of our cells continue to grow and differentiate. These form, for example, the epithelial layers of our lungs and colons and the precursors of the cells of our immune systems. Relatively undifferentiated stem cells produce large numbers of progeny cells to repopulate and renew our worn defensive layers. Through integration of information provided by a complex array of biochemical signals, the new cells are designed to commit themselves to stop dividing and terminally differentiate into a cell type appropriate for their heritage and circumstances (Fig. 11-1).

Occasionally one of these cells will fail to differentiate and will begin to divide without restraint. The descendants of such cells can become the founders of neoplasms, capable of further transformation into invasive, metastatic cancer. Our goals are to understand in detail what has gone wrong in such rogue cells, to detect them very early in their careers, and ultimately to intervene in their development to eliminate them.

▼ **Cells in the body are "programmed" to develop, grow, differentiate, and die in response to a complex system of biochemical signals. Cancer results from the emergence of a clone of cells freed of these developmental programming constraints and capable of inappropriate proliferation. ▲**

CAUSES OF CANCER
Genetic Considerations

Genetic alterations of cell regulatory systems are the primary basis of carcinogenesis. We can create cancer in animal models by damaging specific genes. In cell culture systems, we can reverse a cancer phenotype by introducing normal copies of the damaged genes into the cell. Most of the genetic events that cause cancer occur during the lifetime of the individual, in his or her somatic tissues. The frequency of these events can be altered by exposure to mutagens, thus establishing

FIG. 11-1   In response to environmental signals, a cell may continue to divide or it may differentiate or die (apoptosis).

▼ The basic cause of cancer is damage to specific genes. Usually, mutations in these genes accumulate in somatic cells over the years, until a cell loses a critical number of growth-control mechanisms and initiates a tumor. If damage occurs in cells of the germ line, however, an altered form of one of these genes can be transmitted to progeny and predispose them to cancer. The greatly increased risk of cancer in such individuals is due to the fact that *each* of their cells now carries the first step in a multistep cancer pathway. ▲

a link to environmental **carcinogens** (cancer-causing agents). However, because these genetic events occur in somatic cells, they are not transmitted to future generations. Even though they are *genetic* events, they are not *inherited*.

It is also possible for cancer-predisposing mutations to occur in germline cells. This results in the transmission of cancer-causing genes from one generation to the next, producing families that have a high frequency of specific cancers (Fig. 11-2). Such "cancer families," although rare, demonstrate that inheritance of a damaged gene can cause cancer. In these families, inheritance of one mutant allele seems sufficient to cause a specific form of cancer: almost all individuals who inherit the mutant allele will develop a tumor. This is because each of their cells now carries the altered gene and thus has already taken the first step down the cancer pathway. The childhood cancer of the eye, retinoblastoma, is a good example. As discussed in Chapter 4, those who inherit a mutant version of the retinoblastoma gene have approximately a 90% chance of developing one or more retinoblastoma tumors.

While the transmission of cancer as a single-gene disorder is relatively uncommon, there is good evidence for more frequent clustering of some cancer types in families. For many kinds of cancer, such as breast and colon, the diagnosis of the cancer in one of our first-degree relatives implies a several-fold increase in our risk of developing the cancer. A genetic basis for this familial clustering of cancer is suggested but remains unspecified. However, it is possible that genetic transmission of altered forms of specific genes is responsible.

The extent to which each of these mechanisms— inherited germline mutations versus mutations occurring in somatic cells—contributes to human cancer is an important question. If inherited predispositions are significant determinants of an individual's risk of acquiring a specific form of cancer, it should ultimately be possible to identify individuals whose risk is elevated. More intensive screening of defined high-risk populations could result in early detection and intervention, leading to better prognoses for individuals and lowered morbidity and mortality in the population.

Environmental Considerations

What is the role of the environment in carcinogenesis? At the level of the cell, cancer seems intrinsically genetic. Tumor cells arise when certain changes, or mutations, occur in genes that are responsible for regulating the cell's growth. However, the frequency and consequences of these mutations can be altered by a large number of environmental factors. It is well documented, for example, that many chemicals that cause mutation in experimental animals also cause cancer and are thus carcinogens. Furthermore, other environmental agents may enhance the growth of genetically altered cells without directly causing new mutations. Thus, it is often the interaction of genes with the environment that determines carcinogenesis; both play key roles in this process.

Two additional lines of argument support the idea that exposure to environmental agents can significantly alter an individual's risk of cancer. The first is that a number of environmental agents with carcinogenic properties have been identified. For example, cigarette smoke has been shown to cause lung and other types of cancer, both through epidemiological studies and in laboratory experiments. Roles for other environmental agents in specific cancers are also well documented (e.g., uranium dust in lung cancer among miners and asbestos exposure in lung cancer and mesothelioma).

The second line of argument is based on epidemiological comparisons among populations with differing lifestyles. Many kinds of cancer have quite different frequencies in different populations. Breast cancer, for example, is prevalent among northern Europeans and Americans but relatively rare among women in developing countries. It is usually difficult to determine whether such dissimilarities reflect differences in lifestyle or in gene frequencies.

Examination of genetically similar populations under differing lifestyles, however, provides an opportunity to evaluate the genetic and environmental components of cancer. Epidemiological studies among migrant Japanese populations, for example, have yielded important findings with respect to colon cancer. This type of cancer is relatively rare in the Japanese population

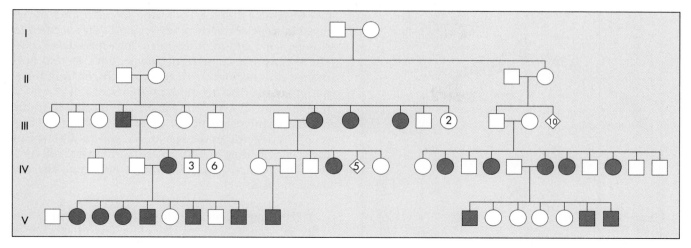

FIG. 11-2   A familial colon cancer pedigree. Darkened symbols represent individuals diagnosed with colon cancer.

living in Japan but is the second most common form of cancer in the United States. Stomach cancer, on the other hand, is frequent in Japan but relatively rare in the United States. These statistics in themselves cannot distinguish environmental from genetic influences in the two populations. However, because large numbers of Japanese have immigrated, first to Hawaii and then to the U.S. mainland, we can observe what happens to the rates of stomach and colon cancer among the immigrants. It is important to note that the Japanese immigrants have maintained a genetic identity, marrying largely among themselves.

In the U.S. population as a whole, the lifetime risk of colon cancer is approximately 5%; in Japan that risk is ten-fold lower, only 0.5%. Among the first-generation Japanese in Hawaii, the frequency of colon cancer rises several-fold—not yet as high as in the U.S. mainland, but higher than in Japan. Among second-generation Japanese on the U.S. mainland, the colon cancer rates are 5%, equal to the U.S. average. At the same time, stomach cancer has become relatively rare among Japanese-Americans. These observations strongly suggest an important role for environment or lifestyle in the etiology of colon cancer.

Are we then to assume that genetic factors play no role in colon cancer? The fact remains that in the North American environment some individuals will get colon cancer and others will not. This distinction can result from differences within this environment (e.g., dietary variation) as well as differences in genetic predisposition: inherited genes that increase the individual's probability of developing cancer. To account for the difference in colon-cancer frequency between Japanese living in the U.S. and those living in Japan, however, we argue that environmental features in Japan render the pre-

disposing genes less penetrant. Furthermore, a genetic component is strongly suggested by the several-fold increase in risk to an individual when a first-degree relative has colon cancer. It is likely, then, that cancer risk is a composite of both genetics and environment, with interaction between the two components.

▼ Environmental factors are known to play important roles in carcinogenesis. However, an individual's overall cancer risk depends on a combination of inherited factors and environmental components. ▲

CANCER GENES
Genetic Control of Cell Growth and Differentiation

Cancers form when a clone of cells emerges that has lost the normal controls over growth and differentiation. More than 100 cancer-causing genes that encode proteins participating in this regulation have now been identified. Characterization of the biochemical activities and interactions of these gene products has revealed an increasingly detailed picture of the normal regulation of cell growth and differentiation and the ways in which these processes become deregulated by the events of carcinogenesis.

Many features of this fundamental process are now well understood (Fig. 11-3). One component of cell regulation is mediated by external signals coming to the cell through polypeptide **growth factors** (e.g., platelet-derived growth factor, epidermal growth factor, steroid hormones) produced in other cells. Each growth factor interacts with a specific **growth factor receptor** located on the cell surface. Binding of a growth factor activates the receptor, triggering molecules that send messages to

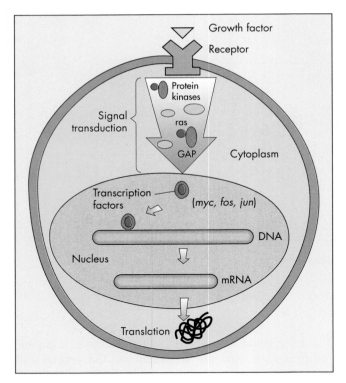

FIG. 11-3 The major features of cellular regulation: external *growth factors* (proteins and steroid hormones such as epidermal growth factor) bind to membrane-spanning *growth factor receptors* on the cell surface. These activate *signal-transduction* pathways, in which genes such as *ras* participate. Components of the signal-transduction pathway in turn interact with *nuclear transcription factors*, such as *myc* and *fos*, which can bind to regulatory regions in DNA.

the cell's nucleus in a process termed **signal transduction.** These signal transduction molecules include **protein kinases,** such as src, mapK, and junK, which can alter the activity of target proteins by tagging them at a specific site with a phosphate molecule (phosphorylation). The ultimate stage of the signal transduction pathway is regulation of DNA transcription in the nucleus. Components of the signal transduction cascade interact with nuclear transcription factors that regulate the activity of specific genes whose protein products influence cellular growth and proliferation. Genes that encode these transcription factors include *myc, fos,* and *jun.* Many other signals and signal transduction pathways have also been identified, including lipid molecules, steroid hormones, cell-cell contacts, and cell-matrix interactions.

Each cell is continually bombarded with these chemical messages and must process and evaluate this information. Processing of the message is at least partially managed by nodes on the signal transduction pathways that receive messages from several sources and give integrated outputs. Following several rounds of cell division, cells normally receive signals that tell them to stop growing and to differentiate into specialized cells. The signals may come from polypeptides, steroid hormones, direct contact with adjacent cells, or from internal programs that define the number of cell divisions that they are allowed. The signals are transduced to the nucleus of the recipient cell. Here, by altering the transcription patterns among genes that govern the steps of the cell cycle, they repress genes that promote cell division and induce genes that inhibit entry into the cell division cycle.

▼ The regulation of cell growth is accomplished by substances that include (1) growth factors that transmit signals from one cell to another; (2) specific receptors for the growth factors; (3) signal transduction molecules that activate a cascade of phosphorylating reactions within the cell; and (4) nuclear transcription factors. The cell integrates and interprets the host of signals it receives from its environment. Decisions to grow and divide, or to stop growing and differentiate, result from processing of the signals. ▲

A cancer cell may emerge from within a population of growing cells through the accumulation of mutations in these regulatory genes. Although such mutations occur only rarely, these cells may fail to respond to differentiation signals and continue to divide instead of undergoing their normal differentiation program. Furthermore, cancers seem usually to result from a *progressive* series of events that incrementally increase the extent of deregulation within a cell lineage; eventually, a cell emerges whose descendants multiply without appropriate restraints. Further changes give these cells the capacity to invade adjacent tissues and form metastases. The requirement for more than one mutation has been characterized as the **multi-hit concept of carcinogenesis.** An example of this concept is given by colorectal cancer, in which a number of genetic events are required to complete the progression from a benign growth to a malignant neoplasm (Fig. 11-4).

▼ Mutations may occur in any of the steps involved in regulating cell growth and differentiation. Accumulation of such mutations within a cell lineage may result in a progressive deregulation of growth, eventually producing a tumor cell. ▲

The Inherited Cancer Gene Versus the Somatically Altered Gene

Although "cancer families" have long been recognized, it was not until the early 1970s that we began to understand the relationship between the inherited genetic

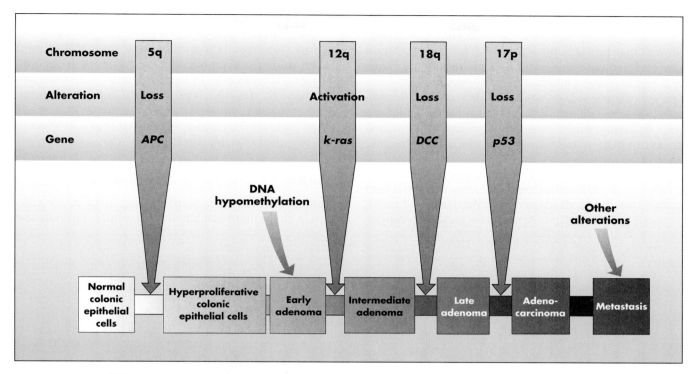

FIG. 11-4 The pathway to colon cancer. Loss of the *APC* gene (adenomatous polyposis coli) transforms normal epithelial tissue lining the gut to hyperproliferating tissue. Hypomethlyation of DNA, activation of the k-*ras* proto-oncogene, and loss of the *DCC* (*d*eleted in *c*olon *c*ancer) gene are involved in the progression to a benign adenoma. Loss of the *p53* gene and other alterations are involved in the progression to malignant carcinoma and metastasis.

(Modified from Vogelstein B, Kinzler KW [1993] Trends Genet. 9:138-141.)

aberrations and the carcinogenic events that occur in somatic tissue. In 1971 A.G. Knudson's analysis of retinoblastoma, a disease already mentioned as a model of inherited cancer, led him to a hypothesis that opened a new window into the mechanism of carcinogenesis. In the genetic form of retinoblastoma (see Chapter 4), a parent is likely to be affected and, if so, there is a 50% chance of genetic transmission to each of the offspring. In the sporadic (noninherited) form, neither parent is affected nor is there additional risk to other progeny. A key distinguishing feature between the two forms is that inherited retinoblastoma is usually bilateral (affects both eyes), whereas sporadic retinoblastoma usually involves only a single tumor and therefore only one eye (unilateral).

Knudson reasoned that at least two mutations may be required to create a retinoblastoma. One of the mutations would alter the retinoblastoma gene; if this happened in the germ line, it would be present in all cells of a child receiving the mutant allele. The second mutation would be an additional, unspecified genetic event in an already-altered cell. The hypothesis of a second event was required to explain why only a tiny fraction

of the retinoblasts of an individual who has inherited a mutant retinoblastoma gene actually give rise to tumors. Knudson's hypothesis is known as the **two-hit model of carcinogenesis**.

Familial retinoblastoma would thus be caused by the inheritance of one of the genetic "hits" as a **constitutional** mutation (i.e., a mutation present in all cells of the body). Individuals who inherited one hit would require only one additional mutational event in a single retinoblast for that cell to seed a tumor clone. In sporadic cases, both mutations would have to occur independently within the same retinoblast, a highly improbable combination of rare events even in the million or so cells of the target tissue. The child who developed a retinoblastoma by this two-hit *somatic* route, therefore, was unlikely to develop more than one tumor. The individual *inheriting* a mutant retinoblastoma gene, however, needed only a single, additional genetic hit to a retinoblast for a tumor clone to develop. Knudson argued that such an event was likely to occur in several of the million or so retinoblasts of each carrier of the inherited mutant gene, thus explaining the bilaterality of inherited retinoblastoma.

An important corollary of this hypothesis is that the genes inherited in mutant form in familial cancer syndromes may be the same as those that generate common cancers by somatic mutation. *By understanding the nature of the mutant alleles inherited in rare cancer families, therefore, we will come to understand more about the somatic pathway to common cancer as well.* The converse is likewise true: understanding the nature of somatically mutated genes can help in understanding the inherited versions.

▼ Alfred Knudson's two-hit theory of carcinogenesis in retinoblastoma became the paradigm for a model to describe how inheritance of an altered gene predisposes the gene carrier to cancer.

The theory states that a cell can initiate a tumor only when it contains *two* damaged alleles; therefore, a person who inherits one copy of a mutant retinoblastoma gene must experience a second, somatic mutation in one or more retinoblasts in order to develop one or more retinoblastomas. Two somatic mutations can also occur in a single retinoblast of a non-predisposed fetus, producing sporadic retinoblastoma. ▲

MAJOR CLASSES OF CANCER GENES

Cancer genes can be classified into three major categories: those that normally inhibit cellular proliferation

FIG. 11-5 Persons inheriting an *RB1* mutation are heterozygous for the mutation in all cells of their body. The second "hit" occurs during embryonic development and may consist of a point mutation, deletion, loss of the normal chromosome and duplication of the abnormal one, or somatic recombination. Each process leads to homozygosity for the mutant *RB1* allele and thus tumor development.

(Modified from Cavenee WK, Dryja TP, Phillips RA, et al. [1983] Nature 305:779-784.)

(tumor suppressors), those that activate proliferation (oncogenes), and those that participate in DNA repair. Each of these categories will be discussed.

Tumor Suppressor Genes

If the first event in the two-hit model is an inherited mutation, what is the nature of the second hit? Again with retinoblastoma as the paradigm, two possibilities seemed plausible at first: (1) the second mutation could affect the function of a gene distinct from the retinoblastoma gene, and the presence of two mutant genes in the same cell would result in the tumor; or (2) the second event could inactivate or alter the remaining (normal) copy of the retinoblastoma gene. If the second possibility were correct, the second hit might sometimes involve the loss of a chromosome or an extensive deletion of a specific chromosome region that contains the retinoblastoma gene. Such large-scale chromosomal losses should be detectable with DNA markers located on the chromosome carrying the retinoblastoma gene.

In fact, losses of marker DNA near the retinoblastoma gene *(RB1)* on chromosome 13 do occur in more than 50% of retinoblastomas. Several mechanisms, including point mutation, deletion, and somatic recombination, can produce such a loss (Fig. 11-5). The observation of DNA loss shows that the second hit, which occurs in the fetus during the period in which retinoblasts are rapidly dividing and proliferating, has re-

moved the remaining normal allele of this gene. This implies that a cell with one mutant *RB1* allele and one normal *RB1* allele cannot form a tumor. Thus, the product of the normal gene, even when present only in a single copy, prevents tumor formation. The term **tumor suppressor** has been coined to describe the *RB1* gene and a growing list of other cancer-associated genes that operate through this mechanism (Table 11-1).

Characteristic of tumor suppressors is the somewhat perplexing feature that inherited mutations are *dominant* alleles at the level of the individual (i.e., heterozygotes usually develop the disease) but *recessive* alleles at the level of the cell (heterozygous cells do not form tumors). This apparent contradiction is resolved by realizing that only a single tumor cell is required, from a population of millions of normal cells, to initiate a tumor in the individual. Thus, in individuals who have inherited the first hit, a second hit that occurs in any one cell will cause a tumor. Because of the large size of the target retinoblast population, heterozygous individuals form, on the average, several retinoblasts homozygous for an *RB1* mutation, each of which leads to a retinoblastoma. Thus, it is the strong *predisposition* to tumor formation (i.e., the first hit) that is inherited as an autosomal dominant trait. The reduced penetrance of the retinoblastoma mutation (90%) is explained by the fact that some individuals who inherit the disease-causing mutation do not experience a second hit in any of their retinoblasts.

TABLE 11-1 Some Examples of Tumor Suppressor Genes and Their Role in Cancer

Gene (related genes in parentheses)	Chromosome location	Function of gene product	Disease caused by germline mutations
RB1 (p107, p130)	13q14	Cell cycle brake; binds to E2F	Retinoblastoma; osteosarcoma
APC	5q21	Interacts with β-catenin in Wnt signaling pathway	Familial adenomatous polyposis
NF1	17q11	Downregulates ras protein	Neurofibromatosis type 1
NF2	22q12	Possible link between cell membrane proteins and cytoskeleton	Neurofibromatosis type 2
p53	17p13	Transcription factor; induces cell cycle arrest or apoptosis	Li-Fraumeni syndrome
VHL	3p25	Regulates transcriptional elongation	Von-Hippel Lindau disease (renal cancer)
WT1	11p13	Transcription factor	Wilms tumor
p16 (p15)	9p21	CDK inhibitor	Familial melanoma
BRCA1	17q21	Interacts with RAD51 DNA repair protein	Familial breast/ovarian cancer
BRCA2	13q12	Interacts with RAD51 DNA repair protein	Familial breast cancer
PTEN	10q23	Phosphatase	Cowden disease (breast and thyroid cancer)
AT	11q22	Cell cycle regulator; responds to DNA damage	Ataxia telangiectasia

A general property of tumor suppressors is that they normally block the uncontrolled cellular proliferation that can lead to cancer. Often, this is done by participating in pathways that regulate the cell cycle. For example, the protein encoded by *RB1* (pRb) is active when it is relatively unphosphorylated but is downregulated when it is phosphorylated by cyclin-dependent kinases just before the S phase of the cell cycle (see Chapter 2). In its active unphosphorylated state, pRb binds to members of the E2F transcription complex, inactivating them (Fig. 11-6). This complex is required for progression into S phase, so its inactivation by pRb halts the cell cycle. pRb thus serves as a cell cycle "brake" that is normally released only when pRb is inactivated through phosphorylation. It becomes reactivated later in the cell cycle when its phosphate groups are removed. However, loss-of-function mutations in *RB1*, and in some cases hypermethylation of its 5′ region, can lead to permanent inactivation. Without this brake on the cell cycle, the cell can proceed unimpeded through numerous uncontrolled divisions.

Loss-of-function mutations of other inhibitory factors can also lead to an unregulated cell cycle. A number of tumor suppressor genes encode **cyclin-dependent kinase inhibitors** (see Fig. 11-6), which inactivate the cyclin-dependent kinases and thus prevent them from phosphorylating and inactivating factors such as pRb. Again, mutations in these genes can lead to unrestricted cell division and ultimately to cancer. Tumor suppressors may also control cell proliferation through their effects on signal transduction, transcription, or cell-cell interactions (examples will be discussed later).

▼ **The discovery that retinoblastoma results when both alleles of the same locus on chromosome 13 are inactivated in the same retinoblast led to the concept of tumor suppressor genes. The products of such genes suppress tumor formation by controlling cell growth and can do so even if a cell contains only one normal version of the gene. Loss-of-function mutations result in inactivation of the tumor suppressor and can lead to uncontrolled cellular proliferation. ▲**

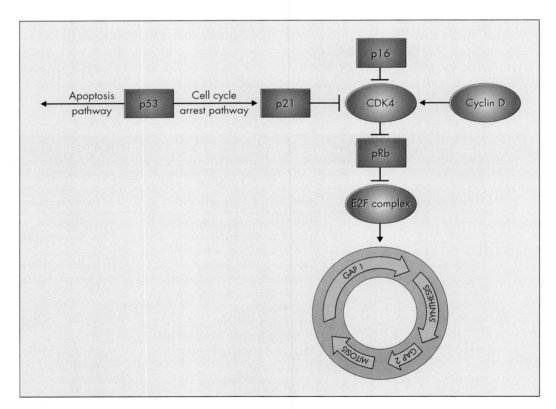

FIG. 11-6 Regulation of the cell cycle is accomplished by a complex series of interactions among activators and repressors of the cycle. pRb acts as a master brake on the cell cycle by binding the E2F transcription complex, halting the cycle before S phase begins. The cyclin D-CDK4 complex inactivates pRb by phosphorylating it, thereby releasing the E2F complex and allowing the cell to progress through S phase. CDK inhibitors, such as p16 and p21, inactivate CDKs, thus acting as another brake on the cycle. p53, acting through p21, can either halt the cell cycle or induce apoptosis in response to DNA damage.

Because of the pivotal role of tumor suppressors in the prevention of tumor formation, their study is of considerable medical significance. By understanding how cancer is naturally suppressed by the body, we can ultimately develop more effective medical therapies for tumor prevention and treatment.

Oncogenes

A second category of genes that can cause cancer is termed **oncogenes** (i.e., "cancer genes"). Most oncogenes originate from **proto-oncogenes**, which are genes that are involved in the four basic regulators of normal cell growth mentioned previously (growth factors, growth factor receptors, signal transduction molecules, and nuclear transcription factors). When a mutation occurs in a proto-oncogene, it can become an oncogene, a gene whose constantly active product can lead to unregulated cell growth and differentiation. When a cell proceeds from regulated to unregulated growth, the cell is said to have been **transformed**.

Unlike tumor suppressor genes, oncogenes are usually dominant at the cellular level: only a single copy of a mutated oncogene is required to contribute to the multi-step process of tumor progression. Whereas tumor suppressors are typically disabled by loss-of-function mutations, oncogenes are typically activated by gain-of-function mutations. Most tumor suppressor genes are known to exhibit germline mutations that cause inherited cancer syndromes (e.g., retinoblastoma, Li-Fraumeni syndrome [LFS]). In contrast, although oncogenes are commonly found in sporadic tumors, germline oncogene mutations that cause inherited cancer syndromes are uncommon (a few exceptions will be noted later in the discussion). In this section we review three approaches that have been used to identify specific oncogenes: retroviral definition, transfection experiments, and mapping in tumors.

▼ Proto-oncogenes encode products that control cell growth and differentiation. When mutated, they may become oncogenes, which can cause cancer. Most oncogenes act as dominant gain-of-function mutations that lead to the deregulation of cell cycle control. In contrast to tumor suppressor genes, most oncogenes do not exhibit germline mutations that cause inherited cancer syndromes. Instead, somatic mutations are seen that lead to sporadic cancers. ▲

Retroviruses

Retroviruses are a type of RNA virus capable of using reverse transcriptase to transcribe RNA into DNA. In this way, the RNA genome of the retrovirus can be converted to DNA, which is inserted into a chromosome of a host cell. The first oncogenes to be identified came from the study of retroviruses that cause cancer in animal systems. These retroviruses carry altered versions of certain growth-promoting genes into cells. In an earlier cycle of infection, a retrovirus may have incorporated a mutant oncogene from the genome of its host. When the retrovirus invades a new cell, it can transfer the oncogene into the genome of the new host, thus transforming the cell.

A number of gene products that receive and interpret extracellular signals for growth or differentiation have been identified through oncogenes carried by transforming retroviruses. For example, the *sis* oncogene, carried by the *simian sarcoma* virus, has been identified as an altered version of the human gene that encodes platelet-derived growth factor (PDGF). Retrovirus studies have likewise identified the gene encoding the receptor molecule for another of the growth factors, epidermal growth factor (EGF), through the *ErbB* oncogene. The *ras* (*rat sarcoma*) oncogenes, Harvey and Kirsten, were first identified through transforming retroviruses. Transforming retroviruses have also identified the nuclear transcription factor genes, *myc*, *jun*, and *fos*, as other molecular components capable of initiating cell transformation. Table 11-2 provides some examples of proto-oncogenes.

▼ Retroviruses are capable of inserting oncogenes into the DNA of a host cell, thus transforming the host into a tumor-producing cell. The study of such retroviral transmission has identified a number of specific oncogenes. ▲

Transfection Experiments

The identification of cellular genes involved in carcinogenesis was complemented by experiments in which mutated forms of cellular proto-oncogenes were transferred from tumor cells to non-tumor cells **(transfection),** causing transformation of the recipients. The prototype experiment was the transfer of DNA from a human bladder-cancer cell line into mouse cells. A few recipient cells became fully transformed; cloning and examination of the human-specific DNA sequences present in the transformed mouse cells revealed that the transforming gene was a mutant allele of the same Harvey *ras* oncogene previously identified by retroviral studies.

Characterization of the protein product of mutant forms of *ras* has revealed an important mechanism for the regulation of signal transduction. The normal *ras* (proto-oncogene) protein product interacts with guanine nucleotide cofactors. The ras protein normally cycles between an *active* form bound to **guanosine triphosphate (GTP)** and an *inactive* form bound to **guanosine diphosphate (GDP).** The biochemical consequence of *ras* mutations is a ras protein unable to shift from the active GTP form, which stimulates growth, to the inactive GDP form. The mutant ras protein cannot quench its growth signal.

TABLE 11-2   Some Examples of Oncogenes and Their Role in Cancer

Oncogene	Chromosome location	Proposed function	Associated tumor
Growth Factors			
HST	11q13	Fibroblast growth factor	Stomach carcinoma
SIS	22q12	B subunit of platelet-derived growth factor	Glioma (brain tumor)
Growth Factor Receptors			
RET	10q	Receptor tyrosine kinase	Multiple endocrine neoplasia
erb-B		Epidermal growth factor receptor	Glioblastoma (brain tumor), breast cancer
erb-A	17q11	Thyroid hormone receptor	Promyelocytic leukemia
NEU		Receptor protein kinase	Neuroblastoma
Signal Transduction Proteins			
H-RAS	11p15	GTPase	Carcinoma of colon, lung, pancreas
K-RAS	12p12	GTPase	Melanoma, thyroid carcinoma, AML
Abl	9q34	Protein kinase	Chronic myelogenous leukemia; acute lymphocytic leukemia
Transcription Factors			
N-myc	2p24	DNA-binding protein	Neuroblastoma; lung carcinoma
MYB	6q22	DNA-binding protein	Malignant melanoma; lymphoma; leukemia
Fos	14q24	Interacts with *jun* oncogene to regulate transcription	Osteosarcoma

▼ The transfection of oncogenes from tumor cells to normal cells can cause transformation of the normal cells. This helps to confirm the role of oncogenes in carcinogenesis. ▲

Mapping in Tumors

The association of chromosomal translocations with human tumors provides a third method for observing the functions of oncogenes. As discussed in Chapter 6, specific chromosomal rearrangements are characteristic of some tumor types. A well-known example is the Philadelphia chromosome, in which a translocation between chromosomes 9 and 22 activates the *abl* proto-oncogene and produces chronic myelogenous leukemia. Recently, close examination of the site on chromosome 17 of the t(15;17)(q22;q11.2-12) translocation characteristic of acute promyelocytic leukemia (APL) has revealed the presence of the gene encoding retinoic acid receptor alpha (*RARA*). Interestingly, retinoic acid was already known as a therapeutic agent for APL. It has been suggested that retinoic acid may be a differentiation signal and that

disruption of the receptor by the translocation may encourage tumor formation by preventing transduction of this signal.

▼ Some oncogenes have been identified when specific rearrangements of chromosomal material were found to be associated with certain cancers. Because these translocations of genetic material are likely to have disrupted genes vital to cellular growth control, the sites of such rearrangements can be investigated to identify new oncogenes. ▲

DNA Repair Genes and Tumorigenesis

Accurate replication of DNA, assisted by repair mechanisms (see Chapter 2), is required for normal cell function. A number of inherited disorders are now recognized in which defective DNA repair leads to **genomic instability** (widespread mutations, including chromosome breaks and aneuploidy, throughout the genome). Some of these disorders, including xeroderma pigmentosum, Bloom syndrome, ataxia telangiectasia, and Werner syndrome, were discussed in Chapter 3. A notable feature common to these diseases is an increased incidence of various types of cancer. This occurs because genomic instability in somatic cells can compromise the regulatory pathways just discussed, leading to tumor formation. Several inherited cancer syndromes, including familial breast cancer and hereditary nonpolyposis colorectal cancer, involve defects in DNA repair and will be treated at greater length later in the chapter.

▼ Inherited defects in DNA repair can lead to a high frequency of somatic mutations. When these mutations affect pathways that regulate cellular proliferation, a tumor may arise. ▲

Genetic Alterations and Cancer Cell Immortality

Even after a tumor cell has escaped regulation by tumor suppressors or DNA repair proteins, it must overcome one more hurdle to unlimited proliferation: the intrinsic limitation on the number of cell divisions allowed to each cell. Ordinarily, the cell is restricted to about 50 to 60 mitotic divisions. After reaching this number, the cell typically becomes **senescent** and cannot continue to divide. Recent research has provided new insights on the mechanisms that count the number of cell divisions and on ways in which tumor cells can circumvent the counting system.

Each time a cell divides, the telomeres of chromosomes shorten slightly as the DNA is replicated during S phase. Once the telomere is reduced to a critical length, a signal is transmitted that causes the cell to become senescent. This process would place severe limitations on the proliferating cells in a tumor, preventing further clonal expansion. Tumor cells overcome the process by activating a gene that encodes **telomerase,** an enzyme that replaces the telomeric segments that are normally lost during cell division. Activation of this enzyme, which is rarely present in normal cells but nearly always present in tumor cells, allows the cell to continue to divide without the restraint ordinarily imposed by telomere shortening. This uninhibited division allows the tumor to become large, and it permits the accumulation of additional mutations that may further contribute to the aggressiveness of the tumor cell.

▼ Normally, progressive shortening of telomeres limits the number of divisions of a cell to about 50 to 60. Tumor cells overcome this limitation by activating telomerase, which replaces the telomere segments that are lost during each cell division. This permits tumor cells to escape the restraint of cellular senescence. ▲

IDENTIFICATION OF INHERITED CANCER GENES

Although the methods described in the previous section were successful in identifying many oncogenes, they did not identify those tumor suppressor genes that cause inherited forms of cancer. This may have been because these methods require dominant expression of the mutant phenotype, whereas the mutant tumor suppressor alleles seem to have a primarily recessive phenotype at the level of the cell. An alternative approach to the identification of these genes was necessary.

When genes responsible for genetically transmitted diseases cannot be identified through known biochemical behavior, they become candidates for investigations based on gene mapping and detection of mutations in patients, as described in Chapter 8. There are two avenues for initial mapping of tumor genes. The primary and most general route is through linkage mapping in families, where the pattern of inheritance of the cancer phenotype defines the genetic transmission of an altered allele. The chromosomal segment bearing this mutation can be identified by linkage with polymorphic markers.

The second basis for mapping takes advantage of the frequent chromosomal losses associated with revealed tumor suppressor genes. As already described, the genetically transmitted mutation is a recessive allele at the cellular level; it does not reveal its tumor phenotype unless both normal copies of the gene are lost. Often an inherited mutant allele is unmasked in the tumor by a deletion of part or all of the homologous chromosome carrying the normal allele. Therefore, the observation that a specific chromosome segment is deleted in a tumor suggests a map location for the inherited mutation. Small deletions can be helpful in pinpointing the subchromosomal location of the gene being sought. As mentioned in Chapter 8, the detection of inherited deletions on chromosome 13q in retinoblastoma patients was an important step in finding the retinoblastoma gene.

The deleted chromosome regions in tumors are pinpointed by examining a series of closely linked marker polymorphisms in the region and determining which of the markers heterozygous in the patient's constitutional DNA have become homozygous in tumor DNA (i.e., which markers have lost an allele in the process of tumorigenesis). This **loss of heterozygosity** in tumor DNA indicates that the normal tumor suppressor gene, as well as polymorphic markers surrounding it, has been lost, leaving only the abnormal copy of the tumor suppressor gene (see Fig. 11-5). This approach was used, for example, to help narrow the locations of the retinoblastoma gene on the long arm of chromosome 13 and a gene for Wilms tumor (nephroblastoma) on 11p.

Although gene mapping studies can often define a region in which an inherited cancer gene is located, they cannot alone identify the disease gene. As discussed in Chapter 8, detection of mutations carried in DNA from patients with the disease is crucial for identifying the specific disease-causing gene.

▼ Map locations of tumor-associated genes can be detected through linkage analysis or by showing that one homolog of a chromosome (or a part of it) is missing in DNA from a tumor. Confirmation of the etiological role of a possible cancer-causing gene is obtained by showing the consistent presence of mutations in the gene in DNA from patients. ▲

Neurofibromatosis Type 1

The initial evidence for mapping of the neurofibromatosis type 1 *(NF1)* gene to chromosome 17 came from linkage studies in families. Subsequently, chromosomal translocations were discovered in the karyotypes of two unrelated neurofibromatosis patients, each with a breakpoint on chromosome 17q at a location indistinguishable from the map location of the *NF1* gene. These translocations were assumed to have caused neurofibromatosis in these individuals by disrupting the *NF1* gene. Located only 50 kb apart, the breakpoints provided the physical clues necessary to define several candidate genes that were screened for mutations in NF1 patients (Fig. 11-7).

The nucleotide sequence of the *NF1* gene provided an early clue to function when its predicted amino acid sequence was compared with amino acid sequences of known gene products found in computerized databases. Extended similarities were observed with the mammalian GTPase-*a*ctivating *p*rotein (GAP). This was an important finding because at least one function of GAP is to increase the rate of hydrolysis of GTP bound to ras protein. As mentioned previously, the ras protein is a key component of the signal transduction pathway, transmitting positive growth signals in its active form. Thus, the closely associated *NF1* gene product, neurofibromin, is also likely to play a role in signal transduction.

By identifying the *NF1* gene product as a component in signal transduction, a picture began to form of how the inheritance of a mutation in one *NF1* allele might contribute to the development of neurofibromas and *café-au-lait* spots. Because neurofibromin downregulates the activity of ras, reduced expression of the *NF1* gene might permit increased ras activity and permit the cell to escape from differentiation and continue its growth. Loss of the remaining allele might further encourage unchecked growth. Discovery of the *NF1* gene has led to identification of a key tumor suppressor that helps to regulate the fundamental process of signal transduction. **WWW**

▼ The gene responsible for NF1 was mapped to chromosome 17q by linkage in families and identi-

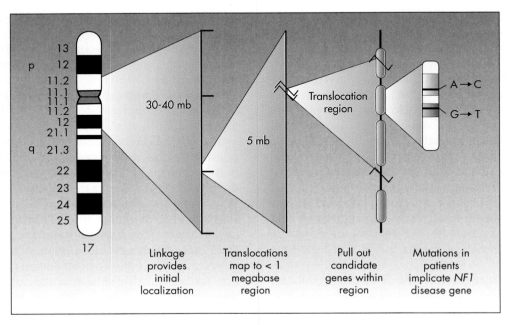

FIG. 11-7 Localization of the *NF1* gene on chromosome 17q involved linkage analysis and identification of two translocation breakpoints that interrupted the disease gene. Candidate genes were isolated from this region and tested for mutations in NF1 patients and normal controls.

fied through translocations and point mutations in patients. DNA sequencing of the gene predicted a protein product with a domain related to GAP, and a similar role in signal transduction was confirmed by biochemical experiments. ▲

The *p53* Gene

Somatic mutations in the *p53* gene are found in approximately 50% of all human tumors, making this the most commonly altered cancer gene. Mutations in the *p53* gene occur in more than 50 different types of tumors, including those of the bladder, brain, breast, cervix, colon, esophagus, larynx, liver, lung, ovary, pancreas, prostate, skin, stomach, and thyroid.

Initially, chromosomal losses and deletions of the short arm of chromosome 17 had been shown to be characteristic of colon carcinoma. Overlapping deletions defined a segment of 17p commonly altered in tumor DNAs. Examination of the genes that had been mapped to this region revealed that *p53* was among them. The numerous mutations found in *p53* in colonic tumors indicate a significant role for this gene in colon tumorigenesis. Indeed, *p53* mutations are seen in approximately 70% of colorectal tumors, and they are seen in 40% of breast tumors and 60% of lung tumors. Approximately 80% to 90% of *p53* mutations are of the missense type, and these are concentrated in the portion of the gene that encodes a DNA-binding domain.

p53 is activated in response to signs of cellular damage. It encodes a transcription factor that interacts with at least six other genes. For example, it binds to the promoter of *p21*, whose protein product is a cyclin-dependent kinase inhibitor that blocks the inactivation of pRb by CDK4 (see Fig. 11-6). As discussed previously, this halts the cell cycle in the G1 phase, before DNA replication occurs in S phase. Arrest of the cell cycle before S phase provides time for repair of damaged DNA. An alternative response of *p53* to damaged DNA is to induce the programmed death of the cell **(apoptosis).** This response is more likely if the pRb pathway for cell cycle arrest is not intact. Lacking the possibility of cell cycle arrest to repair damage, the p53 protein "chooses" cell death. When *p53* is mutated, cells with damaged DNA may evade both repair and destruction, and continued replication of the damaged DNA may lead to tumor formation.

Like *RB1* and *NF1*, *p53* is considered a tumor suppressor gene, and mutations typically lead to a loss of function. However, some *p53* mutations may have a dominant negative effect (see Chapter 3), in which the protein product of the mutated allele interacts with and disables the protein product of the normal allele, inducing cellular transformation. Thus, unlike the typical tumor suppressor mutation, which must be homo-zygous in an individual cell to induce tumorigenesis, these mutations can produce a tumor when present in a single copy.

Carcinogenic substances can induce specific *p53* mutations. For example, dietary ingestion of aflatoxin B_1, which can produce liver cancer, is associated with a G→T mutation that produces an arginine→serine substitution at position 249 of the *p53* gene product. Exposure to benzopyrene, a powerful mutagen and carcinogen found in cigarette smoke, produces mutations in three specific *p53* codons in lung tumors (demonstrating a direct molecular link between cigarette smoking and lung cancer). Thus, examination of the type of *p53* mutation seen in a tumor may provide clues to the identity of the causative carcinogenic agent.

Although tumor-causing *p53* mutations have been observed mostly in somatic cells, germline mutations of *p53* are responsible for an inherited cancer condition known as the Li-Fraumeni syndrome. This rare syndrome is transmitted in autosomal dominant fashion and involves breast and colon carcinomas, soft-tissue sarcomas, osteosarcomas, brain tumors, leukemia, and adrenocortical carcinomas. These tumors usually develop at early ages in LFS family members, and multiple primary tumors are commonly seen in an affected individual. The demonstration of consistent *p53* mutations in the constitutional DNA of LFS patients confirmed the causative role of this gene. As in retinoblastoma, the inheritance of a mutated *p53* gene greatly increases the individual's susceptibility to subsequent cell transformation and tumor development. Among LFS family members who inherit an abnormal *p53* gene, approximately 50% will develop invasive cancer by age 30, and more than 90% will develop invasive cancer by age 70. However, the penetrance with regard to any *specific* tumor type is much lower.

p53 is medically important in at least two ways. First, the presence of *p53* mutations in tumors, particularly those of the breast and colon, often signals a more aggressive cancer with relatively poor survival prospects. It is thus a useful prognostic indicator. Second, *p53* could ultimately prove important in tumor prevention. Laboratory experiments show that the insertion of a normal *p53* gene into tumor cells results in a significant decrease in tumorigenesis. This suggests that insertion of normal *p53* into cancer patients' tumors using gene therapy approaches (see Chapter 13) might, in principle, become a cancer treatment.

▼ Mutant forms of the *p53* gene are found in about 50% of tumors. This gene encodes a transcription factor that can induce either cell cycle arrest or apoptosis in response to damaged DNA. Although *p53* is considered a tumor suppressor gene, some mutations have a dominant cell–transforming effect. ▲

The Familial Polyposis Gene

Familial polyposis (adenomatous polyposis coli, or APC) is characterized by the early appearance of multiple (generally more than 100) adenomas, or polyps, of the colon. Colonic adenomas are now understood to be the immediate precursors to colon cancer. The multiple adenomas of the familial polyposis patient, therefore, present a grave risk of early malignancy. Because early detection and removal of adenomatous polyps can significantly reduce the occurrence of colon cancer, it is important to understand the causative gene and its role in development of polyps (Clinical Commentary 11-1).

The *APC* gene was initially placed on the map of the long arm of chromosome 5 by linkage analysis in families after a microscopically visible chromosomal deletion in a patient with this syndrome provided an important clue to its location. Discovery of small, overlapping deletions in two unrelated patients provided the key to isolation of the gene. Among the genes that lay within the 100-kb region deleted in both patients, one showed apparent mutations in other patients. This mutation was seen in the patient but not in his unaffected parents, confirming the identification of the *APC* gene. **WWW**

Mutations in the *APC* gene have been detected in more than 85% of colon tumors, indicating that, as with retinoblastoma, the inherited gene is also important in the development of the sporadic form of the cancer. A second gene in this region, termed *MCC* (mutated in colon cancer) is also occasionally mutated in colon tumors but seems not to be involved in inherited colorectal cancer.

The *APC* gene encodes a protein product that bears little resemblance to other known proteins. Thus, it has been somewhat difficult to determine its function, although it clearly acts as a tumor suppressor. Recent studies have shown, however, that the *APC* protein product can modulate the levels of β-catenin, a molecule involved in cell adhesion and in nuclear transcription complexes. Examination of several of the relatively few colon carcinomas that do not carry mutations in the *APC* gene has revealed mutations in the β-catenin gene, thus confirming the potential etiological role of this gene in colon cancer and strongly supporting the involvement of this pathway in colon carcinogenesis. This finding is interesting in that β-catenin is already known to be an intermediate in the Wnt signaling pathway, a relatively well-characterized pathway in early development and embryogenesis (see Chapter 10). Furthermore, the mammalian prototype of the Wnt gene family was ascertained as an initiating gene in the pathway to mouse mammary carcinoma induced by mouse mammary tumor virus.

With the exception of several large deletions and one serine→cysteine amino acid substitution, all of the mutations found in *APC* thus far have produced either stop codons (nonsense mutations) or frameshifts in the nucleotide sequence of the gene. Alleles altered in either of these ways would be expected to encode an inactive gene product. Because nonsense mutations should be relatively rare in comparison with missense mutations, the latter probably occur without creating a recognizable polyposis phenotype. An intriguing interpretation is that mutations that result in amino acid substitutions, splice-site variants, or reduced levels of gene expression may produce a distinct phenotype that is relatively subtle, with low expressivity and/or reduced penetrance.

This hypothesis is interesting because pedigree analyses have suggested that there may be common alleles that predispose carriers to develop one to several polyps, which may appear relatively late in life. If such alleles exist, they may define a fraction of our population as predisposed to colon cancer, and frequent screening of these people for polyps might be merited. Support for this hypothesis comes from the characterization of several pedigrees in which an *APC* allele is transmitted that causes an intermediate polyp phenotype. Within each of these families, individuals inheriting the mutant allele can exhibit a variable number of polyps, from one or none to more than a hundred, but with an average of only 10 to 20. Therefore, alleles with markedly reduced expressivity do exist at the polyposis locus. This variant syndrome is called attenuated polyposis, and the alleles are referred to as attenuated *APC* or *AAPC*. Although only a very low frequency of such alleles has thus far been demonstrated, they raise new issues associated with DNA-based diagnosis and counseling, as the attenuated polyposis syndrome may in many cases not be diagnosed on clinical grounds due to a very small number of polyps. In this case, however, the issue of the usefulness of DNA diagnosis is straightforward because there is an effective therapeutic and preventive strategy (either polypectomy or colectomy) for treating affected individuals.

▼ The familial polyposis gene (*APC*), which strikingly predisposes to colon cancer, was ultimately identified by mutations in patients. The inherited gene is also involved in the great majority of sporadic cases of colon polyps and colon cancer. This tumor suppressor gene has been shown to function as a major regulator of the Wnt pathway, a signaling system that is well characterized both biochemically and developmentally. ▲

The Hereditary Nonpolyposis Colon Cancer Genes

Hereditary nonpolyposis colon cancer (HNPCC), a second form of inherited colon cancer, accounts for approximately 1% to 5% of all colorectal cancer cases.

CLINICAL COMMENTARY 11-1
THE *APC* GENE AND COLORECTAL CANCER www

About 1/20 Americans will be diagnosed with colorectal cancer. Currently, the mortality rate for this cancer is approximately one third. Genetic and environmental factors, such as dietary fat and fiber, are known to influence the probability of occurrence of colorectal cancer.

As indicated in the text, familial polyposis coli is an autosomal dominant subtype of colon cancer characterized by a large number of early-onset adenomatous polyps (Fig. 11-8). Germline mutations in the *APC* gene are consistently identified in family members affected with familial polyposis coli. Approximately one third of these cases are the result of new mutations in this gene. Because of the large size of the gene and the large number of disease-causing mutations, it is difficult and expensive to test family members for germline mutations in order to determine whether they inherited the disease gene. However, one test takes advantage of the fact that most *APC* mutations are nonsense or frameshift mutations that yield a truncated protein product. This **protein truncation test** (see Chapter 3) involves the in vitro manufacture of a protein product from *APC* DNA to determine whether the at-risk individual has inherited an *APC* mutation. This is important for family members because it alerts them to the necessity of frequent surveillance and possible colectomy.

Familial polyposis coli, however, is relatively rare, affecting only about 1/8,000 individuals. The broader significance of the *APC* gene derives from the fact that *somatic* mutations in *APC* are seen in approximately 85% of all colon cancers. Furthermore, *APC* mutations occur very early in the development of colorectal malignancies. A better understanding of the *APC* gene product, how it interacts with other proteins, and how it may interact with environmental factors such as diet, may provide important clues for the prevention and treatment of common colon cancer. In this way, the mapping and

FIG. 11-8 A portion of a colon removed from a patient with familial polyposis coli, illustrating a large number of adenomatous polyps covering the colon. Each of these benign neoplasms has the potential to become a malignant tumor.

cloning of a gene responsible for a relatively rare cancer syndrome may have widespread clinical implications.

Treatment for colorectal cancer usually involves surgical resection of the colon. However, because colorectal carcinoma is preceded by the appearance of benign polyps, it is one of the most preventable of cancers. The National Polyp Study Workgroup estimates that colonoscopic removal of polyps could reduce the nationwide incidence of colon cancer by as much as 90%. The importance of early intervention and treatment further underscores the need to understand early events in colorectal cancer, such as somatic mutations in the *APC* gene.

Although this syndrome does not show the very large number of colon polyps characteristic of familial polyposis, small numbers of advanced polyps occur frequently among gene carriers. This is also a high-penetrance cancer syndrome, but with several cancers in addition to colon cancer occurring at high frequency, including endometrial cancer at a frequency of approximately 20%. Four genes have been identified thus far in which mutations can produce HNPCC. Mutations in the *MSH2* gene account for approximately 40% of HNPCC cases, and mutations in the *MLH1* gene account for about 25% of cases. Mutations in two other genes, *PMS1* and *PMS2*, account for a very small proportion of additional cases. An important

clue in pinpointing these loci in the human was the existence of highly similar loci in yeast and bacteria. Remarkably, each of them is known to play an important role in DNA mismatch repair (see Chapter 3); loss of the function of one of these genes leads to substantially elevated rates of spontaneous mutation.

It is very likely, therefore, that this increased rate of mutation results in the induction of mutations in a number of cellular regulatory genes, thus leading to an increased frequency of cancer. Identification and functional analysis of these genes supports the role of genetic mutation in carcinogenesis and demonstrates a new, genetically defined pathway to cancer based on hypermutability rather than deregulation of cell growth. Tumors from HNPCC patients show a high degree of instability of microsatellite loci (see Chapter 3), generating new microsatellite alleles with high frequency.

Such microsatellite instability is also seen in a small proportion of sporadic colorectal carcinomas, but mutations in the HNPCC genes seem to occur only infrequently, suggesting that other DNA repair genes are being damaged in the sporadic pathway. A second type of genomic instability frequently seen in sporadic colorectal tumors is a high incidence of aneuploidy. This may result from defects in proteins that oversee the proper assembly of the mitotic spindle apparatus (in a sense, these proteins perform a mitotic "proofreading" function similar to that of some DNA repair proteins). Mutations in genes that encode these proteins are now being identified and may yield insights on another mechanism of genomic instability and carcinogenesis.

▼ HNPCC is an inherited form of colorectal cancer that is caused by mutations in any of several genes involved in DNA mismatch repair. It represents an example of a cancer syndrome caused by genomic instability. ▲

The Inherited Breast Cancer Genes: *BRCA1* and *BRCA2*

The lifetime prevalence of breast cancer in women is one in eight, and it is estimated that approximately 5% of breast cancer cases result from inherited mutations. Two genes, *BRCA1* and *BRCA2*, have been identified as the cause of the majority of inherited breast cancers. However, the frequencies of *BRCA1* and *BRCA2* mutations, as well as their penetrance, may have been overestimated in early studies because of an emphasis on high-risk families with multiple affected members. A recent population-based study indicated that about 3% of all breast cancer cases result from *BRCA1* mutations; it appears that a slightly smaller percentage are the result of *BRCA2* mutations. Women who inherit mutant alleles of *BRCA1* show an elevated incidence of ovarian cancer in addition to breast cancer. An increased risk in male breast cancer is observed in families in which a *BRCA2* mutation is transmitted (see Chapter 12 for further discussion of breast cancer risk factors).

Each of these genes was identified by linkage analysis in families, followed by positional cloning. Both genes are large: *BRCA1* spans approximately 100 kb and encodes a protein of 1863 amino acids, and *BRCA2* spans 70 kb and encodes a protein of 3418 amino acids. More than 200 *BRCA1* mutations and more than 100 *BRCA2* mutations have been identified. Most of these result in truncated protein products and a consequent loss of function. The large size of these genes, together with extensive allelic heterogeneity, poses challenges for genetic diagnosis (see Chapter 13). As in the *RB1* and *APC*

genes, the normal copy of the *BRCA1* or *BRCA2* gene is lost in tumor cells of individuals who have inherited a *BRCA1* or *BRCA2* mutation (loss of heterozygosity). In contrast to *RB1* and *APC*, somatic mutations affecting these genes are virtually never seen in sporadic (noninherited) breast tumors. **www**

Although *BRCA1* and *BRCA2* share no significant DNA sequence similarity, both genes encode transcription factors. In addition, both protein products interact either directly or indirectly with RAD51, a protein involved in the repair of double-stranded DNA breaks (as with the HNPCC genes, RAD51 has homologs in yeast and bacteria). Both genes thus participate in an important DNA repair pathway, and their inactivation contributes to genomic instability.

▼ Mutations in *BRCA1* and *BRCA2* are responsible for a large proportion of inherited breast cancer cases. These mutations usually result in a truncated protein product and loss of function. The protein products of both of these genes interact with RAD51, a DNA repair protein. ▲

p16 and Familial Melanoma

Largely as a result of increased exposure to ultraviolet radiation, the incidence of melanoma has increased about 20-fold in the United States during the past 70 years. It is now one of the most common cancers, with 37,000 new cases per year. The risk of developing melanoma increases by a factor of two when a first-degree relative is affected. The risk increases further, to approximately 6.5, when the first-degree relative is affected before age 50.

Linkage analysis in families and studies of loss of heterozygosity in melanoma tumor cells mapped a gene for familial melanoma to the short arm of chromosome 9. Subsequent positional cloning and mutation analysis led to the identification of the *p16* gene as a cause of familial melanoma. This gene encodes a cyclin-dependent kinase inhibitor which, like p21, interacts negatively with a cyclin-dependent kinase (CDK4) that phosphorylates and downregulates the pRb protein (see Fig. 11-6). Because active pRb acts as a brake on the cell cycle, loss-of-function mutations in the *p16* tumor suppressor gene result in a lack of cell cycle control that can produce melanomas.

Mutations in the gene that encodes CDK4 can also result in melanoma. These gain-of-function mutations convert the cyclin-dependent kinase from a proto-oncogene to an activated oncogene. The activated CDK4 constantly downregulates pRb, resulting again in a lack of cell cycle control and tumor formation. This system provides an example of a case in which the same tumor type can result from either the activation of a proto-oncogene (*CDK4*) or the loss of a tumor suppressor gene (*p16*).

▼ Familial melanoma can be caused by loss-of-function mutations in the *p16* tumor suppressor gene or by gain-of-function mutations in the target of p16, the *CDK4* proto-oncogene. Both mutations result in a loss of cell cycle control via the pRb pathway. ▲

The *RET* Proto-Oncogene and Multiple Endocrine Neoplasia

As discussed in Chapter 10, the *RET* gene encodes a receptor tyrosine kinase that is involved in embryonic neural crest cell migration. It was initially identified by a transfection assay (see previous discussion). Loss-of-function mutations in *RET* can produce Hirschsprung disease (a lack of enteric nerve cells resulting in severe, chronic constipation and bowel distention). Gain-of-function mutations in the same gene can produce any of three inherited cancer syndromes, depending on the type and location of mutation: (1) multiple endocrine neoplasia 2A (MEN2A, characterized by medullary thyroid carcinomas, parathyroid hyperplasia, and pheochromocytoma [an adrenal tumor]); (2) multiple endocrine neoplasia 2B (MEN2B, similar to MEN2A, but lacks parathyroid hyperplasia and includes multiple mucosal neuromas); (3) familial medullary thyroid carcinoma. Gain-of-function mutations in *RET* result in excess tyrosine kinase activity and increased signal transduction, leading ultimately to cellular proliferation and cancer.

Currently *RET*, *CDK4*, and the *MET* gene (which can cause hereditary papillary renal cancer) are the only known proto-oncogenes in which germline mutations can lead to inherited cancer syndromes (the many other identified proto-oncogenes are involved only in somatic mutations producing sporadic tumors). Somatic alterations of *RET* can produce papillary thyroid carcinomas, the most common type of thyroid tumor. The prevalence of this tumor has increased substantially in areas that were exposed to radioactive fallout from the Chernobyl nuclear reactor accident (see Chapter 3); somatic *RET* alterations are seen in approximately 60% of these tumors.

The *RET* gene provides an example of extraordinary allelic heterogeneity. Loss-of-function mutations in this gene produce defects in the embryonic development of the bowel, while gain-of-function mutations result in increased signal transduction and various forms of endocrine neoplasia. This example illustrates the critical connection between development and cancer: both involve a finely tuned genetic regulation of cell growth and differentiation.

▼ Loss-of-function mutations in the *RET* proto-oncogene can produce Hirschsprung disease, a disorder of embryonic development. Germline gain-of-function mutations in the same gene can lead to any of three different types of inherited cancers. Somatic alterations in *RET* can produce non-inherited papillary thyroid carcinoma. ▲

Other Inherited Cancer Genes

Several other genes associated with inherited cancer syndromes have been mapped to specific chromosomal locations, and some have subsequently been cloned: neurofibromatosis type 2 to chromosome 22; von Hippel-Lindau disease to 3p; and Beckwith-Wiedemann syndrome to 11p. Some of these genes are listed in Table 11-1, and others are discussed in some of the review papers listed at the end of the chapter. With the current generation of genomic resources, such as libraries of yeast and bacterial artificial chromosomes (YACs and BACs) containing human DNA sequences, it is reasonable to expect the identification of more such genes through positional cloning within the next several years.

MOLECULAR BASIS OF CANCER

Each of the identified genes associated with inherited cancer syndromes provides a unique insight into the genetic mechanisms of carcinogenesis. Those that represent important elements in transcriptional regulation of the cell cycle (*RB1*, *p53*), signal transduction (*NF1*), and DNA repair (HNPCC, *BRCA1*, *BRCA2*) promise to make significant contributions to our understanding of these processes. Those genes not yet cloned and characterized promise to be equally revealing.

It is striking that nearly all of the inherited tumor-causing genes described to date seem to have cell-recessive properties, at least at the level of the carcinoma. This observation suggests that an inherited allele that produces a tumor in the heterozygous state would not be tolerated during development. That view is supported by the nearly ubiquitous tissue distribution of the products of these genes. As they are expressed in many if not all cell types, they may each play a fundamental role during embryonic development (see Chapter 10).

From a medical perspective, the characterization of inherited tumor genes can be very fruitful. Presymptomatic diagnosis of at-risk individuals in cancer families may specify those who must undergo close surveillance or even intervention, and it can lift a major medical and psychological burden from those who have not inherited the family's mutant allele. If more subtle, predisposing alleles prove to be important in the incidence of cancer in general, the ability to define an at-risk population might reduce the overall cost of cancer surveillance in the population as a whole. In the future, greater understanding of these genes and their functions will offer hope for the ultimate prevention of tumorigenesis, as these genes are clearly rate-limiting for tumor formation. If their mutant alleles serve as indicators for the appearance of nascent tumors, or if their normal functions can be restored by medical intervention, they will have served an important role in cancer prevention.

Studies of inherited cancer genes have provided many insights, but many important questions remain.

For example, although inherited cancer genes are widely expressed in many tissues, why are most inherited cancer syndromes characterized by very specific tumor types (e.g., retinoblastomas and osteosarcomas for *RB1*, breast and ovarian tumors for *BRCA1*)? Why do the tumor types associated with the inherited alterations of cancer genes often differ from the tumor types associated with somatic alterations of the same genes (e.g., inherited *p53* mutations lead to breast cancer, leukemia, brain tumors, soft tissue sarcoma, and osteosarcoma, but somatic *p53* mutations can produce lung and colon tumors, among others)? To what degree, and in what ways, are inherited cancer genes involved in common, non-inherited cancers?

▼ The continued mapping and cloning of genes for cancer syndromes will provide valuable insights into mechanisms of carcinogenesis and into fundamental biological processes. Presymptomatic diagnosis of family members at risk for cancer, and ultimately the possibility of genetic interventions, are other important goals and potential rewards of such studies. ▲

IS GENETIC INHERITANCE IMPORTANT IN COMMON CANCERS?

The role, or even the significance, of inherited predisposition in the common cancers, such as carcinomas of breast, colon, or prostate, is not yet certain. An apparently increased frequency of common cancers in some families has led some to suggest that common cancer-causing alleles may exist. Familial clustering translates into an increased relative risk of breast cancer, for example, among women with first-degree relatives who have had breast cancer. The genetic basis of this increased risk has not yet been demonstrated. However, evidence indicates that a significant fraction of premenopausal breast cancer cases are associated with the *BRCA1* and *BRCA2* genes. In addition, statistical analysis of large pedigrees has provided support for a genetic component in common colon cancer.

How will we ultimately determine whether common "cancer alleles" exist in the population? One way, perhaps, could exploit new approaches of gene mapping that identify genes involved in cellular pathways to cancer. Each of these becomes a candidate gene that, we hypothesize, may confer a predisposition to cancer. The most critical test of the candidate-gene hypothesis will be to determine whether there are mutations in the gene among cancer patients. Finding them will validate the genetic hypothesis. If no mutations are found, however, we will remain uncertain because a genetic predisposition could still be conferred by an allele of a gene not yet identified and tested.

▼ The question of whether common cancer alleles exist in the population may be approached by seeking mutations among the growing number of identified genes known to be involved in cellular mechanisms leading to cancer. Other candidate genes might include those that function to repair damage to DNA. ▲

A detailed description of the genes and genetic events underlying cancer is rapidly emerging. The identified genes fall into three relatively distinct categories: mutant oncogenes acting as promoters of cell growth, mutant tumor suppressors often failing to inhibit cell growth, and DNA repair gene mutations creating a high frequency of mutant oncogenes and tumor suppressors. These categories share a commonality in that each ultimately affects the genetic regulation of cell growth and development. Although acting at different points, they regulate the same fundamental cell activities and information pathways. New technologies of molecular biology and genetics are now identifying the specific genes associated with specific tumor types. Significant new information is becoming available to researchers and clinicians and can be expected to create a new generation of highly specific diagnostic and therapeutic tools to reduce the cancer burden.

STUDY QUESTIONS

1. The G6PD locus is located on the X chromosome. Studies of G6PD alleles in tumor cells from *women* show that all tumor cells usually express the same single G6PD allele, even though the women are heterozygous at the G6PD locus. What does this finding imply about the origin of the tumor cells?

2. If we assume that the somatic mutation rate at the *RB1* locus is three mutations per million cells, and that there is a population of 2 million retinoblasts per individual, what is the expected frequency of *sporadic* retinoblastoma in the population? What is the expected *number of tumors* per individual among those who *inherit* a mutated copy of the *RB1* gene?

3. Compare and contrast oncogenes and tumor suppressor genes. How have the characteristics of these classes of cancer-causing genes affected our ability to detect them?

4. Members of Li-Fraumeni syndrome families nearly always develop tumors by age 65 to 70, but the probability of developing a *specific* type of cancer, such as a breast or colon carcinoma, is relatively small. Explain this.

SUGGESTED READINGS

Bertwistle D, Ashworth A (1998) Functions of the *BRCA1* and *BRCA2* genes. Curr. Opin. Genet. Dev. 8:14-20

Brown MA (1997) Tumor suppressor genes and human cancer. Adv. Genet. 36:45-135

Brown MA, Solomon E (1997) Studies on inherited cancers: outcomes and challenges of 25 years. Trends Genet. 13:202-206

Cavenee WK, White RL (1995) The genetic basis of cancer. Sci. Amer. 272:72-79

Collins K, Jacks T, Pavletich NP (1997) The cell cycle and cancer. Proc. Natl. Acad. Sci. USA 94:2776-2778

Dunlop MG (1996) Mutator genes and mosaicism in colorectal cancer. Curr. Opin. Genet. Dev. 6:75-80

Fearon ER (1997) Human cancer syndromes: clues to the origin and nature of cancer. Science 278:1043-1050

Gao CY, Zelenka PS (1997) Cyclins, cyclin-dependent kinases and differentiation. BioEssays 19:307-315

Kinzler KW, Vogelstein B (1996) Lessons from hereditary colorectal cancer. Cell 87:159-170

Kinzler KW, Vogelstein B (1997) Cancer-susceptibility genes: gatekeepers and caretakers. Nature 386:761-763

Krontiris TG (1995) Oncogenes. N. Eng. J. Med. 333:303-306

Lengauer C, Kinzler KW, Vogelstein B (1997) Genetic instability in colorectal cancers. Nature 386:623-627

Levine AJ (1997) p53, the cellular gatekeeper for growth and division. Cell 88:323-331

Liggett WH, Sidransky D (1998) Role of the p16 tumor suppressor gene in cancer. J. Clin. Oncol. 16:1197-1206

Marshall CJ, Nigg EA (1998) Cancer genes: lessons from genetics and biochemistry. Curr. Opin. Genet. Dev. 8:11-13

Newman B, Mu H, Butler LM, Millikan RC, Moorman PG, King M (1998) Frequency of breast cancer attributable to *BRCA1* in a population-based series of American women. JAMA 279:915-921

Orr-Weaver TL, Weinberg RA (1998) A checkpoint on the road to cancer. Nature 392:223-224

Pasini B, Ceccherini I, Romeo G (1996) *RET* mutations in human disease. Trends Genet. 12:138-144

Sellers WR, Kaelin WG (1997) Role of the retinoblastoma protein in the pathogenesis of human cancer. J. Clin. Oncol. 15:3301-3312

Sherr CJ (1996) Cancer cell cycles. Science 274:1672-1677

Szabo CI, King M (1997) Population genetics of BRCA1 and BRCA2. Am. J. Hum. Genet. 60:1013-1020

Vogelstein B, Kinzler KW (1998) The Genetic Basis of Human Cancer. McGraw Hill, New York

Weinberg RA (1996) How cancer arises. Sci. Amer. 275:62-70

White RL (1998) Tumor suppressing pathways. Cell 92:591-592

Zhang H, Tombline G, Weber BL (1998) BRCA1, BRCA2, and DNA damage response: collision or collusion? Cell 92:433-436

12

Multifactorial Inheritance and Common Diseases

The focus of previous chapters has been on diseases that are caused by single genes or by abnormalities of single chromosomes. Much progress has been made in identifying specific mutations that cause these diseases, leading to better risk estimates and in some cases more effective treatment. However, these conditions form only a small portion of the total burden of human genetic disease. Most congenital malformations are not caused by single genes or chromosome defects. Many common adult diseases, such as cancer, heart disease, and diabetes, have genetic components, but again they are usually not caused by single genes or by chromosome abnormalities. These diseases, whose treatment collectively occupies the attention of most health care practitioners, are the result of a complex interplay of genetic and environmental factors.

PRINCIPLES OF MULTIFACTORIAL INHERITANCE
The Basic Model

Traits in which variation is thought to be caused by the combined effects of multiple genes are **polygenic** ("many genes"). When environmental factors are also believed to cause variation in the trait, which is usually the case, the term **multifactorial** is used. Many **quantitative traits** (those, such as blood pressure, that are measured on a continuous numerical scale) are multifactorial. Because they are caused by the additive effects of many genetic and environmental factors, these traits tend to follow a normal, or "bell-shaped," distribution in populations.

Let us use an example to illustrate this concept. To begin with the simplest case, suppose (unrealistically) that height is determined by a single gene with two alleles, A and a. Allele A tends to make people tall, whereas allele a tends to make them short. If there is no

dominance at this locus, then the three possible genotypes, AA, Aa, and aa, will produce three phenotypes: tall, intermediate, and short. Assume that the gene frequencies of A and a are each 0.50. If we look at a population of individuals, we will observe the height distribution depicted in Fig. 12-1, A.

Now suppose, a bit more realistically, that height is determined by two loci instead of one. The second locus also has two alleles, B (tall) and b (short), and they affect height in exactly the same way as alleles A and a. There are now nine possible genotypes in our population: aabb, aaBb, aaBB, Aabb, AaBb, AaBB, AAbb, AABb, and AABB. An individual may have zero, one, two, three, or four "tall" alleles, so there are now five distinct phenotypes (Fig. 12-1, B). Although the height distribution in our population is not yet normal, it approaches a normal distribution more closely than in the single-gene case above.

We now extend our example so that many genes and environmental factors influence height, each having a small effect. Then there are many possible phenotypes, each differing slightly, and the height distribution approaches the bell-shaped curve shown in Fig. 12-1, C.

It should be emphasized that the individual genes underlying a multifactorial trait such as height follow the Mendelian principles of segregation and independent assortment, just like any other gene. The only difference is that many of them act together to influence the trait.

Blood pressure is another example of a multifactorial trait. There is a correlation between parents' blood pressures (systolic and diastolic) and those of their children. There is good evidence that this correlation is due in part to genes. But blood pressure is also influenced by environmental factors, such as diet and stress. One of the goals of genetic research is the identification and measurement of the relative roles of genes and environment in the causation of multifactorial diseases.

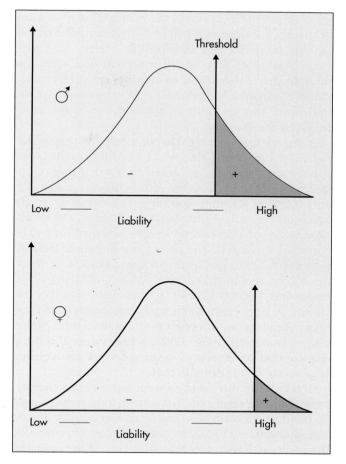

FIG. 12-2   A liability distribution for a multifactorial disease in a population. To be affected with the disease, an individual must exceed the threshold on the liability distribution. This figure shows two thresholds, a lower one for males and a higher one for females (as in pyloric stenosis).

FIG. 12-1   **A,** The distribution of height in a population, assuming that height is controlled by a single locus with genotypes *AA*, *Aa*, and *aa*. **B,** The distribution of height, assuming that height is controlled by two loci. There are now five distinct phenotypes instead of three, and the distribution begins to look more like the normal distribution. **C,** Distribution of height, assuming that multiple factors, each with a small effect, contribute to the trait (the multifactorial model).

▼ Many traits are thought to be influenced by multiple genes as well as environmental factors. These traits are said to be multifactorial. When they can be measured on a continuous scale, they often follow a normal distribution. ▲

The Threshold Model

A number of diseases do not follow the bell-shaped distribution. Instead, they appear to be either present or absent in individuals. Yet they do not follow the patterns expected of single-gene diseases. A commonly used explanation is that there is an underlying **liability distribution** for these diseases in a population (Fig. 12-2). Those individuals who are on the low end of the distribution have little chance of developing the disease in question (i.e., they have few of the alleles or environmental factors that would cause the disease). Those who are closer to the high end of the distribution have more of the disease-causing genes and environmental factors and are more likely to develop the disease. For multifactorial diseases that are either present or absent, it is thought that a **threshold of liability** must be crossed before the disease is expressed. Below the threshold, the individual appears normal; above it, he or she is affected by the disease.

A disease that is thought to correspond to this threshold model is pyloric stenosis, a disorder that presents shortly after birth and is caused by a narrowing or obstruction of the pylorus, the area between the stomach and intestine. Chronic vomiting, constipation, weight loss, and electrolyte imbalance result from the condition, but it sometimes resolves spontaneously or can be corrected by surgery. The prevalence of pyloric stenosis is about 3/1,000 live births in Caucasians. It is much more common in males than females, affecting 1/200 males and 1/1,000 females. It is thought that this difference in prevalence reflects *two* thresholds in the liability distribution, a lower one in males and a higher one in females (see Fig. 12-2). A lower male threshold implies that fewer disease-causing factors are required to generate the disorder in males.

The liability threshold concept may explain the pattern of sibling recurrence risks for pyloric stenosis seen in Table 12-1. Notice that males, having a lower threshold, always have a higher risk than females. However, the recurrence risk also depends on the sex of the proband. It is higher when the proband is female than when the proband is male. This reflects the concept that females, having a higher liability threshold, must be exposed to more disease-causing factors than males in order to develop the disease. Thus, a family with an affected female must have more genetic and environmental risk factors, producing a higher recurrence risk for pyloric stenosis in future offspring. We would expect that the highest risk category would be *male* relatives of *female* probands; Table 12-1 shows that this is indeed the case.

A similar pattern has been observed in a study of infantile autism, a behavioral disorder in which the male-female sex ratio is approximately 4:1. As expected for a multifactorial disorder, the recurrence risks for siblings of male probands (3.5%) was substantially lower than that of siblings of female probands (7%). When the sex ratio for a disease is reversed (i.e., more affected females than males), we would expect a higher recurrence risk when the proband is male.

A number of other congenital malformations are thought to correspond to this model. They include isolated* cleft lip and/or cleft palate (CL/P), neural tube defects (anencephaly and spina bifida), club foot (talipes), and some forms of congenital heart disease. In addition, many of the common adult diseases, such as hypertension, coronary heart disease, stroke, diabetes mellitus (types I and II), and some cancers, are caused by complex genetic and environmental factors and can thus be considered multifactorial diseases.

▼ The threshold model applies to many multifactorial diseases. It assumes that there is an underlying liability distribution in a population and that a threshold on this distribution must be passed before a disease is expressed. ▲

Recurrence Risks and Transmission Patterns

Whereas recurrence risks can be given with confidence for single-gene diseases (50% for typical autosomal dominant diseases, 25% for autosomal recessive diseases, etc.), the situation is more complicated for multifactorial diseases. This is because the number of genes contributing to the disease is usually not known, the precise allelic constitution of the parents is not known, and the extent of environmental effects can vary substantially. For most multifactorial diseases, **empirical risks** (i.e., risks based on direct observation of data) have been derived. To estimate empirical risks, a large series of families is examined in which one child has developed the disease (the proband). Then the siblings of each proband are surveyed in order to calculate the percentage who have also developed the disease. For example, in Great Britain about 5% of siblings of neural tube defect cases also have neural tube defects (Clinical Commentary 12-1). Thus, the recurrence risk for British parents who have had one child with a neural tube defect is 5%. For conditions that are not lethal or severely debilitating, such as cleft lip/palate, recurrence risks can also be estimated for the offspring of affected parents. Because risk factors vary among diseases, empirical recurrence risks are specific for each multifactorial disease.

In contrast to most single-gene diseases, recurrence risks for multifactorial diseases can change substantially from one population to another (notice the differences between the London and Belfast populations in Table 12-1). This is because gene frequencies as well

TABLE 12-1 Recurrence Risks (%) for Pyloric Stenosis*				
Relatives	**Male Probands**		**Female Probands**	
	London	**Belfast**	**London**	**Belfast**
Brothers	3.8	9.6	9.2	12.5
Sisters	2.7	3.0	3.8	3.8

Modified from Carter (1976) Br. Med. Bull. 32:21-26.
*Risks are subdivided by genders of affected probands and relatives. Note that the risks differ somewhat between the two populations.

---

*In this context, the term "isolated" means that this is the *only* observed disease feature (i.e., the feature is not part of a larger constellation of findings, as in cleft lip/palate secondary to trisomy 13).

CLINICAL COMMENTARY 12-1
NEURAL TUBE DEFECTS

Neural tube defects (NTDs) include anencephaly, spina bifida, and encephalocele, as well as several other less common forms. They are one of the most important classes of birth defects, with a newborn prevalence of 1 to 3 per 1,000. There is considerable variation in the prevalence of NTDs among various populations, with an especially high rate among some British and Irish populations (as high as 5 or more per 1,000 births in the 1970s). For reasons that are not fully known, the prevalence of NTDs has been decreasing in many parts of the United States and Europe (including Great Britain) during the past two decades.

Normally the neural tube closes at about the fourth week of gestation. A defect in closure or a subsequent re-opening of the neural tube results in an NTD. Spina bifida (Fig. 12-3, *A*) is the most commonly observed NTD and consists of a protrusion of spinal tissue through the vertebral column (the tissue usually includes meninges,

spinal cord, and nerve roots). About 75% of spina bifida patients have secondary hydrocephalus, which sometimes in turn produces mental retardation. Paralysis or muscle weakness, lack of sphincter control, and club feet are often observed. A study conducted in British Columbia showed that survival rates for spina bifida patients have improved dramatically over the past several decades. Fewer than 30% of cases born between 1952 and 1969 survived to age 10, while 65% of those born between 1970 and 1986 survived to this age. WWW

Anencephaly (Fig. 12-3, *B*) is characterized by partial or complete absence of the cranial vault and calvarium and partial or complete absence of the cerebral hemispheres. At least two thirds of anencephalics are stillborn; term deliveries do not survive more than a few hours or days. Encephalocele (Fig. 12-3, *C*) consists of a protrusion of the brain into an enclosed sac. It is seldom compatible with survival. WWW

NTDs are thought to arise from a combination of genetic and environmental factors. In most populations surveyed thus far, empirical recurrence risks for siblings

FIG. 12-3   The major neural tube defects (NTDs). **A,** An infant with an open spina bifida (meningomyelocele).

(A-C, Courtesy Dr. Edward Klatt, University of Utah Health Sciences Center.)

Continued

FIG. 12-3—cont'd   The major neural tube defects (NTDs). **B,** A fetus with anencephaly. Note the abnormalities of the orbits of the eye and the cranial defect.

CLINICAL COMMENTARY 12-1—cont'd
NEURAL TUBE DEFECTS—cont'd

of affected individuals range from 2% to 5%. Consistent with a multifactorial model, the recurrence risk increases with additional affected siblings. A recent Hungarian study showed that the overall prevalence of NTDs in that country was 1/300 births and that the sibling recurrence risks were 3%, 12%, and 25% after one, two, and three affected offspring, respectively. Recurrence risks tend to be slightly lower in populations with lower NTD prevalence rates, as predicted by the multifactorial

---

as environmental factors can differ among populations. For example, the empirical risk for neural tube defects in North America is about 2% to 3%, somewhat lower than that of the British population.

▼ **Empirical recurrence risks for multifactorial diseases are based on studies of large collections of families. These risks are specific to a given population.** ▲

It is sometimes difficult to distinguish polygenic or multifactorial diseases from single-gene diseases that have reduced penetrance or variable expression. Large data sets and good epidemiological data are necessary to make the distinction. Several criteria are usually used to define multifactorial inheritance:

1. *The recurrence risk is higher if more than one family member is affected.* For example, the sibling recurrence risk for a ventricular septal defect (VSD, a type of congenital heart defect) is 3% if one sibling has had a VSD but increases to approximately 10% if two siblings have had VSDs. In contrast, the recurrence risk for single-gene diseases remains the same regardless of the number of affected siblings. It should be emphasized that this increase does not mean that the family's risk has actually *changed.* Rather, it means that we now have more information about the family's true risk: because they have had two affected children, they are probably located higher on the liability distribution than a family with only one affected child. In other words, they have more risk fac-

C

FIG. 12-3—cont'd The major neural tube defects (NTDs). **C,** An occipital encephalocele.

model. Recurrence risk data support the idea that the major forms of NTDs are caused by similar factors. An anencephalic conception increases the recurrence risk for subsequent spina bifida conceptions, and vice versa.

NTDs can usually be diagnosed prenatally, sometimes by ultrasound and usually by an elevation in alpha-fetoprotein (AFP) in the maternal serum or amniotic fluid (see Chapter 13). A spina bifida lesion can be either open or closed (i.e., covered with a layer of skin). Fetuses with open spina bifida are more likely to be detected by AFP assays.

A major epidemiological finding is that mothers who supplement their diet with folic acid at the time of conception are less likely to produce children with NTDs. This result has been replicated in several different populations and is thus well confirmed. It has been estimated that approximately 50% to 70% of NTDs can be avoided simply by dietary folic acid supplementation. (Traditional prenatal vitamin supplements would not have an effect because administration does not usually begin until well after the time that the neural tube closes.) Since mothers would be likely to ingest similar amounts of folic acid from one pregnancy to the next, folic acid deficiency could well account for at least part of the elevated sibling recurrence risk for NTDs.

Dietary folic acid is an important example of a *nongenetic* factor that contributes to familial clustering of a disease. However, it is likely that there is genetic variation in response to folic acid, which helps to explain why most mothers with folic acid deficiency do not bear children with NTDs and why some who ingest adequate amounts nonetheless do bear children with NTDs.

tors (genetic and/or environmental) and are more likely to produce an affected child. **www**

2. *If the expression of the disease in the proband is more severe, the recurrence risk is higher.* This is again consistent with the liability model because a more severe expression indicates that the affected individual is at the extreme tail of the liability distribution (see Fig. 12-2). His or her relatives are thus at a higher risk to inherit disease genes. For example, the occurrence of a bilateral (both sides) cleft lip/palate confers a higher recurrence risk on family members than does the occurrence of a unilateral (one side) cleft. **www**

3. *The recurrence risk is higher if the proband is of the less commonly affected sex* (see the previous discus-

sion of pyloric stenosis). This is because an affected individual of the less susceptible sex is usually at a more extreme position on the liability distribution.

4. *The recurrence risk for the disease usually decreases rapidly in more remotely related relatives* (Table 12-2). While the recurrence risk for single-gene diseases decreases by 50% with each degree of relationship (e.g., an autosomal dominant disease has a 50% recurrence risk for siblings, 25% for uncle-nephew relationships, 12.5% for first cousins, etc.), it decreases much more quickly for multifactorial diseases. This reflects the fact that many genes and environmental factors must combine to produce a trait. All of the necessary risk factors are unlikely to be present in less closely related family members.

TABLE 12-2   Recurrence Risks (%) for First-, Second-, and Third-Degree Relatives

DISEASE	RISK			
	1st-degree	2nd-degree	3rd-degree	General population
Cleft lip/palate	4.0	0.7	0.3	0.1
Club foot	2.5	0.5	0.2	0.1
Congenital hip dislocation	5.0	0.6	0.4	0.2
Infantile autism	4.5	0.1	0.05	0.04

5. *If the prevalence of the disease in a population is f, the risk for offspring and siblings of probands is approximately √f.* This does not hold true for single-gene traits because their recurrence risks are independent of population prevalence. It is not an absolute rule for multifactorial traits either, but many such diseases do tend to conform to this prediction. Examination of the risks given in Table 12-2 shows that the first three diseases follow the prediction fairly well. However, the observed sibling risk for the fourth disease, infantile autism, is substantially higher than predicted by √f.

▼ Risks for multifactorial diseases usually increase if (1) more family members are affected, (2) the disease has more severe expression, and/or (3) the affected proband is a member of the less commonly affected sex. Recurrence risks decrease rapidly with more remote degrees of relationship. In general, the sibling recurrence risk is approximately equal to the square root of the prevalence of the disease in the population. ▲

Multifactorial Versus Single-Gene Inheritance

It is important to clarify the difference between a multifactorial disease and a single-gene disease in which there is locus heterogeneity. In the former case, a disease is caused by the simultaneous operation of multiple genetic and environmental factors, each of which has a relatively small effect. In contrast, a disease with locus heterogeneity, such as osteogenesis imperfecta, requires only a single mutation for its causation. Because of locus heterogeneity, a chromosome 7 mutation may cause the disease in one family, while a chromosome 17 mutation may cause the disease in another family. There is thus more than one gene that can cause the disease, but *in a given individual* a single gene causes the disease.

In some cases a trait may be influenced by the combination of both a single gene with large effects and a multifactorial "background" in which additional genes and environmental factors have individually

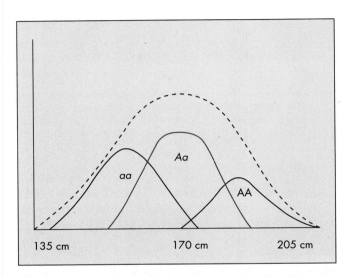

FIG. 12-4   The distribution of height, assuming the presence of a major gene (genotypes *AA*, *Aa*, and *aa*) combined with a multifactorial background. The multifactorial background causes variation in height among individuals of each genotype. If the distributions of each of the three genotypes are superimposed, then the overall distribution of height is approximately normal, as shown by the dotted line.

small effects (Fig. 12-4). Imagine that variation in height, for example, is caused by a single locus (termed a **major gene**) and a multifactorial component. Individuals with the *AA* genotype will tend to be taller, those with the *aa* genotype will tend to be shorter, and those with *Aa* will tend to be intermediate. But additional variation is caused by other factors (the multifactorial component). Thus, those with the *aa* genotype will vary in height from 130 cm to about 170 cm, those with the *Aa* genotype will vary from 150 cm to 190 cm, and those with the *AA* genotype will vary from 170 to 210 cm. There is substantial overlap among the three major genotypes because of the influence of the multifactorial background. The total distribution of height, which is bell-shaped, is caused by the superposition of the three distributions about each genotype.

Many of the diseases to be discussed later can be the result of either a major gene or multifactorial inheritance. Thus, there are subsets of the population in which diseases such as colon cancer, breast cancer, or heart disease are inherited as single-gene disorders (with additional variation in disease susceptibility contributed by other genetic and environmental factors). These subsets usually account for only a small percentage of the total number of disease cases. It is nevertheless important to identify the responsible major genes, since their function can provide important clues to the pathophysiology and treatment of the disease.

▼ Multifactorial diseases can be distinguished from single-gene disorders caused by mutations at different loci (locus heterogeneity). Sometimes a disease may have both single-gene and multifactorial components. ▲

NATURE AND NURTURE: DISENTANGLING THE EFFECTS OF GENES AND ENVIRONMENT

Family members share genes and a common environment. Family resemblance in traits such as blood pressure reflects both genetic and environmental commonality ("nature" and "nurture," respectively). For centuries, people have debated the relative importance of these two types of factors. It is a mistake, of course, to view them as mutually exclusive. Few traits are influenced *only* by genes or *only* by environment. Most are influenced by both. It is useful to try to determine the relative influence of genetic and environmental factors. This can lead to a better understanding of disease etiology. It can also help to plan public health strategies. A disease in which hereditary influence is relatively small, such as lung cancer, may be prevented most effectively through emphasis on lifestyle changes (avoidance of tobacco). When a disease has a relatively larger hereditary component, as in breast cancer, examination of family history should be emphasized in addition to lifestyle modification.

Here we will review two research strategies that are often used to estimate the relative influence of genes and environment: twin studies and adoption studies. We will then discuss methods that aim to delineate the individual genes responsible for multifactorial diseases.

Twin Studies

Twins occur with a frequency of about 1/100 births in Caucasian populations. They are a bit more common in Africans and a bit less common among Asians. **Monozygotic** (MZ, or "identical") twins originate when, for unknown reasons, the developing embryo divides to form two separate but identical embryos. Since they are

genetically identical, MZ twins are an example of natural clones. Their physical appearances can be strikingly similar (Fig. 12-5). **Dizygotic** (DZ, or "fraternal") twins are the result of a double ovulation followed by the fertilization of each egg by a different sperm.* Thus, dizygotic twins are genetically no more similar than other siblings. Because two different sperm cells are required to fertilize the two eggs, it is possible for each DZ twin to have a different father.

Because MZ twins are genetically identical, any differences between them should be due only to environmental effects. MZ twins should thus resemble one another very closely for traits that are strongly influenced by genes. DZ twins provide a convenient comparison because their environmental differences should be similar to those of MZ twins, but their genetic differences are as great as those between siblings. Twin studies thus usually consist of comparisons between MZ and DZ twins. If both members of a twin pair share a trait (e.g., a cleft lip), they are said to be **concordant.** If they do not share the trait, they are **discordant.** For a trait determined totally by genes, MZ twins should always be concordant, while DZ twins should be concordant less often, since they, like siblings, share only 50% of their genes. Concordance rates may differ between opposite-sex DZ twin pairs and same-sex DZ pairs for some traits, such as those that have different frequencies in males and females. For such traits, only same-sex DZ twin pairs should be used when comparing MZ and DZ concordance rates, since MZ twins are necessarily of the same sex.

A concordance estimate would not be appropriate for quantitative traits, such as blood pressure or height. Here the **intraclass correlation coefficient** is used. This statistic varies between -1.0 and 1.0 and measures the degree of similarity in two quantities in a population. The quantities could be height measurements in each member of a twin pair. The measurements are made in a collection of twins, and correlation coefficients are estimated separately for the MZ sample and the DZ sample. If a trait were determined entirely by genes, we would expect the correlation coefficient for MZ pairs to be 1.0. A correlation coefficient of 0.0 would mean that there is no similarity between MZ twins for the trait in question. Because DZ twins share half of their genes, we would expect a DZ correlation coefficient of 0.50 for a trait determined entirely by genes.

▼ Monozygotic (identical) twins are the result of an early cleavage of the embryo, whereas dizygotic (fraternal) twins are caused by the fertilization of

*While MZ twinning rates are quite constant across populations, DZ twinning rates vary somewhat. DZ twinning increases with maternal age until about age 40, after which it declines.

FIG. 12-5 Monozygotic twins, showing a striking similarity in physical appearance. Both twins developed myopia as teenagers.

two eggs by two sperm cells. Comparisons of concordance rates and correlations in MZ and DZ twins help to determine the extent to which a trait is influenced by genes. ▲

Concordance rates and correlation coefficients for a number of traits are given in Table 12-3. The concordance rates for contagious diseases like measles are quite similar in MZ and DZ twins. This is expected, since a contagious disease is unlikely to be influenced markedly by genes. On the other hand, the concordance rates are quite dissimilar for schizophrenia and bipolar affective disorder, indicating a sizable genetic component for these diseases. The MZ correlation for dermatoglyphics (fingerprints), which is determined almost entirely by genes, is close to 1.0.

Correlations and concordance rates in MZ and DZ twins can be used to measure the **heritability** of multifactorial traits. Essentially, heritability is the percentage of population variation in a trait that is due to genes

(statistically, it is the proportion of the total **variance** of a trait that is caused by genes). A simple formula for estimating heritability (h) from twin correlations or concordance rates is: $h = 2(c_{MZ} - c_{DZ})$, where c_{MZ} is the concordance rate (or intraclass correlation) for monozygotic twins and c_{DZ} is the concordance rate (or intraclass correlation) for dizygotic twins.* As this formula illustrates, traits that are largely determined by genes will result in a heritability estimate that approaches 1.0 (i.e., c_{MZ} will approach 1.0, and c_{DZ} will approach 0.5). As the difference between concordance rates becomes smaller, heritability approaches zero. Correlations and concordance rates in other pairs of relatives (e.g., parents and offspring) can also be used to measure heritability.

---

*This formula represents one of the simplest ways of estimating heritability. A description of more complex and accurate approaches can be found in the books by Cavalli-Sforza and Bodmer and Neale and Cardon cited at the end of this chapter.

TABLE 12-3   Concordance Rates in MZ and DZ Twins for Selected Traits and Diseases*

Trait or disease	Concordance rate		Heritability
	MZ twins	DZ twins	
Affective disorder (bipolar)	0.79	0.24	>1.0[‡]
Affective disorder (unipolar)	0.54	0.19	0.70
Alcoholism	>0.60	<0.30	0.60
Autism	0.92	0.0	>1.0
Blood pressure (diastolic)[†]	0.58	0.27	0.62
Blood pressure (systolic)[†]	0.55	0.25	0.60
Body fat percentage[†]	0.73	0.22	>1.0
Body mass index[†]	0.95	0.53	0.84
Cleft lip/palate	0.38	0.08	0.60
Club foot	0.32	0.03	0.58
Dermatoglyphics (finger ridge count)[†]	0.95	0.49	0.92
Diabetes mellitus	0.45-0.96	0.03-0.37	>1.0
Diabetes mellitus (type I)	0.35-0.50	0.05-0.10	0.60-0.80
Diabetes mellitus (type II)	0.70-0.90	0.25-0.40	0.90-1.0
Epilepsy (idiopathic)	0.69	0.14	>1.0
Height[†]	0.94	0.44	1.0
IQ[†]	0.76	0.51	0.50
Measles	0.95	0.87	0.16
Multiple sclerosis	0.28	0.03	0.50
Myocardial infarction (males)	0.39	0.26	0.26
Myocardial infarction (females)	0.44	0.14	0.60
Schizophrenia	0.47	0.12	0.70
Spina bifida	0.72	0.33	0.78

*These figures were compiled from a large variety of sources and represent primarily European and U.S. populations.
[†]Since these are quantitative traits, correlation coefficients are given rather than concordance rates.
[‡]Several heritability estimates exceed 1.0. Since it is impossible for >100% of the variance of a trait to be genetically determined, these values indicate that other factors, such as shared environmental factors, must be operating.

Like recurrence risks, heritability values are specific for the population in which they are estimated. However, there is usually agreement from one population to another regarding the general range of heritability estimates of most traits (e.g., the heritability of height is nearly always high, while the heritability of contagious diseases is nearly always low). The same is true of empirical recurrence risks.

▼ **Comparisons of correlations and concordance rates in MZ and DZ twins allow the estimation of heritability, a measure of the proportion of population variation in a disease that can be attributed to genes.** ▲

At one time, twins were thought to provide a perfect "natural laboratory" in which to determine the relative influences of genetics and environment. But several difficulties arise. One of the most important is the assumption that the environments of MZ and DZ twins are equally similar. MZ twins are often treated more similarly than DZ twins. The eminent ge-

neticist L.S. Penrose once joked that, if one were to study the clothes of twins, it might be concluded that clothes are inherited biologically. A greater similarity in environment can make MZ twins more concordant for a trait, inflating the apparent influence of genes. In addition, MZ twins may be more likely to seek the same type of environment, further reinforcing environmental similarity. On the other hand, it has been suggested that some MZ twins tend to develop personality differences in an attempt to assert their individuality.

Another difficulty is that somatic mutations can occur during mitotic divisions of the cells of MZ twin embryos. Thus, the MZ twins may not be quite "identical." Finally, the uterine environments of different pairs of MZ twins can be more or less similar, depending on whether there are two amnions and two chorions, two amnions and one shared chorion, or one shared amnion and one shared chorion.

Of the various problems with the twin method, the greater degree of environmental sharing among MZ twins is perhaps the most serious. One way to circumvent this problem, at least in part, is to study MZ twins who are raised in separate environments. Concordance among these twin pairs should be caused by genetic, rather than environmental, similarities. As one might expect, it is not easy to find such twin pairs. A major effort to do so has been undertaken by researchers at the University of Minnesota. Their studies have shown a rather remarkable congruence among MZ twins reared apart, even for many behavioral traits. However, these studies must be viewed with caution because the sample sizes are relatively small and because many of the twin pairs had at least some contact with one another before they were studied.

▼ Although twin studies provide valuable information, they are also affected by certain biases. The most serious is greater environmental similarity among MZ twins than among DZ twins. Other biases include somatic mutations that may affect only one MZ twin and differences in the uterine environments of twins. ▲

Adoption Studies

Studies of adopted children are also used to estimate the genetic contribution to a multifactorial trait. Children born to parents who have a disease but adopted by parents lacking the disease can be studied to find out whether they develop the disease. In some cases such children develop the disease more often than a comparative control population (i.e., adopted children who were born to parents who do *not* have the disease). This provides some evidence that genes may be involved in the causation of the disease, since the adopted children do not share an environment with their affected natural parents. For example, about 8% to 10% of adopted children of a schizophrenic parent develop schizophrenia, whereas only 1% of adopted children of unaffected parents become schizophrenics.

As with twin studies, several precautions must be exercised in interpreting the results of adoption studies. First, prenatal environmental influences could have long-lasting effects on an adopted child. Second, children are sometimes adopted after they are several years old, ensuring that some environmental influence would have been imparted by the natural parents. Finally, adoption agencies sometimes try to match the adoptive parents with the natural parents in terms of factors such as background and socioeconomic status. All of these factors could exaggerate the apparent influence of biological inheritance.

▼ Adoption studies provide a second means of estimating the influence of genes on multifactorial diseases. They consist of comparing disease rates among the adopted offspring of affected parents with the rates among adopted offspring of unaf-

fected parents. As with the twin method, certain biases can influence these studies. ▲

These reservations, as well as those summarized for twin studies, underscore the need for caution in basing conclusions upon twin and adoption studies. These approaches do not provide definitive measures of the role of genes in multifactorial disease, nor can they identify specific genes responsible for disease. Instead, they serve a useful purpose in providing a preliminary indication of the extent to which a multifactorial disease may be caused by genetic factors. Methods for the direct detection of genes underlying multifactorial traits are summarized in Box 12-1.

THE GENETICS OF COMMON DISEASES

Having discussed the principles of multifactorial inheritance, we turn next to a discussion of the common multifactorial disorders themselves. Some of these disorders, the congenital malformations, are by definition present at birth. Others, including heart disease, cancer, diabetes, and most psychiatric disorders, are seen primarily in adolescents and adults. Because of their complexity, unraveling the genetics of these disorders is a daunting task. Nonetheless, significant progress is now being made.

Congenital Malformations

Approximately 2% of newborns present with a **congenital** (present at birth) malformation; most of these would be considered multifactorial in etiology. Some of the more common congenital malformations are listed in Table 12-4. In general, sibling recurrence risks for most of these disorders range from 1% to 5%.

Some congenital malformations, such as cleft lip/palate and pyloric stenosis, are relatively easy to repair and thus are not considered to be serious problems. Others, such as the neural tube defects, usually have more severe consequences. While some cases of con-

TABLE 12-4 Prevalence Rates of Common Congenital Malformations in Caucasians

Disorder	Prevalence per 1,000 births (approximate)
Cleft lip/palate	1.0
Club foot	1.0
Congenital heart defects	4.0-8.0
Hydrocephaly	0.5-2.5
Isolated cleft palate	0.4
Neural tube defects	1.0-3.0
Pyloric stenosis	3.0

BOX 12-1
FINDING THE UNDERLYING GENES: QUANTITATIVE TRAIT LOCI

As already mentioned, twin and adoption studies are not designed to reveal specific genes that cause multifactorial diseases. Nevertheless, the identification of specific causative genes is an important goal, since only then can we begin to understand the underlying biology of the disease and undertake to correct the defect. For complex multifactorial traits, this is a formidable task because of locus heterogeneity, the interactions of multiple genes, decreased penetrance, age-dependent onset, and **phenocopies** (individuals who have a phenotype, such as breast cancer, but who do not carry a known disease-causing gene, such as *BRCA1*). Fortunately, recent advances in gene mapping and molecular biology promise to make this goal more attainable. Here, we will discuss several approaches that are used to identify the genes underlying multifactorial traits, often known as **quantitative trait loci (QTLs).**

One way to search for QTLs is to use conventional linkage analysis, as described in Chapter 8. Disease families are collected, a single-gene mode of inheritance is assumed, and linkage analysis is undertaken with a large series of marker polymorphisms that span the genome (this is often termed a **genome scan**). If a sufficiently large LOD score is obtained with a polymorphism, it is assumed that the region around this polymorphism may contain a QTL. This approach is sometimes successful, especially when there are subsets of families in which a single-gene mode of inheritance is seen (e.g., autosomal dominant, autosomal recessive). This was the case, for example, with familial breast cancer, where some families present a clear autosomal dominant mode of inheritance.

With many multifactorial disorders, however, such subsets are not readily apparent. Because of obstacles such as heterogeneity and phenocopies, traditional linkage analysis is impractical. One alternative to traditional linkage analysis is the **affected sib-pair method.** The logic of this approach is simple: if two siblings are both affected by a genetic disease, we would expect to see increased sharing of marker genes in the genomic region that contains a susceptibility gene. To conduct an analysis using this approach, we begin by collecting DNA samples from a large number of sib pairs in which both members of the pair are affected by the disease. Then a genome scan is undertaken, and the proportion of affected sib pairs who share the same allele is estimated for each polymorphism. Because siblings share half their genes (see Chapter 4), we would expect this proportion to be 50% for marker polymorphisms that are not linked to a susceptibility locus. However, if we find that siblings share the same allele for a marker polymorphism more frequently than half the time (say, 75%), this would be evidence that the marker is linked to a susceptibility locus. This approach was used, for example, to show that the HLA region contributes to susceptibility for type I diabetes.

The affected sib-pair method has the advantage that one does not have to assume a specific mode of inheritance. In addition, the method is unaffected by reduced penetrance, since both members of the sib pair must be affected to be included in the analysis. It is especially useful for late age-of-onset disorders, such as prostate cancer, in which it would be difficult to assemble multi-generational families from whom DNA samples could be taken. A weakness of this method is that it tends to require large sample sizes to yield significant results, and it tends to have low resolution (i.e., the genomic region implicated by the analysis tends to be quite large, often 10 cM or more).

Affected sib-pair analyses are sometimes made more powerful by selecting subjects with extreme values of a trait (e.g., sib pairs with very high blood pressure) to enrich the sample for genes likely to contribute to the trait. A variation on this approach is to sample sib pairs that are highly discordant for a trait (e.g., one with very high blood pressure and one with very low blood pressure) and then to look for markers in which there is *less* allele sharing than the expected 50%.

Association tests such as linkage disequilibrium (see Chapter 8) can also be used in the course of a genome scan. These methods are becoming more practical as the Human Genome Project is developing dense sets of polymorphic markers (both microsatellites, and, more recently, single nucleotide polymorphisms, or SNPs). The likelihood of finding QTLs using these approaches, as well as sib-pair and traditional linkage methods, may be enhanced by analyzing isolated populations (e.g., island populations or the populations mentioned in Box 3-1). Because these populations are typically derived from a small number of founders and have experienced little admixture with other populations, it is thought that the number of mutations contributing to a multifactorial disease may be reduced and thus easier to pinpoint.

Another method combines genome scanning and the use of animal models. It consists basically of the following steps (Fig. 12-6):

1. Breeding experiments are carried out with experimental animals, such as rats or mice, to select progeny that have extreme values of a trait (e.g., rats that have high blood pressure levels). These are then crossed with normal animals to produce offspring that each have one normal chromosome and one "affected" chromosome that presumably contains genes that cause high blood pressure. These offspring are in turn mated with the normal animal (a backcross). This produces a third generation of animals in whom one chromosome has only the normal genes and the homologous chromosome has experienced recombinations between the normal and affected chromosomes (as a result of crossovers between the normal and affected chromosomes during meiosis in the parents). This series of matings produces progeny that are useful for linkage analysis.

2. High-resolution genetic maps of the experimental organism must be available. This means that polymorphic markers must be identified at regular intervals (ideally, at least every 10 cM) throughout the organism's genome.

Continued

FIG. 12-6   The basic steps involved in performing a genome scan for QTLs using an animal model (see text for details).

3. Linkage analysis (see Chapter 8) is performed, comparing each polymorphic marker against the trait. Since animals with extreme values have been selected, this procedure should uncover markers that are linked to loci that produce the extreme phenotype.

4. Once a linked marker (or markers) has been found, it may be possible to isolate the actual functional gene responsible for the trait using the techniques outlined in Chapter 8.

5. When a functional gene has been isolated and cloned in the experimental organism, it is used as a probe to search the human genome for a gene with high DNA sequence homology that may have the same function (a candidate gene). This approach is feasible because the DNA sequences of functionally important genes are often similar in humans and experimental animals such as rodents.

This approach has been applied in studies of type I diabetes and hypertension. It has the advantage that animals can easily be selected with extreme values of a trait, and any desired breeding scheme can be used to generate useful recombinants. Animals, of course, do not necessarily model humans accurately. Furthermore, this technique detects only individual genes that cause disease in the animal model; it cannot assess the pattern of *interactions* of these genes. There is evidence that the nature of these interactions may be critically important, and they may well differ in humans and experimental animals. Despite these reservations, this approach demonstrates effectively the way in which new developments in molecular genetics and gene mapping may increase our knowledge of the genes responsible for multifactorial disease.

genital malformations may occur in the absence of any other problems, it is quite common for them to be associated with other disorders. For example, hydrocephaly and club foot are often seen secondary to spina bifida, cleft lip/palate is often seen in babies with trisomy 13, and congenital heart defects are seen in many disorders, including Down syndrome.

Considerable progress is now being made in isolating single genes that can cause congenital malformations. Many of these, including the *HOX, PAX* and *TBX* families of genes, were discussed in Chapter 10. Another example is the *RET* proto-oncogene, which is responsible for some cases of Hirschsprung disease. However, the causes of most cases of this disorder remain undiscovered. Indeed, the genetic factors contributing to many important congenital malformations (e.g., neural tube defects, common congenital heart defects, cleft lip/palate) are as yet unidentified.

Environmental factors have also been shown to cause some congenital malformations. An example is thalidomide, a sedative used during pregnancy in the early 1960s (and recently reintroduced for the treatment of dermatological conditions such as leprosy). When ingested during early pregnancy, this drug often caused phocomelia (severely shortened limbs) in babies. Maternal exposure to retinoic acid, which is used to treat acne, can cause congenital defects of the heart, ear, and central nervous system. Maternal rubella infection can cause congenital heart defects. Other environmental factors that can cause congenital malformations are discussed in Chapter 14.

▼ Congenital malformations are seen in roughly 1/50 live births. Most of them are considered to be multifactorial disorders. Specific genes and environmental causes have been detected for some congenital malformations, but the causes of many congenital malformations remain largely unknown. ▲

Multifactorial Disorders in the Adult Population

Until recently, very little was known about specific genes responsible for common adult diseases. With more powerful laboratory and analytical techniques, this situation is changing. We will next review recent progress in understanding the genetics of the major common adult diseases. Table 12-5 gives approximate prevalence figures for these disorders in the United States.

Coronary Heart Disease

Coronary heart disease (CHD) is the leading killer of Americans, accounting for approximately 25% of all deaths in this country. It is caused by atherosclerosis, a narrowing of the coronary arteries due to the formation of lipid-laden lesions. This narrowing impedes blood flow to the heart and can eventually result in a myocar-

TABLE 12-5 Prevalence Figures for Common Adult Diseases

Disease	Number of affected Americans (approximate)
Alcoholism	10 million
Alzheimer disease	4 million
Bipolar affective disorder	1 million
Cancer (all types)	6 million
Coronary heart disease	5 million
Diabetes (type I)	1 million
Diabetes (type II)	5-10 million
Epilepsy	2 million
Hypertension	25-30 million
Multiple sclerosis	250,000
Obesity*	50 million
Schizophrenia	2 million

*Defined as 20% or more above ideal body weight.

dial infarction (destruction of heart tissue caused by an inadequate supply of oxygen). When atherosclerosis occurs in arteries supplying blood to the brain, a stroke can result. A number of risk factors for heart disease have been identified, including obesity, cigarette smoking, hypertension, elevated cholesterol level, and positive family history (usually defined as having one or more affected first-degree relatives). Many studies have examined the role of family history in CHD, and they show that an individual with a positive family history is two to seven times more likely to suffer from heart disease than is an individual with no family history. Generally, these studies also show that the risk increases if: (1) there are more affected relatives; (2) the affected relative(s) is female (the less commonly affected sex) rather than male; or (3) age of onset in the affected relative is early (before age 55). For example, one study showed that men between the ages of 20 and 39 had a three-fold increase in CHD risk if they had one affected first-degree relative. This risk increased to thirteen-fold if there were two first-degree relatives affected with CHD before age 55.

What part do genes play in the familial clustering of heart disease? Because of the key role of lipids in atherosclerosis, many studies are focusing on the genetic determination of various lipoproteins. An important advance in this area has been the isolation and cloning of the gene for the LDL (low-density lipoprotein) receptor defects that cause familial hypercholesterolemia (Clinical Commentary 12-2). More than a dozen other genes involved in lipid metabolism and transport have been identified, including those that encode various apolipoproteins (these are the protein components of lipoproteins) (Table 12-6). Functional analysis of these genes is leading to an increased understanding, and eventually more effective treatment, of CHD. **www**

CLINICAL COMMENTARY 12-2
FAMILIAL HYPERCHOLESTEROLEMIA

Autosomal dominant familial hypercholesterolemia (FH) is an important cause of heart disease, accounting for approximately 5% of myocardial infarctions in persons under age 60. FH is one of the most common autosomal dominant disorders: in most populations surveyed to date, about 1 in 500 persons is a heterozygote. Plasma cholesterol levels are approximately twice as high as normal (i.e., about 300-400 mg/dl), resulting in substantially accelerated atherosclerosis and the occurrence of distinctive cholesterol deposits in skin and tendons called xanthomas (Fig. 12-7). Data compiled from five studies showed that approximately 75% of men with FH developed coronary disease, and 50% had a fatal myocardial infarction, by age 60. The corresponding percentages for women were lower (45% and 15%, respectively) because women generally develop heart disease at a later age than men.

Consistent with Hardy-Weinberg predictions, about 1/1,000,000 births is homozygous for the FH gene. Homozygotes are much more severely affected, with cholesterol levels ranging from 600 to 1,200 mg/dl. Most experience myocardial infarctions before age 20, and a myocardial infarction at 18 months of age has been reported. If untreated, most FH homozygotes will die before the age of 30.

FIG. 12-7 Xanthomas (fatty deposits) are often seen in patients with familial hypercholesterolemia.

All cells require cholesterol as a component of their plasma membrane. They can either synthesize their own cholesterol, or preferentially they obtain it from the extracellular environment, where it is carried primarily by low-density lipoprotein (LDL). In a process known as **endocytosis**, LDL-bound cholesterol is taken into the cell via LDL receptors on the cell's surface (Fig. 12-8). FH is caused by a reduction in the number of functional LDL receptors on cell surfaces. Lacking the normal number of LDL receptors, cellular cholesterol uptake is reduced, and circulating cholesterol levels increase.

Much of what we know about endocytosis has been learned through the study of LDL receptors. The process of endocytosis and the processing of LDL in the cell is described in detail in Fig. 12-8. These processes result in a fine-tuned regulation of cholesterol levels within cells, and they influence the level of circulating cholesterol as well.

The cloning of the LDL receptor gene in 1984 was a critical step in understanding exactly how LDL receptor defects cause FH. This gene, located on chromosome 19, is 45 kb in length and consists of 18 exons and 17 introns. It encodes a 5.3-kb mRNA transcript that ultimately produces a mature protein of 839 amino acids. More than 150 different mutations, including missense and nonsense substitutions as well as insertions and deletions, have been identified in the LDL receptor gene. These can be grouped into five broad classes, according to their effects on the activity of the receptor.

Class I mutations result in no detectable protein product. Thus, heterozygotes would produce only half the normal number of LDL receptors.

Class II mutations in the LDL receptor gene result in production of the LDL receptor, but it is altered such that it cannot leave the endoplasmic reticulum. It is eventually degraded.

Class III mutations produce an LDL receptor that is capable of migrating to the cell surface but incapable of normal binding to LDL.

Class IV mutations, which are comparatively rare, produce receptors that are normal except that they do not migrate specifically to coated pits and thus cannot carry LDL into the cell.

Class V mutations produce an LDL receptor that cannot disassociate from the LDL particle after entry into the cell. The receptor cannot return to the cell surface and is degraded.

Each class of mutations reduces the number of effective LDL receptors, resulting in decreased LDL uptake and hence elevated levels of circulating cholesterol. The number of effective receptors is reduced by about half in FH heterozygotes, and homozygotes have virtually no functional LDL receptors.

Understanding the defects that lead to FH has helped to develop effective therapies for the disorder. Dietary reduction of cholesterol (primarily through the reduced

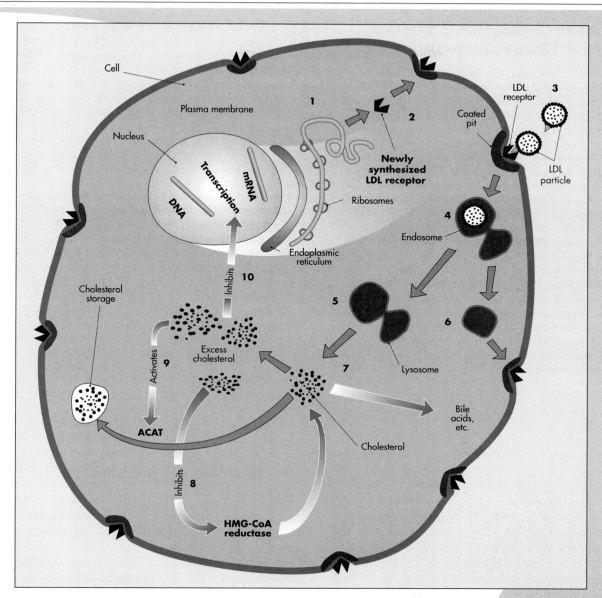

FIG. 12-8 The process of receptor-mediated endocytosis. *1,* The LDL receptors, which are glycoproteins, are synthesized in the endoplasmic reticulum of the cell. *2,* From here, they pass through the Golgi apparatus to the cell surface, where part of the receptor protrudes outside the cell. *3,* The circulating LDL particle is bound by the LDL receptor and localized in cell-surface depressions called "coated pits" (so named because they are coated with a protein called clathrin). *4,* The coated pit invaginates, bringing the LDL particle inside the cell. *5,* Once inside the cell, the LDL particle is separated from the receptor, taken into a lysosome, and broken down into its constituents by lysosomal enzymes. *6,* The LDL receptor is recirculated to the cell surface to bind another LDL particle (each LDL receptor goes through this cycle approximately once every 10 minutes even if it is not occupied by an LDL particle). *7,* Free cholesterol is released from the lysosome for incorporation into cell membranes or metabolism into bile acids or steroids. Excess cholesterol can be stored in the cell as a cholesterol ester or removed from the cell by associating with high-density lipoprotein (HDL). *8,* As cholesterol levels in the cell rise, cellular cholesterol synthesis is reduced by inhibition of the rate-limiting enzyme, HMG-CoA reductase (3-hydroxy-3-methylglutaryl CoA reductase). *9,* Rising cholesterol levels also increase the activity of acyl-CoA:cholesterol acyltransferase (ACAT), an enzyme that modifies cholesterol for storage as cholesterol esters. *10,* In addition, the number of LDL receptors is decreased by lowering the transcription rate of the LDL receptor gene itself. This decreases cholesterol uptake. (Modified from Goldstein JL, Brown MS [1989] In: Scriver CR, Beaudet AL, Sly WS, Valle D (eds) The Metabolic Basis of Inherited Disease, 6th ed. McGraw-Hill, New York.)

Continued

intake of saturated fats) has only modest effects on cholesterol levels in FH heterozygotes. Since cholesterol is reabsorbed into the gut and then recycled through the liver (where most cholesterol synthesis takes place), serum cholesterol levels can be reduced by the administration of bile-acid absorbing resins, such as cholestyramine. The absorbed cholesterol is then excreted. It is interesting to note that reduced recirculation from the gut causes the liver cells to form additional LDL receptors, lowering circulating cholesterol levels. However, the decrease in intracellular cholesterol also stimulates cholesterol synthesis by liver cells, so the overall reduction in plasma LDL is only about 15% to 20%. This treatment is much more effective when combined with agents such as lovastatin, which reduce cholesterol synthesis by inhibiting HMG-CoA reductase (see Fig. 12-8). Decreased synthesis leads to further production of LDL receptors. When these therapies are used in combination, serum cholesterol levels in FH heterozygotes can often be reduced to approximately normal levels.

The picture is less encouraging for FH homozygotes. The therapies mentioned can enhance cholesterol elimination and reduce its synthesis, but they are largely ineffective in homozygotes because these individuals have few or no LDL receptors. Liver transplants, which provide hepatocytes that have normal LDL receptors, have been successful in some cases, but this option is often limited by a lack of donors. Plasma exchange, carried out every 1 to 2 weeks, in combination with drug therapy, can reduce cholesterol levels by about 50%. However, this therapy is difficult to continue for long periods. Somatic cell gene therapy, in which hepatocytes carrying normal LDL receptor genes are introduced into the portal circulation, is now being tested (see Chapter 13). It may eventually prove to be an effective treatment for FH homozygotes.

The FH story illustrates how medical research has made important contributions to both our understanding of basic cell biology and to advancements in clinical therapy. The process of receptor-mediated endocytosis, elucidated largely by research on the LDL receptor defects, is of fundamental significance for cellular processes throughout the body. Equally, this research, by clarifying how cholesterol synthesis and uptake can be modified, has led to significant improvements in therapy for this important cause of heart disease.

Family studies of rare forms of heart disease are also providing important information on the genetics of heart disease. For example, various genes causing inherited cardiomyopathy have been mapped to the X chromosome, the mitochondrial genome, and to several autosomes. One form of familial hypertrophic cardiomyopathy (FHC) is caused by mutations in the β-myosin heavy chain gene on chromosome 14. These mutations may produce abnormal contractile function. Additional mutations responsible for FHC have been found in the genes encoding myosin-binding protein C, α-tropomyosin, and cardiac troponin T. www

In addition, mutations have been identified in several genes that cause the autosomal dominant disorder long QT (LQT) syndrome (describing the characteristically abnormal electrocardiogram profile) (see Table 8-3). This disorder predisposes affected individuals to potentially fatal cardiac arrhythmia. Three of the LQT genes encode potassium channel components, and a fourth encodes a sodium channel. All four ion channels are involved in cardiac repolarization, consistent with the disease phenotype. Because LQT syndrome can be difficult to diagnose accurately, linked markers and mutation detection enable more accurate diagnosis of affected family members. In addition, the identification of disease-causing genes and their protein products is now guiding the development of drug therapy to activate the encoded ion channels. Because cardiac arrhythmias account for most of the 250,000 sudden cardiac deaths that occur annually in the United States, a better understanding of the genetic defects underlying arrhythmia is of considerable public health significance. www

It should be emphasized that environmental factors, many of which are easily modified, are also important causes of coronary heart disease. There is abundant epidemiological evidence that cigarette smoking and obesity increase the risk of coronary heart disease, while exercise and a diet low in saturated fats decrease the risk. Indeed, the approximate 50% decline in CHD incidence in the United States during the past 40 years is usually attributed to a decrease in the proportion of adults who smoke cigarettes, decreased consumption of saturated fats, and an increased emphasis on exercise and a generally healthier lifestyle.

▼ CHD shows familial aggregation. This aggregation is especially strong if there is early age of onset and if there are multiple affected relatives. Specific genes have been identified for some subsets of CHD families, and lifestyle changes (exercise, diet, avoidance of tobacco) can modify CHD risks appreciably. ▲

Hypertension

Systemic hypertension, which is seen in at least 15% of the populations of most developed countries, is a key

TABLE 12-6 Lipoprotein Genes Known to Contribute to Coronary Heart Disease Risk

Gene	Chromosome location	Function of protein product
Apolipoprotein A-I	11q	HDL component; LCAT co-factor
Apolipoprotein A-IV	11q	Component of chylomicrons and HDL; may influence HDL metabolism
Apolipoprotein C-III	11q	Allelic variation associated with hypertriglyceridemia
Apolipoprotein B	2p	Ligand for LDL receptor; involved in formation of VLDL, LDL, IDL, and chylomicrons
Apolipoprotein D	2p	HDL component
Apolipoprotein C-I	19q	LCAT activation
Apolipoprotein C-II	19q	Lipoprotein lipase activation
Apolipoprotein E	19q	Ligand for LDL receptor
Apolipoprotein A-II	1p	HDL component
LDL receptor	19p	Uptake of circulating LDL particles
Lipoprotein(a)	6q	Cholesterol transport
Lipoprotein lipase	8p	Hydrolysis of lipoprotein lipids
Hepatic triglyceride lipase	15q	Hydrolysis of lipoprotein lipids
LCAT	16q	Cholesterol esterification
Cholesterol ester transfer protein	16q	Facilitates transfer of cholesterol esters and phospholipid lipoproteins

Modified from King RA, Rotter JI, Motulsky AG (eds.) (1992) The Genetic Basis of Common Diseases. Oxford University Press, New York.

risk factor for heart disease, stroke, and kidney disease. Studies of blood pressure correlations within families indicate that the heritability of both systolic and diastolic blood pressure is approximately 20% to 40%. Heritability estimates based upon twin studies tend to be higher (about 60%) and may be inflated because of greater similarities in the environments of MZ than DZ twins. The fact that the heritability estimates are substantially less than 100% indicates that environmental factors must also be significant causes of blood pressure variation. The most important environmental risk factors for hypertension are increased sodium intake, decreased physical activity, psychosocial stress, and obesity (but as discussed below, the latter factor is itself influenced both by genes and environment).

Blood pressure regulation is a highly complex process that is influenced by many physiological systems. These include various aspects of kidney function, cellular ion transport, and heart function. Because of this complexity, it is unlikely that family studies of simple blood pressure will reveal much about genes responsible for hypertension. For this reason, most research is now focused on specific components that may influence blood pressure variation, such as angiotensin, angiotensinogen, urinary kallikrein, and sodium-lithium countertransport (Fig. 12-9; Table 12-7). These factors are more likely to be under the control of smaller numbers of genes. For example, linkage and association studies have implicated the gene encoding angiotensinogen in the causation of both hypertension and pre-eclampsia (a form of pregnancy-induced hypertension).

A small proportion of hypertension cases are the result of rare, single-gene disorders, such as Cushing syndrome and Liddle syndrome. At least 10 genes have now been identified that can lead to rare forms of hypertension, and all of them affect the resorption of water and salt by the kidney. It is hoped that isolation and study of these genes will lead to the identification of genetic factors underlying common hypertension.

Large-scale genome scans have been undertaken to identify quantitative trait loci that may underlie common essential hypertension (see Box 12-1). In one application, linkage analysis was undertaken using 181 DNA polymorphisms detected in the offspring of a cross between normal and hypertensive rat strains. Linkage was obtained between hypertension and markers near a gene that is highly similar in DNA sequence to a human gene that encodes the angiotensin converting enzyme (ACE). This enzyme converts angiotensin I to angiotensin II; the latter functions as a vasoconstrictor (it contracts blood vessels) and is also involved in modulating the excretion of sodium in the kidney. While it would thus seem a likely candidate as a hypertension gene, most studies indicate no relationship between variation in the ACE gene and hypertension in human populations. However, there is evidence that mutations in the ACE gene increase susceptibility to myocardial infarction. **www**

▼ **Heritability estimates for systolic and diastolic blood pressure range from 20% to 40%. Several genes influencing blood pressure variation have**

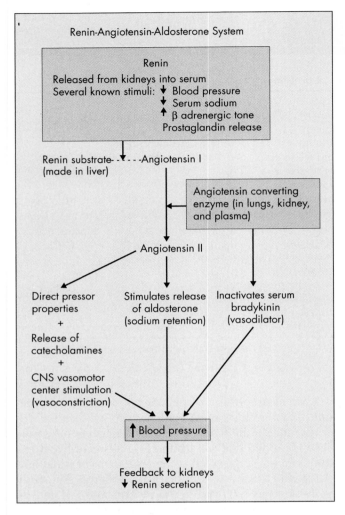

FIG. 12-9 The renin-angiotensin-aldosterone system. (Modified from King RA, Rotter JI, Motulsky AG [eds.] [1992] The Genetic Basis of Common Diseases. Oxford University Press, New York.)

TABLE 12-7 Transport Systems Involved in Blood Pressure Regulation

Laboratory measurement	Positive findings
Sodium-potassium cotransport (red cells)	Decreased in hypertensives and their children
Sodium-lithium counter-transport (red cells)	Increased in hypertensives and their first-degree relatives
Sodium-potassium ATPase (white cells)	Decreased sodium excretion in hypertensives and their relatives

cancer. Diet (i.e., carcinogenic substances and the lack of "anti-cancer" components such as fiber, fruits, and vegetables) is another leading cause of cancer. Since cancer genetics was the subject of Chapter 11, we will confine our attention here to genetic and environmental factors that influence susceptibility to some of the most common cancers.

BREAST CANCER. Breast cancer is the most common cancer among women, affecting approximately 12% of American women who live to age 85 or more. It was formerly the leading cause of cancer death among women, but it has recently been surpassed by lung cancer. Breast cancer can also occur in men, with a lifetime prevalence that is roughly 100 times lower than that of women. The familial aggregation of breast cancer has been recognized for centuries, having been described by physicians in ancient Rome. If a woman has one affected first-degree relative, her risk of developing breast cancer doubles. The risk increases further with more affected relatives, and it increases if these relatives developed cancer at a relatively early age (<45 years of age).

Several genes are now known to predispose women to developing hereditary breast cancer. Most important among these are *BRCA1* and *BRCA2*, two genes involved in DNA repair (see Chapter 11). Germline mutations in the *p53* gene can cause Li-Fraumeni syndrome, which also predisposes to breast cancer. Cowden disease, a rare autosomal dominant condition that includes multiple hamartomas and breast cancer, is caused by mutations in the *PTEN* tumor suppressor gene (see Chapter 11). Ataxia telangiectasia, an autosomal recessive disorder caused by defective DNA repair, includes breast cancer in its presentation. Mutations in the *MSH2* and *MLH1* DNA repair genes, which lead to hereditary nonpolyposis colorectal cancer (HNPCC), also confer an increased risk of breast cancer. Despite the significance of these genes, it should be emphasized that more than 90% of breast cancer cases are not hereditary and are caused instead by somatic mutations in breast cells. **www**

been pinpointed in the human. Other risk factors for hypertension include sodium intake, lack of exercise, psychosocial stress, and obesity. ▲

Cancer

Cancer is the second-leading cause of death in the United States, although it is estimated that it may soon surpass heart disease as the leading cause of death. It is well established that many major types of cancer (e.g., breast, colon, prostate, ovarian) cluster strongly in families. This is due to both shared genes as well as shared environmental factors. While numerous cancer genes are being isolated, environmental factors also play an important role in causing cancer by inducing somatic mutations. In particular, tobacco use is estimated to account for one third of all cancer cases in the United States, making it the most important known cause of

A number of environmental factors are known to increase the risk of developing breast cancer. These include nulliparity (never bearing children), bearing the first child after age 30, high-fat diet, alcohol use, and estrogen replacement therapy.

COLORECTAL CANCER. It is estimated that 1 in 20 Americans will develop colorectal cancer, and roughly one third of those diagnosed with this cancer will die from it. Colorectal cancer is thus second only to lung cancer in the total number of annual cancer deaths (approximately 55,000). Like breast cancer, it clusters in families (in fact, familial clustering of this form of cancer was reported in the medical literature as early as 1881). The risk of colorectal cancer in people with one affected first-degree relative is two to three times higher than that of the general population.

As discussed in Chapter 11, familial colon cancer can be the result of mutations in the *APC* tumor suppressor gene or in one of the four DNA mismatch repair genes (HNPCC). Other (less common) inherited colon cancer syndromes include Peutz-Jeghers syndrome (caused by mutations in a protein kinase gene on chromosome 19). www

As with breast cancer, most colon cancer cases (>90%) are not clearly inherited and are likely to be caused by a complex interaction of somatic gene alterations and environmental factors. The latter risk factors include a lack of physical activity and a high-fat, low-fiber diet.

PROSTATE CANCER. This cancer is the most commonly diagnosed cancer in men, with approximately 320,000 new cases annually in the United States. Prostate cancer is second only to lung cancer as a cause of cancer death in men, with more than 40,000 deaths each year. Having an affected first-degree relative increases the risk of developing prostate cancer by a factor of two to three. It is estimated that about 5% to 10% of prostate cancer cases are the result of inherited mutations.

The relatively late age of onset of most prostate cancer cases (median age = 72 years) makes genetic analysis especially difficult. However, an affected sib-pair analysis (see Box 12-1) has identified linked polymorphisms on chromosome 1q. Loss of heterozygosity has been observed in a number of genomic regions in prostate tumor cells, possibly indicating the presence of genetic alterations in these regions. Thus far, no inherited gene predisposing to prostate cancer has been cloned. Nongenetic risk factors may include a high-fat diet. Because prostate cancer usually progresses slowly and because it is readily diagnosed by digital examination and by the prostate-specific antigen (PSA) test, fatal metastasis can usually be prevented. www

▼ Most common cancers have genetic components. Recurrence risks tend to be higher when there are multiple affected relatives and when they have developed cancer at an early age. Specific genes have been discovered that cause inherited colon and breast cancer in some families. ▲

Diabetes Mellitus

Like the other disorders discussed in this chapter, the etiology of diabetes mellitus is complex and not fully understood. Nevertheless, progress is being made in understanding the genetic basis of this disorder, which is the leading cause of adult blindness, kidney failure, and lower-limb amputation and a major cause of heart disease and stroke. An important advance has been the recognition that diabetes is actually a heterogeneous group of disorders, all characterized by elevated blood sugar. We will focus here on the two major types of diabetes, type I (insulin-dependent diabetes mellitus, or IDDM) and type II (non–insulin-dependent diabetes mellitus, or NIDDM).

TYPE I DIABETES. This form of diabetes, which is characterized by T-cell infiltration of the pancreas and destruction of the insulin-producing cells, usually (though not always) presents before age 40. Patients with type I diabetes must receive exogenous insulin to survive. The pathology of the disorder, together with the common finding of antibodies against pancreatic cells and a strong association with several HLA Class II alleles, indicates that type I diabetes is an autoimmune disorder. Siblings of individuals with type I diabetes face a substantial elevation in risk: approximately 6%, as opposed to a risk of about 0.3% to 0.5% in the general population. The recurrence risk is also elevated when there is a diabetic parent, although this risk varies with the sex of the affected parent. The risk to offspring of diabetic mothers is only 1% to 3%, while it is 4% to 6% for the offspring of diabetic fathers (because type I diabetes affects males and females in roughly equal proportions in the general population, this risk difference is inconsistent with the sex-specific threshold model for multifactorial traits). Twin studies show that the empirical risks for identical twins of type I diabetes patients range from 30% to 50%. The fact that type I diabetes is not 100% concordant among identical twins indicates that genetic factors are not solely responsible for the disorder. There is good evidence that specific viral infections contribute to the causation of type I diabetes in at least some individuals, possibly by activating an autoimmune response. www

The association of specific HLA Class II alleles and type I diabetes has been studied extensively, and it is estimated that the HLA system accounts for about 40% of the familial clustering of type I diabetes. Approximately 95% of Caucasians with type I diabetes have the HLA DR3 and/or DR4 alleles, whereas only about 50% of the general Caucasian population has either of these alleles. If an affected proband and a sibling are both heterozygous for the DR3 and DR4 alleles, the sibling's risk of developing type I diabetes is nearly 20% (i.e., about 40 times higher than the risk in the general population). This association may reflect linkage disequilibrium between alleles of the DR locus and those of the HLA-DQ locus, in which it has been shown that the presence of aspartic acid at position 57 of the DQ chain is strongly associated with resistance to type I diabetes. In fact, those who have this amino acid at position 57 are 100 times less likely to develop the disease than are individuals homozygous for other amino acids (alanine, serine, or valine). It is probable that this particular amino acid is involved in T-cell recognition and that those who lack it are more likely to suffer an autoimmune episode.

The insulin gene, which is located on the short arm of chromosome 11, is another logical candidate for type I diabetes susceptibility. Polymorphisms within and near this gene have been tested for association with type I diabetes. Intriguingly, a strong risk association is seen with allelic variation in a VNTR polymorphism (see Chapter 3) located just 5' of the insulin gene. Differences in the number of VNTR repeat units affect transcription of the insulin gene (possibly by altering chromatin structure), resulting in variation in susceptibility. It is estimated that inherited genetic variation in the insulin region accounts for approximately 10% of the familial clustering of type I diabetes.

Affected sib-pair analysis has been used extensively to map additional genes that can cause type I diabetes. In addition, an animal model, the nonobese diabetic (NOD) mouse, has been used to identify genes that could have homologs in the human (see Box 12-1). These studies have identified at least 20 additional candidate regions that may contain type I diabetes susceptibility genes. Precise identification of such genes is made difficult by the genetic complexity of the disorder (locus heterogeneity, multifactorial background) and by the fact that genes other than insulin and HLA are likely to account for only a small proportion of the genetic susceptibility to type I diabetes. Nonetheless, their further study may aid in understanding this disease.

TYPE II DIABETES. Type II diabetes accounts for more than 90% of all diabetes cases. A number of features distinguish it from type I diabetes. Unlike type I diabetes, there is nearly always some endogenous insulin production in persons with type II diabetes, and the disease can often be treated successfully with dietary modification and/or oral drugs. Type II diabetes patients also suffer from insulin resistance (i.e., their bodies have difficulty using the insulin they produce). This disease typically occurs among people over age 40 and, in contrast to type I diabetes, is seen more commonly among the obese. Neither HLA associations nor autoantibodies are seen commonly in this form of diabetes. Monozygotic twin concordance rates are substantially higher than in type I diabetes, often exceeding 90% (because of age dependence, the concordance rate increases if older subjects are studied). The empirical recurrence risks for first-degree relatives of type II diabetes cases are higher than those for type I, generally ranging from 10% to 15%. The differences between type I and type II diabetes are summarized in Table 12-8.

Linkage studies using affected sib pairs have suggested that type II diabetes susceptibility genes may exist on 2q in a Mexican-American population and on 12q in a Finnish population. However, these results await replication in other populations, and specific genes causing type II diabetes have yet to be cloned.

The two most important risk factors for type II diabetes are positive family history and obesity; the latter increases insulin resistance. The disease tends to rise in prevalence when populations adopt a diet and exercise pattern typical of United States and European populations. Increases have been seen, for example, among Japanese immigrants to the United States and among some native populations of the South Pacific, Australia, and the Americas. Several studies, conducted on both male and female subjects, have shown that regular exercise can substantially lower one's risk of developing type II diabetes, even among individuals with a family history of the disease. This is partly because exercise reduces obesity. However, even in the absence of weight loss, exercise increases insulin sensitivity and improves glucose tolerance.

Approximately 2% to 5% of type II diabetics manifest the disease early in life, typically before 25 years of age. This subset, termed "maturity onset diabetes of the

TABLE 12-8 A Comparison of the Major Features of Type I and Type II Diabetes Mellitus

Feature	Type I diabetes	Type II diabetes
Age of onset	Usually <40 years	Usually >40 years (except MODY)
Insulin production	None	Partial
Insulin resistance	No	Yes
Autoimmunity	Yes	No
Obesity	Not common	Common
MZ twin concordance	0.35-0.50	0.90
Sibling recurrence risk	1%-6%	10%-15%

young" (MODY), can be inherited as an autosomal dominant trait. Studies of MODY pedigrees have shown that about 50% of cases are caused by mutations in the glucokinase gene. Glucokinase is a rate-limiting enzyme in the conversion of glucose to glucose-6-phosphate in the pancreas. MODY can also be caused by mutations in any of three additional genes, all of which encode transcription factors involved in pancreatic development or insulin regulation (hepatocyte nuclear factor 1-α [*HNF1 α*], hepatocyte nuclear factor 4-α [*HNF4 α*], and insulin promoter factor1 [*IPF1*]). Although none of the four MODY genes appear to play a significant role in adult-onset type II diabetes, the study of these genes and their protein products may lead to a better understanding of the pathophysiology of all forms of diabetes.

▼ **Type I (insulin dependent) and type II (non-insulin dependent) diabetes both cluster in families, with stronger familial clustering observed for type II diabetes. Type I has an earlier average age of onset, is HLA-associated, and is an autoimmune disease. Type II is not an autoimmune disorder and is more likely to be seen in obese individuals. Most cases of MODY, a subset of type II diabetes, are caused by mutations in any of four specific genes. ▲**

Obesity

Obesity is often defined as a body weight exceeding 20% of the upper limit of the normal range. Using this criterion, approximately one third of American adults are obese (one of the highest proportions in the world), and the proportion of obese adults and children continues to increase rapidly. Although obesity itself is perhaps not a "disease," it is an important risk factor for several common diseases, including heart disease, stroke, hypertension, and type II diabetes.

As one might expect, there is a strong correlation between obesity in parents and their children. This could easily be ascribed to common environmental effects: parents and children usually share similar dietary and exercise habits. Indeed, it may seem that obesity should be influenced almost exclusively by environmental factors. However, there is good evidence for genetic components as well. Four different adoption studies each showed that the body weights of adopted individuals correlated significantly with their natural parents' body weights but not with those of their adoptive parents. Twin studies also provide evidence for a genetic effect on body weight, with most studies yielding heritability estimates between 0.60 and 0.80.

Recent research has revealed several genes that each play a role in human obesity. This research has been aided substantially by mouse models, in which there are at least five genes that can cause monogenic obesity. Important among these are the genes that encode leptin (Greek, "thin") and its receptor. The leptin hormone is secreted by adipocytes (fat storage cells); increased fat stores lead to increased circulating leptin. Normally, leptin binds to a receptor in the hypothalamus, the site of the body's appetite control center. Higher levels of leptin, sensed by receptors in the hypothalamus, lead to satiety and a loss of appetite; lower levels lead to increased appetite. Mice with loss-of-function mutations in the leptin gene have uncontrolled appetites and become obese. When injected with leptin hormone, these mice lose weight. Mice with mutations in the leptin receptor gene cannot respond to increased leptin levels and also develop obesity.

Cloning of the human homologs of the leptin gene and its receptor led to optimistic predictions that leptin could be a key to weight loss in humans (without the perceived unpleasantness of dieting and exercise). However, most obese humans have high levels of leptin, indicating that the leptin gene is functioning normally. Leptin receptor defects were then suspected, but these are also uncommon in humans. Although mutations in the human leptin gene and its receptor have now been identified in humans with morbid obesity,* they both appear to be extremely rare. Unfortunately, these genes will not solve the problem of human obesity. However, the gene products participate in important interactions with other components of appetite control, such as neuropeptide Y and the melanocortin-4 receptor. Identification of these human genes is thus leading to a better understanding of natural weight control in the human, and it could eventually lead to effective treatments for some cases of obesity.

▼ **Adoption and twin studies indicate that at least half of the population variation in obesity may be caused by genes. Specific genes and gene products involved in appetite control and susceptibility to obesity, including leptin and its receptor, are now being identified. ▲**

Alzheimer Disease

It is estimated that Alzheimer disease (AD) affects approximately 10% of Americans over age 65 and up to half of those over age 85. The cost of caring for AD patients exceeds $40 billion annually. This disorder is characterized by progressive dementia and loss of memory and by the formation of amyloid plaques and neurofibrillary tangles in the brain, particularly in the cerebral cortex and hippocampus. Death usually occurs within 5 to 10 years after the first appearance of symptoms. The risk of developing AD doubles in individuals who have an affected first-degree relative. Although

---

*Morbid obesity is typically defined as a weight exceeding 100 pounds above the upper limit of normal. The individuals identified with leptin gene mutations were extremely obese: more than 55% of their body weight consisted of fat.

most cases of AD do not appear to be caused by single loci, 10% to 15% follow an autosomal dominant mode of transmission. Early-onset AD (before age 60 to 65) accounts for about 10% of AD cases and is much more likely to be inherited in autosomal dominant fashion. **www**

AD is a genetically heterogeneous disorder. Approximately half of early-onset cases can be attributed to mutations in any of three genes, all of which affect amyloid-beta deposition. Two of the genes, *presenilin 1* on chromosome 14 and *presenilin 2* on chromosome 1, are very similar to one another, and their protein products appear to be involved in cleavage of the amyloid precursor protein (posttranslational modification; see Chapter 2). When the protein is not cleaved normally, a long form of it accumulates and is deposited in the brain. This is thought to be a primary cause of AD. A small number of cases of early-onset AD are caused by mutations of the amyloid precursor protein gene itself, located on chromosome 21. These mutations disrupt normal cleavage sites in the protein, again leading to the accumulation of an abnormal protein product. It is interesting that this gene is present in three copies in trisomy 21 individuals, where the extra gene copy is likely to lead to amyloid deposition and the occurrence of AD in Down syndrome patients (see Chapter 6).

An important risk factor for the more common late-onset form of AD is allelic variation in the apolipoprotein E (*APOE*) locus. Many studies conducted in diverse populations have shown that the *APOE4* allele confers increased risk for AD, while the *APOE2* allele has a protective effect. One study showed that, among individuals who are members of late-onset AD families, those who inherit two copies of the *E4* allele had a 90% chance of developing the disease by age 75. Those who inherited one copy of *E4* had a 45% chance, and those who inherited no copies of the allele had only a 20% chance of developing AD (note that, because the study population consisted of families with multiple affected members, the risk estimates for these genotypes do not necessarily apply to the general population). This association is especially interesting because the *E4* protein product binds more rapidly to amyloid protein than does the product of the more common *E3* allele and may thus alter the processing of the amyloid protein. Recently, a genome scan provided evidence for a gene on chromosome 12 that may increase susceptibility to late-onset AD.

AD has several features that make it refractory to genetic analysis. Its genetic heterogeneity has already been described. In addition, because a definitive diagnosis can be obtained only by a brain autopsy, it is difficult to diagnose living family members (although clinical features and brain imaging studies can provide strong evidence that an individual is affected with AD). Finally, because onset of the disease can occur very late in life, individuals carrying a gene for AD could die from an-

other cause before developing the disease. These individuals would then be misdiagnosed as non-carriers. These types of difficulties arise not only in studying AD but in many other common adult diseases as well. Despite these obstacles, further studies of the genes linked to AD will shed light not only on the most common cause of dementia among the elderly, but also on the aging process in general.

▼ **Approximately 10% to 15% of AD cases are caused by autosomal dominant genes. Early-onset cases cluster more strongly in families and are more likely to follow an autosomal dominant inheritance pattern. This disease is genetically heterogeneous: AD susceptibility genes have been identified on chromosomes 1, 14, 19, and 21. All three of the genes that cause early-onset AD affect the cleavage and processing of the amyloid precursor protein.** ▲

Alcoholism

At some point in their lives, alcoholism is diagnosed in approximately 10% of adult males and 3% to 5% of adult females in America. The national cost of alcoholism, in terms of lost productivity and direct medical costs, exceeds $100 billion per year. More than 100 studies have shown that this disease clusters in families. The risk of developing alcoholism among individuals with one affected parent is three to five times higher than for those with unaffected parents. Most twin studies have yielded concordance rates for DZ twins less than 30% and concordance rates for MZ twins in excess of 60%. Adoption studies have shown that the offspring of an alcoholic parent, even when raised by non-alcoholic parents, have a four-fold increased risk of developing the disorder. To control for possible prenatal effects in an alcoholic mother, some studies have included the offspring of alcoholic fathers only. The results have remained the same. One study showed that the offspring of non-alcoholic parents, when reared by alcoholics, did *not* have an increased risk of developing alcoholism. These data argue that there may be genes that predispose some people to alcoholism.

Some researchers distinguish two major subtypes of alcoholism. Type I is characterized by a later age of onset (after age 25), occurrence in both males and females, and greater psychological dependency on alcohol. Type I alcoholics are more likely to be introverted, solitary drinkers. This form of alcoholism is less likely to cluster in families (one study yielded a heritability estimate of 0.21), has a less severe course, and is more easily treated. Type II alcoholism is seen predominantly in males, typically occurs before age 25, and tends to involve individuals who are extroverted and thrill-seeking. This form is more difficult to treat successfully and tends to cluster much more strongly in families, with one study obtaining a heritability estimate of 0.88.

Evidence has been published for an association between alcoholism and a DNA polymorphism linked to the dopamine D2 receptor gene on chromosome 11q. Since the dopamine receptors are part of the brain's reward pathway, this association has some intuitive appeal. However, at least seven additional studies in multiple populations have failed to replicate the association. The inability to replicate this finding reflects some of the difficulties encountered in population association studies (see Chapter 8). It now appears unlikely that this polymorphism contributes importantly to alcoholism susceptibility. Nevertheless, the twin and adoption studies mentioned previously are compelling, and it is quite possible that further studies may reveal genes that do in fact influence susceptibility to this important disease.

It should be underscored that we refer to genes that may increase one's *susceptibility* to alcoholism. This is obviously a disease that requires an environmental component, regardless of one's genetic constitution.

▼ Twin and adoption studies show that alcoholism clusters quite strongly in families, reflecting a possible genetic contribution to this disease. Familial clustering is particularly strong for type II alcoholism (early-onset form primarily affecting males). ▲

Psychiatric Disorders

The major psychiatric diseases, schizophrenia and bipolar affective disorder, have both been the subjects of numerous genetic studies. Twin, adoption, and family studies have shown that both disorders aggregate in families.

SCHIZOPHRENIA. Schizophrenia is a severe emotional disorder characterized by delusions, hallucinations, retreat from reality, and bizarre, withdrawn, or inappropriate behavior (contrary to popular belief, schizophrenia is not a "split personality" disorder). The lifetime recurrence risk for schizophrenia among the offspring of one affected parent is approximately 8% to 10%, which is about 10 times higher than the risk in the general population. As one might expect, the empirical risks increase when more relatives are affected. For example, an individual with an affected sibling and an affected parent has a risk of about 17%, and an individual with two affected parents has a risk of 40% to 50%. The risks decrease when the affected family member is a second- or third-degree relative. Details are given in Table 12-9. On inspection of this table, it may seem puzzling that the proportion of schizophrenic probands who have a schizophrenic parent is only about 5%, which is substantially lower than the risk for other first-degree relatives (e.g., siblings, affected parents, and their offspring). This can be explained by the fact that schiz-

ophrenics are less likely to marry and produce children than are other individuals. There is thus substantial selection against schizophrenia in the population.

Twin and adoption studies indicate that genetic factors are likely to be involved in schizophrenia. Data pooled from five different twin studies show a 47% concordance rate for MZ twins, compared with a concordance rate of only 12% for DZ twins. When the offspring of a schizophrenic parent are adopted by normal parents, their risk of developing the disease is about 10%, which is approximately the same as the risk when raised by a schizophrenic biological parent.

Many linkage studies have been performed to locate genes that may contribute to schizophrenia. Although a number of chromosome regions have been tentatively identified as the possible locations of schizophrenia genes, no specific genes have yet been cloned.

BIPOLAR AFFECTIVE DISORDER. Bipolar affective disorder, also known as manic-depressive disorder, is a form of psychosis in which extreme mood swings and emotional instability are seen. The prevalence of the disorder in the general population is approximately 0.5%, but it rises to 5% to 10% among those with an affected first-degree relative. A study based on the Danish twin registry yielded concordance rates of 79% and 24% for MZ and DZ twins, respectively. The corresponding concordance rates for unipolar disorder (major depression) were 54% and 19%. Thus, it appears that bipolar disorder is more strongly influenced by genetic factors than is unipolar disorder.

As with schizophrenia, many linkage studies have been carried out to identify genes contributing to bipolar affective disorder. Considerable excitement was generated some years ago by a report linking the disorder to a polymorphism on chromosome 11p. This study examined a series of Old Order Amish families in which the disorder is transmitted in autosomal dominant fashion. As discussed in Box 12-1, the use of an isolated population such as this one should increase the likelihood of identifying a single causative gene. Linkage

TABLE 12-9 Recurrence Risks for Relatives of Schizophrenic Probands

Relationship to proband	Recurrence risk (%)
Monozygotic twin	44.3
Dizygotic twin	12.1
Offspring	9.4
Sibling	7.3
Niece/nephew	2.7
Grandchild	2.8
First cousin	1.6
Spouse	1.0

Modified from McGue M et al. (1986) Behav. Genet. 16:75-87.
Figures are based on multiple studies of Western European populations.

analysis initially yielded a LOD score (see Chapter 8) of 4.0. However, the result was later reversed with the addition of another branch of the pedigree and when two initially unaffected family members, who did not carry the marker allele segregating with the disorder, subsequently developed the disorder. This demonstrates the sensitivity of linkage analysis to changes in disease status. Many additional families have been studied since, and the LOD score eventually dropped to -9.0 (i.e., the odds are 1 billion to one *against* linkage to the chromosome 11 marker).

COMMENTS ON PSYCHIATRIC DISORDERS. Large-scale linkage studies involving hundreds of polymorphisms throughout the genome have now been carried out for both schizophrenia and bipolar affective disorder. Although a number of promising regions have been identified, no specific genes have yet been pinpointed. In addition, a number of candidate genes have been tested for linkage or association with both diseases. Most of these candidates were chosen on the basis of the known involvement of certain neurotransmitters, receptors, or neurotransmitter-related enzymes in each disease (e.g., schizophrenia can be treated by drugs that block dopamine receptors, and bipolar affective disorder is sometimes treated with lithium). None of the candidate genes tested thus far, including those for sodium-lithium countertransport, various components of the dopaminergic system, and several neurotransmitter-related enzymes (such as monoamine oxidase, dopamine-β-hydroxylase, and tyrosine hydroxylase), has been shown unequivocally to be linked or associated with either disease.

These results reveal some of the difficulties encountered in doing genetic studies of psychiatric disorders. These diseases are undoubtedly heterogeneous, reflecting the influence of numerous genetic and environmental factors. Also, definition of the phenotype is not always straightforward, and it may change through time. As the bipolar affective disorder linkage story shows, this can be critical. As genetic studies are initiated on traits that are even more ambiguous in their definition (e.g., "criminality"), such difficulties are likely to be magnified even further.

▼ **Marked familial aggregation has been observed for schizophrenia and bipolar affective disorder. Genes for neurotransmitters, receptors, and neurotransmitter-related enzymes have been studied in families, and linkage studies with hundreds of random markers have been carried out. No specific genes predisposing to these diseases have yet been identified.** ▲

Other Complex Disorders

The disorders discussed in this chapter represent some of the most common multifactorial disorders and those for which significant progress has been made in identifying genes. Many other multifactorial disorders are being studied as well, and in some cases specific susceptibility genes have been identified. These include, for example, Parkinson disease, hearing loss, multiple sclerosis, epilepsy, and some forms of blindness.

Some General Principles and Conclusions

Some general principles can be deduced from the results obtained thus far on the genetics of complex disorders. First, the more strongly inherited forms of complex disorders generally have an earlier age of onset (examples include breast cancer, Alzheimer disease, and heart disease). Often, these represent subsets of cases in which there is single-gene inheritance. Second, when there is laterality, bilateral forms sometimes cluster more strongly in families (e.g., cleft lip/palate). Third, while the sex-specific threshold model fits some of the complex disorders (e.g., pyloric stenosis, cleft lip/palate, autism, heart disease), it fails to fit others (e.g., type I diabetes).

There is a tendency, particularly among the lay public, to assume that the presence of a genetic component means that the course of a disease cannot be altered ("if it's genetic, you can't change it"). This is incorrect. Most of the diseases discussed in this chapter have both genetic and environmental components. Thus, environmental modification (e.g., diet, exercise, stress reduction) can often reduce risk significantly. Such modification may be especially important for individuals with a family history of a disease because they are likely to develop the disease earlier in life. Those with a family history of heart disease, for example, can often add many years of productive living with relatively minor lifestyle alterations. By targeting those who can benefit most from intervention, genetics helps to serve the goal of preventive medicine.

In addition, it should be stressed that the identification of a specific genetic lesion can lead to more effective prevention and treatment of the disease. Identification of mutations causing familial colon cancer may enable early screening and prevention of metastasis. Pinpointing a gene responsible for a neurotransmitter defect in a behavioral disorder such as schizophrenia could lead to the development of more effective drug treatments. In some cases, such as familial hypercholesterolemia, gene therapy may be useful. It is important for health care practitioners to make their patients aware of these facts.

While the genetics of common disorders is complex and often confusing, the public health impact of these diseases and the evidence for hereditary factors in their etiology demand that genetic studies be pursued. Substantial progress is already being made. The next decade will undoubtedly witness many further advancements in our understanding and treatment of these disorders.

STUDY QUESTIONS

1. Consider a multifactorial trait that is twice as common in females as in males. Indicate which type of mating is at higher risk for producing affected children (affected father and normal mother versus normal father and affected mother). Is the recurrence risk higher for their *sons* or their *daughters*?

2. Consider a disease that is known to have a 5% sibling recurrence risk. This recurrence risk could be the result of either multifactorial inheritance or a single autosomal dominant gene with 10% penetrance. How would you test which of these possibilities is correct?

3. One member of a pair of monozygotic twins is affected by an autosomal dominant disease, whereas the other member of the pair is not. List two different ways in which this could happen.

4. Suppose that the heritability of body fat is 0.80 when correlations between siblings are studied, but it is only 0.50 when correlations between parents and offspring are studied. Suppose also that a significant positive correlation is observed in the body fat measurements of spouses. How would you interpret these results?

SUGGESTED READINGS

Ackerman MJ (1998) The long QT syndrome: ion channel diseases of the heart. Mayo Clin. Proc. 73:250-269

Baron M (1997) Genes and manic depression. Psychiatr. Genet. 7:49-51

Blacker D, Tanzi RE (1998) The genetics of Alzheimer disease: current status and future prospects. Arch. Neurol. 55:294-296

Boerwinkle E, Ellsworth DL, Hallman DM, Biddinger A (1996) Genetic analysis of atherosclerosis: a research paradigm for the common chronic diseases. Hum. Molec. Genet. 5:1405-1410

Cavalli-Sforza LL, Bodmer WF (1971) The Genetics of Human Populations. W.H. Freeman, San Francisco

Comuzzie AG, Allison DB (1998) The search for human obesity genes. Science 280:1374-1377

Corcoran J (1998) What are the molecular mechanisms of neural tube defects? BioEssays 20:6-8

Darvasi A (1998) Experimental strategies for the genetic dissection of complex traits in animal models. Nature Genet. 18:19-23

Flier JS, Maratos-Flier E (1998) Obesity and the hypothalamus: novel peptides for new pathways. Cell 92:437-440

Ghosh S, Collins FS (1996) The geneticist's approach to complex disease. Ann. Rev. Med. 47:333-353

Hall JG (1996) Twins and twinning. Am. J. Med. Genet. 61:202-204

Hardy J (1997) The Alzheimer family of diseases: many etiologies, one pathogenesis? Proc. Natl. Acad. Sci. USA 94:2095-2097

Hattersley AT (1998) Maturity-onset diabetes of the young: clinical heterogeneity explained by genetic heterogeneity. Diabet. Med. 15:15-24

Hutton M, Hardy J (1997) The presenilins and Alzheimer's disease. Hum. Mol. Genet. 6:1639-1646

Julier C, Hashimoto L, Lathrop GM (1996) Genetics of insulin-dependent diabetes mellitus. Curr. Opin. Genet. Dev. 6:354-360

Kahn BB (1998) Type 2 diabetes: when insulin secretion fails to compensate for insulin resistance. Cell 92:593-596

Keating MT, Sanguinetti MC (1996) Molecular genetic insights into cardiovascular disease. Science 272:681-685

King RA, Rotter JI, Motulsky AG (1992) The Genetic Basis of Common Diseases. Oxford University Press, Oxford

Lifton RP (1996) Molecular genetics of human blood pressure variation. Science 272:676-680

Martin N, Boomsma D, Machin G (1997) A twin-pronged attack on complex traits. Nature Genet. 17:387-392

Mitchell LE (1997) Genetic epidemiology of birth defects: nonsyndromic cleft lip and neural tube defects. Epidemiol. Rev. 19:61-68

Moldin SO (1997) The maddening hunt for madness genes. Nature Genet. 17:127-129

Naggert J, Harris T, North M (1997) The genetics of obesity. Curr. Opin. Genet. Dev. 7:398-404

Neale MC, Cardon LR (1992) Methodology for Genetic Studies of Twins and Families. Kluwer Academic Publishers, Dordrecht, The Netherlands

Perera FP (1997) Environment and cancer: who are susceptible? Science 278:1068-1073

Plomin R, Craig I (1997) Human behavioral genetics of cognitive abilities and disabilities. BioEssays 19:1117-1124

Risch N, Merikangas K (1996) The future of genetic studies of complex human diseases. Science 273:1516-1517

Rutter M, Plomin R (1997) Opportunities for psychiatry from genetic findings. Br. J. Psychiatry 171:209-219

Sherman SL, DeFries JC, Gottesman II, Loehlin JC, Meyer JM, Pelias MZ, Rice J, et al (1997) Behavioral genetics '97: ASHG statement. Recent developments in human behavioral genetics: past accomplishments and future directions. Am. J. Hum. Genet. 60:1265-1275

13

Genetic Screening, Genetic Diagnosis, and Gene Therapy

As we have seen in previous chapters, significant advances have occurred in DNA technology, gene mapping and cloning, cytogenetics, and many other areas of medical genetics. These developments have paved the way for more accurate and efficient diagnosis of genetic disorders. In particular, population screening and prenatal diagnosis of genetic disorders are becoming increasingly widespread. The principles and applications of genetic diagnosis in these contexts are one focus of this chapter.

Another focus is the treatment of genetic disease. Many aspects of disease management involve areas of medicine, such as surgery and drug treatment, that are beyond the scope of this book. However, gene therapy, in which patients' cells are genetically altered to combat specific diseases, falls well within the purview of this text and will be discussed in some detail.

POPULATION SCREENING FOR GENETIC DISEASE

Screening tests represent an important component of routine health care. These tests are usually designed to detect treatable human diseases in their presymptomatic stage. Pap tests for the recognition of cervical dysplasia and population screening for hypercholesterolemia are well-known examples of this public health strategy. **Population screening** has been defined as "the presumptive identification of an unrecognized disease or defect by the application of tests, examinations, or other procedures which can be applied rapidly to sort out apparently well persons who *probably* have a disease from those who *probably do not*" (Mausner and Bahn, 1974). Screening tests are *not* intended to provide definitive diagnoses but rather are aimed at identifying a subset of the population on whom further diagnostic tests should be carried out.

Genetic screening is defined as the "search in a population for persons possessing certain genotypes that: (1) are already associated with disease or predisposition to disease, or (2) may lead to disease in their descendants" (National Academy of Sciences, 1975). Newborn screening for inherited metabolic diseases is a good example of the first type of genetic screening, and heterozygote detection for Tay-Sachs disease (discussed later) exemplifies the second. While these two examples involve screening of populations, genetic screening can also be applied to members of families that have a positive history of a genetic condition. An example would be testing for a balanced reciprocal translocation in families in which one or more members have had a chromosome disorder (see Chapter 6). Box 13-1 lists the various types of genetic screening, including several forms of prenatal diagnosis, that are discussed in this chapter.

▼ The goal of screening is early recognition of a disorder so that intervention will prevent or reverse the disease process (as in newborn screening for inborn errors of metabolism) or so that informed reproductive decisions can be made (as in the prenatal diagnosis of congenital malformations). ▲

Principles of Screening

The basic principles of screening were developed in the 1960s and are still widely applied. The following points should be considered when deciding whether population screening is appropriate:

1. *Disease characteristics.* The condition should be serious and relatively common. This ensures that the benefits to be derived from the screening program will justify its costs. The natural history of the disease should be clearly understood. There should be an acceptable and effective treatment or, in the case of

3. *System characteristics.* The resources for diagnosis and treatment of the disorder must be accessible. A strategy for communicating results efficiently and effectively must be in place.

As summarized in Clinical Commentary 13-1, the phenylketonuria (PKU) screening program meets these criteria quite well.

Screening programs typically use tests that are widely applicable and inexpensive in order to identify an at-risk population. Members of this population are then targeted for subsequent tests that are more accurate but also more expensive and time consuming. In this context, the **validity** of a screening test deserves emphasis. Validity refers to the ability of a test to separate individuals who have the disease from those who do not. It involves two components: sensitivity and specificity. **Sensitivity** is defined as the ability to correctly identify those *with* the disease. It is measured as the proportion of affected individuals in whom the test is positive (i.e., **true positives**). **Specificity** is the ability to correctly identify those *without* the disease. It is measured as the proportion of unaffected individuals in whom the test is negative (i.e., **true negatives**). Sensitivity and specificity are determined by comparing the screening results with those of a definitive diagnostic test (Table 13-1).

Screening tests are seldom, if ever, 100% sensitive and 100% specific. This is because the range of test values in the disease population overlaps that of the unaffected population (Fig. 13-1). Thus, a screening test (as opposed to the definitive follow-up diagnostic test) will diagnose some members of the population incorrectly. Usually a cutoff value for separating the diseased and non-diseased portions of the population is designated. A balance exists between the impact of non-detection or low sensitivity (i.e., an increased **false-negative** rate) versus low specificity (an increased **false-positive** rate). If the penalty for missing affected individuals is high (as in untreated PKU), then the cutoff level is lowered so that nearly all disease cases will be detected (higher sensitivity). This also increases the number of non-disease cases (lower specificity) targeted for subsequent diagnosis. If confirmation of a positive test is expensive and/or hazardous, then false-positive rates are minimized (i.e., the cutoff level is increased, producing high specificity at the expense of sensitivity).

▼ The basic elements of a test's validity include its sensitivity (proportion of true positives detected) and specificity (proportion of true negatives detected). When sensitivity is increased, specificity decreases, and vice versa. ▲

A primary concern in the clinical setting is the accuracy of a positive screening test. One needs to know the proportion of persons with a positive test who truly have the disease in question (i.e., $a/(a+b)$ in Table 13-1).

some genetic conditions, prenatal diagnosis should be available.

2. *Test characteristics.* The screening test should be acceptable to the population, easy to perform, and relatively inexpensive. The screening test should be valid and reliable.

CLINICAL COMMENTARY 13-1
NEONATAL SCREENING FOR PHENYLKETONURIA

DISEASE CHARACTERISTICS

Population screening of newborns for phenylketonuria (PKU) represents the best example of the application of the screening model to genetic disease. As discussed in Chapter 4, the prevalence of this autosomal recessive disorder of phenylalanine metabolism is about 1 in 10,000 to 15,000 Caucasian births. The natural history of PKU is well understood. More than 95% of untreated PKU patients become moderately to severely mentally retarded. The condition is not identified clinically in the first year of life, as the physical signs are subtle and PKU usually manifests only as developmental delay. Dietary restriction of phenylalanine, when begun before 4 weeks of age, is highly effective in altering the course of the disease. Virtually all individuals with classical PKU will have normal intelligence when treated (an important exception is those who have a defect in biopterin metabolism and in whom a different therapy is used). The diet, while not particularly palatable, is effective in treating the disease.

SCREENING CHARACTERISTICS

PKU is detected by the measurement of blood phenylalanine using a bacterial inhibition assay, the Guthrie test. Blood is collected in the newborn period, usually by heel stick, and placed on filter paper. The dried blood is placed on an agar plate and incubated with a bacterial strain (*Bacillus subtilis*) that requires phenylalanine for growth. Measurement of bacterial growth permits quantification of the amount of phenylalanine in the blood sample. Positive test results are usually repeated and followed by a quantitative assay of plasma phenylalanine and tyrosine.

If the test is performed after 2 days of age and after regular feeding on a protein diet, the detection rate (sensitivity) is about 98%. If performed at less than 24 hours of age, the sensitivity is about 84%. Thus, early discharge from the nursery requires a repeat test a few weeks after birth. Specificity is close to 100%.

SYSTEM CHARACTERISTICS

Because of the requirement of normal protein in the diet, many states request rescreening at 2 to 4 weeks of age. At that point, sensitivity approaches 100%. Because of the impact of a misdiagnosis, a high sensitivity level is desirable.

Phenylalanine levels in children with classical PKU typically exceed 20 mg/dl. For every 20 positive PKU screens, only one infant will have classical PKU. The others will either be false positives (usually due to a transient reversible tyrosinemia) or will have a form of hyperphenylalaninemia (elevated phenylalanine) not due to classical PKU.

The cost of a Guthrie test is about $1.25. Several studies have shown that the cost of nationwide PKU screening is significantly less than the savings it achieves by avoiding institutionalization costs and lost productivity.

TABLE 13-1 Definitions of Sensitivity and Specificity*

Screening test	Disease state	
	Affected	Unaffected
Results positive (+)	a (true positive)	b (false positive)
Results negative (−)	c (false negative)	d (true negative)

*Sensitivity = a/(a+c); specificity = d/(b+d).

This quantity is defined as the **positive predictive value.**

The concepts of sensitivity, specificity, and positive predictive value can be illustrated by an example. Congenital adrenal hyperplasia (CAH) due to a deficiency of 21 hydroxylase is an inborn error of steroid biosynthesis that may produce ambiguous genitalia in females and adrenal crises in males and females. The screening test, a 17-hydroxyprogesterone assay, has a sensitivity of about 95% and a specificity of 99% (Table 13-2). The prevalence of CAH is about 1/10,000 in most Caucasian populations but rises to about 1/400 in the Yupik Eskimo population. www

Let us assume that a screening program for CAH has been developed in both of these populations. In a population of 500,000 Caucasians, the false positive rate (1 − specificity) is 1%. Thus, about 5,000 normal individuals will have a positive test. With 95% sensitivity, 47 of the 50 individuals who have CAH will be detected through a positive test. Note that the great majority of people who have a positive test result would *not* have CAH: the positive predictive value is 47/(47 + 5,000), or less than 1%. Suppose that 10,000 members of the Yupik population are screened for CAH. As Table 13-2 shows, 24 of 25 individuals with CAH will test positive, and 100 without CAH will test positive. Here, the positive predictive value is much higher than in Caucasians: 24/(24 + 100) = 19%. This example illustrates an important principle: *the positive predictive value of a test increases as the prevalence of the disease increases.*

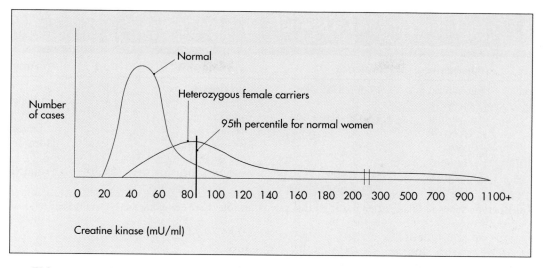

FIG. 13-1 The distribution of creatine kinase (CK) in normal women and in women who are heterozygous carriers for a mutation in the Duchenne muscular dystrophy gene. Note the overlap in distribution between the two groups: about two thirds of carriers have CK levels that exceed the 95th percentile in normal women. If the 95th percentile is used as a cutoff to identify carriers, then the sensitivity of the test is 67% (i.e., two thirds of carriers will be detected), and the specificity is 95% (95% of normal women will be correctly identified).

TABLE 13-2 Hypothetical Results of Screening for Congenital Adrenal Hyperplasia in a Low-Prevalence Caucasian Population and a High-Prevalence Yupik Population*

Screening test	CAH present		CAH absent	
	Positive	Negative	Positive	Negative
Caucasian	47	3	5,000	494,950
Yupik	24	1	100	9,875

*Caucasian positive predictive value = 47/(47 + 5,000) = 1%.
Yupik positive predictive value = 24/(24 + 100) = 19%.

▼ The positive predictive value of a screening test is defined as the proportion of positive tests that are true positives. It increases as the prevalence of the target disorder increases. ▲

Newborn Screening

Newborn screening programs represent an ideal opportunity for presymptomatic detection and prevention of genetic disease. At present, all states in the United States screen newborns for PKU, galactosemia (see Chapter 7), and hypothyroidism. All of these conditions fulfill the previously stated criteria for population screening. Each is a disorder in which the individual is at significant risk

for mental retardation, which can be prevented by early detection and effective intervention.

In recent years, many parts of the United States and other nations have instituted screening programs to identify neonates with hemoglobin disorders (e.g., sickle cell disease). These programs are justified by the fact that up to 15% of children with sickle cell disease will die from infections before age 5 (see Chapter 3). Effective treatment, in the form of prophylactic antibiotics, is available.

Some communities have begun screening for Duchenne muscular dystrophy (DMD) by measuring creatine kinase levels in newborns. The objective is not presymptomatic treatment; rather it is identification of families who should receive genetic counseling in order to make informed reproductive decisions. Conditions for which newborn screening is commonly performed are summarized in Table 13-3.

▼ Newborn screening is an effective public health strategy for treatable disorders such as PKU, hypothyroidism, galactosemia, and sickle cell disease. ▲

Heterozygote Screening

The aforementioned principles of population screening can be applied to the detection of unaffected carriers of disease-causing genes. The target population is a group known to be at risk. The "intervention" consists of the

TABLE 13-3   Characteristics of Selected Newborn Screening Programs

Disease	Inheritance	Prevalence	Screening Test	Cost	Treatment
Phenylketonuria	Autosomal recessive	1/10,000-1/15,000	Guthrie test	$1.25	Dietary restriction of phenylalanine
Galactosemia	Autosomal recessive	1/50,000-1/100,000	Transferase assay	$1.00	Dietary restriction of galactose
Congenital hypothyroidism	Usually sporadic	1/5,000	Measurement of T4 or TSH	$1.50	Hormone replacement
Sickle cell disease	Autosomal recessive	1/400-1/600 African-Americans	Isoelectric focusing or DNA diagnosis	$1.50	Prophylactic penicillin

Modified from American Academy of Pediatrics Committee on Genetics. (1989) Newborn Screening Fact Sheets. Pediatrics 83:449-464.

presentation of risk figures and the option of prenatal diagnosis. Genetic diseases amenable to heterozygote screening are typically autosomal recessive disorders for which prenatal diagnosis and genetic counseling are available, feasible, and accurate.

An example of a highly successful heterozygote screening effort is the Tay-Sachs screening program in North America. Infantile Tay-Sachs disease is an autosomal recessive lysosomal storage disorder in which the lysosomal enzyme β-hexosaminidase A (HEX A) is deficient (see Chapter 7). This causes a buildup of the substrate, GM_2 ganglioside, in neuronal lysosomes. The accumulation of this substrate damages the neurons and leads to blindness, seizures, hypotonia and death by about the age of 5. **www**

Tay-Sachs disease is especially common among Ashkenazi Jews, with a heterozygote frequency of about 1 in 30. Thus, this population is a reasonable candidate for heterozygote screening. Accurate carrier testing is available (assays for HEX A or, in some populations, direct testing for mutations). Because the disease is uniformly fatal, options such as pregnancy termination or artificial insemination by non-carrier donors are acceptable to most couples. A well-planned effort was made to educate members of the target population about risks, testing, and available options. As a result of screening, the number of Tay-Sachs disease births in the United States and Canada has declined by 90%, from 40 to 50 per year before 1970 to 3 to 5 per year in the 1990s.

Cystic fibrosis is another autosomal recessive disorder for which carrier screening is possible. However, the relative costs and benefits of such a screening program are less clear-cut than those of Tay-Sachs disease (Clinical Commentary 13-2). Table 13-4 presents a list of selected conditions in which heterozygote screening programs have been developed in industrial countries.

In addition to the criteria for establishing a population screening program for genetic disorders, guidelines have been developed regarding the ethical and legal aspects of heterozygote screening programs. These are summarized in Box 13-2.

▼ Heterozygote screening consists of testing (at the phenotype or genotype level) a target population to identify unaffected carriers of a disease gene. The carriers can then be given information about risks and reproductive options. ▲

Presymptomatic Diagnosis

With the development of genetic diagnosis through linkage analysis and direct mutation detection, presymptomatic diagnosis has become feasible for some genetic diseases. Individuals known to be at risk for a disorder can be tested to determine whether they have inherited a disease-causing mutation before they develop clinical symptoms of the disorder. Presymptomatic diagnosis is available, for example, for Huntington disease, adult polycystic kidney disease, hemochromatosis, and autosomal dominant breast cancer. By informing individuals that they do or do not carry a disease-causing gene, presymptomatic diagnosis can aid in making reproductive decisions. It can provide reassurance to those who learn that they do not carry a disease-causing gene. In some cases, early diagnosis may improve health supervision. For example, persons who inherit an autosomal dominant breast cancer gene can undergo mammography at an earlier age to detect a tumor while it is still small. Those who inherit genes that cause some forms of familial colon cancer (APC and HNPCC; see Chapter 11) can also benefit from early diagnosis and treatment.

Because most genetic diseases are relatively uncommon in the general population, universal presymptomatic screening is currently impractical. It is usually recommended only for individuals who are known to be at risk for the disease, generally because of a positive family history.

CLINICAL COMMENTARY 13-2
POPULATION SCREENING FOR CYSTIC FIBROSIS

There are now more than 700 known cystic fibrosis-causing mutations at the CFTR locus. Clearly, it would be technologically impractical to test for all of them in a population carrier screening program. However, among the mutations that can cause cystic fibrosis in Caucasians, about 70% are the three-base deletion termed ΔF508 (see Chapter 4). Carrier screening using PCR-based detection of this mutation alone would detect approximately 90% of Caucasian couples in which one or both members of the couple are heterozygous carriers of this mutation ($1-0.30^2$, where 0.30^2 represents the frequency of carrier couples in which *neither* member of the couple carries the ΔF508 mutation). It is now common to test simultaneously for the 12 mutations that are most common in Caucasian populations. This will detect approximately 90% of CFTR mutations. Then, 99% of couples would be recognized in which one or both members carry a CF mutation (i.e., $1-0.10^2$), yielding a high level of sensitivity.

These carriers would define a subset of the population in which prenatal diagnosis for CF might be offered. Given the CF heterozygote frequency of about 1/25 (see Chapter 4), only about one in every 600 couples would consist of two heterozygotes ($1/25^2$). Only some of these couples would produce a child affected with cystic fibrosis. Considering the cost of these tests and the large number of tests required to identify one affected fetus, it has been estimated that the cost of identifying an affected fetus through carrier screening would be about $1,000,000.

Moreover, an enormous amount of counseling time would be required to explain the complexities of these results to the at-risk families identified by screening (in this context, it is important that one study of the parents of children with CF showed that only 64% could accurately state the recurrence risk for their future children). It is estimated that *half* of all board-certified geneticists and genetic counselors in the United States would have to devote all of their time to CF screening in order to meet this need. Obviously this is impractical.

For these reasons, the professional community does not recommend general population screening for CF. Carrier screening is appropriate for individuals with a positive family history of CF or for couples in which one member is a known carrier. Screening for couples planning a pregnancy has been recommended by some bodies (see NIH Consensus Statement, 1997), but this recommendation remains controversial.

TABLE 13-4 Selected Examples of Heterozygote Screening Programs in Specific Ethnic Groups

Disease	Ethnic group	Carrier frequency	At-risk couple frequency	Disease incidence in newborns
Sickle-cell disease	African-Americans	1/12	1/150	1/600
Tay-Sachs disease	Ashkenazi Jews	1/30	1/900	1/3,600
β-Thalassemia	Greeks, Italians	1/30	1/900	1/3,600
α-Thalassemia	Southeast Asians and Chinese	1/25	1/625	1/2,500
Cystic fibrosis	Northern Europeans	1/25	1/625	1/2,500

Modified from McGinniss MJ, Kaback MM (1997) Carrier screening. In Rimoin DL, Connor JM, Pyeritz RE (eds.) Emery and Rimoin's Principles and Practice of Medical Genetics, Churchill Livingstone, New York, pp. 535-543.

▼ Genetic testing can sometimes be performed to identify individuals who have inherited a disease-causing gene before they develop symptoms. This is termed "presymptomatic testing." ▲

Psychosocial Implications of Genetic Screening and Diagnosis

Screening for genetic diseases has many social and psychological implications. The burden of anxiety, cost, and potential stigmatization surrounding a positive test must be weighed against the need for detection. Often, screening tests are misperceived as diagnostically definitive. The concept that a positive screening test does not necessarily indicate disease presence must be emphasized to those who undergo screening.

The initial screening programs for sickle cell trait in the 1970s were plagued by misunderstandings about the implications of carrier status. Occasionally, carrier detection led to cancellation of health insurance or employer discrimination. Such experiences underscore the need for effective genetic counseling and public education. Other issues include the right to choose *not* to be tested and the potential for invasion of privacy.

The social, psychological, and ethical aspects of genetic screening will become more complicated as newer techniques of DNA diagnosis become more accessible. For example, even though presymptomatic diagnosis of Huntington disease is available, only about 20% of at-risk individuals elect this option. Largely, this reflects the fact that no effective treatment is presently available for this disorder. Presymptomatic diagnosis of *BRCA1* and *BRCA2* carrier status in breast/ovarian cancer families has also met with mixed responses. In part, this is a reaction to the cost of the test: because of the large number of different mutations in each gene, testing typically consists of sequencing both genes entirely, an expensive procedure. It also reflects the fact that periodic mammography, which may be indicated for gene carriers, will detect a tumor but not prevent it. Furthermore, there is some concern that the radiation from mammography could induce a somatic second hit leading to tumor formation. Preventive measures such as prophylactic mastectomy and oophorectomy (removal of the breasts and ovaries, respectively) are known to reduce cancer risk but do not completely eliminate it.

For some genetic diseases, such as autosomal dominant colon cancer syndromes or hemochromatosis, early diagnosis can lead to improved survival because effective preventive treatments are readily available (polypectomy or colectomy for precancerous colon polyps; phlebotomy to reduce iron levels in hemochromatosis). In addition, at-risk individuals will often find that they do not carry the disease-causing gene, allowing them to avoid unpleasant (and possibly hazardous) diagnostic procedures such as sigmoidoscopy or mammography. However, as screening for such diseases becomes more common, the issues of privacy and confidentiality, and the need for accurate communication of risk information, must also be addressed.

MOLECULAR TOOLS FOR SCREENING AND DIAGNOSIS

Until recently, genetic screening usually relied on assays of the disease phenotype, such as a β-hexosaminidase assay for Tay-Sachs disease or a creatine kinase assay for Duchenne muscular dystrophy. Advances in DNA technology have led to diagnosis at the level of the genotype. In some cases linkage analysis can determine whether an individual has inherited a disease gene, and in other cases direct assays of disease-causing mutations have been developed. Genetic diagnosis at the DNA level is now supplementing, and in some cases supplanting, screening tests based on phenotypic assays.

Linkage analysis and/or direct mutation diagnosis have been used for diagnostic testing within families, for prenatal diagnosis of genetic disorders, and more recently in population screening. Improved technology and an increased demand for testing have led to the establishment of clinical molecular laboratories in many medical centers in North America and Europe.

Linkage Analysis

DNA polymorphisms (RFLPs, VNTRs, and, most commonly, microsatellite repeat polymorphisms) can be used as markers in linkage analysis as described in Chapter 8. Once linkage phase is established in a family, the marker locus can be assayed to determine whether an individual has inherited a chromosome (or, more precisely, a chromosome segment) containing a disease gene or one containing a normal gene (Fig. 13-2). Because this approach uses linked markers but does not involve direct examination of the disease-causing mutation(s), it is a form of **indirect diagnosis.**

Linkage analysis has been employed successfully in diagnosing many of the genetic diseases discussed in this text. In principle, it can be used to diagnose any mapped genetic disease. It has the advantages that the disease gene and its product need not be known. The marker simply tells us which chromosome the at-risk individual has inherited.

The disadvantages of this approach are: (1) multiple family members must be tested in order to establish linkage phase, (2) not all markers are informative (sufficiently heterozygous) in all families, and (3) recombination may occur between the marker and the disease-causing mutation, introducing a source of diagnostic error.

As discussed in Chapter 8, the highly polymorphic microsatellite loci greatly increase the likelihood that a marker will be informative in a family. Informativeness

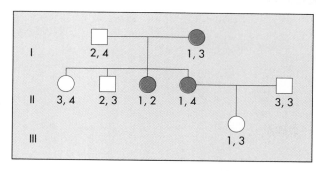

FIG. 13-2 In this pedigree for autosomal dominant breast cancer, the analysis of a closely linked marker on chromosome 17 shows that the mutation is on the same chromosome as marker allele 1 in the affected mother in generation II. This indicates that the daughter in generation III has inherited the mutation-bearing chromosome from her mother and is highly likely to develop a breast tumor.

can also be increased by using multiple marker polymorphisms, all of which are closely linked to the disease locus. Particularly useful are markers flanking both sides of the disease locus. This often enables the investigator to determine that a recombination has occurred.

▼ Linkage analysis, a form of indirect genetic diagnosis, uses linked markers to determine whether an individual has inherited a chromosome containing a disease gene from his or her parent. The need for typing multiple family members, and the possibilities of recombination and uninformative matings, are disadvantages of this approach. ▲

Direct Mutation Analysis

Sometimes the mutation causing a disease happens to alter a recognition sequence for a restriction enzyme. In this case the mutation itself creates a restriction site polymorphism that can be detected after digestion with this enzyme. An example is given by the sickle-cell disease mutation, which alters an *Mst*II recognition site in the β-globin gene (see Chapter 3, Fig. 3-16). Because the resulting RFLP reflects the disease-causing mutation directly, RFLP analysis in this context is an example of **direct diagnosis** of the disease. Direct diagnosis has the advantages that family information is not needed (the mutation is viewed directly in each individual), uninformative matings are not a problem, and there is no error due to recombination. The primary disadvantage of using RFLPs for direct diagnosis is that only about 5% of disease-causing mutations happen to affect known restriction sites.

▼ Direct genetic diagnosis is accomplished by typing the disease-causing mutation itself. It is poten-

tially more accurate than indirect diagnosis and does not require family information. RFLP techniques can be used for direct diagnosis if the mutation affects a restriction site. ▲

Allele-Specific Oligonucleotides

If the DNA sequence surrounding a mutation is known, an oligonucleotide probe can be synthesized that will hybridize (undergo complementary base pairing) only to the mutated sequence (such probes are often termed **allele-specific oligonucleotides,** or ASOs). A second probe that will hybridize to the normal DNA sequence is also synthesized. Stringent hybridization conditions are used so that a one-base mismatch will prevent hybridization. DNA from individuals homozygous for the mutation will hybridize only with the ASO containing the mutated sequence, whereas DNA from individuals homozygous for the normal sequence will hybridize with the normal ASO. DNA from heterozygotes will hybridize with both probes (Fig. 13-3). The length of the ASO probes, usually about 18 to 20 nucleotides, is critical. Probes of shorter length would not be unique in the genome and would therefore hybridize to other regions. Longer probes are more difficult to synthesize correctly and could hybridize both to the normal and mutated sequence.

The ASO method of direct diagnosis has the same advantages that were listed for direct diagnosis using RFLPs. It has the additional advantage that it is not limited to mutations that cause alterations in restriction sites. However, it does require that at least part of the disease gene has been cloned and sequenced. In addition, each disease-causing mutation requires a different oligonucleotide probe. For this reason, this approach, while powerful, becomes impractical unless a disease is caused by a limited number of relatively common mutations.

▼ Direct diagnosis can be performed by hybridization of an individual's DNA with allele-specific oligonucleotide probes. This approach is feasible if the DNA sequence causing a genetic disease is known and if the number of disease-causing mutations is limited. ▲

Examples of diseases caused by a limited number of mutations include sickle cell disease and α1-antitrypsin deficiency (Clinical Commentary 13-3). Although more than 700 cystic fibrosis mutations have been identified, the dozen or so most common ones account for the great majority of mutations in most populations (see Clinical Commentary 13-2). Thus, direct diagnosis can be used to identify most CF homozygotes and heterozygous carriers. Prenatal diagnosis is also possible. Direct diagnosis, using PCR or Southern blotting, can also be used to detect deletions or duplications in the dystrophin gene

FIG. 13-3 Hybridization of allele-specific oligonucleotide (ASO) probes corresponding to normal DNA sequence and a mutation (R117H) that can produce cystic fibrosis. In this "dot blot," the DNA from individuals A and B hybridizes only to the normal sequence; they are normal homozygotes. Individual C's DNA hybridizes to both ASO probes, so he is a heterozygous carrier.

(Courtesy Lesa Nelson and Dr. Kenneth Ward, University of Utah Health Sciences Center.)

CLINICAL COMMENTARY 13-3
THE GENETIC DIAGNOSIS OF α1-ANTITRYPSIN DEFICIENCY

α1-Antitrypsin (α1-AT) deficiency is one of the most common autosomal recessive disorders among Caucasians, affecting approximately 1 in 2,500. α1-AT, synthesized primarily in the liver, is a serine protease inhibitor. It does bind trypsin, as its name suggests. However, α1-AT binds much more strongly to neutrophil elastase, a protease that is produced by neutrophils (a type of leukocyte) in response to infections and irritants. It carries out its binding and inhibitory role primarily in the lower respiratory tract, where it prevents elastase from digesting the alveolar septi of the lung. WWW

Individuals with less than 10% to 15% of the normal level of α1-AT activity will experience significant lung damage and typically develop emphysema during their 30s, 40s or 50s. In addition, at least 10% develop liver cirrhosis as a result of the accumulation of variant α1-AT molecules in the liver; α1-AT deficiency accounts for nearly 20% of all non-alcoholic liver cirrhosis in the United States. An important feature of this disease is that cigarette smokers with α1-AT deficiency develop emphysema much earlier than do nonsmokers. This is because cigarette smoke irritates lung tissue, increasing secretion of neutrophil elastase. At the same time, it inactivates α1-AT, so there is also less inhibition of elastase. One study showed that the median age of survival of nonsmokers with α1-AT deficiency was 62 years, whereas it was only 40 years for smokers with this disease. Because the combination of cigarette smoking (an environmental factor) and an α1-AT mutation (a genetic factor) produces more severe disease than either factor alone, it is known as an example of a **gene-environment interaction.**

The α1-AT gene has been localized to chromosome 14q32, and it has been cloned and sequenced. While there are more than 75 known α1-AT mutations, the only common one with clinically significant effects is a missense mutation in exon 5 that produces an allele known as "Z." The gene frequency of the Z allele is as high as 0.02 in Scandinavia and decreases to less than 0.01 in Southern European populations. It is virtually absent in Japanese and Chinese populations. Because it is the result of a single base-pair substitution, the Z mutation can be diagnosed directly by using ASO probes. Typically, PCR is used to amplify the individual's DNA from this region of the gene, and the amplified DNA is blotted onto a membrane. The amplified DNA is hybridized with an ASO probe that has a DNA sequence corresponding to the mutation and a second ASO probe that has the normal DNA sequence. This permits direct determination of the individual's genotype. Thus, rapid, direct diagnosis is possible for this important and common genetic disease.

that cause most cases of Duchenne muscular dystrophy. The most common DNA diagnostic tests performed in a clinical molecular laboratory are presented in Table 13-5.

Other Methods of Direct Diagnosis

The ASO method, often implemented as a "dot blot" (see Fig. 13-3), is commonly used in direct mutation detection. Many other techniques can also be used for mutation detection, including several discussed in Chapter 3 (e.g., direct sequencing, SSCP, DGGE, and mismatch cleavage analysis). One of the most promising new methods for large-scale mutation detection is the use of DNA chips, also discussed in Chapter 3. DNA chips have many convenient properties, including miniaturization and automated computerized processing. In one application, the entire 16.6-kb sequence of the mitochondrial DNA genome was analyzed for polymorphic variation by placing 135,000 different 16-bp oligonucleotide probes on a single chip. Mitochondrial DNA from study subjects was then hybridized with the probes on the chip to test simultaneously for 180 distinct polymorphisms. DNA chips can be designed to test large numbers of disease-causing mutations in a single, rapid analysis, and the results can readily be analyzed and archived by a computer.

Mass spectrometry, a method commonly used in chemistry, is also being explored as a means of rapid mutation detection. This technique detects minute differences in the mass of PCR-amplified DNA molecules. These differences represent variations in DNA sequence. Mass spectrometry, which offers the advantages of high speed and great accuracy, has been used to detect mutations in the cystic fibrosis and apolipoprotein E genes.

▼ New methods of direct mutation detection, including the use of DNA chips and mass spectrometry, promise to increase the speed and accuracy of genetic diagnosis. ▲

PRENATAL DIAGNOSIS OF GENETIC DISORDERS AND CONGENITAL DEFECTS

Prenatal diagnosis is a major focus of genetic diagnosis, and several important areas of technology have evolved to provide this service. The principal aim of prenatal diagnosis is to supply at-risk families with information so that they can make informed choices during pregnancy. The potential benefits of prenatal testing include: (1) providing reassurance to at-risk families when the result is normal; (2) providing risk information to couples who, in the absence of such information, would not choose to begin a pregnancy; (3) allowing the couple to prepare psychologically for the birth of an affected baby; (4) helping the health care professional to plan delivery, management, and care of the infant when the fetus is diagnosed with a disease; and (5) providing risk information to couples for whom pregnancy termination is an option.

TABLE 13-5 Selected Single-Gene Disorders for Which Family Screening and Prenatal Diagnosis by DNA are Available

Disease	DNA analysis
Neurofibromatosis type 1	Linkage analysis/ direct mutation analysis
Myotonic dystrophy	Direct mutation analysis
Cystic fibrosis	Direct mutation analysis
Sickle-cell disease	Direct mutation analysis
Fragile X syndrome	Direct mutation analysis
Hemophilia A	Direct mutation analysis/ linkage analysis
Huntington disease	Direct mutation analysis
Duchenne muscular dystrophy	Direct mutation analysis/ linkage
Familial breast cancer	Direct sequencing/linkage
Hemochromatosis	Direct mutation analysis

Given the controversy surrounding the issue of pregnancy termination, it should be emphasized that 98% of prenatal diagnoses yield a normal test result. Thus, the great majority of families receive reassurance, and only a small minority must face the issue of termination.

Prenatal diagnosis includes both screening and diagnostic tests. An example of a population screening test is an assay of maternal serum α-fetoprotein (AFP) at 15 weeks' gestation. An abnormal result identifies a subgroup for further testing. **Amniocentesis** (the withdrawal of amniotic fluid during pregnancy) and **chorionic villus sampling** (CVS, the biopsy of chorionic villus tissue) represent diagnostic tests. Another example of the distinction between screening and diagnosis is given by amniocentesis for pregnancies in advanced maternal age: the selection of women 35 years of age or older is the screening strategy, and amniocentesis is the diagnostic test. Primarily because of the increased risk of trisomies with advanced maternal age (see Chapter 6), approximately half of North American women over age 35 currently undergo amniocentesis or CVS during pregnancy.

Prenatal diagnostic methods can be divided into two major types: (1) analysis of fetal tissues (amniocentesis, chorionic villus sampling, cordocentesis, and in vitro fertilization diagnosis) and (2) visualization of the fetus (ultrasonography). In this section, each of these procedures is described, and their accuracy, safety, and feasibility are discussed.

Amniocentesis

Amniocentesis is traditionally performed at 15 to 17 weeks after a pregnant woman's last menstrual period (LMP). A needle is inserted through the abdominal wall

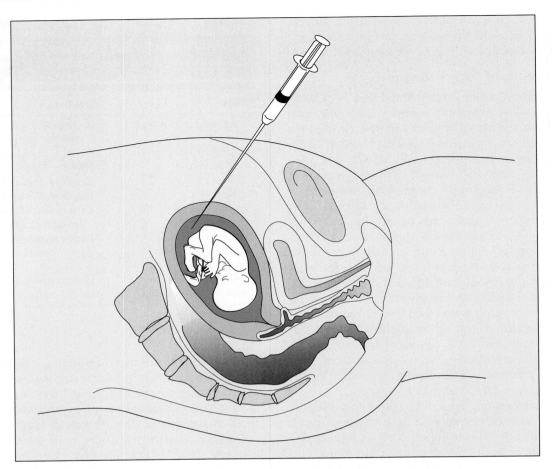

FIG. 13-4 A schematic illustration of an amniocentesis, in which 20 to 30 ml of amniotic fluid is withdrawn transabdominally (with ultrasound guidance), usually at 15 to 17 weeks' gestation.

into the amniotic sac after real-time ultrasound localizes the placenta and determines the position of the fetus (Fig. 13-4). Twenty to thirty milliliters of amniotic fluid is withdrawn; this fluid contains living cells (**amniocytes**) shed by the fetus. Standard cytogenetic studies are carried out after culturing the amniocytes to increase their number. In addition, cells can be grown for biochemical assays, FISH, or DNA diagnosis. α-Fetoprotein, which is used to test for the presence of a neural tube defect (see Chapter 12), is also measured in the amniotic fluid. The results of cytogenetic studies are typically completed in 10 to 12 days. Indications for prenatal diagnosis by amniocentesis are listed in Box 13-3.

The safety and accuracy of amniocentesis have been established by several large collaborative studies. The risk of maternal complications is very low. Transient fluid leakage occurs in about 1% of mothers, and maternal infections are extremely rare. The risk of primary concern is fetal loss. Amniocentesis increases the risk of fetal loss by no more than 0.5% above the background risk at 15 to 17 weeks post-LMP.

BOX 13-3

INDICATIONS FOR PRENATAL DIAGNOSIS BY AMNIOCENTESIS

Maternal age >35 years
Previous child with chromosome abnormality
History of structural chromosome abnormality in one of the parents
Family history of genetic defect that is diagnosable by biochemical or DNA analysis
Risk of neural tube defect (NTD)

One must weigh the risk of fetal loss against the probability that the fetus is affected with a diagnosable condition. For women younger than 35 years, the former risk usually outweighs the latter. After age 35, the risk of bearing an aneuploid fetus increases considerably, and the latter risk outweighs the former. Thus,

CLINICAL COMMENTARY 13-4
THE AMNIOCENTESIS DECISION

During the medical care of a pregnant woman older than 35 years, a common discussion with the primary care practitioner involves the decision to undergo amniocentesis. Several factors enter into this decision. First is the age-specific risk for Down syndrome and other chromosomal disorders. A second factor is the risk of fetal loss from the procedure (about 0.5% above the background risk). A third issue is the cost of an amniocentesis with ultrasound and cytogenetic analysis, which ordinarily ranges from $1,000 to $2,000. These factors must be weighed in terms of their relative costs and benefits for the woman and her family.

As this decision is explored in greater depth, other considerations often arise. If a woman has had previous miscarriages, the 0.5% risk of fetal loss may be weighed more heavily. In addition, the seriousness of bearing a child with disabilities may be perceived differently from family to family. Some couples are uncomfortable with the amount of time that elapses before test results are available (usually 10 to 12 days). Here, the possibility of CVS, which can be performed earlier and which usually yields results more rapidly, may be explored. The possibility of an ambiguous result (e.g., mosaicism) also deserves discussion. Finally, it is important for the clinician to specify that a typical amniocentesis in a woman older than 35 years detects only a specific class of disorders (i.e., chromosome abnormalities and NTDs) and not the entire range of congenital malformations and genetic disorders.

amniocentesis is not recommended for women under age 35 unless they have a previous indication of risk for a genetic disease, such as a positive family history (Clinical Commentary 13-4).

Although amniocentesis provides highly accurate results, chromosomal mosaicism can lead to misdiagnosis. Most apparent mosaicism is caused by the generation of an extra chromosome during in vitro cell culture and is labeled as **pseudomosaicism.** This can be distinguished easily from true mosaicism if techniques are used in which all cells in a colony are the descendants of a single fetal cell. If only some cells in the colony have the extra chromosome, it is assumed that pseudomosaicism exists. If, however, consistent aneuploidy is visualized in all cells of multiple colonies, then true fetal mosaicism is diagnosed. Further confirmation of fetal mosaicism (which is generally a rare condition) can be obtained by fetal blood sampling, as described later.

Recently, some centers have been evaluating amniocentesis performed earlier in pregnancy, at about 12 to 14 weeks post-LMP. Since less amniotic fluid is present at this time, the risk of fetal loss or injury may be higher. A number of large-scale evaluations have indicated significantly higher rates of fetal loss for **early amniocentesis,** and some studies have shown increased rates of specific congenital anomalies (club foot in particular).

▼ Amniocentesis, the withdrawal of amniotic fluid during pregnancy, is performed at about 16 weeks post-LMP and is used to diagnose many genetic diseases. The rate of fetal loss attributable to this procedure is approximately 1/200. Amniocentesis can also be performed earlier in the pregnancy; some studies indicate an elevated rate of fetal loss after early amniocentesis. ▲

Chorionic Villus Sampling

Chorionic villus sampling (CVS) is performed by aspirating fetal trophoblastic tissue (chorionic villi) by either a transcervical or transabdominal approach (Fig. 13-5). Since it is usually performed at 10 to 11 weeks post-LMP, CVS has the advantage of providing a diagnosis much earlier in pregnancy than second-trimester amniocentesis. This is beneficial for those couples who consider pregnancy termination an option.

Cell culture (as in amniocentesis) and direct analysis from rapidly growing trophoblasts can provide material for cytogenetic analysis. When chorionic villi are successfully obtained, CVS provides diagnostic results in more than 99% of cases. **Confined placental mosaicism** (mosaicism in the placenta but not in the fetus itself) is seen in about 1% to 2% of cases in which direct analysis of villus material is performed. This confuses the diagnosis because the mosaicism observed in placental (villus) material is not actually present in the fetus. This problem can usually be resolved by a follow-up amniocentesis. A disadvantage of CVS is that amniotic fluid AFP cannot be measured. Women who undergo CVS may have their serum AFP level measured at 15 to 16 weeks post-LMP as a screen for neural tube defects.

CVS, like amniocentesis, is generally a safe procedure. Several collaborative studies revealed a post-CVS fetal loss rate to be 0.5% to 1% higher than that of amniocentesis (i.e., a fetal loss rate of approximately 1% to 1.5% above the background rate, compared with 0.5% for amniocentesis). The most important factors increasing the risk of fetal loss are a lack of experience with the procedure and an increase in the number of transcervical passages to obtain the villus sample. In experienced hands, transcervical and transabdominal procedures appear to entail similar risk levels.

Some studies have indicated that CVS may increase the risk of limb reduction defects. Although other investigations have not corroborated this result, the apparent

FIG. 13-5 A schematic illustration of a transcervical chorionic villus sampling (CVS) procedure. With ultrasound guidance, a catheter is inserted, and several milligrams of villus tissue are aspirated.

association has been of concern because the proposed mechanism (vascular insult leading to hypoperfusion of the limb) is biologically plausible. The risk is greatest when CVS is performed earlier than 10 weeks post-LMP and decreases to no more than one in several thousand when the procedure is performed at 10 to 11 weeks post-LMP. Accordingly, many professionals now recommend against performing CVS prior to 10 weeks post-LMP.

▼ **CVS is performed earlier than amniocentesis (at 10 to 11 weeks post-LMP) using either a transcervical or transabdominal approach. The risk of fetal loss attributable to CVS is approximately 1% to 1.5%. Confined placental mosaicism can confuse the diagnosis. There is some evidence that CVS may increase the risk of limb reduction defects; this risk is greatest when the procedure is performed before 10 weeks post-LMP.** ▲

Inborn errors of metabolism (see Chapter 7), which are usually autosomal or X-linked recessive diseases, can be diagnosed prenatally by amniocentesis or CVS if the specific metabolic defect is expressed in amniocytes or trophoblastic tissue. Table 13-6 lists selected inborn errors of metabolism and single gene disorders for which amniocentesis or CVS is available. A comprehensive summary of conditions that may be prenatally diagnosed is provided by Weaver (1992).

Other Methods of Fetal Tissue Sampling

Cordocentesis, or **percutaneous umbilical blood sampling** (PUBS), has become the preferred method to access fetal blood, replacing the riskier procedure of fetal blood sampling by **fetoscopy** (direct visualization of the fetus by insertion of an endoscope through the abdominal wall). PUBS is usually carried out after the sixteenth week of gestation and is accomplished by ultrasound-guided puncture of the umbilical cord and withdrawal of fetal blood. The fetal loss rate attributable to PUBS is low, but it is slightly higher than that of amniocentesis or CVS. The primary applications of PUBS are as follows:

1. Cytogenetic analysis of fetuses with structural anomalies detected by ultrasound when rapid diagnosis is required. Cytogenetic analysis from fetal blood sampling is completed in 2 to 3 days, while diagnosis following amniocentesis requires 10 to 12 days because of the necessity of culturing amniocytes. This time difference can be critical in the later stages of a pregnancy.
2. Diagnosis of hematological diseases that are analyzed most effectively in blood samples or diagnosis of immunologic disorders such as chronic granulomatous disease (see Chapter 9).
3. Rapid distinction between true fetal mosaicism and false mosaicism caused by maternal contamination of an amniotic fluid sample.

TABLE 13-6 Selected Inborn Errors of Metabolism That Are Diagnosable Through Amniocentesis and/or CVS

Disease	Measurable enzyme
Disorders of Amino Acid/Organic Acid Metabolism	
Maple syrup urine disease	Branched-chain ketoacid decarboxylase
Methylmalonic acidemia	Methylmalonic CoA mutase
Multiple carboxylase deficiency	Biotin responsive carboxylase
Disorders of Carbohydrate Metabolism	
Glycogen storage disease, type 2	α-Glucosidase
Galactosemia	Galactose-1-uridyl transferase
Disorders of Lysosomal Enzymes	
Gangliosidosis (all types)	β-Galactosidase
Mucopolysaccharidosis (all types)	Disease-specific enzyme (see Chapter 7)
Tay-Sachs disease	Hexosaminidase A
Disorders of Purine and Pyrimidine Metabolism	
Lesch-Nyhan syndrome	Hypoxanthine-guanine phosphoribosyl transferase
Disorders of Peroxisomal Metabolism	
Zellweger syndrome	Long-chain fatty acids

▼ Percutaneous umbilical blood sampling (PUBS, or cordocentesis) is a method for the direct sampling of fetal blood and is used to obtain a sample for rapid cytogenetic or hematological analysis or for confirmation of mosaicism. ▲

Ultrasonography

Technological advances in real-time **ultrasonography** have made this an important tool in prenatal diagnosis. A transducer placed on the mother's abdomen sends pulsed sound waves through the fetus. The fetal tissue reflects the waves in patterns corresponding to tissue density. The reflected waves are displayed on a monitor, allowing real-time visualization of the fetus. Ultrasonography has become the most widely used form of fetal visualization and is useful in the detection of many fetal malformations. It also assists in the effectiveness of amniocentesis, CVS, and PUBS. Box 13-4 lists some of the congenital malformations diagnosable by fetal ultrasound (a more comprehensive list is provided by Weaver, 1992).

Ultrasonography is sometimes used to test for a specific condition in an at-risk fetus (e.g., a short-limb skeletal dysplasia). More often, fetal anomalies are detected during the evaluation of obstetrical indicators such as uncertain gestational age, poor fetal growth, or amniotic fluid abnormalities. Several European nations

BOX 13-4
SELECTED DISORDERS DIAGNOSED BY ULTRASOUND IN THE SECOND TRIMESTER*

Symptom Complex

Hydrops
Oligohydramnios
Polyhydramnios
Intrauterine growth
  retardation

Central Nervous System

Anencephaly
Encephalocele
Holoprosencephaly
Hydrocephalus

Craniofacial

Cleft lip

Chest

Congenital heart disease
Diaphragmatic hernia

Abdomen/Pelvis

Gastrointestinal atresias
Gastroschisis
Omphalocele
Renal agenesis
Cystic kidneys
Hydronephrosis

Skeletal System

Limb reduction defects
Many chondrodystrophies,
  including thanatophoric
  dysplasia and osteo-
  genesis imperfecta

*Detection rate varies by condition.

FIG. 13-6 **A,** Photograph of an ultrasound result, revealing the presence of a fetus with anencephaly. **B,** Ultrasound result for a normal fetus (note the clear presence of the cranial vault in the normal fetus).

perform routine second-trimester ultrasound screening in all pregnancies. Studies of ultrasound screening suggest that sensitivity for the detection of most major congenital malformations ranges from 30% to 50%. Specificity, however, approaches 99%.

The sensitivity of ultrasonography is higher for some congenital malformations. In particular, ultrasound can detect virtually all fetuses with anencephaly (Fig. 13-6) and 85% to 90% of those with spina bifida. It may also sometimes identify a fetus with a chromosome abnormality by detecting a congenital malformation, intrauterine growth retardation, hydrops (abnormal accumulation of fluid in the fetus), or an alteration of the amniotic fluid volume.

Ultrasonography is by far the most common technique now used for fetal visualization, but other techniques are also used. They include radiography and occasionally magnetic resonance imaging (MRI).

▼ **Prenatal diagnosis includes invasive techniques designed to analyze fetal tissue (CVS, amniocen-**

tesis, or PUBS) and non-invasive procedures that visualize the fetus (ultrasonography). ▲

α-Fetoprotein Measurement in Amniotic Fluid and Maternal Serum

α-Fetoprotein (AFP) is a fetal protein similar to albumin; it is produced initially by the yolk sac and subsequently by the liver. The AFP level normally increases in amniotic fluid until about 10 to 14 weeks' gestation and then decreases steadily. Amniotic fluid AFP is significantly higher in pregnancies in which the fetus has a neural tube defect (NTD). When an amniotic fluid AFP assay is used with ultrasonography in the second trimester, more than 98% of fetuses with an open spina bifida and probably all with anencephaly can be recognized. It is routine for all women having an amniocentesis for cytogenetic analysis to also have their amniotic fluid AFP level measured.

In addition to a fetal NTD, there are several other causes of elevated (or apparently elevated) amniotic fluid AFP. These include underestimation of gestational age, fetal death, presence of twins, blood contamination, and several specific malformations (e.g., omphalocele or gastroschisis, which are abdominal wall defects). Usually, targeted ultrasonography can distinguish among these alternatives.

▼ The amniotic α-fetoprotein level is elevated when the fetus has a neural tube defect and provides a reliable prenatal test for this condition. ▲

Soon after the link between elevated amniotic fluid AFP and NTDs was recognized, an association between elevated levels of **maternal serum AFP** (MSAFP) and NTDs was identified. AFP diffuses across the fetal membranes into the mother's serum, so MSAFP levels are correlated with amniotic fluid AFP levels. Thus, it is possible to measure amniotic fluid AFP noninvasively by obtaining a maternal blood sample.

Because 90% to 95% of NTD births occur in the absence of a family history of the condition, a safe, noninvasive population screening procedure for NTDs is highly desirable. However, there is considerable overlap of MSAFP levels in women carrying NTD and normal fetuses (Fig. 13-7). Thus, the issues of sensitivity and specificity must be considered. Typically, an MSAFP level is considered to be elevated if it is 2 to 2.5 times higher than the normal median level (adjustments for maternal weight, presence of diabetes mellitus, and race are included in these calculations). Approximately 1% to 2% of pregnant women will exhibit MSAFP levels above this cutoff level. They may choose to undergo amniocentesis to determine whether in fact they are carrying a fetus with an NTD. After adjustment for advanced gestational age, fetal demise, and presence of twins, about 1 in 15 of these women will have an elevated amniotic fluid AFP. Thus, the positive predictive value of the MSAFP screening test is rather low, approximately 6% (1/15). However, the sensitivity of the test is fairly high: MSAFP screening will identify approximately 90% of anencephaly cases and about 80% of open spina bifida cases. Although this sensitivity level is lower than that of amniotic fluid AFP testing, the risk of the MSAFP measurement is also much lower.

An association has also been found between *low* MSAFP and the presence of a fetus with Down syndrome. Previously, population screening for Down syndrome consisted of amniocentesis for women over 35 years of age. This screening strategy has a detection rate (sensitivity) of only 20% because only about 20% of all babies with trisomy are born to mothers older than age 35. MSAFP measurement has expanded the option of population screening for Down syndrome.

As indicated in Fig. 13-7, MSAFP levels overlap considerably in normal and Down syndrome pregnancies.

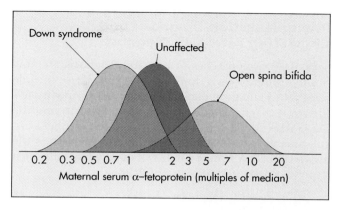

FIG. 13-7 Maternal serum α-fetoprotein (MSAFP) levels in mothers carrying normal fetuses and in mothers carrying fetuses with Down syndrome and open spina bifida. MSAFP is somewhat lowered when the fetus has Down syndrome, and it is substantially elevated when the fetus has an open spina bifida.

(From Milunsky A [1998] Genetic Disorders and the Fetus: Diagnosis, Prevention, and Treatment. Ed 4. Johns Hopkins University Press, Baltimore.)

The risk for Down syndrome in women younger than age 35 increases by a factor of 3 to 4 when the adjusted MSAFP value is lower than 0.5 multiples of the normal population median. In deriving a risk estimate, complex formulas take into account the mother's weight, age, and MSAFP level. A woman who is 25 years of age ordinarily has a risk of about 1/1250 for producing a fetus with Down syndrome, but if she has a weight-adjusted MSAFP of 0.35 multiples of the median, her risk increases to 1 in 171. This risk is higher than that of a 35-year-old woman in the general population. Most screening programs use a risk factor of 1 in 380 (equivalent to the average risk for a 35-year-old woman to produce a newborn with Down syndrome) as an indication for amniocentesis.

The accuracy of Down syndrome screening can be increased by measuring the serum levels of unconjugated estriol and human chorionic gonadotropin in addition to MSAFP **(triple screen).** While MSAFP alone identifies only about 40% of Down syndrome pregnancies, the three indicators together can identify approximately 70%. Additional indicators that may increase this detection rate are being evaluated.

▼ MSAFP has provided a screening approach that increases the ability to prenatally detect fetuses with various abnormalities, including NTDs and Down syndrome. This noninvasive procedure entails virtually no risk, but its sensitivity for detecting NTDs is lower than that of amniotic AFP diagnosis. Use of the "triple screen" increases sensitivity for detecting Down syndrome. ▲

New Diagnostic Techniques: Preimplantation Diagnosis and Circulating Fetal Cell Diagnosis

Several new approaches to prenatal diagnosis are now in the testing or early application stages. These include two preimplantation diagnostic approaches, in vitro fertilization diagnosis and polar body diagnosis, and the diagnosis of fetal cells obtained from the mother's circulation. Because each of these methods involves the analysis of DNA from a single cell or very few cells, each depends critically on the use of PCR.

In Vitro Fertilization Diagnosis

In vitro fertilization diagnosis begins with the removal of a single cell from an 8- or 16-cell blastomere that has been generated through in vitro fertilization (the procedure can also be done slightly later, using cells from the trophoectoderm of the blastocyst). The removal of one cell does not adversely affect the development of the blastomere. Using PCR, DNA from the single cell can be amplified, leading to the diagnosis of single-gene conditions. Also, FISH analysis (see Chapter 6) can be used to diagnose aneuploidy. If the disease-causing mutation is not detected, the blastomere is implanted into the mother's uterus. A number of genetic diseases, including cystic fibrosis, Tay Sachs disease, β-thalassemia, myotonic dystrophy, Huntington disease, and Duchenne muscular dystrophy, have been tested using this approach. To date, more than 100 normal babies have been born after in vitro fertilization diagnosis.

An occasional problem with this procedure is that an allele may be undetectable. This occurs because of partial PCR amplification failure when using DNA from only a single cell. Because this has led to misdiagnosis in a small number of cases, more sensitive techniques are being developed to avoid non-detection.

Polar Body Diagnosis

Polar body diagnosis involves an examination of the polar body shed at the same time as the ovum. The polar body's DNA is tested to determine whether it contains a disease-causing mutation. If it does, it is assumed that the egg does not contain the mutation. This egg is then fertilized and implanted using the usual in vitro techniques. Polar body and blastomere diagnosis both offer the advantage of very early detection of genetic disorders, and they avoid the issue of pregnancy termination. These approaches, however, are costly and technologically challenging, and their availability is still limited.

▼ In vitro fertilization diagnosis consists of PCR amplification of DNA from a single cell taken from a blastomere or blastocyst. Diagnosis of genetic conditions permits implantation of only the unaffected embryos and avoids the issue of pregnancy termination. ▲

Diagnosis Using Fetal Cells Isolated from Maternal Blood

During pregnancy, a small number of fetal cells find their way into the mother's circulation. One such cell type is the nucleated red blood cell, which is common in the fetus but very rare in the adult circulation. These cells can be isolated as early as 6 to 8 weeks post-LMP and are identified using cell-sorting techniques. Further specificity for fetal cells can be achieved by testing cells for receptors expressed only in early erythrocytes but not mature erythrocytes. FISH analysis of these cells has been used to diagnose fetal conditions such as trisomy 21 and trisomy 18. PCR has been used to diagnose a limited number of single-gene disorders, although this remains a challenge because of the difficulty of sorting pure populations of fetal cells. The major advantage of this approach is that it requires only a blood sample from the mother and thus poses no risk for the fetus. Its accuracy and feasibility are being evaluated.

▼ Fetal cells that enter the maternal circulation can be isolated and evaluated for mutations using PCR or FISH. This experimental procedure poses no risk to the fetus. ▲

FETAL TREATMENT

A goal of prenatal diagnosis is treatment of the affected fetus. Although this is not currently possible for most conditions, some examples can be cited. Many of these procedures are experimental.

Two of the best-established forms of in utero intervention are treatment for rare inborn errors of metabolism and treatment for hormone deficiencies. An important example of a biochemical disorder for which treatment is available is biotin-responsive multiple carboxylase deficiency. This autosomal recessive enzyme deficiency can be diagnosed by amniocentesis. In one case report oral administration of biotin to the mother was initiated at 23 weeks of pregnancy. This resulted in the birth of a normal baby.

Congenital adrenal hyperplasia (CAH) is a second example of a condition for which in utero treatment has been successful. Because of excessive androgen secretion by the enlarged fetal adrenal glands, female fetuses with CAH become masculinized. Administration of dexamethasone to the mother beginning at 10 weeks post-LMP diminishes or prevents this masculinization.

Surgical treatment of fetuses, primarily for conditions involving urinary tract obstruction, has met with moderate success. Surgical correction of diaphragmatic hernia at 20 weeks' gestation has also been attempted. Preliminary results have been discouraging, but work is continuing. In utero correction of fetal hydrocephalus was halted after initial results showed no beneficial effects.

GENE THERAPY

As we have seen, the isolation and cloning of disease genes provide opportunities for improved understanding and diagnosis of genetic diseases. In addition, the possibility of genetic alteration of the cells of individuals with genetic diseases **(gene therapy)** emerges. Although gene therapy is still in its infancy and has only begun to affect the lives of patients, the potential for curing genetic diseases through recombinant DNA techniques has excited a great deal of interest in both professional and lay circles. As of 1998, more than 200 gene therapy protocols have been approved for experimental trials (see Table 13-7 for some examples), and more than 2,000 patients are enrolled in these trials. In this section we review gene therapy techniques and discuss their application to genetic disease.

Somatic Cell Therapy

Somatic cell gene therapy, which has been the focus of gene therapy research in humans, consists of the alteration of genes in human somatic cells to treat a specific disorder. The patient's cells may be extracted and manipulated outside the body (ex vivo therapy), or in some cases the cells may be treated while they are in the body (in vivo therapy). Some types of somatic cells are more amenable to gene therapy than others. Good candidates should be easily accessible and should have a long life span in the body. Proliferating cells are preferred for some gene delivery systems, since the vector carrying the gene can then integrate into the cell's replicating DNA. The bone marrow stem cell meets all of these qualifications and thus has been a prime candidate cell for somatic therapy. However, these cells are difficult to manipulate and to isolate from bone marrow (the great majority of bone marrow cells are not stem cells). Consequently, many other cell types have been investigated as potential targets, including skin fibroblasts, muscle cells, vascular endothelial cells, hepatocytes, and lymphocytes. A disadvantage of using such cells is that their life span is relatively short. Thus, therapy using them requires repeated treatment and administration of genetically altered cells.

Gene Replacement Therapy

Most current gene therapy techniques involve the replacement of a missing gene product by inserting a normal gene into a somatic cell. This approach is best suited to recessive diseases that involve a nonfunctional or missing gene product; the insertion of a normal gene will supply the missing product. Many recessive enzyme deficiency disorders can potentially be corrected when only about 10% of the normal enzyme amount is produced. Thus, even a partially effective gene therapy strategy may provide significant health benefits.

There are many techniques for introducing genes into cells, including cell fusion, calcium phosphate coprecipitation (the chemical disturbs the cell membrane, allowing negatively charged DNA to overcome the natural chemical repulsion of the negatively charged cell membrane), microinjection, electroporation (electrically shocking the cell so that foreign DNA can pass through the membrane), liposome fusion, and the direct introduction of "naked" DNA. Because viruses have evolved clever methods for inserting their genes into cells, they have thus far received the most attention as gene therapy vectors. They will be discussed first, following by a discussion of some potentially effective non-viral delivery systems.

TABLE 13-7	Partial List of Diseases for Which Somatic Cell Gene Therapy Protocols Are Being Tested	
Disease	**Target cell**	**Inserted gene**
ADA deficiency	Circulating lymphocytes, bone marrow stem cells	Adenosine deaminase
Hemophilia B	Hepatocytes, skin fibroblasts	Factor IX
Familial hypercholesterolemia	Hepatocytes	LDL receptor
Cystic fibrosis	Airway epithelial cells	CFTR
Malignant melanoma	Melanoma tumor cells	HLA-B7 gene
Duchenne muscular dystrophy	Myoblasts	Dystrophin; also upregulation of utrophin
Gaucher disease (lysosomal storage disorder)	Macrophages	Glucocerebrosidase
Lung cancer	Lung cancer cells	Normal p53
Brain tumors	Brain cells	Herpes thymidine kinase
Ovarian cancer	Ovarian cancer cells	Herpes thymidine kinase
AIDS	Helper T lymphocytes	Dominant negative retrovirus mutations

RETROVIRAL VECTORS. As mentioned in Chapter 11, retroviruses are able to insert copies of their genomes into host cells after reverse-transcribing their viral RNA into DNA. They integrate into the host DNA with a high degree of efficiency, making them a reasonable choice as a gene-delivery vector (Fig. 13-8). The retrovirus must be modified so that it cannot replicate and infect the host. This is done by using recombinant DNA techniques to delete most of the retroviral genome, replacing it with a normal copy of a human gene, its regulatory elements, and a polyadenylation signal (the human genetic material is termed the "insert"). Retroviruses are capable of accepting inserts as large as 8 kb.

These replication-defective retroviruses are propagated in **packaging cells** (sometimes called helper cells) that compensate for the missing replicative machinery of the retrovirus. This allows the production of multiple copies of retroviruses that contain the human gene but cannot replicate themselves. Retrovirus-containing particles are then incubated with the patient's somatic cells (e.g., human bone marrow stem cells or lymphocytes). The modified retrovirus inserts the normal human gene into the DNA of the host cell. Ideally, the inserted gene will then encode a normal gene product in the patient's somatic cells. This type of protocol has been used to treat several diseases, including adenosine deaminase deficiency (Clinical Commentary 13-5).

Although retroviruses offer the advantages of stable and efficient integration into the genome, they also present specific disadvantages. Because it integrates randomly into the host's DNA, the retrovirus could locate near a proto-oncogene, activating it and thus causing tumor formation. The retroviral promoters are altered to minimize this possibility, and thus far no cases of oncogenesis directly attributable to retrovirus insertion have been observed in humans. Because most retroviruses can only enter the cell when its membrane dissolves during cell division, they can typically infect only dividing cells and are ineffective in nondividing or slowly dividing cells (e.g., neurons).

ADENOVIRUS VECTORS. Because of the inability of most retroviruses to invade nondividing cells, other delivery systems have been explored that are not limited in this way. An important example is the **adenovirus,** a double-stranded DNA virus that is often used in vaccine

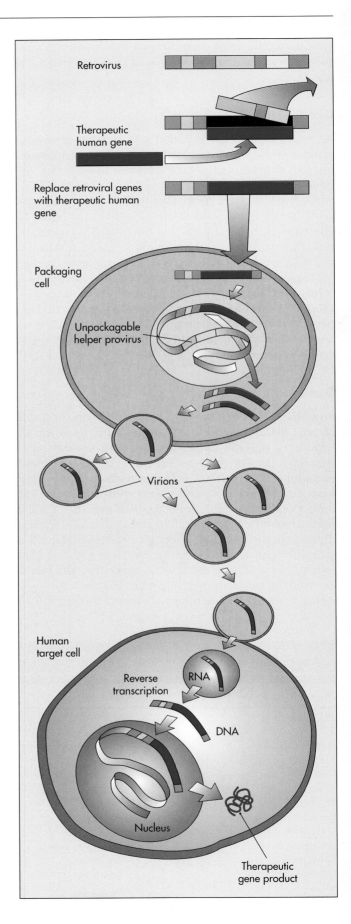

FIG. 13-8 Gene therapy using a retroviral vector. The retrovirus is prevented from replicating by removing most of its genome, a normal human gene is inserted into the retrovirus, and the retrovirus is propagated in a packaging cell. Virions from the packaging cell are incubated with human somatic cells, allowing the retrovirus to insert copies of the normal human gene into the cell. Once integrated into the cell's DNA, the inserted gene produces normal gene product.

CLINICAL COMMENTARY 13-5
ADENOSINE DEAMINASE DEFICIENCY AND GENE THERAPY

Adenosine deaminase (ADA) is produced primarily in lymphoid tissues. It is an important component of the purine salvage pathway, catalyzing the deamination of adenosine into inosine as well as deoxyadenosine (dAdo) into deoxyinosine. ADA deficiency, an autosomal recessive disorder, results in the accumulation of dAdo and its metabolites. This inhibits DNA synthesis in cells and is especially toxic to T lymphocytes. Subsequently, B lymphocytes are also reduced in function and number. The resulting severe combined immune deficiency (SCID; see Chapter 9) is usually fatal by the age of 2 years if untreated. It is estimated that approximately 25% to 30% of SCID cases are caused by ADA deficiency.

The preferred treatment for ADA deficiency is a bone marrow transplant. However, complications of bone marrow transplants increase patient morbidity and are sometimes fatal. In addition, MHC-compatible sibling donors are available for fewer than 30% of ADA deficiency patients. Patients may be treated with polyethylene glycol (PEG)-conjugated ADA (administered once to twice weekly by intramuscular injection), but the response to this treatment is variable, and some patients develop antibodies against PEG-ADA.

Because it is a systemic autosomal recessive disorder caused by an enzyme deficiency, ADA deficiency represents a good candidate for gene replacement therapy. Ideally, proliferating bone marrow stem cells would be modified by retroviral vectors containing the normal ADA gene, resulting in a permanent cure for the disorder. Because of difficulties in dealing with bone marrow stem cells, gene therapy for ADA deficiency has been initiated instead by retroviral insertion of ADA genes into lymphocytes that have been extracted from patients and artificially stimulated to replicate. After retroviral insertion, the lymphocytes are injected back into the patient's peripheral circulation.

This therapy has been applied in more than a dozen patients with ADA deficiency, and the results have been encouraging. Following gene therapy, ADA levels typically increase to about 25% of the normal level. T lymphocyte counts improve dramatically, and the number of infections decreases. Because of the limited life span of T lymphocytes, these patients must be re-injected with modified T cells once every several months (however, the treated lymphocytes have displayed surprising longevity, surviving in the circulation for well over a year in some cases).

There are potential concerns associated with this procedure. For example, there is a possibility of retrovirally induced oncogenesis in a T cell. Also, because only a sample of mature T cells is treated, the immune systems of these patients are likely to be incomplete (i.e., there would be less T-cell receptor diversity than in a normal individual). Finally, the patients continue to be treated with PEG-ADA, so gene therapy is not entirely responsible for their improvement. Nonetheless, the results thus far are promising, particularly after a 50% reduction of PEG-ADA dosage showed no decline in immune function. These protocols may eventually lead to effective treatment, and they provide invaluable information for the development of gene therapy protocols for other genetic diseases.

---

preparations. The adenovirus can accept an insert of approximately 30 kb. It must be made replication-defective before use in gene therapy. Because of their ability to target nondividing cells, adenoviruses are being used in trials in which the normal CFTR gene (see Chapter 4) is delivered by an aerosol method to epithelial cells (in vivo gene therapy). It is hoped that this treatment may alter chloride ion channel activity in cystic fibrosis patients.

Adenoviruses do not integrate into the host cell's DNA, which provides the advantage that they will not activate a proto-oncogene or otherwise disturb the genome. However, lack of integration is also a disadvantage because adenoviruses are soon eliminated from the nucleus. This results in transient gene expression and the necessity for reintroduction of the vector. A current difficulty in clinical trials for CF is that adenoviruses often induce inflammatory responses in patients. This problem increases with repeated introduction of the adenovirus, which stimulates further immune response to the foreign protein.

OTHER VIRAL VECTORS. Adeno-associated viruses, which are a type of parvovirus, offer several advantages, including stable integration into DNA and no known association with a human disease. These vectors, however, can accept a DNA insert of only about 5 kb in size. Disabled herpesviruses are also being investigated because of their ability to invade neurons, a cell type that is inaccessible to many other vectors.

Although viral gene therapy holds considerable promise, there are several important obstacles:

1. *Transient and low-level expression.* The gene product may be expressed at subtherapeutic levels, often less than 1% of the normal amount. In part, this reflects the fact that only some of the target cells successfully incorporate the normal gene. In addition, random insertion of the virus into the host's genome may affect gene regulation (e.g., enhancer sequences

required for normal expression levels are not present). Transcription of the gene often ceases after a few weeks or months.

2. *Difficulties in reaching target tissue.* While some systemic disorders may be relatively easy to target by modifying lymphocytes or possibly bone marrow stem cells, others present formidable challenges. It is often difficult, for example, to target affected neurons responsible for central nervous system disorders.

3. *Necessity for precise regulation of gene activity.* Accurate regulation of gene activity is not a concern for some diseases (e.g., a 50-fold over-expression of adenosine deaminase has no clinically significant effects). However, it is critical for diseases such as thalassemia, in which the number of α-globin and β-globin chains must be closely balanced (see Chapter 3). It is difficult to achieve such precision using viral gene therapy.

Considerable research is being devoted to overcoming these and other problems. In particular, methods for targeted insertion of genes are being explored, and ways to increase the levels and permanence of gene expression are being developed. In addition, specific types of retroviruses capable of infecting nondividing cells are now being studied.

▼ **Viral vectors offer highly efficient transfer of therapeutic genes into somatic cells. However, they have several drawbacks, including low or transient expression of the gene product, limited insert size, generation of immune responses, difficulty in precise regulation, and, for some vectors, a lack of ability to invade nondividing cells and the (remote) potential for oncogenesis.** ▲

NON-VIRAL VECTORS. Although viral vectors provide the advantage of efficient gene transfer into cells, the disadvantages just listed have prompted researchers to investigate several types of non-viral vectors. One of the most extensively studied is the **liposome,** a fat body that can accept large DNA inserts. Liposomes will sometimes fuse with cells, allowing the DNA insert to enter the cell. Because the liposome has no peptides, it does not elicit an immune response. Its primary disadvantage is that it lacks the transfer efficiency of viruses; only a tiny proportion of target cells accept modified DNA. Various approaches are being tested to overcome this deficiency.

Surprisingly, it is possible to insert DNA directly into cells without using any delivery vector at all. Although most "naked" DNA is repelled by the cell membrane, the DNA will, for unknown reasons, occasionally enter the cell and temporarily encode proteins. Attempts are under way to use naked DNA as a "vaccine" that would encode a pathogenic protein to which the body mounts an immune response.

An intriguing development with potential for somatic cell therapy is the recent synthesis of **human artificial chromosomes.** Because these synthetically constructed chromosomes contain functional centromeres and telomeres, they should be able to integrate and replicate in human cell nuclei. They can reach 5 to 10 Mb in total size, which means they could accept huge inserts of therapeutic DNA. Human artificial chromosomes may help to overcome many of the limitations of current viral and non-viral gene delivery systems.

▼ **Non-viral gene therapy delivery, including liposomes, human artificial chromosomes, and naked DNA, offer some advantages over viral vectors, but they currently lack the transfer efficiency of viral vectors.** ▲

Gene Blocking Therapies

Gene replacement techniques would not be effective in correcting gain-of-function or dominant negative mutations (e.g., Huntington disease, Marfan syndrome). Here, the defective gene product must be disabled in some way. Although not as well developed as gene replacement therapy methods, gene blocking methods are being developed and some show promise.

ANTISENSE THERAPY. The principle behind **antisense therapy** is simple: an oligonucleotide is engineered whose DNA sequence is complementary to that of the mRNA sequence produced by a gain-of-function mutation. This "antisense" oligonucleotide binds to the abnormal mRNA, preventing its translation into a harmful protein (Fig. 13-9).

RIBOZYME THERAPY. Ribozymes are enzymatic RNA molecules, some of which can cleave mRNA. They can be engineered to cleave specific mRNA sequences that contain an unwanted mutation, destroying them before they can be translated into protein.

▼ **Gene blocking techniques may be used to counter the effects of dominant-negative or gain-of-function mutations. They include the use of antisense molecules and RNA-cleaving ribozymes.** ▲

Gene Therapy for Non-Inherited Diseases

As indicated in Table 13-7, the application of gene therapy techniques is by no means limited to inherited diseases. Indeed, about two thirds of the gene therapy protocols now under way involve non-inherited cancers, and approximately 10% involve AIDS therapy. For example, the *p53* tumor suppressor gene, which is lost in about half of all cancers (see Chapter 11), is inserted into lung tumors in an effort to halt tumor progression. As discussed in Chapter 9, some tumors evade immune system detection by discarding Class I HLA molecules. Liposomes containing DNA that will encode the HLA-B7 molecule have been

FIG. 13-9 Gene therapy using an antisense technique. Binding the abnormal mRNA with the antisense molecule prevents it from being translated into an abnormal protein.

introduced into malignant melanoma cells, resulting in HLA-B7 expression on the cell surface and subsequent cell destruction by cytotoxic T cells. In some cases, this has led to regression of the melanoma.

A variety of gene therapy approaches are being directed at the human immunodeficiency virus (HIV). Most of these efforts are aimed at halting replication of the virus or preventing its spread to healthy cells. For example, a dominant-negative mutation introduced into HIV-infected T cells produces a protein that interferes with proteins produced by HIV, blocking their normal action.

Germline Therapy

Somatic cell therapy consists of the alteration of only specific somatic cells and thus differs little in principle from many other types of medical intervention (e.g., bone marrow transplants). In contrast, **germline gene therapy** involves the alteration of all cells of the body, including those giving rise to the gametes. Thus, this type of gene therapy would affect not only the patient but all of his or her descendants.

Germline therapy was first achieved in the mouse in 1983, when copies of a human growth hormone gene were successfully introduced into mouse embryos by microinjection (the gene is inserted directly into the embryo using a very small needle). Among the minority of embryos in which the gene integrated, the gametes were also modified, and the human growth hormone gene was transmitted to future generations (the mice, incidentally, were abnormally large).

While germline therapy is, in principle, possible in humans, it presents significant problems. First, injected embryos usually die, and some develop tumors and malformations. Second, even in an autosomal dominant disorder, half of the embryos will be genetically normal. If it is possible to distinguish the genetically normal embryos (e.g., through PCR diagnosis of in vitro fertilization products), then it would be simpler to implant the normal embryos than to alter the abnormal ones. Finally, there are numerous ethical questions associated with the permanent alteration of a human's genetic legacy. For these reasons, it appears unlikely that human germline therapy would be useful or desirable.

Gene Therapy: A Perspective

Although gene therapy represents a highly active and widely publicized area of research, critics often point out that nobody has yet been *cured* by gene therapy. Undeniably, gene therapy has boosted immune function in patients with ADA deficiency (see Clinical Commentary 13-5) and has decreased cholesterol levels in patients with familial hypercholesterolemia. However, these patients continued to receive other therapy (e.g., PEG-ADA or cholesterol-lowering drugs) as well. It is also unclear at this time whether gene therapy will ever provide a safe treatment or cure for a reasonable cost.

Despite these reservations, gene therapy research is providing many new insights of fundamental biological significance. Somewhat unexpectedly, it is showing perhaps the most promise in treating diseases that are not inherited at all. As with many avenues of biomedical research, the potential of gene therapy research is considerable, and current progress suggests strongly that it may yet provide efficacious treatment of some important human diseases.

STUDY QUESTIONS

1. A newborn screening program for a metabolic disease has just been initiated. Of 100,000 newborns, 100 were shown by a definitive test to have been affected with the disease. The screening test identified 93 of these individuals as affected and 7 as unaffected. It also identified 1,000 individuals as affected who were later shown to be unaffected. Calculate the sensitivity, specificity, and positive predictive value of the screening test, and specify the rate of false positives and false negatives.

2. Study the family shown in the pedigree in Fig. 13-10. Individual 3 has PKU, an autosomal recessive disease. A two-allele RFLP closely linked to the PKU locus has been assayed for each family member, and the figure shows the genotypes of each individual. The marker alleles are 5 kb and 3 kb in size. Based on the genotypes of the linked marker, is individual 6 affected, a heterozygous carrier, or a normal homozygote?

FIG. 13-11 Pedigree to accompany Study Question 3.

4. In the pedigree for an autosomal dominant disorder shown in Fig. 13-12, a tightly linked two-allele RFLP has been typed in each family member. Based on this information, what can you tell the family about the risk that the offspring in generation III will develop the disorder? How might diagnostic accuracy be improved in this case?

5. Compare the advantages and disadvantages of amniocentesis and chorionic villus sampling (CVS).

6. What type of gene therapy would be most appropriate for Huntington disease? Why?

FIG. 13-10 Pedigree to accompany Study Question 2.

3. Study the family shown in the pedigree in Fig 13-11. The affected individuals have neurofibromatosis type 1 (NF1), an autosomal dominant condition. A four-allele microsatellite system closely linked to the NF1 locus has been typed for each family member. Based on the genotypes shown in the accompanying figure, will individual 6 develop NF1?

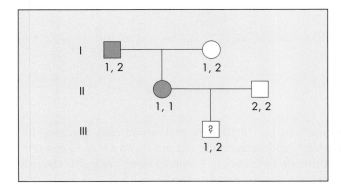

FIG. 13-12 Pedigree to accompany Study Question 4.

SUGGESTED READINGS

American Academy of Pediatrics Committee on Genetics (1989) Newborn screening fact sheets. Pediatrics 83:449-464

Anderson WF (1998) Human gene therapy. Nature 392(suppl.):25-30

Bank A (1996) Human somatic cell gene therapy. BioEssays 18:999-1007

Cao A, Saba L, Galanello R, Rosatelli MC (1997) Molecular diagnosis and carrier screening for β-thalassemia. JAMA 278:1273-1277

Couture LA, Stinchcomb DT (1996) Anti-gene therapy: the use of ribozymes to inhibit gene function. Trends Genet. 12:510-515

Elias S, Simpson JL (1997) Prenatal diagnosis. In: Rimoin DL, Connor JM, Pyeritz RE (eds) Emery and Rimoin's Principles and Practice of Medical Genetics. Vol. 1. Churchill Livingstone, New York, pp 563-580

Eng CM, Schechter C, Robinowitz MS, Fulop G, Burgert T, Levy B, Zinberg R, Desnick RJ (1997) Prenatal genetic carrier testing using triple disease screening. JAMA 278:1268-1272

Felgner PL (1997) Nonviral strategies for gene therapy. Sci. Amer. 276(6):102-106

Ferrari M, Cremonesi L, Carrera P, Bonini PA (1996) Molecular diagnosis of genetic diseases. Clin. Biochem. 29:201-208

Friedmann T (1997) Overcoming the obstacles to gene therapy. Sci. Amer. 276(6):96-101

Graber JH, O'Donnell MJ, Smith CL, Cantor CR (1998) Advances in DNA diagnostics. Curr. Opin. Biotechnol. 9:14-18

Hall SJ, Chen S-H, Woo SLC (1997) The promise and reality of cancer gene therapy. Am. J. Hum. Genet. 61:785-789

Handyside AH, Delhanty JDA (1997) Preimplantation genetic diagnosis: strategies and surprises. Trends Genet. 13:270-275

Harrington JJ, Van Bokkelen G, Mays RM, Gustashaw K, Willard HF (1997) Formation of de novo centromeres and construction of first-generation human artificial microchromosomes. Nature Genet. 15:345-355

Holtzman NA (1998) Bringing genetic tests into the clinic. Hosp. Pract. 33:107-128

Karpati G, Gilbert R, Petrof BJ, Nalbantoglu J (1997) Gene therapy research for Duchenne and Becker muscular dystrophies. Curr. Opin. Neurol. 10:430-435

Lapham EV, Kozma C, Weiss JO (1996) Genetic discrimination: perspectives of consumers. Science 274:621-624

Lissens W, Sermon K (1997) Preimplantation genetic diagnosis: current status and new developments. Hum. Reprod. 12:1756-1761

Mausner JS, Bahn AK (1974) Epidemiology: An Introductory Text. W.B. Saunders, Philadelphia

Milunsky A (1998) Genetic Disorders and the Fetus: Diagnosis, Prevention, and Treatment, 4th ed. Johns Hopkins University Press, Baltimore

Motulsky A (1997) Screening for genetic diseases. N. Eng. J. Med. 336:1314-1316

National Academy of Sciences (1975) Genetic Screening: Programs, Principles and Research. National Academy of Sciences, Washington, DC

National Institutes of Health (1997) NIH Consensus Statement: Genetic Testing for Cystic Fibrosis. National Institutes of Health, Bethesda, MD

Robbins PD, Tahara H, Ghivizzani SC (1998) Viral vectors for gene therapy. Trends Biotechnol. 16:35-40

Russell DW, Hirata RK (1998) Human gene targeting by viral vectors. Nature Genet. 18:325-330

The Canadian Early and Mid-Trimester Amniocentesis Trial (CEMAT) Group (1998) Randomised trial to assess safety and fetal outcome of early and midtrimester amniocentesis. Lancet 351:242-247

Verma IM, Somia N (1997) Gene therapy—promises, problems and prospects. Nature 9:239-242

Wald NJ, Kennard A (1997) Prenatal screening for neural tube defects and Down syndrome. In: Rimoin DL, Connor JM, Pyeritz RE (eds) Emery and Rimoin's Principles and Practice of Medical Genetics. Vol. 1. Churchill Livingstone, New York, pp 545-562

Weaver D (1992) Catalog of Prenatally Diagnosed Conditions, 2nd ed. Johns Hopkins University Press, Baltimore

Wilson JM (1996) Adenoviruses as gene-delivery vehicles. N. Eng. J. Med. 334:1185-1187

14
Clinical Genetics and Genetic Counseling

Medical genetics has recently emerged as a true specialty in medicine. In the 1960s the fields of biochemical genetics, clinical cytogenetics, and **dysmorphology** (the study of abnormal physical development) developed. The 1970s witnessed the establishment of the techniques necessary for the prenatal diagnosis of genetic disorders. By the end of the 1970s, discussions about the formation of an American Board of Medical Genetics had occurred, and in 1981 the first certification examination was administered. Ten years later the American Board of Medical Specialties recognized this new field.

Whereas medical genetics is the study of the genetics of human disease, **clinical genetics** deals with the direct clinical care of persons with genetic diseases. The diagnostic, counseling, and management issues surrounding genetic disease are the principal foci of clinical genetics.

In this chapter we summarize the principles of clinical genetics and the process of genetic counseling. In addition, this chapter will provide an overview of the field of dysmorphology, since the growth of this area has influenced and paralleled the emergence of clinical genetics.

THE PRINCIPLES AND PRACTICE OF CLINICAL GENETICS

As mentioned in Chapter 1, genetic conditions as a group are common and are a significant cause of human mortality and morbidity. Typically, genetic disorders are complex, multi-organ, systemic conditions. The care of persons with these disorders often involves multiple specialties. Thus, genetic disorders are part of the differential diagnosis of most symptoms and clinical presentations. For example, when evaluating an infant with a blistering skin disease, the ability to distinguish between one of the many forms of epidermolysis bullosa (an inherited disorder of keratinocytes in which skin blisters develop after mild trauma) and staphylo-

coccal skin disease must be part of the clinician's repertoire. WWW

Because of the complexity and number of human genetic diseases, their clinical diagnosis and treatment can seem overwhelming. To help manage this information, we provide an overview of the most important concepts. These include the importance of accurate diagnosis, the application of the tenets of medical genetics to medical practice, and the role of genetic counseling in the care of persons with genetic disease.

Accurate Diagnosis

The significance of this basic medical principle cannot be overemphasized. The process of genetic counseling, one of the central services of medical genetics, begins with correct diagnosis. All discussions of natural history, prognosis, management, risk determination, options for prenatal diagnosis, and referral to support groups depend on an accurate diagnosis. For example, genetic counseling for a family who has a son with mental retardation usually involves questions of risk for this condition in future offspring. An accurate answer requires the clinician to identify a condition of known etiology. If a specific diagnosis (e.g., fragile X syndrome) is made, then the rest of the genetic counseling process starts: current information can be shared and management initiated (Clinical Commentary 14-1).

▼ In clinical genetics, as in all of medicine, accurate diagnosis is the most important first step in patient care. ▲

The process of diagnosing a genetic disorder is a complex sequence of events. It depends upon diagnostic decision making, biochemistry, dysmorphology, laboratory diagnosis, and the basic principles of medical genetics. For diseases in which the diagnostic criteria

CLINICAL COMMENTARY 14-1
REASONS FOR MAKING A DIAGNOSIS OF A SYNDROME

The long list of syndromes associated with congenital malformations is overwhelming to the clinician. More than 400 conditions are listed in *Smith's Recognizable Patterns of Human Malformations,* and more than 1,000 are accessible through the POSSUM computerized database. This number imparts a sense that the diagnosis of a malformation syndrome lies in the arena of "academic trivia." However, this is not the case.

Consider, for example, the child who is large for gestational age and has a number of physical abnormalities: omphalocele (intestinal protrusion at the umbilicus), large tongue, facial hemangioma, flank mass, and asymmetrical limb length (Fig. 14-1). His family has questions such as, "What does he have?", "How will he do?", "Will he look different?", "Will he have mental retardation?", "What is the chance of his condition occurring again in another child?"

By putting these features together and making the pattern recognition diagnosis of the Beckwith-Wiedemann syndrome, the clinician is able to answer all of the parents' questions fairly precisely. Beckwith-Wiedemann syndrome is an autosomal dominant condition with variable expression and incomplete penetrance. In addition, the gene is thought to exhibit imprinting (see Chapter 4). When there is no family history, however, the sibling recurrence risk is less than 5%. When there is a family history, the recurrence risk is much higher, and linkage or mutation analysis may provide a more precise risk estimate. In future pregnancies, prenatal diagnosis using ultrasound can test for an omphalocele in the second trimester and for large size for gestational age, excessive amniotic fluid (polyhydramnios), and large tongue. If a fetus is thought to have Beckwith-Wiedemann syndrome, then the delivery plan would change and the baby should be born in a tertiary care center. WWW

Children with the Beckwith-Wiedemann syndrome do not usually have mental retardation. Although the large tongue can cause orthodontic problems, speech difficulties, and occasionally upper airway problems, these conditions usually improve as the child gets older. The facial appearance is not strikingly abnormal in later childhood.

Chromosomes should probably be studied, although most Beckwith-Wiedemann patients do not have the chromosome 11 abnormality that has been reported in a small number of cases. Otherwise, the main emphases of the medical care plan include periodic ultrasound to look

FIG. 14-1 A child with Beckwith-Wiedemann syndrome. Note the prominent eyes and large, protruding tongue.

(Courtesy Dr. David Viskochil, University of Utah Health Sciences Center)

for intraabdominal malignancies, especially Wilms tumor and hepatoblastoma. Children with Beckwith-Wiedemann syndrome have a 5% to 10% risk of developing these tumors, and both types are treatable if detected early.

In this example, it was important to diagnose the Beckwith-Wiedemann syndrome. The correct label led to precise information for genetic counseling, prediction of natural history (including reassurance), organization of appropriate laboratory studies, a health maintenance plan, and referral to a support group. Diagnosis was helpful to the parents, the family physician, and the child.

are well established, the practitioner has guidelines for making a diagnosis. An example of such criteria would be those recommended by the National Institutes of Health Consensus Development Conference for the diagnosis of neurofibromatosis type 1 (NF1; see Chapter 4). For conditions that are defined by a specific laboratory marker, such as an abnormal karyotype or biochemical assay, the diagnostic procedure is generally straightforward. For many genetic diseases, however, there are no well-established criteria, and the definition and delineation of the disorder are not clear-cut.

Dysmorphic syndromes require knowledge and skills in the recognition of mild malformations, minor anomalies, and phenotypic variations. The diagnosis of other genetic diseases may require expertise from a variety of disciplines. For instance, the diagnosis of any of the forms of retinitis pigmentosa (see Chapter 8) requires input from an ophthalmologist who is familiar with this group of retinal degenerative conditions. The diagnostic process is further complicated by the variable expression, incomplete penetrance, and heterogeneity of many genetic diseases. These concepts were discussed in Chapter 4.

Application of the Principles of Medical Genetics

Developing a genetic approach to human disease in the clinical setting requires the application of all of the basic principles of medical genetics discussed in this book. For example, making or excluding the diagnosis of NF1 requires knowledge of the clinical variability and age of onset of certain features of the condition (Clinical Commentary 14-2). Recognition of the various forms of neurofibromatosis (i.e., heterogeneity) is also important.

Knowledge of the other formal principles of medical genetics is also necessary in the care of persons with genetic conditions. The accumulation of family history data and the interpretation of pedigree information are important in answering a family's questions of risk. An understanding of the different modes of inheritance is important in any explanation of recurrence risk. Discussion of the concepts of new mutation and pleiotropy are commonplace in reviewing the cause and pathogenesis of a genetic disease with a family. Even an understanding of meiosis is a requirement for discussions of etiology with the family of a newborn with Down syndrome.

Genetic Counseling
Definition and Principles

Genetic counseling represents one of the central foci of medical genetics. At first glance, use of the term "counseling" implies that this service lies in the domain of mental health, social work, or psychotherapy. In fact, genetic counseling is based on the conventional medical model because it depends significantly on accurate diagnosis and knowledge of medical genetics. As a tradition, genetic counseling grew out of the field of human genetics rather than from behavioral science, unlike other counseling disciplines.

In 1975 the American Society of Human Genetics adopted a definition of genetic counseling that has stood the test of time:

Genetic counseling is a communication process which deals with the human problems associated with the occurrence or risk of occurrence of a genetic disorder in a family. This process involves an attempt by one or more appropriately trained persons to help the individual or family to: 1) comprehend the medical facts including the diagnosis, probable course of the disorder, and the available management; 2) appreciate the way heredity contributes to the disorder and the risk of recurrence in specified relatives; 3) understand the alternatives for dealing with the risk of recurrence; 4) choose a course of action which seems to them appropriate in their view of their risk, their family goals, and their ethical and religious standards and act in accordance with that decision; and 5) make the best possible adjustment to the disorder in an affected family member and/or to the risk of recurrence of that disorder.

This definition illustrates the complex tasks that face the practitioner. The first task involves establishing the diagnosis and discussing the natural history and management of the condition. In this regard the treatment of a genetic disease does not differ from that of any other type of disease.

The second task requires an understanding of the basic tenets of medical genetics, especially risk determination. For chromosomal and multifactorial disorders, empirical risks are used to estimate recurrence. Inheritance patterns are used to predict the recurrence risk of Mendelian disorders. However, the clinical issues are frequently complicated by incomplete penetrance, variable expression, delayed age of onset, and allelic and locus heterogeneity. In some cases, incorporation of additional information using the Bayesian probability approach can significantly alter risk estimates (Clinical Commentary 14-3).

The third and fourth objectives of the genetic counseling process underlie the primary differences between the genetic model and the traditional biomedical approach. These tasks involve the discussion of reproductive options and the facilitation of decision making. Implicit in the fourth part of the definition is the notion of respect for the family's autonomy and their perceptions of risk and of the disorder itself. This approach has been called **nondirectiveness**: the counselor leaves all decisions about future reproduction up to the family. This differs somewhat from the more traditional medical approach in which *recommendations* for treatment or intervention are made.

This is an important issue, since nondirectiveness sometimes conflicts with the broader view of preventive medicine that might suggest that the principal goal of genetic counseling should be the reduction of the incidence of genetic diseases. If prevention or reduction of occurrence is the primary goal, then one's approach might be more directive. However, the main goal of genetic counseling is to help families understand and cope with genetic disease, not to reduce the incidence of genetic disease.

CLINICAL COMMENTARY 14-2
THE NEGATIVE FAMILY HISTORY

One of the common discussions on ward rounds is the notation that a person's family history is "negative" or "noncontributory." This is often thought to rule out a genetic disorder. However, the *majority* of individuals who have a genetic disease will not have a "positive" family history. A quick review of the mechanisms of Mendelian, chromosomal, and multifactorial disease inheritance shows that a lack of other affected persons in the family is common and does not by any means rule out the presence of a genetic disease. For example, the sibling recurrence risk is 25% for diseases with autosomal recessive inheritance. Thus, a significant number of families with multiple offspring will have only one affected child and no family history. Even some well-established autosomal dominant disorders may often present a negative family history because of high proportions of new mutations (examples include Marfan syndrome, neurofibromatosis type 1 [NF1], and achondroplasia, where the proportions of cases caused by new mutations are 30%, 50%, and 80%, respectively). Chromosomal syndromes usually have a low recurrence risk. Even when a parent carries a balanced chromosome rearrangement, the recurrence risk among the offspring is usually less than 15%. The sibling recurrence risks for multifactorial conditions are usually 5% or less.

CASE

A family comes in with a 6-year-old boy who has 10 *café-au-lait* spots exceeding 0.5 cm in diameter and an optic glioma (Fig. 14-2). The family has questions about the diagnosis and recurrence risk in future pregnancies. On initial telephone contact it is learned that there is no history of a family member with similar features.

There are several possible explanations for this finding. Exploring them underscores the implications of a negative family history:

1. *New mutation of the NF1 gene*. Because of the relatively high proportion of new mutations for this disorder, this is the most likely explanation.
2. *Variable expression*. It is also possible that one of the parents carries the gene but has mild expression of the phenotype. Occasionally a parent has multiple *café-au-lait* spots and a few neurofibromas, but a diagnosis of NF1 has never been made.
3. *Incomplete penetrance*. This is a possibility; however, it is unlikely for NF1, in which penetrance is close to 100%. If a family has two children with NF1 and neither parent has the gene, germline mosaicism would be the more likely explanation.
4. *Incorrect diagnosis*. One of the assumptions and basic principles of medical genetics is accurate diagnosis. This patient meets the NIH established criteria for

NF1 (see Chapter 4). However, if this individual had only *café-au-lait* spots, then the diagnosis would have been an issue. One would need to know the differential diagnosis of multiple *café-au-lait* spots.

5. *False paternity*. While relatively unlikely, this possibility must be kept in mind.

We began with an individual having a classical autosomal dominant disorder with no family history. This can be explained in a number of ways. The statement that there is "a negative family history" should not be considered conclusive evidence against the presence of a heritable condition.

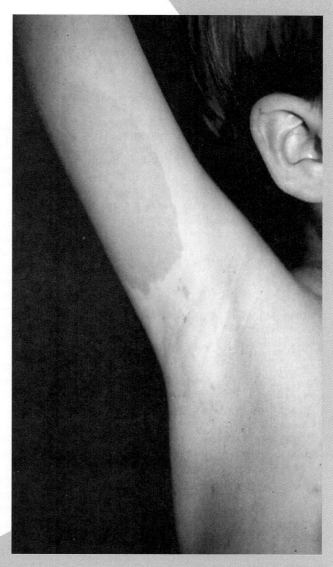

FIG. 14-2 A 6-year-old boy with multiple *café-au-lait* spots and axillary freckling.

CLINICAL COMMENTARY 14-3
RECURRENCE RISKS AND BAYES THEOREM

The estimation of recurrence risks was treated at some length in Chapters 4 and 5. A typical example of recurrence risk estimation would be a case in which a man affected with hemophilia A, an X-linked recessive disorder, produces a daughter (individual II-1 in Fig. 14-3). Because the man can transmit only the X chromosome carrying the hemophilia A mutation to his daughter, she must be a carrier. The carrier's daughter, individual III-6, has a 50% chance of receiving the X chromosome carrying the mutation and being herself a carrier. Even though the daughter in generation III has five normal brothers, her risk remains 50% because we know that the mother in generation II is a carrier.

Suppose now that the woman in generation III produces three sons (generation IV), none of whom has hemophilia A. Intuitively, we might begin to suspect that she is not a carrier after all. How can we incorporate this new information into our recurrence risk estimate?

A statistical principle that allows us to make use of such information is called **Bayes theorem** (the application of Bayes theorem is often termed Bayesian analysis or Bayesian inference). The table below summarizes the basic steps involved in Bayesian analysis. We begin with the **prior probability** that the woman in generation III is a carrier. As its name suggests, the prior probability denotes the probability that she is a carrier *before* we account for the fact that she has produced three normal sons. Because we know her mother is a carrier, this prior probability must be 1/2. Then the prior probability that she is not a carrier is also 1/2.

FIG. 14-3

	She is a carrier	She is not a carrier
Prior probability	1/2	1/2
Conditional probability	1/8	1
Joint probability	1/16	1/2
Posterior probability	1/9	8/9

Next we take into account her three normal sons by estimating the probability that all three of them would be normal, given that she is a carrier. Because this probability is *conditioned* on her carrier status, it is termed a **conditional probability**. If she is a carrier, the conditional probability that all three of her sons are normal would be $(1/2)^3$, or 1/8. We also estimate the probability that all of her sons are normal, given that she is *not* a carrier. This conditional probability is, of course, very close to 1.

Next we want to find the probability that the woman is a carrier *and* that she is a carrier with three normal sons. To obtain the probability of the co-occurrence of these two events, we multiply the prior probability times the conditional probability to derive **a joint probability** (i.e., the probability of *both* events occurring together, a concept discussed in Chapter 4). The joint probability that she is a carrier is then $1/2 \times 1/8 = 1/16$. Similarly, the joint probability that she is not a carrier is $1/2 \times 1 = 1/2$. These joint probabilities indicate the woman is 8 times more likely *not* to be a carrier than to be a carrier.

The final step is to standardize the joint probabilities so that the two probabilities under consideration (i.e., being a carrier versus not being a carrier) sum to 1. To do this, we simply divide the joint probability that the woman is a carrier (1/16) by the sum of the two joint probabilities $(1/16 + 1/2)$. This yields a **posterior probability** of 1/9 that she is a carrier and 8/9 that she is not a carrier. Notice that this standardization process allows us to provide a risk estimate (1/9, or 11%), while preserving the odds of non-carrier versus carrier status indicated by the joint probabilities.

Having worked through the Bayesian analysis, we see that our intuition was confirmed: the fact that the woman in question produced three normal sons reduced her risk of being a carrier substantially, from an initial estimate of 50% to a final probability of only 11%.

Prior to the advent of disease diagnosis through linked markers or mutation detection, Bayesian analysis was often the only way to derive a risk estimate in a situation such as this one. Now, of course, one would attempt to identify the factor VIII mutation that causes hemophilia A in this family directly, or, failing this, linked markers would be used. This is a much more direct and accurate approach for determining carrier status. However, as discussed in Chapter 13, it is not always possible to identify the responsible mutation, particularly when a large number of mutations can cause the disorder (as is the case for hemophilia A). In addition, linkage analysis is not always informative. Thus, Bayesian analysis is still sometimes a useful tool for refining risk estimates.

CLINICAL COMMENTARY 14-3—cont'd
RECURRENCE RISKS AND BAYES THEOREM—cont'd

The additional information incorporated in Bayesian analysis is not confined to the assessment of health status in relatives, as shown in this example. Another type of information is a biochemical assay, such as factor VIII activity level, that could help to indicate carrier status. Because there is usually overlap between carriers and normal homozygotes for such tests, the assay cannot determine carrier status with certainty but gives us a *probability* estimate for incorporation into Bayesian analysis. In diseases with delayed age of onset, such as adult polycystic kidney disease, the probability of being affected at a certain age can be used in a Bayesian analysis. Here, one considers the fact that the at-risk individual is less and less likely to possess the disease gene if he or she remains normal beyond a certain age.

CLINICAL COMMENTARY 14-4
TALKING TO THE PARENTS OF A NEWBORN WITH DOWN SYNDROME

The birth of a newborn with Down syndrome presents many challenges. Typically the infant is not acutely ill, and the parents will not be aware of the diagnosis. Thus, the practitioner has to approach the parents, oftentimes strangers, with disappointing news. The family experiences a series of emotions that are somewhat similar to the reactions after a loss: anger, denial, sadness, and then usually reorganization and adaptation. Families face these situations with markedly different backgrounds: varying attitudes toward crisis, varied demographic and socioeconomic circumstances, and even a wide range of differences in the cultural meaning of a disability or defect. All of these variables, plus the fact that physicians are often not trained in being the bearers of bad news, can make this a difficult situation. Parents remember in detail the way in which the news is presented. The practitioner has both the opportunity and the challenge to help the family through these events.

From studies that have investigated the recommendations of parents who have experienced this event, we can provide a number of practical suggestions:

1. *Talk to both parents together whenever possible.* This is sometimes not practical, but when it can be accomplished it is critical.
2. *Communicate the diagnosis as soon as possible.* All studies of parental interviews show that they prefer early communication of the diagnosis.
3. *Choose a place that is private and quiet where both the parents and the professionals can sit down.* Avoid standing up with the parents seated. Always be sure to introduce yourself. Structure the interview from the beginning.
4. *Humanize the situation as much as possible.* Learn the baby's first name if it has been decided on, and always know the baby's gender. Refer to the infant as a son or daughter, and be aware of the use of all language. Phrases like "mental retardation" have great impact. Terms like "mongolism" are not appropriate as they are stigmatizing, pejorative, and incorrect.
5. *Develop a sense of realistic positivism.* It is important to discuss the developmental limitations in a patient with Down syndrome, but it is also important to have an optimistic and positive attitude. This suggestion comes from the self-help and parents' organizations that have developed in the last two decades.
6. *Answer the parents' questions, but avoid technical overload.* It is important to be accurate and current on the biological and medical aspects of the disease under discussion. When an answer is not known, mention that it can be reviewed or referred to a consultant.
7. *Listen actively.* Assume that almost all feelings are natural and that parents will be wrestling with their own guilt and shame. Validate all feelings that arise. Most parents will meet this challenge quite effectively and will not require psychiatric consultation.
8. *Refer the family to the appropriate resources early.* This would include parents' support groups or even individual parents who have a child with Down syndrome. Share any written material that is available, but make certain it is accurate and current.

Above all, be aware of the unique plight of families in such a situation, and make an effort to spend time with them. While it is difficult to present in written form how one can develop attributes such as kindness and empathy, it is important for physicians in training to learn from their mentors and utilize their own personality style as a strength.

Although most geneticists subscribe to the principles of autonomy and nondirectiveness, it may sometimes be impossible to be entirely nondirective simply because of the limited options that the counselor has in a time-restricted session. In addition, information may be presented quite differently in different contexts. Information about Down syndrome, for example, may be communicated differently depending on whether a diagnosis has been made prenatally or following the birth of an affected newborn (Clinical Commentary 14-4).

▼ The majority of clinical geneticists subscribe to the principle of nondirectiveness: information about risks, natural history, treatment, and outcome are presented in a balanced and neutral manner, but decisions about reproduction are left to the family. ▲

The facilitation of discussion about reproductive decision-making is central to the task of genetic counseling. Several factors are involved in a family's decision about future pregnancies when there is an increased risk. The obvious ones are the magnitude of the risk figure and the burden or impact of the disorder. However, these are not the only significant issues. A family's individual perception of the impact of the condition is probably more important in their decision making than the professional's perception of the burden. The meaning of children to the individual family, according to their own cultural, religious, or personal preferences, is weighed heavily in the reproductive decision-making process. In addition, families frequently play out the scenario of coping with a recurrence of the condition in another child. Identification of these issues for a family often helps to stimulate their own discussions. Some families perceive risk qualitatively rather than quantitatively: they consider themselves to be either "at risk" or not, with the actual risk estimate being a secondary consideration. The fact that there is so much variation in the importance people assign to each of these factors (perception of risk, perception of impact, meaning of children, and the possibility of recurrence) underscores

---

BOX 14-1
BIRTH OF A CHILD WITH TRISOMY 18

Our daughter Juliett arrived on a beautiful summer afternoon in 1984. Late in my pregnancy, an ultrasound had showed an enlarged heart, dilated left kidney, and possible malformation of the cerebellum. During labor, our daughter's heart rate decelerated significantly, and we were given the option of an emergency C-section. Without hesitation, we opted for the C-section. A drape was hung so that I could not see, and I only knew the baby was born when the pediatrician ran out of the room with something in his arms. My husband quickly followed, and then I waited for what seemed an eternity.

Juliett weighted 4 pounds, 6 ounces and was 18 inches long. I had graduated as an RN just before Juliett was conceived and had worked in a pediatric ICU. I had just enough experience to pick up a few of her obvious problems, but many escaped me. She was clearly much too thin, and her rib cage looked too short and prominent. But compared to the mental images I had formed after the ultrasound, I was relieved to see how beautiful she was. Her most striking feature was her incredible blue eyes, which were wide open and very alert. Her nose and mouth were beautifully formed and very petite. As my husband and I sat in awe over her, a neonatalogist entered the room. He pointed out several characteristics, the only one of which I clearly remember was the clenched fist with the index finger lying over the middle finger. He concluded that she probably had trisomy 18. Of the grim things he rattled off, the only thing I remembered was that he said she would be a vegetable and that she would most likely die within the next couple of days. He then walked away, and we sat there, stunned. In this state of grief and turmoil I tried to understand how this clenched fist could lead to death, and how these bright, alert eyes could belong to a vegetable.

In the days that followed, I often opened up her fist and lay her fingers straight, hoping that the blood tests would not confirm the doctor's suspicions. Our bonding with Juliett had been instant, and our great desire was to be able to take her home before she died. As she began to tolerate feedings and was weaned away from oxygen, our pleas to take her home were granted.

We left with no follow-up or care plan. Each time she went to sleep, we prayed she would wake up again and that we could complete another feeding. At 3 months of age, she started to smile at us, and our hopes brightened. We have been fortunate to see her outlive the grim statistics, and we have learned that there is no clear explanation why some children with this condition live longer than others. Juliett's heart was enlarged because of a defect similar to a tetralogy of Fallot. Mild scoliosis at birth has now progressed to a 100-degree lumbar curve and a 90-degree thoracic curve. Despite her many physical challenges, Juliett has continued at her slower pace to learn and develop new skills. Her personality is delightful, and people are often surprised to see how responsive and interactive she is.

We have often been asked if we were afraid to have more children. Perhaps we were crazy, but we felt that another like Juliett would be great. We have had four more girls. To everyone's surprise, our fifth child, Camille, was born with Down syndrome. With Juliett, the grieving process had been covered up with the gratitude we felt that she was even alive. With Camille, we experienced the more typical grieving process.

On the day of Juliett's birth, a pediatrician came forward, put his arms around us, and told us he thought she was beautiful and to love her for as long as she could be with us. He turned her into a human being with a life to be highly valued. In the 13 years that have followed, Juliett has seen many doctors. Most of them, although they could not cure her problems, gave us the most important thing we needed: to know that our daughter's life was of great worth and that, if they could, they would do anything to help her.

the point that the professional should be a facilitator and not the decision maker.

The final task of genetic counseling is to help the family cope with the presence of the disorder and/or its risk of recurrence. This task is similar to the physician's support of a family that deals with any chronic disease and/or disability. What is unique, perhaps, is the family's perception of the *meaning* of a genetic disorder (Boxes 14-1 and 14-2). In many acquired conditions, such as infections or accidents, the ultimate meaning of the condition is externalized. In genetic disorders, the condition is more intrinsic to the individual and the family; it thus often presents a complex personal dilemma. Validation of the plight of families is vital and is probably more effective than simplistic attempts to wipe away guilt. Feelings of guilt and shame are natural to the situation and also need acknowledgment.

The primary care practitioner plays a vital role in the ongoing support of families in which a member has a genetic disease. Additional support strategies include referral of the family to a genetics support group, distribution of written information on the disorder, referral to mental health professionals for ongoing counseling, and frequent follow-up visits that include time for discussions of feelings and thoughts.

▼ Genetic counseling includes five themes: medical management, risk determination, risk options, reproductive decision making, and support services. ▲

Numerous studies in the past two decades have attempted to evaluate the effectiveness of genetic counseling. The methodology of these studies is complicated, and the evaluation of the results depends on one's interpretation of the goal of genetic counseling. A few general points, however, can be made. Families tend to recall recurrence risks relatively well. A letter sent to them after the visit improves this recall. Families who perceive their offspring's condition as being serious and

---

BOX 14-2
RAISING A CHILD WITH BLOOM SYNDROME

Tommy was born via an emergency Caesarean section because 1 week before his delivery date, his fetal movements markedly decreased. At birth, he weighed only 4 pounds, and the first time that I saw him, he was in an incubator connected to all sorts of tubes. He spent his first month of life in the neonatal intensive care unit so that his weight gain could be closely monitored . Since he was so small, he was fed through a feeding tube for many months, and as a consequence, he refused to drink from a bottle. Eventually, he overcame his aversion to using his mouth to eat but only after substantial training. Nevertheless, despite our care, Tommy remained small for his age.

The following summer, Tommy developed dark red marks on his cheeks and under his eyes. Our pediatrician referred us to a dermatologist who suspected that the marks on Tommy's face were related to his growth failure. We were very surprised. How could these two findings be related? That is when we were told that Tommy might have a genetic disorder called Bloom syndrome. We hoped that the doctor was wrong, but soon thereafter Tommy had a genetic test that measured the number of sister chromatid exchanges per cell (see Chapter 2). This test confirmed that Tommy had Bloom syndrome. Although I insisted that it was a false-positive result, I learned to accept that our son had a very rare cancer syndrome.

We were barraged by questions from family, friends, and doctors. As a result, we became very protective of our son and his privacy. Nevertheless, there was only so much we could do to protect him because he is such a social little boy, loving to play with family and friends. This also made choosing an appropriate elementary school a very difficult decision for us. We expected that children would pick on him because of his small size. However, to our surprise, he easily developed friendships and adjusted well to his classmates. In fact, the problems that he did develop were largely because of his misbehavior. Thus, we struggled to find a balance between protecting Tommy while not permitting him special privileges because of his small stature.

In our home, we try to treat Tommy like any of our other children. One challenge for us is that because of Tommy's small size, people wrongly perceive that he is much younger than his chronological age. This is very frustrating for Tommy, yet we occasionally reinforce this image because of our concern for his safety. For example, although Tommy is 6 years old, he weighs only 21 pounds. Thus, he must sit in an infant seat when he travels in a car and we explain to Tommy's friends that it helps him see through the windows. Another safety problem is that many of the sensors for the automatic doors at supermarkets cannot detect his presence and easily slam into him.

Overall, Tommy has adapted well. He climbs or jumps in order to reach things. To keep up with his peers, he often runs, hops, or jumps instead of walking. We constantly worry about his safety, but we cannot control all that happens to him. To date, he has been healthy, and although it seems like we have been riding an emotional roller-coaster, we wouldn't trade our experiences for anything.

one of "burden" recall risk figures better. Most studies suggest that genetic counseling is relatively effective in providing information about the medical aspects and genetic risks of the condition. Issues surrounding decision making and psychosocial support require additional investigation.

The Delivery of Genetic Counseling: Genetic Counselors and Support Groups

As genetic counseling evolved in the 1970s, it became clear that the delivery of this service is complex and time consuming. Not only did the geneticist need to have skills in most specialties of medicine, but facilita-

---

BOX 14-3

AN INSIDER'S VIEW OF GENETIC COUNSELING

What Is a Genetic Counselor?

In its most general usage, the term "genetic counselor" refers to any medical professional who is professionally qualified to provide genetic counseling. Typically, a genetic counselor is a genetics professional with a master's or Ph.D. degree in genetic counseling. Degree programs in genetic counseling provide education and clinical training in medical genetics and counseling. A certified genetic counselor has also passed a certification examination administered by the American Board of Genetic Counseling or the American Board of Medical Genetics.

What Do Genetic Counselors Do?

Some of the primary responsibilities of a genetic counselor are to interview individuals and families with genetic disorders and to answer questions about the possibilities of a genetic disorder. A genetic counselor often works as part of a team that may include medical geneticists, other physicians (e.g., obstetricians, oncologists, neurologists), social workers, psychologists, nutritionists, or nurses. Genetic counselors help to collect and assess medical information leading to a diagnosis, provide patient education, provide psychosocial support and counseling, provide genetic counseling and risk assessment for genetic testing, and help physicians with the management of genetic conditions. They often triage inquiries and/or referrals to the genetics service in which they practice. They may manage or coordinate clinics and/or personnel. They are active in genetic education programs for medical professionals and the lay public.

In What Settings Do Genetic Counselors Work?

Genetic counselors often work in general genetics settings in pediatrics and adult medicine. They also work in obstetrical settings, providing counseling for prenatal diagnosis and screening, genetic testing for couples with multiple pregnancy loss, diagnosis and management of pregnancies affected with abnormalities detected by radiological imaging, and, most recently, alternative reproductive technologies. They work in multidisciplinary specialty clinics for groups of diseases (e.g., metabolic, craniofacial, bone dysplasia, neurogenetic) or single diseases (e.g., Down syndrome, neurofibromatosis, hemophilia). More recently, genetic counselors are becoming increasingly integrated into cancer genetics clinics.

Many counselors participate in research related to clinical genetics and genetic counseling. For example, predictive testing for disorders such as Huntington disease and hereditary cancers has occurred mainly in research studies aimed at assessing its medical, ethical, legal, and social consequences. Within this research setting, genetic counselors provide counseling and help to design, implement, and evaluate research protocols.

Some genetic counselors work in laboratories to provide an interface between the laboratory and its clients and to help develop laboratory protocols. A small percentage of genetic counselors are in private practice, and some work in administrative positions for the state or federal government. Many genetic counselors are active at the regional and/or national level in professional organizations, and some counselors help to start, maintain, or advise support groups for genetic disorders.

What Skills and Personal Qualities Make a Good Genetic Counselor?

A good genetic counselor needs both a strong background in the biological sciences and genetics and training in the theory and practice of psychosocial techniques (e.g., family systems, crisis counseling, interviewing skills). Since most genetic counselors provide direct patient service, it is essential to work well with people. Genetic counselors must work well both independently and on a team. There is a high level of responsibility involved in patient care aspects, and counselors must successfully learn to handle the stress of the difficult situations of the families with whom they work.

What Is the Future of Genetic Counseling?

It is difficult to predict the extent to which medical genetics will continue to move into mainstream medicine. Will geneticists and genetic counselors increase in number, or will genetics professionals remain small in number and limit their role to advising generalists and seeing only the most complicated cases? In either case, there is clearly a need for an increase in the genetic education of medical professionals and the public. Many observers think that medical genetics and genetic counseling have a high potential for expansion. What is undisputed is the striking emergence of medical genetics from an obscure medical subspecialty to an area of knowledge that is fast becoming integrated into every field of medicine.

Courtesy Bonnie J. Baty, MS.

tion of decision making and provision of psychological support were also necessary. As a need for genetics professionals other than the physician became apparent, a number of genetic counseling training programs were initiated. Currently, more than 20 accredited programs in North America provide master's or doctoral degree training in genetic counseling. Genetic counselors have become an integral part of the delivery of medical genetic services. From this growth evolved a professional society, The National Society of Genetic Counselors, and more recently the certifying and accrediting board, the American Board of Genetic Counseling. Although the range of skills is wide and job descriptions vary in different medical centers, genetic counselors have established themselves as experts in risk determination, reproductive decision making, and psychosocial support (Box 14-3).

The importance of support groups in assisting families in which a member has a genetic disorder is becoming increasingly obvious. These volunteer groups provide the family with the sense of the "fellow traveler" in a way that the professional is not able to do. The sense of isolation that frequently accompanies genetic disorders (and rare conditions in general) is often alleviated by meeting someone else in the same situation. Immediate bonds are formed that often assist in the coping process. In the last few decades, a clear partnership of professionals and persons with genetic disorders and disabilities has developed. Not only have these groups provided a needed service, but they have also promoted the establishment of databases and research studies. Referral to a support group and distribution of their written information are now a routine part of the care and management of persons with genetic disorders. **www**

▼ Genetic counseling involves a partnership of physicians, genetic counselors, and genetics support groups. ▲

Clinical Genetics Evaluation and Services

With the development of medical genetics as a medical specialty, clinical genetics services have become part of the health care delivery system. Most university medical centers in North America include a genetics clinic whose major objective is the provision of genetic diagnosis and counseling services.

As in all medical visits, evaluation of a person or family for a potential genetic condition requires a thorough history and physical examination. The history includes information about the family's concerns, the prenatal period, labor, delivery, and documentation of the family relationships (the pedigree). The physical examination should focus on the physical variations or minor anomalies that provide clues to a diagnosis. Additional family members may need evaluation for the presence or ab-

sence of a genetic disorder. Photographs and recording of certain physical measurements are a standard component of the genetic evaluation. Ancillary tests may be required to document specific physical features (e.g., an echocardiogram for aortic dilatation in Marfan syndrome or x-rays to diagnose achondroplasia).

An important type of clinical data gathered in this process is the family history (Box 14-4). The data obtained in a family history are often useful in obtaining an accurate diagnosis of a condition. For example, a strong family history of early-onset coronary disease may indicate the presence of an LDL-receptor defect causing familial hypercholesterolemia. A family history of early-onset colon cancer could indicate that a gene for familial adenomatous polyposis or hereditary nonpolyposis colorectal cancer is present in the family. Family history information can also guide the estimation of recurrence risks by helping to determine whether

---

BOX 14-4
THE FAMILY HISTORY

A thorough, accurate family history is an indispensable part of a medical evaluation. At a minimum, the following items should be included:

1. The gender of each individual and his or her relationship to other family members. This information should be indicated using standard pedigree symbols (see Chapter 4).
2. *At least* all first-degree relatives (parents, siblings, and offspring) of the proband. Preferably, a three-generation family history should be obtained. For example, male relatives on the mother's side of the family will be especially important when considering an X-linked recessive disorder.
3. The age of each individual. A record must be kept of whether each individual is affected with the disease in question, and inquiries should be made about diseases that may be related to the disease in question (e.g., ovarian cancer in a family being seen for familial breast cancer).
4. All known miscarriages and stillbirths.
5. If possible, the ethnic origin of the family. This is important because many diseases vary considerably in prevalence among different ethnic groups.
6. Information about consanguinity. While relatively rare in most Western populations, consanguinity is common in many of the world's populations, and immigrant populations will often maintain relatively high rates of consanguinity (see Chapter 4).
7. Changes in family histories. Family members develop newly diagnosed diseases, and additional children are born. These changes can affect diagnosis and risk estimation, so the family history must be kept current.

a genetic disease has been transmitted by one's parents or has occurred as a new mutation (this is especially important for diseases with reduced penetrance). The knowledge and skills required to take an accurate and thorough family history are important for all clinicians, not only clinical geneticists.

Routinely, the clinician sends the family a letter summarizing the diagnosis, natural history, and risk information regarding the condition. This letter is a valuable resource for the family, as it helps to document the risk information for later review. Information regarding genetics support groups, including pamphlets, booklets, and brochures, is frequently provided. Follow-up visits are recommended depending on the individual situation. Box 14-5 provides a list of clinical genetics services.

▼ Clinical genetic evaluations include physical examination, detailed family history, ancillary tests as needed, and the communication of information to the family through letters and the distribution of published literature. ▲

In recent years the care of persons with genetic disease has included the development of guidelines for follow-up and routine care. Knowledge of the natural history of a condition, coupled with a critical review of screening tests and interventions, can provide a framework for health supervision and anticipatory guidance. The management plan can subsequently be used by the primary care provider. It is primarily for this purpose that many of the specialized clinics, such as those for NF1 or hemophilia, have been established. An example of this approach is the management checklist for the health maintenance of infants and children with Down syndrome (see Chapter 6).

Traditionally, genetic counseling involves the family who comes in with questions about the diagnosis, management, and recurrence risk of the condition in question. Thus, in the majority of situations, genetic counseling is carried out retrospectively. With the increased availability of prenatal, carrier, and presymptomatic testing, "prospective" genetic counseling will become more common. Box 14-6 lists common reasons for referral for genetics evaluation.

DYSMORPHOLOGY AND CLINICAL TERATOLOGY

Dysmorphology was defined at the beginning of this chapter as the study of abnormal physical development **(morphogenesis).** Congenital defects are caused by altered morphogenesis. Although the term "dysmorphology" may seem synonymous with **teratology,** the latter term usually implies the study of the environmental

---

BOX 14-5

TYPES OF CLINICAL GENETIC SERVICES AND PROGRAMS

Center-based Genetics Clinics
Outreach Clinics
Inpatient Consultations
Specialty Clinics
    Metabolic Clinic
    Spina bifida Clinic
    Hemophilia Clinic
    Craniofacial Clinic
    Other single-disorder clinics (e.g., NF1 clinic)
Prenatal Diagnosis Program: Perinatal Genetics
    Amniocentesis/CVS clinic
    Ultrasound program
    Maternal serum AFP program
Genetic Screening
    Newborn screening program/follow-up clinic
    Other population screening programs (e.g., Tay-Sachs disease)
Education/Training
    Health care professionals
    General public
    School system
    Teratology information services

BOX 14-6

COMMON INDICATIONS FOR GENETICS REFERRAL

1. Evaluation of a person with mental retardation or developmental delay
2. Evaluation of a person with single or multiple malformations; question of a dysmorphic syndrome
3. Evaluation of a person with a possible inherited metabolic disease
4. Presence of a possible single-gene disorder
5. Presence of a chromosomal disorder, including balanced rearrangements
6. Person at risk for a genetic condition, including questions of presymptomatic diagnosis
7. Person or family with questions about the genetic aspects of any medical condition
8. Couples with a history of recurrent miscarriages
9. Consanguinity in a couple, usually first cousin or closer relationship
10. Teratogen counseling
11. Preconceptional counseling and risk factor counseling, including advanced maternal age and other potential indications for prenatal diagnosis

causes of congenital anomalies, even though its literal meaning does not refer to etiology. (The term "teratology" is derived from the Greek word for "monster," *teras*. The newer term "dysmorphology" was partly a reaction to the pejorative connotation of teratology.)

As mentioned previously, congenital defects represent an important cause of infant mortality and morbidity. Current studies indicate that the frequency of medically significant malformations diagnosed in the newborn period is 2% to 3%. Investigations that have followed children for a longer period demonstrate that this frequency increases to 3% to 4% by the age of 1 year. In the United States, congenital malformations represent the most frequent cause of mortality during the first year of life. Table 14-1 lists some of the most common and important malformation syndromes.

There are several ways in which congenital defects can be classified. The most common classification approach is by organ system or body region (e.g., craniofacial, limb, heart). More clinically useful systems of classification include: (1) single defect vs. multiple congenital anomaly syndrome, (2) major (medically

or surgically significant defects) vs. minor anomalies, (3) categorization by pathogenic process, and (4) an etiological classification.

Table 14-2 lists the causes of main defects in a major study conducted in Boston. Three key messages emerged from these data: (1) the etiology of two thirds of congenital defects is unknown or multifactorial; (2) environmental causes of congenital malformations are infrequent; and (3) a known genetic component is identified in approximately 30% of cases.

Principles of Dysmorphology

In discussing the basic principles of dysmorphology, it is important to define certain key terms. The following definitions, based on pathogenic processes, are used in clinical practice:

1. **Malformation**, a primary morphologic defect of an organ or body part resulting from an intrinsically abnormal developmental process (e.g., cleft lip or polydactyly).
2. **Dysplasia**, a primary defect involving abnormal organization of cells into tissue (e.g., hemangioma).
3. **Sequence** (formerly **anomalad**), a primary defect with its secondary structural changes (e.g., Pierre Robin sequence, a disorder in which a primary defect in mandibular development produces a small jaw, glossoptosis, and cleft palate).
4. **Syndrome**, a pattern of multiple primary malformations due to a single etiology (e.g., trisomy 13 syndrome).
5. **Deformation**, alteration of the form, shape, or position of a normally formed body part by mechanical forces; usually occurs in the fetal period, not in embryogenesis; a secondary alteration; can be extrinsic as in oligohydramnios (reduced amniotic fluid) or intrinsic as in congenital myotonic dystrophy.

TABLE 14-1 The Most Common Multiple Congenital Anomaly/Dysplasia Syndromes

Syndrome	Etiology
Down syndrome	Chromosomal
NF1	Single gene (AD)
Oligohydramnios sequence	Heterogeneous
Amnion disruption sequence	Unknown
Osteogenesis imperfecta	Single gene; heterogeneous; type I collagen
Trisomy 18	Chromosomal
VATER association	Unknown
Marfan syndrome	Single gene (AD)
Prader-Willi syndrome	Microdeletion of chromosome 15q; disomy
Noonan syndrome	Single gene (AD)
Williams syndrome	Microdeletion of chromosome 7
Achondroplasia	Single gene (AD)
Trisomy 13	Chromosomal
Turner syndrome	Chromosomal (45,X)
Rubinstein-Taybi syndrome	Single gene (AD)
Klippel-Trenaunay-Weber syndrome	Unknown
Fetal alcohol syndrome	Excessive alcohol
Cornelia de Lange syndrome	Unknown

Modified from Hall BD (1981) In Genetic Issues in Pediatrics and Obstetrics Practice. Year Book, Chicago.

TABLE 14-2 Causes of Malformations Among Affected Infants

Genetic causes	Number	Percent
Chromosome abnormalities	157 (45)*	10.1
Single mutant genes	48	3.1
Familial	225 (3)	14.5
Multifactorial inheritance	356 (23)	23.0
Teratogens	49	3.2
Uterine factors	39 (5)	2.5
Twinning	6 (2)	0.4
Unknown cause	669 (24)	43.2
TOTAL	1549 (102)	

From Nelson K, Holmes LB (1989) Malformations due to spontaneous mutations in newborn infants. N. Eng. J. Med. 320: 19-23.
*Values in parentheses denote therapeutic abortions. Of the 69,277 infants studied, 1,549 had malformations, for an incidence of 2.24%

6. **Disruption**, a morphological defect of an organ, part of an organ, or a larger region of the body resulting from the extrinsic breakdown of, or an interference with, an originally normal developmental process; a secondary malformation (e.g., secondary limb defect resulting from a vascular event).

Note that malformations and dysplasias are primary events in embryogenesis and histogenesis, whereas disruptions and deformations are secondary.

The first question asked in diagnosing a congenital malformation is whether the abnormality represents a single, isolated anomaly or is instead one component of a broader, organized pattern of malformation (i.e., a syndrome). An example is given by the evaluation of a baby with a cleft lip. If a baby has an isolated, nonsyndromic cleft lip and no other malformations, the discussion of natural history, genetics, prognosis, and management is markedly different than if the baby's cleft lip is one feature of the trisomy 13 syndrome (see Chapter 6). The former condition can be repaired surgically and has a relatively low recurrence risk (see Chapter 12) and few associated medical problems. Trisomy 13 is a serious chromosomal disorder. In addition to oral-facial clefts, these infants often have congenital heart disease and central nervous system malformations. More importantly, 50% of children with trisomy 13 die in the newborn period, and 90% die before 1 year of age.

Another example is a child with cleft lip who also has pits or fistulas of the lower lip. The combination of oral-facial clefts and lip pits signifies an autosomal dominant condition called the van der Woude syndrome. Although the natural history of this condition differs little from that of nonsyndromic cleft lip, the discussion of genetic recurrence risks is much different. In the evaluation of a child with van der Woude syndrome, it is very important to determine if one of the parents carries the gene. If so, the sibling recurrence risk is 50%. This is much greater than the 4% sibling recurrence risk usually given for nonsyndromic cleft lip. Because van der Woude syndrome has highly variable expression and frequently manifests itself only by lip fistulas, it is quite commonly overlooked. Thus, a careful physical examination, combined with a knowledge of the genetics of isolated malformations and syndromes, is necessary in determining accurate recurrence risks.

▼ **The first question to ask when evaluating a child with a congenital malformation is whether or not the defect is isolated or part of a syndrome pattern.** ▲

The increasing knowledge of the pathogenesis of human congenital defects has led to a better understanding of the developmental relationship of the defects in multiple congenital anomaly patterns. Some well-established conditions that appear to be true syndromes at first glance are really a constellation of defects consisting of a primary malformation with its secondary effects (i.e., a sequence). In a sequence, the pattern is a developmental unit in which the cascade of secondary pathogenic events is well understood. In contrast, the pathogenic relationship of the primary malformations in a syndrome is poorly understood. It is likely that some conditions now called syndromes will be recognized eventually as sequences.

One of the best examples of a sequence is the so-called Potter phenotype or oligohydramnios sequence. It is currently believed that any significant and persistent condition leading to oligohydramnios can produce this sequence, whether it be intrauterine renal failure due to kidney malformations or chronic leakage of amniotic fluid. The fetus will develop a pattern of secondary growth deficiency, joint contractures, facial features, and pulmonary hypoplasia (Fig. 14-4). Before the cause of these features was understood, the phenotype was termed the "Potter syndrome." Now, with the understanding that all of the features are secondary to oligohydramnios, the disorder is more properly called the oligohydramnios sequence. As in any malformation, the renal defect can occur *by itself*, or it can be a part of any number of syndromes in which renal malformations are component features (e.g., in autosomal recessive Meckel-Gruber syndrome or the more common nonsyndromic disease, bilateral renal agenesis). Distinguishing between syndromes and sequences can often improve our understanding of the underlying cause of a disorder. **www**

▼ **It is important to distinguish between a sequence, which is a primary defect with secondary structural changes, and a syndrome, which is a collection of malformations whose relationship to one another tends to be poorly understood.** ▲

Etiology	Pathogenesis	Phenotype
Bilateral renal agenesis		Fetal compression
		Immobility
Polycystic kidneys, type 1	Oligohydramnios	Facial, limb deformities (club foot)
Urethral obstruction		Breech presentation
		Growth deficiency
Chronic leakage of amniotic fluid		Pulmonary hypoplasia

FIG. 14-4 The oligohydramnios sequence. Oligohydramnios can arise from a number of distinct causes. It produces a constellation of secondary phenotypic features.

TABLE 14-3   Well-Established Human Teratogens*

Drug	Potential defect	Critical exposure period	% of exposed who are affected
ACE inhibitors	Renal dysgenesis; oligohydramnios; skull ossification defects	Second to third trimester	Not established
Alcohol, chronic	Craniofacial dysmorphology; CNS abnormalities; heart defects	<12 weeks	10-15
	Low birth weight; developmental delay	>24 weeks	
Aminopterin	Spontaneous abortion	<14 weeks	Not established
	Craniofacial dysmorphology; limb defects; craniosynostosis; neural tube defects	First trimester	
	Low birth weight	>20 weeks	
Androgens/ norprogesterones	Masculinization of external female genitalia	>10 weeks	0.3
Carbamazepine	Spina bifida	<30 days postconception	1
Carbimazole/ methimazole	Hypothyroidism; goiter	Not established	Not established
Cocaine	Abruptio placentae	Second to third trimester	Not established
	Intracranial hemorrhage; premature labor/delivery	Third trimester	
Diethylstilbestrol	Uterine abnormalities; vaginal adenosis; vaginal adenocarcinoma; cervical ridges; male infertility	<12 weeks	Not established
Fluconazole (high-dose IV)	Limb and craniofacial defects	First trimester	Not established
Isotretinoin	Fetal death; hydrocephalus; CNS defects; microtia/ anotia; small or missing thymus; conotruncal heart defects; micrognathia	>15 days postconception	45-50
Lithium	Ebstein abnormality	<8 weeks	<1
Methotrexate	Craniosynostosis; underossified skull; craniofacial dysmorphology; limb defects	6 to 9 weeks postconception	Not established
Penicillamine	Cutis laxa	Not established	Not established
Phenytoin	Craniofacial dysmorphology; hypoplastic phalanges/nails	First trimester	10-30
Solvents, abuse (entire pregnancy)	Small size for gestational age; developmental delay	Not established	Not established
Streptomycin	Hearing loss	Third trimester	Not established
Tetracycline	Stained teeth and bone	>20 weeks	Not established
Thalidomide	Limb reduction defects; limb hypoplasia; ear anomalies	38-50 days post-LMP	15-25
Thiouracil	Spontaneous abortion	First trimester	Not established
	Stillbirth	>20 weeks	
	Goiter		
Trimethadione	Developmental delay; V-shaped eyebrows; low-set ears; irregular teeth	First trimester	Not established
Valproic acid	Spina bifida	<30 days postconception	<1
	Craniofacial dysmorphology; preaxial defects	First trimester	
Warfarin	Nasal hypoplasia; stippled epiphyses	6 to 9 weeks	Not established
	CNS defects secondary to cerebral hemorrhage	>12 weeks	

Courtesy Lynn Martinez, Pregnancy Risk Line, Utah State Department of Health.

*Other established teratogens include maternal infections (rubella, cytomegalovirus, toxoplasmosis, varicella, Venezuela equine encephalitis, syphilis, parvovirus), maternal disease states (diabetes mellitus, phenylketonuria, systemic lupus erythematosus, Graves disease), and ionizing radiation.

Clinical Teratology

A **teratogen** is an agent external to the fetus's genome that induces structural malformations, growth deficiency, and/or functional alterations during prenatal development. Although teratogens cause only a small percentage of all birth defects, the preventive potential alone makes them worthy of study. Table 14-3 lists the well-established human teratogens, of which there are actually very few.

It is important to understand the reasoning process that leads to the designation of a substance as a teratogen. This process is based upon an evaluation of epidemiological, clinical, biochemical, and physiological evidence. Animal studies may also help to establish whether an agent is teratogenic.

Some of the issues involved in determining whether an agent is teratogenic are summarized in Clinical Commentary 14-5. A key clinical point is that it is common for families to ask their doctors questions about the risks of certain exposures during pregnancy. When faced with such a question, the physician has a number of options. One is to review the human literature on a particular exposure, make a judgment regarding the degree of risk, and then provide counseling. An alternative is to refer the patient or family to a clinical genetics unit or to a teratology information service. Because of the complexity of these issues, teratology information services have sprung up throughout the United States, Canada, and Europe.

▼ Teratogens are external agents that cause a small but important proportion of congenital malformations. It is often difficult to prove conclusively that a substance is teratogenic. ▲

Prevention of Congenital Malformations

Because the majority of structural defects have no obvious cause, their prevention presents a challenge (see Clinical Commentary 14-6, which discusses fetal alcohol syndrome, one of the more common preventable causes of human malformation). The institution of rubella immunization programs and, recently, the preconceptional administration of folic acid are both examples of successful prevention (Clinical Commentary 14-7).

Preconceptional counseling is a model for primary prevention. Women who have diabetes mellitus, PKU,

or systemic lupus erythematosus (an autoimmune disorder involving production of autoantibodies that affect multiple organs) can decrease their risk of producing an infant with a structural defect through appropriate preconceptional management. Secondary and tertiary levels of prevention occur, respectively, with newborn screening and with the provision of quality medical care for infants and children with congenital malformations. The institution of appropriate guidelines for health maintenance and anticipatory guidance can decrease some of the complications of these disorders. Also important are public education regarding the limitations of scientific knowledge and the emotional difficulties of families in which a child has a congenital defect. They have the potential to diminish anxiety, improve the family's coping process, and reduce the stigma that surrounds congenital malformations and genetic disorders.

CLINICAL COMMENTARY 14-6
FETAL ALCOHOL SYNDROME

Among the human teratogens, one of the most common and potentially preventable exposures is excessive alcohol consumption. Women who are chronic alcoholics are at significant risk of bearing a child with the fetal alcohol syndrome (FAS). This condition consists of prenatal and postnatal growth deficiency, microcephaly (small head), a wide range of developmental disabilities, and a constellation of facial alterations (Fig. 14-5). The more distinctive and consistent facial features include short palpebral fissures, low nasal root, upturned nose, simple/flat philtral folds, and a thin upper lip. Although most of these signs are not specific for FAS, their mutual occurrence in the context of maternal alcohol abuse allows the clinician to make the diagnosis. www

In addition to these findings, infants and children with FAS are at risk for a number of structural defects, including congenital heart defects, neural tube defects, and renal malformations. Most children with FAS have a mild degree of developmental delay, ranging from mild mental retardation to learning disabilities.

There are still many unanswered questions regarding alcohol use in pregnancy. These include the extent of genetic predisposition to FAS, the risk of binge drinking, the role of moderate and social drinking, and the safe level of alcohol in pregnancy. While there is no conclusive evidence that light to moderate drinking in early pregnancy is harmful, avoidance of alcohol during pregnancy is the most cautious approach.

FIG. 14-5 A 2-year-old child with fetal alcohol syndrome. Note the low nasal root, short palpebral fissures, smooth philtrum, and thin upper lip.

CLINICAL COMMENTARY 14-7
FOLATE AND THE PREVENTION OF NEURAL TUBE DEFECTS

The primary prevention of congenital malformations is an important goal of clinical genetics. Because the ultimate cause of most congenital malformations is currently unknown, there are relatively few opportunities for primary prevention. A recent approach to the prevention of congenital defects is the periconceptional use of folate and multivitamin regimens to prevent the occurrence and recurrence of neural tube defects (NTDs).

NTDs consist of malformations of the developing neural tube and express themselves as anencephaly, encephalocele, and spina bifida (see Chapter 12). Their impact is serious: anencephaly is invariably fatal, and the medical complications of spina bifida (lower limb paralysis, hydrocephalus, urinary obstruction) are significant. Because of the potential influence of nutritional elements on embryogenesis, a series of epidemiological studies were performed in the 1970s and 1980s. With one exception, they demonstrated that the use of vitamins and folate in the periconceptional period reduced the recurrence risk of spina bifida and anencephaly in families that had previously had a child with one of these conditions. In 1991 the Medical Research Council of the United Kingdom published a double-blind study*

*A **double-blind** study is one in which, during the treatment phase of the study, neither the subjects nor the investigator knows which subjects are receiving an active ingredient and which are receiving placebos.

in which 4 mg of folate with or without vitamins was administered to women who had had a child with an NTD. The group receiving folate alone experienced a 70% reduction in the recurrence of these malformations in their offspring. In 1992 a Hungarian group demonstrated the usefulness of vitamins and folic acid in preventing the initial occurrence of neural tube defects. In this study, two groups of women, one receiving vitamins and folic acid and the others not, were followed for the duration of their pregnancies. The vitamin/folic acid regimen significantly decreased the occurrence of neural tube defects.

While it is still not clear whether the purported protective effect is due to folic acid or a combination of folic acid and other vitamins, these data suggest that periconceptional vitamin use is an effective prevention strategy. The mechanism for the apparent effect remains unknown. Nonetheless, the encouraging results of these studies have prompted the Centers for Disease Control and Prevention to publish two recommendations regarding the use of folate. The first is that all women who have had a previous child with an NTD should take 4 mg/day of folic acid if they are planning to become pregnant. The second recommendation is that all women of reproductive age take 0.4 mg/day of folic acid (the amount available in a typical multivitamin tablet) throughout their reproductive years. The latter recommendation is prudent in light of the fact that approximately half of pregnancies in the United States are unplanned. These recommendations have led to the folic acid fortification of wheat and other grain products in the United States.

STUDY QUESTIONS

1. Allen, a 40-year-old male, comes to your office because he is concerned about his family history of heart disease. His father had a fatal myocardial infarction (MI) at the age of 45, and his grandfather (father's father) had a fatal MI at the age of 47. Allen's father had two brothers and two sisters. One of the brothers had an MI at the age of 44, and one of the sisters had an MI at age 49. Allen's mother had a brother and sister, both of whom are still alive. Allen's mother's parents both survived into their 80s and died of "natural causes." Draw a pedigree summarizing the information you have taken about Allen's family, and make a recommendation for further study and/or treatment.

2. Mary's two brothers and her mother's brother all had Duchenne muscular dystrophy (DMD) and are now dead. Based on only this information, what is the probability that Mary is a heterozygous carrier for this disorder? What is the probability

that she will produce affected offspring? She then has a serum creatine kinase test and is told that her level is above the 95th percentile for homozygous normal individuals. Approximately two thirds of DMD carriers have CK levels above the 95th percentile. Given this information, use Bayes' theorem to calculate the probability that Mary is a carrier and the probability that she will produce affected offspring.

3. Bob's father had Huntington disease and is now deceased. Bob is now 51 years old and has no symptoms of Huntington disease. Age-of-onset curves show that approximately 85% of individuals with an affected father show symptoms by this age (this percentage is slightly lower, about 80%, if the mother is affected). Based on this information, use Bayes' theorem to estimate the probability that Bob inherited the Huntington disease mutation from his father.

SUGGESTED READINGS

Aase J (1992) Dysmorphologic diagnosis for the pediatric practitioner. Pediatr. Clin. North Am. 39:135-156

Brent RL (1983) The Bendectin saga: an American tragedy. Teratology 27:283-286

Carey JC (1992) Health supervision and anticipatory guidance for children with genetic disorders (including specific recommendations for trisomy 21, trisomy 18, and neurofibromatosis I). Pediatr. Clin. North Am. 39:25-53

Carey JC, Viskochil DH (1996) Current status of the human malformation map. Birth Defects Original Series 32:13-33

Cohen MM (1997) The Child with Multiple Birth Defects. Oxford University Press, New York

Daly LE, Kirke PN, Molloy A, Weir DG, Scott JM (1995) Folate levels and neural tube defects: implications for prevention. JAMA 274:1698-1702

Epstein CJ (1995) The new dysmorphology: application of insights from basic developmental biology to the understanding of human birth defects. Proc. Natl. Acad. Sci. USA 92:8566-8573

Friedman JM, Polifka JE (1994) Teratogenic effects of drugs: a resource for clinicians (TERIS). Johns Hopkins University, Baltimore

Gorlin RJ, Cohen MM, Levin LS (1990) Syndromes of the Head and Neck, 3rd ed. Oxford University Press, New York

Hall BD (1982) The 25 most common multiple genetical anomaly syndromes. In: Kaback MM (ed) Genetic Issues in Pediatrics and Obstetrics Practice. Year Book, Chicago

Harper PS (1993) Practical Genetic Counselling, 4th ed. Butterworth Heineman, Oxford

Jones KL (1996) Smith's Recognizable Patterns of Human Malformation, 5th ed. W.B. Saunders, Philadelphia

Jones KL, Jones MC (1997) A clinical approach to the dysmorphic child. In: Rimoin DL, Connor JM, Pyeritz RE (eds) Emery and Rimoin's Principles and Practice of Medical Genetics. Vol. 1. Churchill Livingstone, New York, pp 687-696

Kessler S (1979) Genetic Counseling: Psychological Dimensions. Academic Press, New York

Koren G, Pastuszak A, Ito S (1998) Drugs in pregnancy. N. Eng. J. Med. 338:1128-1137

Nelson K, Holmes LB (1989) Malformations due to presumed spontaneous mutations in newborn. N Eng J Med 320:19-23

Ptacek JT, Eberhardt TL (1996) Breaking bad news—a review of the literature. JAMA 276:496-503

Robinson A, Linden MG (1993) Clinical Genetics Handbook, ed. 2. Blackwell Scientific Publications, Boston

Schneider KA (1994) Counseling About Cancer: Strategies for Genetic Counselors. Graphic Illusions, Dennisport, MA

Walker AP (1997) Genetic counseling. In: Rimoin DL, Connor JM, Pyeritz RE (eds) Emery and Rimoin's Principles and Practice of Medical Genetics. Vol. 1. Churchill Livingstone, New York, pp 595-618

Weiss JO (1992) Support groups for patients with genetic disorders and their families. Pediatr. Clin. North Am 39:13-23

Weiss JO, Mackta JS (1996) Starting and Sustaining Genetic Support Groups. Johns Hopkins University Press, Baltimore

Winter RM (1996) Analysing human developmental abnormalities. BioEssays 18:965-997

Answers to Study Questions

CHAPTER 2

1. The mRNA sequence is: 5'-CAG AAG AAA AUU AAC AUG UAA-3' (remember that transcription moves along the 3'-5' DNA strand, allowing the mRNA to be synthesized in the 5' to 3' direction). This mRNA sequence is translated in the 5' to 3' direction to yield the amino acid sequence: Gln-Lys-Lys-Ile-Asn-Met-STOP.

2. The *genome* is the sum total of our genetic material. It is composed of 23 pairs of nuclear *chromosomes* and the mitochondrial chromosome. Each chromosome contains a number of *genes*, the basic unit of heredity. Genes are composed of one or more *exons*; exons alternate with introns. Exons encode mRNA *codons*, which consist of three *nucleotides* each. It is important to remember that DNA coiling patterns also produce a hierarchy: chromosomes are composed of 100-kb chromatin loops, which are in turn composed of solenoids. Each solenoid contains approximately six nucleosomes. Each nucleosome contains about 150 DNA base pairs and may or may not include coding material.

3. Approximately 25% of our DNA consists of repetitive sequences whose function is unknown. Single-copy DNA includes protein-coding genes, but it consists mostly of extragenic sequences and introns that do not encode proteins. Because individual cells have specialized functions, most make only a limited number of protein products. Thus only a small percentage of the cell's coding DNA is transcriptionally active at any given time. This activation is controlled by elements such as transcription factors, enhancers, and promoters.

4. Mitosis is the cell division process whereby one diploid cell produces two diploid daughter cells. In meiosis, a diploid cell produces haploid cells (gametes). Meiosis produces haploid cells because the centromeres are not duplicated in meiosis I and because there is no replication of DNA in the interphase stage between meiosis I and meiosis II. Another difference between mitosis and meiosis is that the homologous chromosomes form pairs and exchange material (crossing over) during meiosis I. Homologs do not pair during mitosis, and mitotic crossing over is very rare.

5. Each mitotic division doubles the number of cells in the developing embryo. Thus the embryo proceeds from 1 to 2 to 4 to 8 cells, and so on. After n cell divisions, there are 2^n cells. For example, after 10 divisions, there are 2^{10}, or 1,024 cells. We want a value of n that satisfies the simple relationship $2^n = 10^{14}$. One way to our answer is simply to "plug in" values of n until we get 10^{14}. A more elegant approach is to take the common logarithms of both sides of this equation, yielding $n\log(2) = 14\log(10)$. Since the common logarithm of 10 is 1, we obtain the relationship $n = 14/\log(2)$. Thus, $n = 46.5$. It should be emphasized that this result, approximately 46 to 47 cell divisions, is only an *average* value. Some cell lineages divide more times than others, and many cells are replaced as they die.

6. A total of 400 mature sperm and 100 mature egg cells will be produced. Each primary spermatocyte will produce four mature sperm cells, while each primary oocyte will produce only one mature egg cell (the other products of meiosis are polar bodies, which degenerate).

CHAPTER 3

1. Mutation 1 is a nonsense mutation in the fourth codon, producing premature termination of translation. Mutation 2 is a frameshift mutation in the third codon, and mutation 3 is a missense mutation in the second codon.

2. Transcription mutations generally lower the production of a gene product, but often they do not eliminate it completely. Transcription mutations in the β-globin gene usually produce β$^+$-thalassemia, a condition in which there is some production of β-globin chains. β$^+$-thalassemia tends to be less severe than β^0-thalassemia. Missense mutations alter only a single amino acid in a polypeptide chain and, when they occur in the β-globin chain, can produce β$^+$-thalassemia (however, keep in mind that sickle cell disease, which is relatively severe, is also caused by a missense mutation). In contrast, frameshift mutations alter many or all codons downstream from the site of the mutation, so a large number of amino acids may be changed. Frameshifts can also produce a stop codon. Nonsense mutations produce truncated polypeptides, which are often useless (especially if the nonsense mutation occurs near the 5' end of the gene, eliminating most of the polypeptide chain). Donor-acceptor mutations can delete whole exons or large portions of them. This can substantially alter the amino acid composition of the polypeptide. Nonsense, frameshift, and donor-acceptor mutations all tend to produce the more severe β^0-thalassemia, in which no β-globin chains are present.

3. In thalassemia conditions, one of the chains, α- or β-globin, is reduced in quantity. Most of the harmful

consequences are caused by the relative *excess* of the chain that is produced in normal quantity. If both chains are reduced in quantity, there may be a rough balance between the two, resulting in less accumulation of excess chains.

4. Restriction site polymorphisms (RSPs) reflect the presence or absence of a restriction site. They thus can have only two alleles. They are detected using RFLP technology. VNTRs are also a type of RFLP, but here the polymorphism is in the number of tandem repeats that lie between two restriction sites, rather than in the presence or absence of a restriction site. Because the number of tandem repeats can vary considerably, VNTRs can have many different alleles in populations. VNTRs are found in minisatellite regions. Microsatellite repeat polymorphisms consist of variations in the number of shorter microsatellite repeats (usually dinucleotides, trinucleotides, and tetranucleotides). They are usually detected using the polymerase chain reaction (PCR). However, it should be noted that RSPs and VNTRs can also be detected using PCR (instead of Southern blotting technology), provided that the DNA sequences flanking the polymorphism are known. The autoradiogram represents a microsatellite repeat polymorphism. This is indicated by the fact that there are multiple alleles (distinguishing it from an RSP) and by the fact that the various alleles differ in size by only 4 bp (recall from Chapter 2 that the tandem repeat units in minisatellite regions are generally 20 to 70 bp long).

5. Because the disease mutation destroys a recognition site, those who have the disease allele will have a longer restriction fragment. This fragment will migrate more slowly on the gel and will be seen higher on the autoradiogram. Individual A has only the longer fragment and thus has two copies of the disease mutation. This individual has α-1-antitrypsin deficiency. Individual B has only the short fragment and will be genetically and physically unaffected. Individual C has both fragments and is thus a clinically unaffected heterozygote.

CHAPTER 4

1. In this sample of 100 individuals, there are 88 × 2 HbA alleles in the HbA homozygotes and 10 HbA alleles in the heterozygotes. There are thus 186 HbA alleles in the population. The frequency of HbA, p, is 186/200 = 0.93. Then the frequency of HbS, q, is 1 − 0.93 = 0.07. The genotype frequencies in the population are 88/100 = 0.88, 10/100 = 0.10, and 2/100 = 0.02. Assuming Hardy-Weinberg proportions, the expected genotype frequencies are given by p^2, $2pq$, and q^2. This yields expected genotype frequencies of $(0.93)^2$ = 0.865, 2 × 0.93 × 0.07 = 0.130, $(0.07)^2$ = 0.005. In this population, the observed and expected genotype frequencies are fairly similar to one another.

2. For an autosomal recessive disease, the prevalence (1/10,000) equals the recessive genotype frequency, q^2. Then the PKU gene frequency, q, is given by $\sqrt{q^2}$ = $\sqrt{1/10,000}$ = 1/100 = 0.01. The carrier frequency is given by $2pq$, which is approximately $2q$, or 0.02 (1/50).

3. Because this is an autosomal dominant disorder, and because affected homozygotes die early in life, the man is a heterozygote and has a 50% chance of passing the disease gene to each of his offspring. The probability that all four will be affected is given by the product of each proba-

bility: $1/2^4$ = 1/16. The probability that none will be affected (1/16) is obtained in exactly the same way.

4. The probability that the offspring will inherit the retinoblastoma susceptibility gene is 0.50, since familial retinoblastoma is an autosomal dominant disease. However, we must also consider the penetrance of the disorder. The probability of inheriting the disease gene (0.50) *and* expressing the disease phenotype (0.90) is given by multiplying the two probabilities together: 0.90 × 0.50 = 0.45.

5. Since the woman's sister had Tay-Sachs disease, both parents must be heterozygous carriers. This means that, at birth, one fourth of their offspring will be affected, one half will be carriers, and one fourth will be genetically normal. However, note that the woman in question is 30 years old. She cannot possibly be an affected homozygote because affected individuals die by age 6. There are thus three equally likely possibilities: (1) the disease allele was inherited from the mother and a normal allele was inherited from the father; (2) the disease allele was inherited from the father and a normal allele was inherited from the mother; (3) normal alleles were inherited from both parents. Because two of these three possibilities lead to the carrier state, the woman's probability of being a heterozygous carrier is 2/3.

6. The probability that the woman's disease gene is transmitted to her offspring is 1/2, and the probability that this offspring in turn transmits the disease gene to his or her offspring (i.e., the grandchild) is again 1/2. Thus, the probability that one grandchild has inherited the disease gene is 1/2 × 1/2, or 1/4. Similarly, the probability that the other grandchild has inherited the gene is 1/4. The probability that *both* inherit the gene is 1/4 × 1/4 = 1/16.

7. This is explained by genomic imprinting. For normal development, differential expression of genes inherited from the father and mother is necessary. If the expression pattern from only one parent is inherited, the embryo cannot develop normally and dies. The experiment works in amphibians because genomic imprinting does not occur in these animals.

8. The coefficient of relationship is 2^6 = 1/64. This gives the probability that the woman also carries the PKU gene. Then, the probability that two carriers produce an affected offspring is 1/4. The overall probability that this couple will produce a baby affected with PKU is given by multiplying the probability that the woman carries the gene (1/64) by the probability that they both transmit the gene to their offspring (1/4). 1/64 × 1/4 = 1/256. This demonstrates that the probability of producing an affected offspring in this consanguineous mating is actually quite small.

9. The frequency of the heterozygote genotype in the general population is given by $2pq$, according to the Hardy-Weinberg law. Thus, the frequency of the first genotype in the general population is predicted to be 2 × 0.05 × 0.10 = 0.01. Similarly, for the second system, the frequency of heterozygotes in the general population is 2 × 0.07 × 0.02 = 0.0028. The perpetrator was a homozygote for the third system; the frequency of the homozygote genotype in the general population is given by p^2, or 0.08^2 = 0.0064. If we can assume independence of the three VNTR systems in the general population, we can

then multiply the frequencies of the three genotypes together to get the probability that somebody in the general population would have the same genotypes as the perpetrator. We thus multiply $0.01 \times 0.0028 \times 0.0064$ to obtain a probability of 0.000000179, or 1/5,580,357. This probability can be made smaller by typing additional systems.

10. As in question 5, we assume independence of the four microsatellite systems. In this case, we multiply the four allele frequencies together to get the probability: $0.05 \times 0.01 \times 0.01, \times 0.02 = 0.0000001 = 1/10,000,000$. Notice a key difference between question 9 and question 10: in the paternity case, the father has contributed only half of the baby's genotype at each locus, the other half being contributed by the mother. Thus, we examine only a single allele for each locus. In contrast, the rapist has contributed *both* alleles of each genotype to the evidentiary sample, so we include both alleles in the analysis.

CHAPTER 5

1. There are four Barr bodies, always one less than the number of X chromosomes.

2. This is most likely a result of X inactivation. The heterozygotes with muscle weakness are the ones with relatively large proportions of active X chromosomes containing the mutant allele.

3. The disease frequency in males is q, while in females it is q^2. The male/female ratio is thus q/q^2 or $1/q$. Thus, as q decreases, the male/female ratio increases.

4. Since the male's grandfather is affected with the disorder, his mother must be a carrier. His father is phenotypically normal, so he does not have the disease gene. Thus, the male in question has a 50% risk of developing hemophilia A. His sister's risk of being a heterozygous carrier is 50%. Her risk of being affected with the disorder is close to zero (barring a new mutation on the X chromosome transmitted by her father).

5. Male-male transmission can be observed in autosomal dominant inheritance, but it will not be observed in X-linked dominant inheritance. Thus, males affected with X-linked dominant disorders must always have affected mothers, unless a new mutation has occurred. Males and females are affected in approximately equal proportions in autosomal dominant inheritance, but there are twice as many affected females as males in X-linked dominant inheritance (unless the disorder is lethal prenatally in males, in which case *only* affected females are seen). In X-linked dominant inheritance, *all* of the sons of an affected male are normal, and *all* of the daughters are affected. In X-linked dominant diseases, heterozygous females tend to be more mildly affected than are hemizygous males. In autosomal dominant inheritance, there is usually no difference in severity of expression in male and female heterozygotes.

6. In mitochondrial inheritance, the disease can be inherited *only* from an affected mother. In contrast to all other types of inheritance, *no* descendants of affected fathers can be affected. Note that males affected with an X-linked recessive disease who mate with normal females cannot transmit the disease to their offspring, but their grandsons can be affected with the disease.

7. Since Becker muscular dystrophy is relatively rare, it is reasonable to assume that the woman is a normal homo-

zygote. Thus, she can transmit only normal X chromosomes to her offspring. Her male offspring, having received a Y chromosome from the father and a normal X from the mother, will all be unaffected. The female offspring of this mating, receiving a mutated X chromosome from the father, will all be heterozygous carriers of the disorder.

8. If the man is phenotypically normal, his X chromosome cannot carry a Duchenne muscular dystrophy mutation. The female will transmit her mutation-carrying chromosome to half of her offspring, on average. Thus, half of the sons will be affected with the disorder, and half of the daughters will be heterozygous carriers.

9. The boys' mother must be a heterozygous carrier for a factor VIII mutation. Thus, one of the mother's parents must also have carried the mutation. Consequently, the probability that the mother's sister is a carrier is 1/2.

CHAPTER 6

1. Euploid cells have a multiple of 23 chromosomes. Haploid (n = 23), diploid (n = 46), and polyploid (triploid and tetraploid) cells are all euploid. Aneuploid cells do not have a multiple of 23 chromosomes and would include trisomies (47 chromosomes in a somatic cell) and monosomies (45 chromosomes in a somatic cell).

2. Conventional FISH analysis involves the hybridization of a fluorescently labeled probe to denatured metaphase chromosomes and is most useful in detecting aneuploidy, deletions, and chromosome rearrangements. FISH can also be extended to use multiple differently colored probes, allowing the detection of several different aneuploidies simultaneously. Spectral karyotyping is an extension of FISH in which each chromosome can be visualized as a different color. This enables accurate and easy characterization of aneuploidy, loss or duplication of chromosome material, and (especially) chromosome rearrangements such as translocations. CGH is particularly useful in detecting the gain or loss of chromosome material, but it cannot detect balanced rearrangements of chromosomes, such as reciprocal translocations. This is because, despite the rearrangement, the test sample and the reference sample each have the same amount of DNA from each chromosome region.

3. A normal egg can be fertilized by two sperm cells (dispermy, the most common cause of triploidy). An egg and polar body can fuse, creating a diploid egg, which is then fertilized by a normal sperm cell. Diploid sperm or egg cells can be created by meiotic failure; subsequent union with a haploid gamete would produce a triploid zygote.

4. The difference in incidence of various chromosome abnormalities reflects the fact that embryos and fetuses with chromosome abnormalities are spontaneously lost during pregnancy. The rate and timing of loss varies among different types of chromosome abnormalities.

5. A karyotype will establish whether the condition is the result of a true trisomy or a translocation. If the latter is the case, the recurrence risk in future pregnancies is greatly elevated. A karyotype will also help to establish whether the patient is a mosaic. This may help to predict and explain the severity of expression of the disorder.

6. The ranking, from lowest risk to highest, would be: (1) 25-year-old female with one previous Down syndrome child

(approximately 1%); (2) 25-year-old male carrier of a 21/14 translocation (1% to 2%); (3) 45-year-old female with no family history (approximately 3%); (4) 25-year-old female carrier of a 21/14 translocation (10% to 15%).

7. Nondisjunction of the X chromosome can occur in both meiosis I and meiosis II. If these two nondisjunctions occur in the same cell, an ovum with four X chromosomes can be produced. If fertilized by an X-bearing sperm cell, the zygote will have the 49,XXXXX karyotype.

8. The meiotic error must have occurred in the father, since his X chromosome carries the gene for hemophilia A. Since the daughter has normal factor VIII activity, she must have inherited her single X chromosome from her mother.

9. Since a loss of genetic material usually produces more severe consequences than does a gain of material, one would expect the deletion (46,XY,del(8p)) patient to be more severely affected than the duplication patient.

10. A translocation may place a proto-oncogene near a sequence that activates it, producing a cancer-causing oncogene. It may also interrupt a tumor-suppressor gene (see Chapter 11), inactivating it. Because these genes encode tumor-suppressing factors, their inactivation can also lead to cancer.

CHAPTER 7

1. In consanguineous matings, a higher proportion of genes in the offspring are identical by descent. The identical proportion is measured by the coefficient of relationship. The carrier frequency of autosomal recessive inborn errors of metabolism such as alkaptonuria decreases as the prevalence of the disorder diminishes. Thus, the carrier frequency of very rare disorders is very low. If a child is diagnosed with alkaptonuria, it would be reasonable to suspect that parents who might be related are more likely to share an individual's alkaptonuria gene than two individuals chosen at random from the population.

2. Many metabolic reactions can proceed in the complete absence of an enzyme. For example, a hydroxide ion can combine with carbon dioxide to form bicarbonate. Yet this reaction occurs much more efficiently in the presence of a catalyst, in this case the enzyme carbonic anhydrase. Although many reactions in the human body would continue in the absence of an enzymatic catalyst, they would not do so at a rate high enough to support normal metabolism and physiology.

3. Although most inborn errors of metabolism are rare, in aggregate they contribute substantially to the morbidity and mortality of children and adults. Additionally, understanding the pathogenetic basis of rare metabolic disorders has the potential to help physicians and scientists understand similar processes that contribute to common diseases. For example, by understanding how mutations in *glucokinase* cause hyperglycemia, we may better understand the pathogenesis of diabetes mellitus.

4. Metabolic disorders have been classified in many different ways. In Chapter 7, we have categorized them by the types of metabolic processes that are affected. Some examples include: carbohydrate metabolism (e.g., galactosemia, hereditary fructose intolerance, glycogen storage disorders); amino acid metabolism (e.g., PKU, MSUD, tyrosinemia);

lipid metabolism (e.g., MCAD, LCAD); degradative pathways (e.g., Hurler syndrome, OTC deficiency, Gaucher disease); energy production (e.g., OXPHOS defects); and transport systems (e.g., cystinosis, cystinuria).

5. Mutations in *GAL-1-P uridyl transferase* are the most common cause of galactosemia. However, mutations encoding other enzymes necessary for the metabolism of galactose such as galactokinase and uridine diphosphate galactose-4-epimerase can also result in galactosemia. This is an example of genetic heterogeneity. That is, indistinguishable phenotypes may be produced by mutations in different genes. Other examples of metabolic disorders that are genetically heterogeneous include hyperphenylalanemia, maple syrup urine disease, and cystinuria.

6. The prevalence rates for many inborn errors of metabolism vary widely between ethnic groups. In many instances this is due to founder effect and genetic drift (see Chapter 3). For example, in Finland more than 30 autosomal recessive disorders are found at an unusually high prevalence compared to closely related populations. A similar scenario partly explains the finding of only a single or few disease-causing mutations in Ashkenazic Jews (lysosomal storage disorders), Mennonites (MSUD), and French Canadians (tyrosinemia type 1). In other cases, it appears that there may be a selective advantage for carriers of a recessive allele (remember that heterozygotes for recessive disorders are unaffected). This may explain the varying frequency distribution of *LAC*P*, which confers persistent lactase activity and may have been advantageous in populations in which dairy products were a valuable nutritional source.

7. Although the mitochondrial genome is inherited only from the mother, most of the proteins in the mitochondria are encoded by genes in the nuclear genome. Thus, disorders of mitochondrial fatty acid oxidation are inherited in an autosomal recessive pattern. Given the age of this young woman, it is unlikely that she is affected with a mitochondrial fatty acid oxidation disorder, so we can assume that she is either a heterozygous carrier or is homozygous for the normal allele. Consequently, the probability that she is a carrier is 0.67. The probability that her mate is a carrier is given by the carrier rate for MCAD in the general population: 1 in 70 (~0.014). In a carrier × carrier mating, there is a 25% chance of having an affected child (probability of two gametes bearing mutant alleles uniting); then her risk of having an affected child is $0.67 \times 0.014 \times 0.25 = 0.002$ or 1/500. Note that her risk of being a carrier (0.67/0.014) is 48 times higher than in the general population.

8. Five different enzymes control the urea cycle pathway. Deficiencies of four of these enzymes (AS, AL, arginase, and CPS) are inherited in an autosomal recessive pattern. OTC deficiency is X-linked recessive. Most women who are carriers for an X-linked recessive disorder are not symptomatic. However, there are at least two explanations for a symptomatic female. First, one X chromosome is normally inactivated (lyonized) at random in each somatic cell. Sometimes, inactivation is skewed and more normal X chromosomes than abnormal X chromosomes are inactivated and a woman becomes symptomatic. Testing for skewed inactivation is not commonly performed in diag-

nostic laboratories. A second possible explanation is that only a single X chromosome is present in each somatic cell (Turner syndrome; see Chapter 6). Thus, lyonization does not take place because each cell must contain one functional copy of the X chromosome. If this X chromosome contains a mutated gene (e.g., *OTC*), a woman will be symptomatic. The simplest test to confirm this diagnosis would be a karyotype.

9. A functioning OXPHOS is necessary to metabolize pyruvate aerobically. Defects of the OXPHOS system cause pyruvate to be metabolized anaerobically into lactate, increasing the level of circulating lactate. Thus, an elevated level of circulating lactate may signal the presence of a disorder of energy production. Elevated levels of lactate are also produced by decreased tissue oxygenation due to decreased circulation (e.g., strenuous exercise, shock). Often there are other biochemical abnormalities that suggest a defect of OXPHOS; however, the diagnosis can be challenging.

10. Polymorphisms in the genes controlling the metabolism of drugs (e.g., *CYP2D6*) may affect a patient's therapeutic response as well as the profile of side effects. Natural foods contain thousands of chemical compounds, many of which have pharmacological properties similar to, but less potent than, contemporary drugs used by health care providers. Thus, polymorphisms in the genes may have enabled some groups of hunter-gatherers to utilize resources that other groups found inedible. Over time this may have been enough of a selective advantage that the size of one group grew more quickly than others.

CHAPTER 8

1. The affected male in generation II inherited the disease allele and marker allele 1 from his affected father, and he inherited a normal allele and marker allele 2 from his mother. Therefore, the disease allele must be on the chromosome that contains marker allele 1 in this male (linkage phase). Because he married a female who is heterozygous for marker alleles 3 and 4, we expect to observe allele 1 in the affected offspring under the hypothesis of linkage. Individual III-5 has the 2,4 marker genotype but is affected, and individual III-7 has the 1,3 genotype but is normal. They both represent recombinants. Thus, there are two recombinations observed in eight meioses, giving a recombination frequency of 2/8 = 25%.

2. For marker A, the affected mother in generation II must carry allele 2 on the same chromosome as the Huntington disease allele. Under the hypothesis that $\theta = 0.0$, all of her children must also inherit allele 2 if they are affected. Marker A shows a recombinant with the disease allele in individual III-5 and thus produces a likelihood of zero for a recombination frequency of 0.0. The LOD score is -∞ (the logarithm of 0). For marker B, the disease allele is on the chromosome bearing marker allele 1 in the affected mother in generation 2. All offspring inheriting allele 1 also inherit the disease allele, so there are no recombinants. Under the hypothesis that $\theta = 0.0$, the affected mother can transmit only two possible haplotypes: the disease allele with marker allele 1 and the normal allele with marker allele 2. The probability of each of these events is 1/2. Thus, the probability of observing six off-

spring with the marker genotypes shown is $(1/2)^6 = 1/64$. This is the numerator of the likelihood ratio. Under the hypothesis that $\theta = 0.5$ (no linkage), four possible haplotypes can be transmitted, each with probability 1/4. The probability of observing six children with these haplotypes under the hypothesis of no linkage is then $(1/4)^6 = 1/4096$. This is the denominator of the likelihood ratio. The ratio is then $(1/64)/(1/4096) = 64$. The LOD score is given by the common logarithm of 64, 1.8.

3. The table shows a maximum LOD score, 3.5, at a recombination frequency of 10%. Thus, the two loci are most likely to be linked at a distance of approximately 10 cM. The odds in favor of linkage at this θ value versus nonlinkage are 3162 ($10^{3.5}$) to 1.

4. Linkage phase can be established in both families, and no recombinants are observed in either family. Thus the estimated recombination frequency is 0.0. The LOD score for $\theta=0.0$ in the first family is given by $\log_{10}(1/2)^5/(1/4)^5 = \log_{10}(32) = 1.5$. In the second family the LOD score for $\theta=0.0$ is $\log_{10}(1/2)^6/(1/4)^6 = \log_{10}(64) = 1.8$. These two LOD scores can then be added to obtain an overall LOD score of 3.3.

5. These matings allow us to establish linkage phase in individuals II-2 and II-3, the parents of the individuals in generation III. The disease allele is on the same chromosome as marker 4 in individual II-2, and the disease allele is on the same chromosome as marker 5 in individual II-3. Under the hypothesis of linkage, we would predict that offspring who inherit markers 4 and 5 will be homozygous affected, offspring who inherit 4 *or* 5 will be heterozygous carriers, and offspring who inherit neither 4 nor 5 will be homozygous normal. Note a key difference between autosomal recessive and autosomal dominant pedigrees in estimating recombination frequencies: here, *both* parents in generation II contribute informative meioses because both parents carry a disease-causing allele. Thus, we can evaluate all 10 meioses contributing to generation III for recombination between the disease and marker loci. No recombinations are seen in the first four offspring, but individual III-5 is homozygous normal but has inherited allele 5 from his mother. Thus, one recombination in five meioses has occurred in the mother, and no recombinations in five meioses have occurred in the father. One recombination in 10 meioses yields a recombination frequency of 1/10 = 10%.

6. These matings allow us to establish linkage phase in individual II-1. Under the hypothesis of linkage, she carries the disease-causing allele (labeled *D*) on the same chromosome as marker allele 1. Her haplotypes are thus *D1/d2*. Based on her haplotypes and on those of her unaffected mate, we can predict that the offspring who inherit the 1,1 genotype will be affected while those who inherit the 1,2 genotype will not be affected. We see that this is the case for all but one of the offspring (III-5). This means that the likelihood that $\theta=0.0$ is zero, so the LOD score for this recombination frequency is -∞. To assess the LOD score for $\theta = 0.1$, we consider that the probability that the father passes each recombinant haplotype (*D2* or *d1*) is $\theta/2 = 0.45$. The probability that he transmits each nonrecombinant haplotype (*D1* or *d2*) is $(1-\theta)/2 = 0.05$ (see Box 8-1 for the details of this reasoning process).

There is one recombinant and seven nonrecombinants among the offspring. The probability of observing these eight events is $0.05 \times 0.45^7 = 0.00019$. This is the numerator of the likelihood ratio. For eight offspring, the probability that $\theta = 0.5$ is $(1/4)^8 = 0.000015$. This is the denominator of the ratio. The logarithm of the odds ratio is given by $\log_{10}(12.2) = 1.09$. This is the LOD score for $\theta = 0.1$.

7. The mating in generation II is uninformative because the father is a homozygote for the marker allele. It will be necessary to type the family for another closely linked marker (preferably one with more alleles) before any risk information can be given. At this point the only risk information that can be given is that each child has a 50% risk of inheriting the disease gene from the affected father.

8. Synteny refers to loci that are on the same chromosome. Linkage refers to loci that are less than 50 cM apart on a chromosome; alleles at these loci tend to be transmitted together within families. Linked loci are thus syntenic, but syntenic loci are not necessarily linked. Linkage disequilibrium is the nonrandom association of alleles at linked loci, observable when chromosome haplotypes are examined in populations. Association indicates that two traits are observed together in a population more often than expected by chance; the traits may or may not be genetic. Association thus does not necessarily have anything to do with linkage, *unless* we are referring to linkage disequilibrium.

9. Linkage disequilibrium can arise when a disease mutation occurs on a specific chromosome. If there are multiple disease mutations, they are likely to occur on chromosomes with different marker alleles, and little association will be observed between the disease genotype (which actually consists of a *collection* of different mutations at the disease locus) and a specific marker allele.

10. A hybridization signal is seen consistently in clones that include chromosome 5. This indicates that this is the chromosome most likely to contain the cDNA segment.

CHAPTER 9

1. The class I molecules present peptides at the surfaces of nearly all of the body's cells. The peptide-class I molecule complex is recognized by cytotoxic T cells, which kill the cell if the class I MHC molecule presents foreign peptide. The class II MHC molecules also present peptides at the cell surface, but only in antigen-presenting cells of the immune system (e.g., dendritic cells, macrophages, and B cells). If the class II molecule presents foreign peptide derived from an invading microbe, they are bound by the receptors of helper T cells, which in turn stimulate appropriate B cells to proliferate and produce antibodies that will help to kill the microbes.

2. Immunoglobulins differ among B cells within individuals so that a large variety of infections can be combated. MHC molecules are identical on each cell surface within an individual, but they vary a great deal between individuals. This inter-individual variability may have evolved to prevent infectious agents from spreading easily through a population.

3. T-cell receptors and immunoglobulins are similar in that they are both cell surface receptors that bind to foreign peptides as part of the immune response. Diversity in both types of molecules is generated by multiple germline genes, VDJ recombination, and junctional diversity. They differ in that immunoglobulins are secreted into the circulation (as antibodies) and can bind directly to foreign peptide, while T-cell receptors are not secreted and must "see" foreign peptide in conjunction with MHC molecules to recognize them. Also, somatic hypermutation generates diversity in immunoglobulins but not in T-cell receptors.

4. Somatic recombination alone could produce $30 \times 6 \times 80 = 14,400$ different heavy chains of this class.

5. The probability that a sibling will be HLA-identical is 0.25. This is because the probability that two siblings share one gene or haplotype is 0.50 (this is the coefficient of relationship for siblings; see Chapter 4). Then, the probability that they share two haplotypes and are HLA-identical is $0.50 \times 0.50 = 0.25$.

6. If a homozygous Rh-positive (*DD*) man marries an Rh-negative woman, all of the offspring will be Rh-positive heterozygotes (*Dd*) and incompatible with the mother. If the man is an Rh-positive heterozygote (*Dd*), half of the children, on average, will be incompatible Rh-positive heterozygotes. However, if the couple is ABO-incompatible, this will largely protect against Rh incompatibility.

CHAPTER 10

1. Animals such as roundworm, fruit fly, frog, zebra fish, chick, and mouse are commonly used to model human development. Each of these organisms has a relatively short generation time and can be selectively bred, and large populations can be maintained in captivity. Furthermore, embryos from each of these animals can be manipulated either in vitro or in vivo using a variety of techniques (e.g., surgical ablation or transplantation of cells or tissues, ectopic expression of native genes or transgenes, knockouts). Of course, each organism has advantages and disadvantages that must be considered when choosing an appropriate model. In some animals, naturally occurring mutant strains have proved to be valuable models of human genetic disease. For example, mutations in murine *Pax6* produce an abnormally small eye. Mutations in the human homolog, *PAX6*, cause hypoplasia or absence of the iris. Most of what we understand about axis determination and pattern formation has been learned from studies of non-human animal models.

2. Although identical mutations in a developmental gene may produce different birth defects, the defects are usually the same within each family. One possible explanation is that other genes may be modifying the phenotype differently in each family. In other words, the same mutation is occurring in different genetic backgrounds, resulting in different phenotypes. To date, only a few examples of different human conditions caused by identical mutations are known. However, strain-dependent phenotypic effects are well described in other organisms such as mice and fruit flies.

3. Transcription factors commonly activate or repress more than a single gene. Often they affect the transcription of many genes that may be members of different developmental pathways. This maintains developmental flexibility and genomic economy. These developmental path-

ways are used to build many different tissues and organs. Thus, a mutation in a transcription factor can affect the growth and development of many body parts. For example, mutations in *TBX5* cause defects of both the limbs and the heart in a pleiotropic disorder called Holt-Oram syndrome.

4. Pattern formation is the process by which ordered spatial arrangements of differentiated cells create tissues and organs. Initially, the general pattern of the animal body plan is established. Then, semi-autonomous regions are formed that will pattern specific organs and appendages. Thus, pattern formation requires that complex temporal-spatial information be available to different populations of cells at different periods during development. This information is communicated between cells by signaling molecules. Mutations in the genes encoding these signaling molecules can disrupt signaling pathways, leading to abnormal pattern formation. For example, Sonic hedgehog (SHH) is widely used in many different patterning processes, including that of the brain. Mutations in *SHH* can cause failure of the forebrain to divide (holoprosencephaly). Patterning defects are also produced by mutations in genes encoding transcription factors (e.g., HOX, T-box) that are activated in response to signals from other cells.

5. Because of the tight constraints on developmental programs, the role of some elements in developmental pathways can be played by more than one molecule. This is known as functional redundancy. Hox paralogs appear to act in some developmental pathways in just this manner. For example, mice with *Hoxa-11* or *Hoxd-11* mutations have only minor abnormalities, whereas *Hoxa-11/Hoxd-11* double mutants exhibit a marked reduction in the size of the radius and ulna. Thus, *Hoxa-11* and *Hoxd-11* may be able to partially compensate for one another in some developmental programs.

6. There are many reasons why it may be impractical to use an organism to study loss-of-function mutations by creating knockouts. For example, baboons have small nuclear families and long generation times and are expensive to maintain in captivity. A short generation time is critical because complete loss of function is achieved by back-crossing chimeras and subsequently mating heterozygotes with a genetic modification to produce animals homozygous for a genetic modification (e.g., a knockout). One way to circumvent the problem of long generation times would be to produce sperm from the model animal (e.g., baboon) in an organism with a short generation time (e.g., mouse). In this technique, immature sperm-making cells from an infant baboon would be placed in the testicles of mice in order to make mature sperm. These sperm could be used for in vitro fertilization with eggs harvested from female baboons with a genetic modification (i.e., chimeras or heterozygotes). Thus, the generation time would be substantially reduced. This type of experiment has not yet been successfully completed, although the technology is forthcoming.

7. Cells communicate with each other through many different signaling pathways. Signaling requires that a ligand bind to a receptor molecule. This generates a response that may activate and/or inhibit a variety of processes within a cell. Mutations in fibroblast growth factor receptor (FGFR) genes cause a variety of craniosynostosis syndromes. How-

ever, mutations in FGFR ligands, fibroblast growth factors, have not been described. Mutations in the genes encoding endothelin-3 and its receptor, endothelin-B, cause defects of the enteric cells of the gastrointestinal tract, leading to severe, chronic constipation (Hirschsprung disease). This demonstrates that a mutation in a ligand or its receptor may produce the same phenotype.

8. There are many obstacles to treating birth defects with gene therapy. Many developmental genes are expressed early in development. Thus, the phenotype would have to be identifiable at a very early age. This is certainly feasible (e.g. via pre-implantation testing) in the gametes or zygotes of a known carrier. Since many of these genes encode axis, pattern, or organ-specific information, gene therapy would have to be initiated very early in the developmental process. In addition, the therapy might have to be targeted to specific areas, at critical times during development, and at appropriate levels required for interacting with other developmental genes. Consequently, it will be challenging to develop strategies that may be useful for treating birth defects with gene therapy.

CHAPTER 11

1. G6PD is on a portion of the X chromosome that is inactivated in one copy in normal females. Thus, any single cell will express only one G6PD allele. If *all* tumor cells express the same G6PD allele, this indicates that they all arose from a single ancestral cell. This evidence was used to support the theory that most tumors are monoclonal.

2. The probability that a single cell will experience two mutations is given by the square of the mutation rate per cell (i.e., the probability of one mutation *and* a second mutation in the same cell): $(3 \times 10^{-6})^2 \approx 10^{-11}$. We then multiply this probability times the number of retinoblasts to obtain the probability that an individual will develop sporadic retinoblastoma: $10^{-11} \times 2 \times 10^6 = 2 \times 10^{-5}$. We would thus expect 2 in 100,000 individuals to develop sporadic retinoblastoma, which is consistent with observed prevalence data (i.e., retinoblastoma is seen in about 1/20,000 children, and about half of these cases are sporadic). If an individual has inherited one copy of a mutant retinoblastoma gene, then the number of tumors is given by the somatic mutation (second hit) rate per cell times the number of target cells: $3 \times 10^{-6} \times 2 \times 10^6 = 6$ tumors per individual.

3. Oncogenes are produced when proto-oncogenes, which encode substances that affect cell growth, are altered. Oncogenes usually act as dominant genes at the level of the cell and help to produce transformation of a normal cell into one that can give rise to a tumor. Tumor suppressor genes are also involved in growth regulation, but they usually act as recessive genes at the level of the cell (i.e., both copies of the gene must be altered before progression to a tumor can proceed). Because only a single oncogene need be altered to initiate the transformation process, oncogenes have been detected by using transfection and retroviral assays and by observing the effects of chromosome translocations. Such methods are less effective for uncovering tumor suppressors because two altered copies of these genes must be present before their effects can be observed in a cell. As a consequence, most tumor

suppressor genes have been detected by studying relatively rare cancer syndromes in which one mutant copy of the tumor suppressor is inherited and the second alteration occurs during somatic development.

4. Li-Fraumeni syndrome is caused by the inheritance of a mutation in the *p53* gene. The inherited mutation is present in all cells and greatly increases predisposition to tumor formation. However, because of the multi-step nature of carcinogenesis, this inherited event is not sufficient to produce a tumor. Other events, occurring in somatic cells, must also take place. These somatic events are rare, so the probability of their occurrence in any given cell is small, explaining the low frequency of any specific tumor type. The involvement of many different tumor types in Li-Fraumeni syndrome is explained by the fact that normal *p53* activity is required for growth regulation in many different tissues. Thus, the likelihood that an individual will develop at least one primary tumor, in one of many tissues, is very high.

CHAPTER 12

1. Since the trait is more common in females than in males, we infer that the threshold is lower in females than in males. Thus, an affected father is at greater risk for producing affected offspring than is an affected mother. The recurrence risk is higher in daughters than in sons.

2. For a multifactorial trait, the recurrence risk will decrease rapidly in more remote relatives of a proband (as shown in Table 12-2). In contrast, for an autosomal dominant gene, the recurrence risk will be 50% smaller with each degree of relationship, reflecting the coefficient of relationship (see Chapter 4). Recall that first-degree relatives (parents and offspring, siblings) share 50% of their genes, second-degree relatives (uncles and nieces, grandparents and grandchildren) share 25% of their genes, and so on. Thus, for a gene with 10% penetrance, the recurrence risk is obtained by multiplying the penetrance times the percentage of shared genes between relatives: 5% (10% × 50%) for first-degree relatives, 2.5% (10% × 25%) for second-degree relatives, 1.25% (10% × 12.5%) for third-degree relatives, and so on. In addition, if the disease is multifactorial, the recurrence risk should increase in populations in which the disease is more common. There will be no relationship between disease frequency and recurrence risk for an autosomal dominant disease.

3. (1) The disease gene may have reduced penetrance. (2) A somatic mutation may have occurred following cleavage of the embryo, such that one twin is affected by the disorder while the other is not.

4. These results imply that shared environmental factors are increasing the correlations among siblings, since siblings tend to share a more common environment than do parents and offspring. The spouse correlation reinforces the interpretation of a shared environment effect, although it is also possible that individuals with similar body fat levels may marry preferentially.

CHAPTER 13

1. The sensitivity of the test is 93% (93 of the 100 true disease cases were detected). The specificity is 99% (98,900 of 99,900 unaffected individuals were correctly identified). The positive predictive value is 8.5% (93 of the 1093 individuals with positive tests actually had the disease). The false-positive rate is 1% (1 - specificity, or 1,000 of 99,900), and the false-negative rate is 7% (1 - sensitivity, or 7 of 100).

2. Based on the fact that individual 3 is homozygous for the 5 kb allele, we infer that the disease gene is on the same chromosome as the 5 kb allele in both parents. Thus, individual 6, who inherited both copies of the 5 kb allele, also inherited both copies of the PKU disease gene and is affected.

3. The NF1 disease gene is on the same chromosome as allele 1 in the affected father. Thus, individual 6, who inherited allele 2 from his father, should be unaffected. Note that our degree of confidence in both answers 2 and 3 depends on how closely linked the marker and disease loci are.

4. The mating in generation I is uninformative, so we cannot establish linkage phase in the female in generation II. Thus, the risk estimate for her daughter cannot be improved from the usual 50% figure used for autosomal dominant disease genes. Diagnostic accuracy could be improved by assaying another, more polymorphic marker (e.g., a microsatellite repeat polymorphism, which would more likely permit the accurate definition of linkage phase).

5. The primary advantages of amniocentesis are a lower rate of fetal loss (approximately 0.5% versus 1% to 1.3% for CVS) and the ability to do an AFP assay for the detection of neural tube defects. CVS offers the advantages of diagnosis earlier in the pregnancy and a more rapid laboratory diagnosis. The CVS diagnosis may be complicated by confined placental mosaicism, and there is limited evidence for an association between early (before 10 weeks post-LMP) CVS and limb reduction defects.

6. Huntington disease (HD) is a poor candidate for gene replacement therapy because it is caused by a gain-of-function mutation. Thus, simple gene insertion is unlikely to correct the disorder. It would be a better candidate for antisense or ribozyme treatment, in which the defective gene product would be disabled. An additional consideration is that this disorder affects primarily neurons, which are relatively difficult to manipulate or target. The fact that HD has a delayed age of onset, however, is encouraging because identification of the action of the HD gene may lead to drug therapy to block the gene product's effects before neuronal damage occurs.

CHAPTER 14

1. Allen's family includes several members who have had myocardial infarctions at a relatively young age. The pedigree (p. 317) suggests that an autosomal dominant gene predisposing family members to heart disease *may* be segregating in this family. This could be caused by autosomal dominant familial hypercholesterolemia, or possibly another disorder of lipid metabolism. Allen should be encouraged to have his serum lipid levels tested (total cholesterol, LDL, HDL, and triglyceride). If his LDL level is abnormally high, intervention may be necessary (e.g., dietary modification and/or cholesterol-lowering drugs).

2. Based on the fact that Mary's brothers and uncle are all affected, we can be quite certain that her mother is a carrier of the Duchenne muscular dystrophy (DMD) gene (if only one of Mary's brothers were affected, we would have to consider the possibility that he was the product of a new mutation). If Mary's mother is a carrier, then there is a probability of 1/2 that Mary is a carrier. As we saw in Chapter 5, a female carrier will transmit the disease gene to half of her sons, on average. Thus, the probability that one of her son's will be affected with DMD is $1/2 \times 1/2 = 1/4$. The creatine kinase test contributes additional information. We can set up the Bayesian calculation as follows:

	Mary is a carrier	Mary is not a carrier
Prior probability	1/2	1/2
Conditional probability that her CK is in the 95th percentile	2/3	0.05
Joint probability	1/3	0.025
Posterior probability	0.93	0.07

It should be clear that the conditional probability of being a carrier given a CK level above the 95th percentile is 2/3. The conditional probability of *not* being a carrier with this CK level must be 0.05, because only 5% of normal individuals will lie above the 95th percentile. Thus, the information derived from the CK test has increased Mary's probability of being a carrier from 1/2 to 0.93. Since the probability that she would transmit the DMD gene to her male offspring is 1/2, the probability of producing an affected male increases from 0.25 to 0.47. Currently, it is likely that additional tests, such as screening for DMD mutations and a dystrophin assay, would yield even more precise information.

3. The prior probability that Bob has inherited the gene from is father is 1/2. Because 85% of gene carriers manifest symptoms by age 51 if they inherited the gene from an affected father, the conditional probability that Bob is 51 years old and unaffected, *given* that he inherited the gene, is 0.15. The probabilities can be set up as in the table below. In this example, the incorporation of age-of-onset information decreased Bob's chance of inheriting the disease gene from 50% to only 13%. With the cloning of the Huntington disease gene, Bob would likely be given a DNA diagnostic test to determine with certainty whether he inherited an expanded repeat mutation from his father.

	Bob carries the Huntington disease gene	Bob does not carry the Huntington disease gene
Prior probability	1/2	1/2
Conditional probability that Bob is normal at age 51	0.15	1
Joint probability	0.075	1/2
Posterior probability	0.13	0.87

Glossary

5′ cap   A chemically modified guanine nucleotide added to the 5′ end of a growing mRNA molecule.

acceptor site   AG sequence that defines the splice site at the 3′ end of an intron.

acrocentric   A chromosome whose centromere is close to the end of one arm.

activator   A **specific transcription factor** that binds to **co-activators** and to **enhancers** to help regulate the transcriptional activity of certain genes.

adaptive immune system   The portion of the immune system that is capable of changing its DNA sequence to bind foreign particles more effectively. Includes the humoral and cellular components. Compare with **innate immune system.**

addition rule   A law of probability that states that the probability of one event *or* another event occurring is derived by adding the probabilities of the two events together, assuming the events occur independently of one another.

adenine   One of the four DNA bases (abbrev.: A).

adeno-associated virus   A type of parvovirus sometimes used as a vector for somatic cell gene therapy.

adenovirus   A double-stranded RNA virus that is sometimes used in gene therapy.

adjacent segregation   A meiotic segregation pattern in which the pairing of translocated chromosomes leads to unbalanced gametes. Compare with **alternate segregation.**

affected sib-pair method   Linkage analysis method in which sib pairs both affected with a disease are assessed for the extent to which they share alleles at various marker loci. If alleles are shared significantly more often than the expected 50%, linkage of the disease to the marker is indicated.

affinity   The binding power of an antibody with an antigen (low affinity indicates poor binding; high affinity indicates precise binding).

allele   Conventional abbreviation for "allelomorph." Refers to the different forms, or DNA sequences, that a gene may have in a population.

allele-specific oligonucleotide   A short DNA sequence, usually 18 to 20 nucleotides, that can hybridize with either disease-causing or normal DNA sequences. Used in **direct diagnosis** of mutations.

alpha-fetoprotein   Albumin-like protein produced by the fetus. The level of alpha-fetoprotein is elevated in pregnancies with neural tube defects and may be decreased in pregnancies with Down syndrome.

alpha-satellite DNA   A type of repetitive DNA sequence found near centromeres.

alternate segregation   A meiotic segregation pattern in which the pairing of translocated chromosomes leads to balanced gametes. Compare with **adjacent segregation.**

alternative splice site   A variation in the location of intron-exon splice sites in some genes that allow one gene to produce multiple different protein products.

Alu **family**   A major group of dispersed repetitive DNA sequences.

amino acids   The major building blocks of polypeptides. Each of the 20 amino acids is encoded by one or more mRNA codons.

amniocentesis   Prenatal diagnostic technique in which a small amount of amniotic fluid is withdrawn transabdominally at about 16 weeks post-LMP. Fetal cells can then be tested for some genetic diseases.

amniocentesis, early   Amniocentesis carried out at approximately 12 to 14 weeks post-LMP.

amniocyte   Fetal cell found in the amniotic fluid.

anaphase   One of the stages of cell division in which sister chromatids separate and move toward opposite sides of the cell.

aneuploid   Condition in which the number of chromosomes is not a multiple of 23, as in trisomy and monosomy. Compare with **euploid**.

antibody   Molecule produced by plasma cells; antibodies bind to invading antigens.

anticipation   A feature of pedigrees in which a disease is seen at earlier ages or with increased severity in more recent generations.

anticodon   A three-nucleotide DNA sequence in a tRNA molecule that undergoes complementary base pairing with an mRNA codon.

antigen   Molecule that provokes antibody formation (from *anti*body *gene*rator).

antigen presenting cell   A cell that engulfs foreign bodies, digests them, and then displays the foreign antigens on its cell surface for recognition by T lymphocytes.

antisense therapy   A type of somatic cell gene therapy in which an **oligonucleotide** is synthesized, which can hybridize with a mutant mRNA sequence, blocking its translation into protein.

apoptosis Programmed cell death.

association The co-occurrence of two traits or events more often than expected by chance.

autoimmunity Condition in which one's immune system attacks one's own cells.

autoradiogram The image produced by exposing a radioactively labeled substance, such as a probe, to x-ray film (used, for example, in detecting RFLPs and in performing in situ hybridization).

autosomes The 22 pairs of chromosomes excluding the sex chromosomes (X and Y).

axis specification Definition, during embryonic development, of the major axes of the embryo: ventral/dorsal and anterior/posterior.

B lymphocyte (also, **B cell**) A component of the adaptive immune system that produces antibodies.

bacterial artificial chromosome (BAC) A recombinant plasmid inserted in bacteria that serves as a cloning **vector** capable of accepting DNA inserts of 50 to 200 kb.

bacteriophage Viruses that infect bacteria. In recombinant DNA technology, they are used as vectors to carry inserted DNA sequences.

bacteriophage P1 artificial chromosome (PAC) A cloning **vector** that consists of bacteriophage P1 and is inserted into a plasmid; accepts DNA inserts up to 100 kb in size.

bands 1. Visibly darkened areas on **autoradiograms** that represent the location of alleles on a gel. 2. Alternating dark and light areas visible on chromosomes after certain types of stains are used.

Barr body The inactive X chromosome, visible as a densely staining chromatin mass in the somatic cells of normal females. Also known as **sex chromatin**.

base One of the four nitrogenous substances (adenine, cytosine, guanine, or thymine) that makes up part of the DNA molecule. Combinations of bases specify amino acid sequences.

base analog A substance that can mimic the chemical behavior of one of the four DNA bases. Base analogs are a type of **mutagen.**

base pair A unit of complementary DNA bases in a double-stranded DNA molecule (A-T, C-G).

base pair substitution The replacement of one base pair by another. A type of mutation.

Bayes theorem A statistical procedure in which prior and conditional probabilities are used to derive an improved estimate of probability or risk.

benign Describes a neoplasm (tumor) that does not invade surrounding tissue or **metastasize** to other parts of the body. Compare with **malignant.**

bivalent A pair of intertwined homologous chromosomes seen in prophase I of meiosis. Synonymous with **tetrad.**

blood group Molecules found on the surfaces of erythrocytes, some of which (ABO and Rh) determine blood transfusion compatibility.

body plan The pattern and arrangement of body segments during embryonic development.

bp Abbreviation for **base pair**.

breakpoint The location on a chromosome at which a translocation has occurred.

C-banding A type of chromosome staining that highlights the constitutive heterochromatin that lies at and near centromeres.

candidate gene A gene that, on the basis of known properties or protein product, is thought to be the gene causing a specific genetic disease.

carcinogen Substance that can produce cancer (adj.: carcinogenic).

carcinogenesis The process of cancer development.

carrier An individual who has a copy of a disease-causing gene but does not express the disease. The term is usually used to denote heterozygotes for a recessive disease gene.

catalyst A substance that increases the rate of a chemical reaction. Enzymes are an example of a catalyst.

cDNA Complementary DNA, formed by reverse transcribing mRNA purified from a collection of cells. This type of DNA corresponds only to coding sequence (**exons**).

cDNA library A collection of segments of complementary DNA (cDNA) cloned into vehicles such as phage or plasmid. Compare with **genomic library**.

cell adhesion molecule Cell-surface molecule that participates in the interaction of T cells and their targets.

cell cycle The alternating sequence of mitosis and interphase.

cell fate The location and function of cells, programmed during embryonic development.

cellular immune system The T-cell component of the adaptive immune system.

centiMorgan (cM) A unit of measure of the frequency of recombination between two loci, also known as a map unit. One cM corresponds to a recombination frequency of 1%.

centriole Structure in cells that helps to pull chromosomes apart during meiosis and mitosis.

centromere The region of a chromosome that separates the two arms; centromeres are the sites of attachment of spindle fibers during cell division.

CG islands Unmethylated CG sequences that are found near the 5' ends of many genes.

chiasma (pl. **chiasmata**) The location of a **crossover** between two homologous chromosomes during meiosis.

chorionic villus sampling A prenatal diagnostic technique in which a small sample of chorionic villi is aspirated. Usually performed at 10 to 12 weeks' gestation.

chromatin The combination of proteins (e.g., **histones**) and nucleic acids that makes up chromosomes.

chromatin loop A unit of DNA coiling consisting of a group of **solenoids**. Each loop is approximately 100 kb in size.

chromatin opener Regulatory element that is capable of decondensing or "opening" regions of chromatin.

chromosome Threadlike structure (literally "colored body") consisting of **chromatin**. Genes are arranged along chromosomes.

chromosome abnormalities A major group of genetic diseases, consisting of microscopically observable alterations of chromosome number or structure.

chromosome banding The process of applying specific stains to chromosomes in order to produce characteristic patterns of **bands** (example: G-banding).

chromosome breakage The fracture of chromosomes; breakage is increased in the presence of **clastogens**.

chromosome instability syndrome Diseases characterized by the presence of large numbers of chromosome breaks or exchanges, such as **sister chromatid exchange** (example: Bloom syndrome).

chromosome-specific library   A collection of DNA fragments from a single chromosome.

chromosome walking   A process in which overlapping clones are used to progress along a chromosome toward a gene of interest.

class switching   The process in which heavy chains of B lymphocytes change from one class, or **isotype**, to another (e.g., IgM to IgG).

clastogen   A substance that can induce **chromosome breakage** (example: radiation).

clone   A series of identical DNA fragments created by recombinant DNA techniques. Clones also refer to identical cells that are descended from a single common ancestor.

cloning, functional   A method of isolating genes in which a gene whose protein product's function is already known is evaluated as a **candidate gene** responsible for a trait or disease.

cloning, positional   The isolation and cloning of a disease gene after determining its approximate physical location; the gene product is subsequently determined. Formerly termed "reverse genetics."

co-activator   A type of **specific transcription factor** that binds to **activators** and to the **general transcription factor** complex to regulate the transcription of specific genes.

codominant   Alleles that are both expressed when they occur together in the heterozygous state (example: A and B alleles of the ABO blood group system).

codon   A group of three mRNA bases, each of which specifies an amino acid when translated.

coefficient of relationship   A statistic that measures the proportion of genes shared by two individuals as a result of descent from a common ancestor.

co-factor   Substances that interact with enzymes to produce chemical reactions, such as various metabolic processes (examples: dietary trace elements, vitamins).

colcemid or **colchicine**   A spindle poison that arrests cells in metaphase, making them easily discernible microscopically.

comparative genomic hybridization   Cytogenetic technique in which a mixture of DNA from a test source (e.g., a tumor) and a normal control are differentially labeled, mixed, and hybridized with normal metaphase chromosomes. Differences in color reveal chromosome losses or duplications in the test DNA.

complement system   A component of the immune system, encoded by genes in the Class III MHC region, that can destroy invading organisms. The complement system also interacts with other components of the immune system, such as antibodies and phagocytes.

complementary base pairing   A fundamental process in which adenosine pairs only with thymine and guanine pairs only with cytosine. Also sometimes known as "Watson-Crick pairing."

compound heterozygote   An individual who is heterozygous for two different disease-causing mutations at a locus. Compare with **homozygote**. Compound heterozygotes for recessive disease mutations are usually affected with the disorder.

concordant   When two individuals have the same trait (e.g., monozygotic twins may be concordant for a disease such as diabetes). Compare with **discordant.** (n.: concordance).

conditional probability   The probability that an event will occur, *given* that another event has already occurred. Conditional probabilities are used, for example, in **Bayes theorem.**

confined placental mosaicism   A form of **mosaicism** that is observed in the placenta but not in the fetus.

congenital   Present at birth.

consanguinity   The mating of related individuals.

consensus sequence   A sequence that denotes the DNA bases most often seen in a region of interest. The sequences that are found near **donor** and **acceptor splice sites** are a type of consensus sequence.

conservation   The preservation of highly similar DNA sequences among different organisms; conserved sequences are usually found in functional genes.

conserved   see **conservation.**

constitutional or **constitutive**   Pertaining to DNA in normal cells of the body, usually used in contrast to tumor DNA.

constitutive heterochromatin   See **heterochromatin, constitutive.**

contig map   A physical map of a chromosome region constructed by isolating overlapping (contiguous) DNA segments.

contiguous gene syndrome   A disease caused by the deletion or duplication of multiple consecutive genes. *See also* **microdeletion.**

cordocentesis   See **percutaneous umbilical blood sampling (PUBS)**

cosmid   A phage-plasmid hybrid capable of accepting larger DNA inserts (up to 40 to 50 kb) than either phage or plasmids.

costimulatory molecule   Cell-surface molecule that participates in the binding of T-cell receptors to MHC-antigen complexes.

cross   Mating between organisms in genetic studies.

cross-reaction   The binding of an antibody to an antigen *other* than the one that originally stimulated antibody formation. Such antigens are usually very similar to the original antibody-generating antigen.

crossing over or **crossover**   The exchange of genetic material between homologous chromosomes during meiosis (also occurs rarely during mitosis); produces **recombination.**

cryptic splice site   Site at which intron-exon splicing may occur when the usual splice site is altered.

cyclin-dependent kinases   Enzymes that form complexes with specific **cyclins** to phosphorylate regulatory proteins (such as pRb) at specific stages of the cell cycle.

cyclin-dependent kinase inhibitors   Proteins that inactivate **cyclin-dependent kinases**. Many of these are tumor suppressors (examples: p16, p21).

cyclins   Proteins that interact with specific **cyclin-dependent kinases** to regulate the cell cycle at specific stages.

cytogenetics   The study of chromosomes and their abnormalities. Combines cytology, the study of cells, and genetics.

cytokine   Growth factor that causes cells to proliferate (example: interleukins).

cytokinesis   Cytoplasmic division that occurs during mitosis and meiosis.

cytosine   One of the four DNA bases (abbrev.: C).

cytotoxic T lymphocyte   A type of T lymphocyte that destroys a cell when the cell presents a complex of MHC Class I molecule and foreign peptide. Part of the cellular immune system.

daughter cells   Cells that result from the division of a parent cell.

deformation   Alteration of the form, shape, or position of a normally formed body part by mechanical forces (example: oligohydramnios sequence).

delayed age of onset   Describes phenotypes that are not seen at birth, but later in life (examples: Huntington disease, familial breast cancer).

deletion   The loss of chromosome material. May be terminal or interstitial. Compare with **duplication.**

deletion, interstitial   Deletion that removes part of the interior of the chromosome.

deletion, terminal   Deletion that removes part of a chromosome, including one telomere.

denaturing gradient gel electrophoresis (DGGE)   See **electrophoresis, denaturing gradient gel.**

derivative chromosome   A chromosome that has been altered as a result of a translocation (example: derivative 9, or der(9)).

dideoxy method   A technique for sequencing DNA in which dideoxynucleotides, which terminate replication, are incorporated into replicating DNA strands.

diploid   Having two copies of each chromosome. In humans, the diploid number is 46. Compare with **haploid, polyploid.**

direct cDNA selection   Method of exon detection in which a genomic DNA fragment inserted into a vector such as a YAC is hybridized with cDNA; hybridization and selection identify the regions of the genomic DNA fragment that correspond to cDNA (i.e., exon-containing DNA).

direct diagnosis   A form of DNA-based disease diagnosis in which the mutation itself is examined directly. Compare with **indirect diagnosis.**

discordant   When two individuals do not share the same trait. Compare with **concordant.** (n.: discordance)

dispermy   Fertilization of a single ovum by two sperm cells.

dispersed repetitive DNA   A class of repeated DNA sequences in which single repeats are scattered throughout the genome. Compare with **tandem repeats.**

disruption   Morphological defect that results from a breakdown of an otherwise normal developmental process (example: limb reduction defect resulting from poor vascularization).

dizygotic   A type of twinning in which each twin is produced by the fertilization of a different ovum. Synonymous with "fraternal" twin. Compare with **monozygotic.**

DNA (deoxyribonucleic acid)   A double-helix molecule that consists of a sugar-phosphate backbone and four nitrogenous bases (A, C, G, and T). DNA bases encode messenger RNA (mRNA), which in turn encodes amino acid sequences.

DNA-binding motifs   Portions of transcription factors that allow them to interact with specific DNA sequences (examples: helix-loop-helix motif, zinc finger motif).

DNA chips   Computer chips that contain arrays of DNA sequences, such as oligonucleotides consisting of normal and mutated sequences. These oligonucleotides can be hybridized to labeled DNA from subjects to conduct computer-aided mutation analysis or to sequence DNA.

DNA looping   The formation of looped structures in DNA; sometimes permits the interaction of various regulatory elements.

DNA mismatch repair   A type of **DNA repair** in which nucleotide mismatches (i.e., violations of the G-C, A-T complementary base-pairing rule) are corrected by specialized enzymes.

DNA polymerase   An enzyme involved in DNA replication and repair.

DNA profile   A series of DNA polymorphisms (usually VNTRs or microsatellites) typed in an individual. Because these polymorphisms are highly variable the combined genotypes are useful in identifying individuals for forensic purposes.

DNA repair   A process in which mistakes in the DNA sequence are altered to represent the original sequence.

DNA sequence   The order of DNA bases along a chromosome.

DNA sequencing, automated   DNA sequencing techniques in which automated procedures such as computer-guided laser scanning are used to provide more rapid, accurate DNA sequence results.

dominant   Allele that is expressed in the same way in single copy (heterozygotes) as in double copy (homozygotes). Compare with **recessive.**

dominant negative   A type of mutation in which the altered protein product in a heterozygote forms a complex with the normal protein product produced by the homologous normal gene, thus disabling it.

donor site   GT sequence that defines the splice site at the 5' end of an intron.

dosage compensation   As a consequence of X inactivation, the amount of X chromosome–encoded gene product in females is roughly equal to that in males.

dosage mapping   A technique for mapping genes in which excess or deficient gene product is correlated with a chromosomal duplication or deletion.

dosage sensitivity   Condition in which alteration of the level of a gene product (e.g., a **deletion** resulting in 50% expression or a **duplication** resulting in 150% expression of the gene product) causes a substantial alteration of the phenotype (including disease).

double helix   Describes the "twisted ladder" shape of the double-stranded DNA molecule.

double-stranded DNA breaks   A type of DNA breakage in which both strands are broken at a specific location.

duplication   The presence of an extra copy of chromosome material. Compare with **deletion.**

dysmorphology   The study of abnormal physical development.

dysplasia   A defect in which cells are abnormally organized into tissue (example: bone dysplasia).

ectopic expression   Expression of a gene product in an abnormal location or tissue type.

electrophoresis   A technique in which charged molecules are placed in a medium and exposed to an electrical field, causing them to migrate through the medium at different rates, according to charge, length, or other attributes.

electrophoresis, denaturing gradient gel (DGGE)   A method of mutation detection in which DNA fragments are electrophoresed through a gel in which there is a changing denaturing factor, such as temperature.

empirical risk   Risk estimate based on direct observation of data.

endocytosis   Process in which molecules are transported into the interior of cells.

enhancer Regulatory DNA sequence that interacts with **specific transcription factors** to increase the transcription of genes. Compare with **silencer.**

equational division The second major cycle of meiosis: meiosis II. Compare with **reduction division.**

equatorial plane The middle of the cell's spindle, along which homologous chromosomes are arranged during metaphase.

erythroblast A nucleated red blood cell; precursors of erythrocytes.

erythrocyte A red blood cell.

euchromatin Chromatin that is light-staining during interphase and tends to be transcriptionally active. Compare with **heterochromatin.**

eukaryotes Organisms whose cells have true nuclei.

euploid Cells whose chromosome number is a multiple of 23 (in humans).

exons Portions of genes that encode amino acids and are retained after the primary mRNA transcript is spliced. Compare with **intron.**

exon trapping Method for isolating exons in a fragment of genomic DNA by using an in vitro cell system to artificially splice out the introns.

expanded repeat A type of mutation in which a tandem trinucleotide repeat increases in number (example: Huntington disease).

expressed sequence tag (EST) Several hundred bp of known cDNA sequence, flanked by PCR primers. Because they are derived from cDNA libraries, these sequences represent portions of expressed genes.

false negative A test result in which an affected individual is incorrectly identified as being unaffected with the disease in question. Compare with **false positive.**

false positive A test result in which an unaffected individual is incorrectly identified as being affected with the disease in question. Compare with **false negative.**

fetoscopy A fetal visualization technique in which an endoscope is inserted through the abdominal wall. Sometimes used in prenatal diagnosis.

fiber FISH See **fluorescence in situ hybridization, fiber.**

fibrillin Connective tissue component; mutations in the fibrillin gene can cause Marfan syndrome.

flow cytometry A technique whereby chromosomes can be individually sorted.

fluorescence in situ hybridization (FISH) A molecular cytogenetic technique in which labeled probes are hybridized with chromosomes and then visualized under a fluorescence microscope.

fluorescence in situ hybridization, fiber (fiber FISH) A version of the **FISH** technique in which fluorescent probes are hybridized to interphase chromosomes that have been manipulated so that the chromatin fibers are stretched, allowing high-resolution visualization and mapping.

founder effect A large shift in gene frequencies that results when a small "founder" population, which contains limited genetic variation, is derived from a larger population. Founder effect can be considered a special case of **genetic drift**.

frameshift mutation An alteration of DNA in which a duplication or deletion occurs that is not a multiple of three base pairs.

fusion gene A gene that results from a combination of two genes, or parts of two genes.

gain of function A class of mutations that results in a protein product that is either increased in quantity or has a novel function. Compare with **loss of function**.

gamete The haploid germ cell (sperm and ova).

gametogenesis The process of gamete formation.

gastrulation Embryonic stage in which cells of the blastula are arranged to become a three-layer structure consisting of endoderm, mesoderm, and ectoderm.

gene The fundamental unit of heredity.

gene-environment interaction A mutual phenotypic effect of a gene and an environmental factor that is greater than the single effect of either factor alone (example: the effect of α-1-antitrypsin deficiency and cigarette smoking on pulmonary emphysema).

gene family A group of genes that are similar in DNA sequence and have evolved from a single common ancestral gene; may or may not be located in the same chromosome region.

gene flow The exchange of genes between different populations.

gene frequency In a population, the proportion of chromosomes that contain a specific gene.

gene therapy The insertion or alteration of genes to correct a disease.

gene therapy, germline Gene therapy that alters all cells of the body, including the germ line. Compare with **gene therapy, somatic cell.**

gene therapy, somatic cell Gene therapy that alters somatic cells but not cells of the germ line. Compare with **gene therapy, germline.**

genetic code The combinations of mRNA **codons** that specify individual amino acids.

genetic counseling The delivery of information about genetic diseases (risks, natural history, and management) to patients and their families.

genetic drift An evolutionary process in which gene frequencies change as a result of random fluctuations in the transmission of genes from one generation to the next. Drift is greater in smaller populations.

genetic engineering The alteration of genes; typically involves **recombinant DNA** techniques.

genetic mapping The ordering of genes on chromosomes according to recombination frequency. Compare with **physical mapping**.

genetic screening The large-scale testing of defined populations for a genetic disease or disease-causing gene.

genome The totality of an organism's DNA.

genome scan A gene mapping approach in which markers from the entire human genome are tested for linkage with a disease phenotype.

genomic library A collection of DNA fragments from an organism's entire genome. Includes cDNA as well as noncoding DNA. Compare with **cDNA library.**

genomic instability Abnormal condition in which there is a substantial increase in mutations throughout the genome. Can occur, for example, when a DNA repair system is disabled.

genotype An individual's allelic constitution at a locus.

genotype frequency The proportion of individuals in a population that carry a specific genotype.

germ line Cells responsible for the production of gametes.

Giemsa A type of staining that produces G-bands in chromosomes.

globin Major component of the hemoglobin molecule. Globin is also found in the vertebrate myoglobin molecule.

growth factor A substance capable of stimulating cell proliferation.

growth factor receptor Structure on cell surfaces to which growth factors can bind.

guanine One of the four DNA bases (abbrev.: G).

guanosine diphosphate (GDP) Partially dephosphorylated form of **guanosine triphosphate**.

guanosine triphosphate (GTP) A molecule required for the synthesis of peptide bonds during translation.

haploid Cells having one copy of each chromosome, the typical state for gametes. In humans, the haploid number is 23.

haploinsufficiency Describes the situation in which 50% of the normal level of gene expression (i.e., in a heterozygote) is not sufficient for normal function.

haplotype The allelic constitution of multiple loci on a single chromosome. Derived from "haploid genotype."

Hardy-Weinberg principle Specifies an equilibrium relationship between gene frequencies and genotype frequencies in populations.

heavy chain A major structural component of an antibody molecule, having a higher molecular weight than the other major component, the light chain. There are five major types of heavy chains in the human: γ, μ, α, δ, and ε.

helper T lymphocyte A type of T lymphocyte whose receptors bind to a complex of MHC class II molecule and foreign peptide on the surfaces of antigen presenting cells. Part of the cellular immune system.

heme Iron-containing component of the hemoglobin molecule; binds with oxygen.

hemizygous A gene present in only a single copy (hemi = "half"). Most commonly, refers to genes on the single male X chromosome, but can refer to other genes in the haploid state, such as the genes homologous to a deleted region of a chromosome.

heritability The proportion of population **variance** in a trait that can be ascribed to genetic factors.

heterochromatin Dark-staining chromatin that is usually transcriptionally inactive and consists mostly of repetitive DNA. Compare with **euchromatin.**

heterochromatin, constitutive Heterochromatin that consists of **satellite DNA**; located near centromeres and on the short arms of acrocentric chromosomes.

heterodisomy The presence in a cell of two chromosomes derived from a single parent and none from the other parent (disomy). In *hetero*disomy, the two chromosomes are the nonidentical homologous chromosomes. Compare with **isodisomy.**

heterogeneity, allelic Describes conditions in which different alleles at a locus can produce variable expression of a disease. Depending on phenotype definition, allelic heterogeneity may cause two distinct diseases, as in Duchenne and Becker muscular dystrophy.

heterogeneity, locus Describes diseases in which mutations at distinct loci can produce the same disease phenotype (examples: osteogenesis imperfecta; retinitis pigmentosa).

heteromorphism Variation in the microscopic appearance of a chromosome.

heteroplasmy The existence of differing DNA sequences at a locus within a single cell. Often seen in mitochondrial genes.

heterotetramer A molecule consisting of four (tetra) subunits, at least one of which differs from the others. Compare with **homotetramer.**

heterozygote An individual who has two different alleles at a locus. Compare with **homozygote.**

high-resolution banding **Chromosome banding** using prophase or prometaphase chromosomes, which are more extended than metaphase chromosomes and thus yield more bands and greater resolution.

histone The protein core around which DNA is wound in a chromosome.

holandric Y-linked inheritance; a transmission exclusively from father to son.

homeodomain A DNA-binding portion of transcription factor proteins that are involved in embryonic development.

homologous 1. DNA or amino acid sequences that are highly similar to one another. 2. Describes chromosomes that pair during meiosis, one derived from the individual's father and the other derived from the mother.

homologs Chromosomes that are **homologous.**

homotetramer Molecule consisting of four (tetra) identical subunits. Compare with **heterotetramer.**

homozygote An individual in whom the two alleles at a locus are the same. Compare with **heterozygote.**

housekeeping genes Genes whose protein products are required for cellular maintenance or metabolism. Because of their central role in the life of the cell, housekeeping genes are transcriptionally active in all cells.

human artificial chromosome A synthetic chromosome consisting of an artificial centromere and telomeres and an insert of human DNA that can be 5 to 10 Mb in size.

human leukocyte antigen (HLA) Older term for **major histocompatibility complex (MHC)**.

humoral immune system The B-cell component of the adaptive immune system, termed humoral because antibodies are secreted into the circulation.

immunodeficiency disease A class of diseases characterized by insufficiencies in the immune response (example: severe combined immune deficiency, SCID).

immunodeficiency disease, primary Disorder of the immune system that is caused directly by defects (usually genetic) in components or cells of the immune system.

immunodeficiency disease, secondary Disorder of the immune system that is a consequence of an agent or defect that originates outside the immune system (e.g., infection, radiation, drugs).

immunogenetics The study of the genetic basis of the immune system.

immunoglobulin Receptor found on the surfaces of B cells. When secreted into the circulation by B cells that have matured into plasma cells, immunoglobulins are known as **antibodies.**

imprinting, genomic Describes process in which genetic material is expressed differently when inherited from the mother than when inherited from the father.

in situ hybridization Molecular gene mapping technique in which labeled probes are hybridized to stained metaphase chromosomes and then exposed to x-ray film to reveal the position of the probe.

in vitro fertilization (IVF) diagnosis A form of genetic diagnosis in which DNA from a single embryonic cell (obtained by IVF) is amplified by PCR so that disease-causing mutations can be tested.

incest The mating of closely related individuals, usually describing the union of first-degree relatives.

independence A principle, often invoked in statistical analysis, indicating that the occurrence of one event has no effect on the probability of occurrence of another. (adj.: independent)

independent assortment One of Mendel's fundamental principles; dictates that alleles at different loci are transmitted independently of one another.

index case See **proband.**

indirect diagnosis A form of genetic diagnosis in which the disease-causing mutation is not directly observed; usually refers to diagnosis using linked markers. Compare with **direct diagnosis.**

induction The influence or determination of development of one group of cells by a second group of cells.

innate immune system Portion of the immune system that does not change its characteristics to respond to infections. Major part of the initial immune response. Compare with **adaptive immune system.**

insert A DNA sequence that is placed into a vector, such as a plasmid or cosmid, using recombinant DNA techniques.

interphase Portion of the cell cycle that alternates with **meiosis** or **mitosis** (cell division). DNA is replicated and repaired during this phase.

intraclass correlation coefficient A statistical measure that varies between -1 and 1 and specifies the degree of similarity of two quantities in a sample or population.

intron DNA sequence found between two **exons.** Transcribed into primary mRNA but spliced out in the formation of the mature mRNA transcript.

inversion A structural rearrangement of a chromosome in which two breaks occur, followed by the reinsertion of the chromosome segment, but in reversed order. May be either paracentric or pericentric. See also **inversion, paracentric** and **inversion, pericentric.**

inversion, paracentric An inversion that does not include the centromere.

inversion, pericentric An inversion that includes the centromere.

isochromosome A structural chromosome rearrangement caused by the division of a chromosome along an axis perpendicular to the usual axis of division; results in chromosomes with either two short arms or two long arms.

isodisomy The presence in a cell of two identical chromosomes derived from one parent and none from the other parent. Compare with **heterodisomy.**

isotype Classes of immunoglobulin molecules (e.g., IgA, IgE, IgG), determined by the type of heavy chain present in the molecule.

joint probability The probability of two events *both* occurring.

karyotype A display of chromosomes, ordered according to length.

kilobase (kb) One thousand DNA base pairs.

knockout Animal model in which a specific gene has been disabled.

light chain A major structural component of the antibody molecule, consisting of either a κ or a λ chain. The light chain has a lower molecular weight than the other major component, the heavy chain.

likelihood A statistic that measures the probability of an event or a series of events.

LINEs (long interspersed elements) A class of dispersed repetitive DNA in which each repeat is relatively long, up to 7 kb. Compare with **SINEs.**

linkage Describes two loci that are located close enough on the same chromosome that their **recombination frequency** is less than 50%.

linkage disequilibrium Nonrandom association of alleles at linked loci in populations. Compare with **linkage equilibrium**.

linkage equilibrium Lack of preferential association of alleles at linked loci. Compare with **linkage disequilibrium.**

linkage phase The arrangement of alleles of linked loci on chromosomes.

liposome A fat body sometimes used as a vector for somatic cell gene therapy.

locus The chromosome location of a specific gene. (pl.: loci)

locus control region DNA sequence in the 5' region of the globin gene clusters that is involved in transcriptional regulation.

LOD score Common logarithm of the ratio of the likelihood of linkage at a specific recombination fraction to the likelihood of no linkage.

loss of function A class of mutation in which the alteration results in a non-functional protein product. Compare with **gain of function**.

loss of heterozygosity Describes a locus or loci at which a deletion or other process has converted the locus from heterozygosity to homozygosity or hemizygosity.

Lyon hypothesis A proposal (now verified) that one X chromosome is randomly inactivated in each somatic cell of the normal female embryo (Lyonization).

macrophage A type of **phagocyte** that ingests foreign microbes and displays them on its surface for recognition by T-cell receptors.

major gene A single locus responsible for a trait (sometimes contrasted with a polygenic component).

major histocompatibility complex (MCH), class I A membrane-spanning glycoprotein, found on the surfaces of nearly all cells, that presents antigen for recognition by cytotoxic T lymphocytes. Compare with **MHC class II.**

major histocompatibility complex (MHC), class II A membrane-spanning glycoprotein, found on the surfaces of **antigen-presenting cells**, that presents antigen for recognition by helper T cells.

malformation A primary morphologic defect resulting from an intrinsically abnormal developmental process (example: polydactyly).

malignant Describes a tumor that is capable of invading surrounding tissue and metastasizing to other sites in the body. Compare with **benign.**

manifesting heterozygote An individual who is heterozygous for a recessive trait but displays the trait. Most often used to describe females heterozygous for an X-linked trait who display the trait.

markers Polymorphisms, such as RFLPs, VNTRs, microsatellite repeats, and blood groups, that are linked to a disease locus.

mass spectrometry Analysis of the mass/charge ratio of molecules; can be used to sequence DNA and detect mutations.

maternal serum alpha-fetoprotein (MSAFP) Alpha-fetoprotein present in the serum of pregnant women; used in the prenatal screening of fetal disorders such as neural tube defects and Down syndrome.

mature transcript Describes mRNA after the introns have been spliced out. Prior to splicing, the mRNA is referred to as a **primary transcript**.

maximum likelihood estimate A statistical procedure in which the likelihoods of a variety of parameter values are estimated and then compared to determine which likelihood is the largest. Used, for example, in evaluating LOD scores to determine which recombination frequency is the most likely.

megabase (Mb) One million base pairs.

meiosis Cell division process in which haploid gametes are formed from diploid germ cells.

meiotic failure Aberrant **meiosis** in which a diploid gamete is produced rather than the normal haploid gamete.

memory cells A class of high-affinity-binding B cells that remains in the body after an immune response has ended; provides a relatively rapid, high-affinity response should the same disease antigen be encountered a second time.

mendelian Referring to Gregor Mendel, describes a trait that is attributable to a single gene.

mesenchyme Tissue that forms connective tissues and lymphatic and blood vessels during embryonic development.

messenger RNA (mRNA) RNA molecule that is formed from the **transcription** of DNA. Prior to intron splicing, mRNA is termed a **primary transcript**; after splicing, the **mature transcript** (or mature mRNA) proceeds to the cytoplasm where it is translated into an amino acid sequence.

metacentric A chromosome in which the centromere is located approximately in the middle of the chromosome arm.

metaphase A stage of mitosis and meiosis in which homologous chromosomes are arranged along the equatorial plane, or metaphase plate, of the cell. This is the mitotic stage at which chromosomes are maximally condensed and most easily visualized.

metastasis The spread of malignant cells from one site in the body to another (v.: metastasize).

methylation The attachment of methyl groups; in genetics, refers especially to the addition of methyl groups to cytosine bases, forming 5-methylcytosine. Methylation is correlated with reduced transcription of genes.

MHC restriction The limiting of immune response functions to MHC-mediated interactions (e.g., the binding of T-cell receptors is MHC restricted because it requires the presentation of antigen by MHC class I or MHC class II molecules).

microdeletion A chromosome deletion too small to be visible under a microscope (examples: DiGeorge syndrome; Prader-Willi syndrome). See also **contiguous gene syndrome**.

microsatellite A type of **satellite DNA** that consists of small repeat units (usually two, three, four, or five bp) that occur in tandem.

microsatellite repeat polymorphism A type of genetic variation in populations consisting of differing numbers of **microsatellite** repeat units at a locus.

minisatellite A type of **satellite DNA** that consists of tandem repeat units that are each about 20 to 70 bp in length. Variation in the number of minisatellite repeats is the basis of VNTR polymorphisms.

mismatch The presence in one chain of double-stranded DNA of a base that is not complementary to the corresponding base in the other chain. Also known as mispairing.

missense A type of mutation that results in a single amino acid change in the translated gene product. Compare with **nonsense mutation.**

mitochondria Cytoplasmic organelles that are important in cellular respiration. The mitochondria have their own unique DNA.

mitosis Cell division process in which two identical progeny cells are produced from a single parent cell. Compare with **meiosis.**

mobile elements DNA sequences that are capable of inserting themselves into other locations in the genome.

modifier gene A gene that alters the expression of a gene at another locus.

molecular genetics Study of the structure and function of genes at the molecular level.

monoclonal A group of cells that consist of a single clone (i.e., all cells are derived from the same single ancestral cell).

monogenic Describing a single-gene, or mendelian, trait.

monosomy An aneuploid condition in which a specific chromosome is present in only a single copy, giving the individual a total of 45 chromosomes.

monozygotic Describing a twin pair in which both members are derived from a single zygote. Synonymous with "identical" twin. Compare with **dizygotic.**

morphogenesis The process of development of a cell, organ, or organism.

mosaic The existence of two or more genetically different cell lines in an individual.

mosaic, germline A type of **mosaic** in which the germ line of an individual contains an allele not present in the somatic cells.

multi-hit concept of carcinogenesis The principle that most tumors arise from a series of errors, or "hits," occurring in a cell.

multifactorial Describes traits or diseases that are the product of the interaction of multiple genetic and environmental factors (example: neural tube defects).

multiplication rule A law of probability that states that the probability of co-occurrence of two or more independent events can be obtained by multiplying the individual probabilities of each event.

multipoint mapping A type of genetic mapping in which the recombination frequencies among three or more loci are estimated simultaneously.

mutagen A substance that causes a **mutation.**

mutation An alteration in DNA sequence.

mutation, induced A mutation that is caused by an exogenous factor, such as radiation. Compare with **mutation, spontaneous.**

mutation, spontaneous A mutation that is not known to be the result of an exogenous factor. Compare with **mutation, induced.**

natural killer cell A type of lymphocyte that is involved in the early phase of defense against foreign microbes and tumors and is not MHC restricted.

natural selection An evolutionary process in which individuals with favorable genotypes produce relatively greater numbers of surviving offspring.

neoplasm or **tumor** A group of cells characterized by unregulated proliferation (may be **benign** or **malignant**).

neurofibromin The protein product of the neurofibromatosis type 1 gene.

neurulation Formation of the neural tube during embryonic development.

new mutation An alteration in DNA sequence that appears for the first time in a family as the result of a mutation in one of the parents' germ cells.

nondirectiveness Describes genetic counseling approach in which information is provided to a family, while leaving decisions about reproduction to the family.

nondisjunction Failure of homologous chromosomes (in mitosis or meiosis I) or sister chromatids (in meiosis II) to separate properly into different progeny cells. Can produce **aneuploidy.**

nonsense mutation A type of mutation in which an mRNA stop codon is produced or removed, resulting in premature termination of translation or an elongated protein product, respectively. Compare with **missense mutation.**

Northern blotting A gene expression assay in which mRNA on a blot is hybridized with a labeled probe.

nucleosome A structural unit of chromatin in which 140 to 150 bp of DNA are wrapped around a core unit of eight histone molecules.

nucleotide A basic unit of DNA or RNA, consisting of one deoxyribose (or ribose in the case of RNA), one phosphate group, and one nitrogenous base.

nucleotide excision repair A type of **DNA repair** in which altered groups of nucleotides, such as pyrimidine dimers, are removed and replaced with properly functioning nucleotides.

obligate carrier An individual who is known to possess a disease-causing gene (usually on the basis of pedigree examination) but may or may not be affected with the disease phenotype.

occurrence risk The probability that a couple will produce a child with a genetic disease. Refers to couples who have not yet produced a child with the disease in question. Compare with **recurrence risk.**

oligonucleotide DNA sequence consisting of a small number of nucleotide bases.

oncogene A gene that can transform cells into a highly proliferative state, causing cancer.

oogenesis The process in which ova are produced.

oogonium The diploid germline stem cell from which ova are ultimately derived.

organogenesis The formation of organs during embryonic development.

packaging cells or **helper cells** Cells in which replication-deficient viruses are placed so that the replication machinery of the packaging cell can produce viral copies.

palindrome A DNA sequence whose complementary sequence is the same if read backwards (e.g., 5′ AATGCGCATT 3′).

panmixia Describes a population in which individuals mate at random with respect to a specific genotype.

paralog Within a species, a member of a set of homologous genes (example: *HOXA-13* and *HOXD-13*).

partial trisomy Chromosome abnormality in which a portion of a chromosome is present in three copies; may be produced by reciprocal translocation or unequal crossover. See also **translocation, reciprocal** and **crossover, unequal.**

pattern formation The spatial arrangement of differentiated cells to form tissues and organs during embryonic development.

pedigree A diagram that describes family relationships, gender, disease status, and other attributes.

penetrance In a population, the proportion of individuals possessing a disease-causing genotype who express the disease phenotype. When this proportion is less than 100%, the disease genotype is said to have reduced or incomplete penetrance.

percutaneous umbilical blood sampling (PUBS) Prenatal diagnostic technique in which fetal blood is obtained by puncturing the umbilical cord. Also called cordocentesis.

phagocyte A cell that engulfs foreign particles.

pharmacogenetics Study of genetic variation in drug response.

phenocopy A **phenotype** that resembles the phenotype produced by a specific gene but is due instead to a different, typically nongenetic, factor.

phenotype The observed characteristics of an individual, produced by the interaction of genes and environment.

Philadelphia chromosome A reciprocal translocation between the long arms of chromosomes 9 and 22 in somatic cells; produces chronic myelogenous leukemia.

physical mapping The determination of physical distances between genes using cytogenetic and molecular techniques. Compare with **genetic mapping**, in which recombination frequencies are estimated.

plasma cell Mature B lymphocyte capable of secreting antibodies.

plasmid Circular double-stranded DNA molecule found in bacteria; capable of independent replication. Plasmids are often used as cloning vectors in recombinant DNA techniques.

pleiotropy Describes genes that have multiple phenotypic effects (examples: Marfan syndrome, cystic fibrosis). (adj.: pleiotropic)

polar body Cell produced during oogenesis that has a nucleus but very little cytoplasm.

polar body diagnosis Prenatal diagnostic technique in which DNA from a polar body is subjected to PCR amplification and assayed using molecular methods.

polarity Direction (e.g., definition of anterior versus posterior in **axis specification**).

poly-A tail The addition of several adenine nucleotides to the 3′ end of a primary mRNA transcript.

polygenic Describes a trait caused by the combined additive effects of multiple genes.

polymerase chain reaction (PCR) A technique for amplifying a large number of copies of a specific DNA sequence flanked by two oligonucleotide primers. The DNA is alternately heated and cooled in the presence of DNA polymerase and free nucleotides so that the specified DNA segment is denatured, hybridized with primers, and extended by DNA polymerase.

polymorphism   A locus in which two or more alleles have gene frequencies greater than 0.01 in a population. When this criterion is not fulfilled, the locus is monomorphic.

polypeptide   A series of amino acids linked together by peptide bonds.

polyploidy   Chromosome abnormality in which the number of chromosomes in a cell is a multiple of 23 but is greater than the diploid number (examples are **triploidy** [69 chromosomes in the human] and **tetraploidy** [92 chromosomes in the human]).

population genetics   Branch of genetics dealing with genetic variation and genetic evolution of populations.

population screening   The large-scale testing of populations for a disease.

positional candidate   A gene mapping approach in which linkage analysis is used to define a gene's approximate location. Known **candidate genes** in the region are then evaluated for their possible role in causing the trait or disease being analyzed.

positional cloning   See **cloning, positional.**

positive predictive value   Among the individuals identified by a test as having a disease, the proportion that actually have the disease.

posterior probability   In Bayesian analysis, the final probability of an event after taking into account prior, conditional, and joint probabilities.

posttranslational modification   Various types of additions and alterations of a polypeptide that take place after the mature mRNA transcript is translated into a polypeptide (e.g., hydroxylation, glycosylation, cleavage of portions of the polypeptide).

prenatal diagnosis   The identification of a disease in a fetus or embryo.

presymptomatic diagnosis   The identification of a disease before the phenotype is clinically observable.

primary oocyte   The diploid product of an oogonium. All primary oocytes are produced in the female during prenatal development; they undergo meiosis I to produce secondary oocytes when ovulation begins.

primary spermatocyte   The diploid progeny cell of a spermatogonium, which then undergoes meiosis I to produce secondary spermatocytes.

primary transcript   The mRNA molecule directly after transcription from DNA. A mature mRNA transcript is formed from the primary transcript when the introns are spliced out.

primer   An oligonucleotide sequence that flanks either side of the DNA to be amplified by **PCR.**

primer extension   Part of the **PCR** process, in which DNA polymerase extends the DNA sequence beginning at an oligonucleotide primer.

primitive streak   A structure formed during mammalian **gastrulation**, consisting of thickened epiblast tissue along the anterior/posterior axis.

prior probability   In Bayesian analysis, the probability that an event will occur *before* any additional information, such as a biochemical carrier test, is incorporated.

probability   The proportion of times that a specific event occurs in a series of trials.

proband   The first person in a pedigree to be identified clinically as having the disease in question. Synonymous with **propositus** and **index case**.

probe   In molecular genetics, a labeled substance, such as a DNA segment, that is used to identify a gene, mRNA transcript, or gene product (usually through hybridization of the probe with the target).

promoter   A DNA sequence located 5' of a gene to which RNA polymerase binds in order to begin transcription of the DNA into mRNA.

proofreading   The correction of errors that occur during replication, transcription, or translation.

prophase   The first stage of mitosis and meiosis.

propositus   See **proband.**

protein electrophoresis   A technique in which amino acid variations are identified on the basis of charge differences that cause differential mobility of polypeptides through an electrically charged medium.

protein kinase   An enzyme that phosphorylates serine, threonine, or tyrosine residues in proteins.

protein truncation test   A mutation detection test in which the encoded protein product is artificially translated to reveal the presence of truncation-causing mutations (e.g., **nonsense** or **frameshift** mutations).

proto-oncogene   A gene whose protein product is involved in the regulation of cell growth. When altered, a proto-oncogene can become a cancer-causing **oncogene.**

pseudoautosomal region   The distal tip of the Y chromosome short arm, which undergoes crossover with the distal tip of the X chromosome short arm during meiosis in the male.

pseudogene   A gene that is highly similar in sequence to another gene or genes but has been rendered transcriptionally or translationally inactive by mutations.

pseudomosaicism   A false indication of fetal mosaicism, caused by an artifact of cell culture.

pulsed field gel electrophoresis   A type of electrophoresis suitable for relatively large DNA fragments; the fragment is moved through a gel by alternating pulses of electricity across fields that are 90 degrees in orientation from one another.

Punnett square   A table specifying the genotypes that can arise from the gametes contributed by a mating pair of individuals.

purine   The two DNA (also RNA) bases, adenine and guanine, that consist of double carbon-nitrogen rings. Compare with **pyrimidine.**

pyrimidine   The bases (cytosine and thymine in DNA, and cytosine and uracil in RNA) that consist of single carbon-nitrogen rings. Compare with **purine.**

quantitative trait   Characteristics that can be measured on a continuous scale (e.g., height, weight).

quantitative trait locus methods   Methods for finding genes (quantitative trait loci, QTLs) underlying complex multifactorial traits.

quasidominant   A pattern of inheritance that appears to be autosomal dominant but is actually autosomal recessive. Usually the result of a mating between an affected homozygote and a heterozygote.

quinacrine banding (Q-banding) Chromosome staining technique in which a fluorochrome dye (quinacrine compound) is added to chromosomes, which are then viewed under a fluorescence microscope.

radiation hybrid mapping Ionizing radiation is used to break human chromosomes into small pieces that are then hybridized with rodent chromosomes. The physical distance between loci is estimated by assessing how frequently two loci are found together on the same human chromosome fragment.

radiation, ionizing A type of energy emission that is capable of removing electrons from atoms, thus causing ion formation (example: x-rays).

radiation, non-ionizing A type of energy emission that does not remove electrons from atoms, but can change their orbits (example: ultraviolet radiation).

random mating See **panmixia.**

receptor A cell-surface structure that binds to extracellular particles.

recessive An allele that is phenotypically expressed only in the homozygous or hemizygous state. The recessive allele is masked by a dominant allele when the two occur together in a heterozygote. Compare with **dominant.**

recognition site See **restriction site.**

recombinant DNA A DNA molecule that consists of components from more than one parent molecule (e.g., a human DNA insert placed in a plasmid vector).

recombinase An enzyme that helps to bring about somatic recombination in B and T lymphocytes.

recombination The occurrence among offspring of new combinations of alleles, resulting from crossovers that occur during parental meiosis.

recombination frequency The proportion of meioses in which recombinants between two loci are observed. Used to estimate genetic distances between loci. See also **centiMorgans.**

recombination hot spot A region of a chromosome in which the recombination frequency is elevated.

recurrence risk The probability that another affected offspring will be produced in families in which one or more affected offspring have already been produced. Compare with **occurrence risk.**

reduction division The first stage of meiosis (meiosis I), in which the chromosome number is reduced from diploid to haploid.

redundancy, genetic The existence of alternate genetic mechanisms or pathways that can compensate when another mechanism or pathway is disabled.

repetitive DNA DNA sequences that are found in multiple copies in the genome. They may be dispersed or repeated in **tandem.**

replication The process in which the double-stranded DNA molecule is duplicated.

replication bubble Replication structures that occur in multiple locations on a chromosome, allowing replication to proceed more rapidly.

replication origin The point at which replication begins on a DNA strand; in eukaryotes, each chromosome has numerous replication origins.

replicative segregation Refers to changes in the proportions of different mitochondrial DNA alleles as the mitochondria reproduce.

restriction digest Process in which DNA is exposed to a restriction enzyme, causing it to be cleaved into **restriction fragments.**

restriction endonuclease Bacterial enzyme that cleaves DNA at a specific DNA sequence (restriction site).

restriction fragment A piece of DNA that has been cleaved by a restriction endonuclease.

restriction fragment length polymorphism (RFLP) Variations in DNA sequence in populations, detected by digesting DNA with a restriction endonuclease, electrophoresing the resulting restriction fragments, transferring the fragments to a solid medium (blot), and hybridizing the DNA on the blot with a labeled probe.

restriction site A DNA sequence that is cleaved by a specific restriction endonuclease.

restriction site polymorphism (RSP) A variation in DNA sequence that is due to the presence or absence of a restriction site. This type of polymorphism is the basis for most traditional RFLPs.

retrovirus A type of RNA virus that can reverse transcribe its RNA into DNA for insertion into the genome of a host cell; useful as a vector for gene therapy.

reverse banding (R-banding) A chromosome banding technique in which chromosomes are heated in a phosphate buffer; produces dark and light bands in patterns that are the reverse of those produced by G-banding.

reverse transcriptase An enzyme that transcribes RNA into DNA (hence "reverse").

ribonucleic acid (RNA) A single-stranded molecule that consists of a sugar (ribose), phosphate group, and a series of bases (adenine, cytosine, guanine, and uracil). There are three basic types of RNA: **messenger RNA, ribosomal RNA,** and **transfer RNA.**

ribosomal RNA (rRNA) In conjunction with protein molecules, composes the **ribosome.**

ribosome The site of translation of mature messenger RNA into amino acid sequences.

ribozyme An mRNA molecule that has catalytic activity. Some ribozymes can be used to cleave mRNA in somatic cell gene therapy.

ring chromosome A structural chromosome abnormality formed when both ends of a chromosome are lost and the new ends fuse together.

RNA polymerase Enzyme that binds to a promoter site and synthesizes messenger RNA from a DNA template.

satellite DNA A portion of the DNA that differs enough in base composition so that it forms a distinct band on a cesium chloride gradient centrifugation; usually contains highly repetitive DNA sequences.

secondary oocyte A cell containing 23 double-stranded chromosomes, produced from a primary oocyte after meiosis I in the female.

secondary spermatocyte A cell containing 23 double-stranded chromosomes, produced from a primary spermatocyte after meiosis I in the male.

segregation The distribution of genes from homologous chromosomes to different gametes during meiosis.

senescent Aged (as in an aged, or senescent, cell).

sensitivity The proportion of affected individuals who are correctly identified by a test (**true positives**). Compare with **specificity.**

sequence (formerly "anomalad")   A primary defect with secondary structural changes in development (examples: oligohydramnios sequence, Pierre-Robin sequence).

sequence tagged sites (STSs)   DNA sequences of several hundred bp in size that are flanked by PCR primers. Their chromosome location has been established, making them useful as indicators of physical positions on the genome.

sex chromatin   See **Barr body.**

sex chromosomes   The X and Y chromosomes in humans. Compare with **autosomes.**

sex-influenced   A trait whose expression is modified by the gender of the individual possessing the trait.

sex-limited   A trait that is expressed in only one sex.

signal transduction   Process in which biochemical messages are transmitted from the cell surface to the nucleus.

silencer   A DNA sequence that binds to **specific transcription factors** to decrease or repress the activity of certain genes. Compare with **enhancer.**

silent substitution   DNA sequence change that does not change the amino acid sequence because of the degeneracy of the genetic code.

SINEs (short interspersed elements)   A class of dispersed repetitive DNA in which each repeat is relatively short. Compare with **LINEs.**

single-strand conformation polymorphism (SSCP)   A technique for detecting variation in DNA sequence by running single-stranded DNA fragments through a non-denaturing gel. Fragments with differing secondary structure (conformation) caused by sequence variation will migrate at different rates.

single-copy DNA   DNA sequences that occur only once in the genome. Compare with **repetitive DNA.**

single-gene disorder or trait   A feature or disease that is caused by a single gene. Compare with **polygenic** and **multifactorial.**

single nucleotide polymorphisms (SNPs)   Polymorphisms that result from variation at a single nucleotide. Compare with **microsatellites** and **VNTRs.**

sister chromatid exchange   Crossover between **sister chromatids**; can occur either in the sister chromatids of a tetrad during meiosis or between sister chromatids of a duplicated somatic chromosome.

sister chromatids   The two identical strands of a duplicated chromosome, joined by a single centromere.

solenoid   A structure of coiled DNA, consisting of approximately six **nucleosomes.**

somatic cell   Cell other than those of the gamete-forming germ line. In humans, most somatic cells are diploid.

somatic cell hybridization   A physical gene mapping technique in which somatic cells from two different species are fused and allowed to undergo cell division. Chromosomes from one species are selectively lost, resulting in clones with only one or a few chromosomes from one of the species.

somatic hypermutation   An extreme increase in the mutation rate of somatic cells; observed in B lymphocytes as they achieve increased binding affinity for a foreign antigen.

somatic recombination   The exchange of genetic material between homologous chromosomes during mitosis in somatic cells; much rarer than meiotic recombination.

Southern transfer (also, **Southern blot**)   Laboratory procedure in which DNA fragments that have been electro-phoresed through a gel are transferred to a solid membrane, such as nitrocellulose. The DNA can then be hybridized with a labeled probe and exposed to x-ray film (an **autoradiogram**).

specificity   The proportion of unaffected individuals who are correctly identified by a test (**true negatives**). Compare with **sensitivity.**

spectral karyotype   A chromosome display (**karyotype**) in which combinations of fluorescent probes are used with special cameras and image-processing software so that each chromosome has a unique color.

spermatid   One of the four haploid cells formed from a primary spermatocyte during spermatogenesis. Spermatids mature into spermatozoa.

spermatogenesis   The process of male gamete formation.

spermatogonia   Diploid germline stem cells from which sperm cells (spermatozoa) are ultimately derived.

spindle fiber   One of the microtubular threads that form the spindle in a cell.

splice site mutation   DNA sequence alterations in **donor** or **acceptor sites** or in the consensus sites near them. Produces altered intron splicing, such that portions of exons are deleted or portions of introns are included in the mature mRNA transcript.

sporadic   The occurrence of a disease in a family with no apparent genetic transmission pattern (often the result of a new mutation).

stop codon   mRNA base triplets that specify the point at which translation of the mRNA ceases.

structural genes   Genes that encode protein products.

submetacentric   A chromosome in which the centromere is located closer to one end of the chromosome arm than the other. Compare with **metacentric** and **acrocentric.**

synapsis   The pairing of homologous chromosomes during prophase I of meiosis.

syndrome   A pattern of multiple primary malformations or defects all due to a single underlying cause (examples: Down syndrome, Marfan syndrome).

syntenic   Describes two loci located on the same chromosome; they may or may not be linked.

T lymphocyte or **T cell**   A component of the adaptive immune system whose receptors bind to a complex of MHC molecule and foreign antigen. There are two major classes of T lymphocytes, **helper T lymphocytes** and **cytotoxic T lymphocytes**.

tandem repeat   DNA sequences that occur in multiple copies located directly next to one another. Compare with **dispersed repetitive DNA.**

targeted disruption   The disabling of a specific gene so that it is not expressed.

telomerase   A transferase enzyme that replaces the DNA sequences in **telomeres** during cell division.

telomere   The tip of a chromosome.

telophase   The final major stage of mitosis and meiosis, in which daughter chromosomes are located on opposite edges of the cell and new nuclear envelopes form.

template   A strand of DNA that serves as the model for replication of a new strand. Also denotes the DNA strand from which mRNA is transcribed.

teratogen   A substance in the environment that can cause a birth defect.

teratology The study of environmental factors that cause birth defects or congenital malformations.

termination sequence DNA sequence that signals the cessation of transcription.

tetrad The set of four homologous chromatids (two sister chromatids from each homologous chromosome) observed during meiotic prophase I and metaphase I. Synonymous with **bivalent**.

tetraploidy A polyploid condition in which the individual has four copies of each chromosome in each cell, for a total of 92.

thymine One of the four DNA bases (abbrev.: T).

tissue-specific mosaic A **mosaic** in whom the mosaicism is confined to only specific tissues of the body.

transcription The process in which an mRNA sequence is synthesized from a DNA template.

transcription factor Protein that binds to DNA to influence and regulate transcription.

transcription factor, general A class of transcription factors that are required for the transcription of all structural genes.

transcription factor, specific A class of transcription factors that activate only specific genes at specific points in time.

transfection The transfer of a DNA sequence into a cell.

transfer RNA (tRNA) A class of RNA that helps to assemble a polypeptide chain during translation. The anticodon portion of the tRNA binds to a complementary mRNA codon, and the 3′ end of the tRNA molecule attaches to a specific amino acid.

transformation The oncogenic conversion of a normal cell to a state of unregulated growth.

transgenic Refers to an organism into which a gene has been introduced from an organism of another species (e.g., a transgenic mouse could contain an inserted human gene).

translation The process in which an amino acid sequence is assembled according to the pattern specified by the mature mRNA transcript.

translocation The exchange of genetic material between nonhomologous chromosomes.

translocation, reciprocal A translocation resulting from breaks on two different chromosomes and a subsequent exchange of material. Carriers of reciprocal translocations maintain the normal number of chromosomes and normal amount of chromosome material.

translocation, Robertsonian A translocation in which the long arms of two acrocentric chromosomes are fused at the centromere; the short arms of each chromosome are lost. The translocation carrier has 45 chromosomes instead of 46 but is phenotypically normal because the short arms contain no essential genetic material.

transposon See **mobile element.**

triploidy A polyploid condition in which the individual has three copies of each chromosome in each cell, for a total of 69.

trisomy An aneuploid condition in which the individual has an extra copy of one chromosome, for a total of 47 chromosomes in each cell.

true negative Individual who is correctly identified by a test as not having a disease. See also **specificity.**

true positive Individual who is correctly identified by a test as having a disease. See also **sensitivity.**

tumor See **neoplasm.**

tumor suppressor A gene whose product helps to control cell growth and proliferation; mutations in tumor suppressors can lead to cancer (example: retinoblastoma gene, *RB1*).

two-hit model A model of carcinogenesis in which both copies of a gene must be altered before a neoplasm can form.

ultrasonography A technique for fetal visualization in which sound waves are transmitted through the fetus and their reflection patterns are displayed on a monitor.

unequal crossover Crossing over between improperly aligned DNA sequences; produces deletions or duplications of genetic material.

uninformative mating A mating in which **linkage phase** cannot be established.

uniparental disomy Condition in which two copies of one chromosome are derived from a single parent, and no copies are derived from the other parent. May be either **heterodisomy** or **isodisomy.**

variable expression A trait in which the same genotype may produce phenotypes of varying severity or expression (example: neurofibromatosis type 1).

variable number of tandem repeats (VNTRs) A type of polymorphism created by variations in the number of minisatellite repeats in a defined region.

variance Statistical measure of variation in a quantity: estimated as the sum of the squared differences from the average value.

vector The vehicle used to carry a DNA insert (e.g., phage, plasmid, cosmid, BAC, or YAC).

X inactivation Process in which genes from one X chromosome in each cell of the female embryo are rendered transcriptionally inactive.

X inactivation center The location on the X chromosome from which the X inactivation signal is transmitted (includes the *XIST* gene).

X-linked Refers to genes that are located on the X chromosome.

yeast artificial chromosome (YAC) A synthesized yeast chromosome capable of carrying a large DNA insert (up to 1,000 kb).

zygote The diploid fertilized ovum.

Index

Mutations—cont'd
  in hemoglobin disorders, *33*, 33-36, *34, 34t, 35*
  in Huntington disease, 71*b*
  in hyperphenylalaninemias, 141-142
  in isolated growth hormone deficiency, 68-69
  of LDL receptor gene, 254*b*
  locus heterogeneity and, 74-75
  in Marfan syndrome, 74, 77*b*
  in metabolic disorders, 137
  in mitochondrial inheritance, 106-107
  molecular consequences of, 31-33
  in mutation, 139
  in myotonic dystrophy, 80-84, *82*
  in neurofibromatosis type 1, 75*b*
  new; *see* New mutation
  in osteogenesis imperfecta, 21*b*
  in phenylketonuria, 63-64
  in Prader-Willi syndrome, 78-79, *79-80*
  rates of, 38-40, *40, 41*
  in retinoblastoma, 72*b*
  screening for, 179-181
  in transcription, 15, 15*t*
  in Turner syndrome, 120
  types of, 29-31, *30, 32*
  in tyrosinemia, 144
  in variable expression, 73-74
  in Williams syndrome, 128-129
Mutation hot spots, 40
Myasthenia gravis, 199*t*
myb transcription factor, 230*t*
myc gene, 229
  in Burkitt lymphoma, 133-134, 134*t*
  cancer and, 224, *224*
Myocardial infarction, 249*t*
Myoclonic epilepsy
  mapping and cloning in, 182*t*
  mutation in, 106
  prevalence of, 2*t*
  repeat expansion in, 84
Myopia, 76*b*
Myotonic dystrophy, 80-84, *81, 82,* 83*t*
  appearance in, 81, *81*
  in vitro fertilization diagnosis in, 282
  knockout models in, 216*b*
  linkage disequilibrium in, 166, *167*
  mapping and cloning in, 182*t*
  prevalence of, 2*t*
MZ twins; *see* Monozygotic twins

N

N-acetylglutamate synthetase, *150*
NADH-CoQ reductase deficiency, 138*t*
NAGS; *see* N-acetylglutamate synthetase

Naked DNA, 286
Narcolepsy, 198, 199*t*
Nathans, Jeremy, 103*b*
National Society of Genetic Counselors, 299
Natural killer cells
  in innate immune system, 188
  major histocompatibility complex and, 197
  in pregnancy, 198*b*
Natural selection, *54,* 54-55*b,* 70
Neanderthal specimen, 51
Neck
  in Down syndrome, 114, *114*
  muscles and bones of, 218
  in Turner syndrome, 119, 120, *120*
Negative family history, 292, *293,* 293*b*
Neoplasia, multiple endocrine, 237
Neoplasm, 221; *see also* Tumors
Nephews; *see* Second-degree relatives
Nephrolithiasis, 151
Nerve cells, enteric tract, 212*b*
Nervous system
  abnormalities of
    in Patau syndrome, 118
    polyploidy in, 112
    teratogens in, 303*t*
  in Charcot-Marie-Tooth disease, 30-31
  in chromosome abnormalities, 132-133
  formation of, 218
  in Huntington disease, 70, 71*b*
  in phenylketonuria, 64
NEU growth factor receptor, 230*t*
Neural crest cells
  in craniofacial development, 218
  in DiGeorge anomaly, 130*b*
  formation of, 210, *212,* 212*b*
Neural hearing loss, 115, 116*b*
Neural tube closure, 210
Neural tube defects, *243-245,* 243-245*b,* 250-253
  α-fetoprotein in, 280, 281, *281*
  prevalence of, 2*t,* 250*t*
  prevention of, 306*b*
  recurrence risks in, 242
  teratogens in, 303*t*
  threshold model in, 242
Neural tube formation, 210
Neurodegeneration, 144
Neurofibrillary tangles, 261
Neurofibroma, *74,* 74-75*b*
Neurofibromatosis type 1
  diagnosis of, 292, *293,* 293*b*
  etiology of, 301*t*
  1F10 polymorphism in, 157, *159, 159, 161,* 161-162*b*

Neurofibromatosis type 1—cont'd
  gene for, *NF1* gene
  germline mosaicism in, 70
  knockout models in, 216*b*
  linkage analysis in, 163
  management plan in, 300
  mapping and cloning in, 182*t*
  mobile elements in, 31
  negative family history and, 293*b*
  prevalence of, 2*t*
  segmental, 75*b*
  tumor suppressor genes in, 227*t*
Neurofibromatosis type 2, 75*b*
  gene in, 237
  mapping and cloning in, 182*t*
Neurofibromin gene product, 75*b*
Neurofibrosarcoma, 75*b*
Neurological impairment, 150
Neuroma, bilateral acoustic, 75*b*
Neurons
  cell division in, 23
  in Huntington disease, 71*b*
Neuropathy
  in Charcot-Marie-Tooth disease, 30-31
  mutations in, 31
  optic
    mitochondrial inheritance in, 106
    prevalence of, 2*t*
Neurospora, 3
Neurotransmitters, 264
Neurulation, 210, *212,* 212*b*
New genetics, 45*b*
New mutation, 69
  in Huntington disease, 71*b*
  negative family history and, 292, 293*b*
  in neurofibromatosis type 1, 75*b*
  trisomy 21 as, 116
Newborn
  chromosomal abnormalities in, 124*t*
  cystic fibrosis in, 61*b,* 63
  Down syndrome in, 114
  galactosemia in, 139
  hemolytic disease of, 200
  Hirschsprung disease in, 212*b*
  holoprosencephaly in, 209, *209*
  isochromosomes in, 131-132
  Marfan syndrome in, 77*b*
  metabolic disorders in, 146*b*
  phenylketonuria in, 63-64
    dietary management of, 142-143*b, 143,* 143*t*
  screening for, 267, 268*b*
  screening of, 268*b,* 269, 270*t*
  thalassemia in, 34*t,* 35
NF1; *see* Neurofibromatosis type 1
NF2; *see* Neurofibromatosis type 2